Building a Medical Vocabulary

with SPANISH TRANSLATIONS

Building *a* Medical Vocabulary

with SPANISH TRANSLATIONS

Sixth Edition

Peggy C. Leonard, MT, MEd
St. Louis County, Missouri

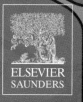

ELSEVIER
SAUNDERS

ELSEVIER
SAUNDERS

11830 Westline Industrial Drive
St. Louis, Missouri 63146

BUILDING A MEDICAL VOCABULARY WITH   ISBN 0-7216-0464-1
SPANISH TRANSLATIONS, ED 6
Copyright © 2005, Elsevier Inc.

NOTICE

Medicine is an ever-changing field. Standard safety precautions must be followed, but as new research and clinical experience broaden our knowledge, changes in treatment and drug therapy may become necessary or appropriate. Readers are advised to check the most current product information provided by the manufacturer of each drug to be administered to verify the recommended dose, the method and duration of administration, and contraindications. It is the responsibility of the licensed prescriber, relying on experience and knowledge of the patient, to determine dosages and the best treatment for each individual patient. Neither the publisher nor the author assumes any liability for any injury and/or damage to persons or property arising from this publication.

Previous editions copyrighted 1983, 1988, 1993, 1997, 2001.

International Standard Book Number 0-7216-0464-1

Publishing Director: Andrew Allen
Executive Editor: Jeanne Wilke
Developmental Editor: Carolyn Kruse
Publishing Services Manager: Melissa Lastarria
Book Design Manager: Julia Dummitt
Artist: Jeanne Robertson

Printed in Canada
Last digit is the print number: 9 8 7 6 5 4 3 2 1

REVIEWERS

Ruth Ann Ehrlich, RT (R)
Senior Instructor in Radiology
Western States Chiropractic College
Portland, Oregon

Gertrude Frangipani, RN, BS, MBA
Instructor
Learning Tree University
Chatsworth, California

Mary Rahr, MS, RN, CMA-C
Medical Assistant Program Director
Northeast Wisconsin Technical College
Green Bay, Wisconsin

Jackie Rothweil, MLT (ASCP)
Barnes Hospital
St. Louis, Missouri

Susan E. Saullo, RN, MT
RN Instructor
Webster College
Ocala, Florida

Steven J. Thurlow, BS, MS
Professor
Jackson Community College
Jackson, Michigan

Dedicated to the instructors and students whose enthusiasm and influence have helped shape this book.

ACKNOWLEDGMENTS

Several individuals have contributed to the refreshing approach of the sixth edition of *Building a Medical Vocabulary*. Suggestions from instructors and students have been incorporated, as well as in-depth analyses by an outstanding group of reviewers.

The new pharmacological appendix was made possible by James F. McCalpin, RPh. I am also indebted to the companies who have allowed the use of illustrations that vividly enhance the written word and bring life to the explanations of medical terms.

The production of this book would not have been possible without the producers, editors, proofreaders, and all others whose expertise has produced a book that I am sure will be valuable to students in their search for an understanding of the medical language.

Peggy Leonard, MT, MEd

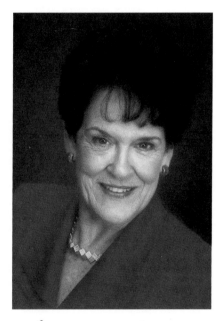

TO THE INSTRUCTOR

The sixth edition of *Building a Medical Vocabulary* is now even easier to use than previous editions! This easy-to-use, interactive text, first published in 1983, is designed to help students learn medical vocabulary, and instructors have depended on it for years. Although each profession and each specialty has its own particular terminology, much of the medical language is understood by all members of the health team and that is the focus of this book.

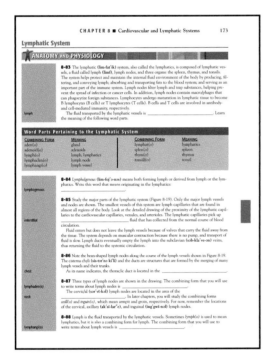

New Organization within Chapters!

A logical, step-by-step learning method is presented. After learning the meaning of word parts and how they are combined, the student begins recognizing and writing new terms in the first chapter! Immediate involvement and feedback within the programmed method provide intrinsic motivation that is not found in other systems, and your students will have fun using this book. You will especially appreciate the new organization of systems chapter material: anatomy and physiology, diagnostic tests and procedures, pathologies, and surgical and therapeutic interventions.

Systems' chapters begin with a new "Function First" section that provides a quick overview of each system's purpose to help students understand the importance of what they are studying.

Chapters 1 Through 7 Provide a Foundation for Chapters about the Body Systems.

It is important that students study Chapters 1 through 7 in the sequence that they are presented. Students will learn many word parts, as well as concepts pertaining to body structure and fluids in the foundation material. For instructors who have used previous editions, you will be delighted to find an even stronger foundation for the other chapters.

Body Systems (Chapters 8 through 17) Can Be Taught and Studied in Any Sequence.

The book is useful in a medical terminology course or as self-paced material for anyone pursuing a career in the allied health professions. Although terminology is given primary emphasis, the book can also be used as an introductory anatomy and physiology book. Because instructors can easily change the sequence of the "body systems" chapters, the book adapts well for study of terminology in conjunction with anatomy, physiology, or introductory medical science courses.

Healthcare Reports Add Real Life Dimension to Study.

Students are inspired by healthcare documents that reflect on the diagnosis and treatment of the patient using terms and abbreviations they just learned. Records include the history and physical, consultation, and pathology reports.

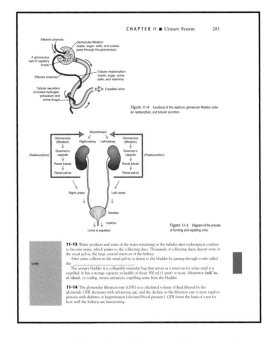

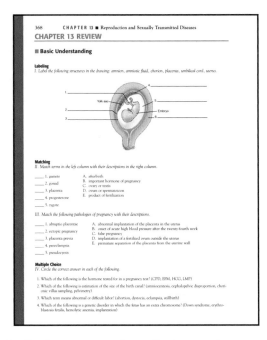

Even More Full Color Illustrations and Photos in the 6th Edition

Full color art throughout the book enhances learning and makes difficult concepts easier to understand.

Caution Boxes key the student to discriminate between similar terms.

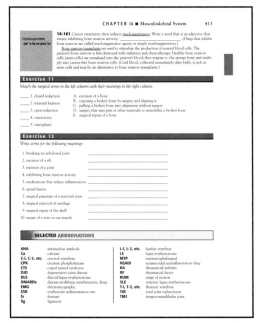

Each Chapter has Section Exercises for Learning Reinforcement.

Section exercises reinforce learning by helping students recall the meaning of word parts they just learned.

End-of-Chapter Reviews help Students Measure How Much They Learned.

A variety of question types are included in comprehensive end-of-chapter reviews, including labeling diagrams, fill in the blanks, medical record exercises, writing terms, and multiple-choice questions.

Pharmacology by Chapter in an Appendix

Drug classes are presented within applicable chapters. If more information on pharmacology is desired, it is now available in an appendix, separated by chapter to coordinate with each lesson.

Software is Fun and Challenging.

The software introduces a gaming aspect and provides another way for the student to determine how much they have learned. The new testing mode (in addition to the study mode) offers you the option of having students print their results as proof of completion.

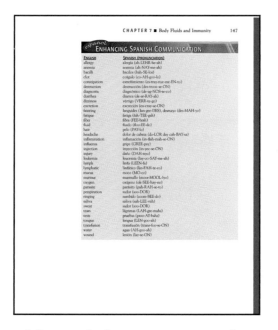

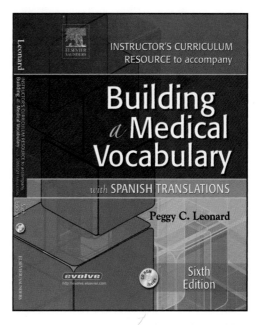

Spanish Translations Are Presented.

I lived in Venezuela several years ago and learned the Spanish language. I am pleased to offer a translation of many medical terms. This edition's instructor's curriculum resource also has matching exercises for the Spanish translations, if you wish to use them for extra credit assignments.

Instructor's Curriculum Resource with CD

A comprehensive curriculum resource is available to instructors by contacting Elsevier Health Sciences. It includes both printed material and software with access to over 2000 questions that can be used to produce your own tests. Several types of questions are included, along with classroom exercises, art from the text, transparency masters, and several summary tables designed especially for classroom use.

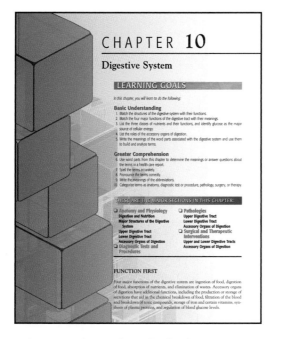

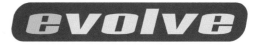

Evolve Course Management

The Evolve website provides a course management platform for instructors who want to post course materials online. Elsevier Health Sciences provides hosting and technical support. Student area includes study tips, updates, and links. Faculty area includes the Instructor's Curriculum Resource, the Computerized Test Bank, and the Electronic Image Collection.

Learning Goals and End-of-Chapter Exercises Are Classified as "Basic" or "Greater Comprehension"

Basic understanding requires labeling or simple recall of the meaning of word parts and medical terms. Greater comprehension includes spelling, pronunciation, abbreviations, reading health care reports, and categorizing terms (an application exercise). You determine and inform the students of your expectations. Instructors often have the students work all of the review questions, then exercise more specificity when choosing questions for the examination.

TO THE STUDENT

Here's Your Blueprint for Learning Medical Terminology!

Imagine being able to read and write medical words the first day you begin studying. You will have this experience as you begin studying *Building a Medical Vocabulary*. You will soon be breaking medical terms down into easier parts that will help you understand their meaning.

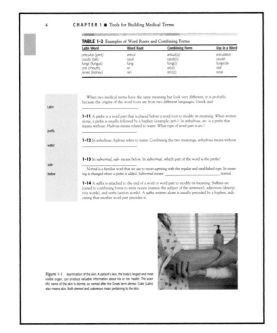

You'll Have Lots of Tools to Make Learning Easy.

Frames make learning easy! You will find the readability of a textbook, even though it's organized into frames. It is important to write your answers in the blanks, because writing increases retention of the material.

A Good Foundation Is Essential.

Be sure to study Chapters 1 through 7 in the order that they are presented, because each chapter builds on the material learned in the previous chapter. Read all material within a chapter, including the tables and illustrations. Chapters 8 through 17 can be studied in any order. Chapter 18 is a review of the whole text.

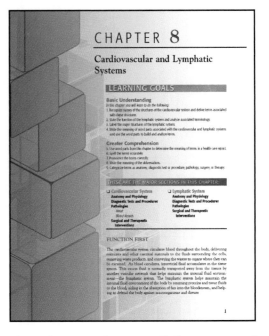

Function First Sections Explain WHY Each System Is Important.

Each of the body systems chapters (8 through 17) opens with a "Function First" section that gives you an overview of what each body system accomplishes and why it is so important for you to know its medical terms.

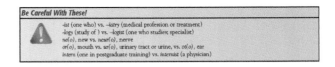

Caution! Students at Work!

Be careful of similar terms. The Caution Boxes help you distinguish between terms that look alike but have different meanings.

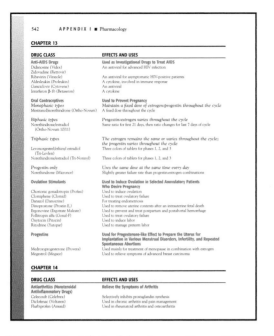

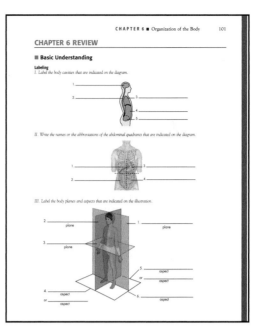

Don't Be Intimidated by Long Drug Names!

Your instructor will expect you to remember material presented within the chapter. However, you are not expected to remember the names of drugs in the pharmacological sections in the appendix. Since new drugs are introduced and other drugs are removed each year, it is important to consult current drug reference materials. Sources like Mosby's *Drug Consult*, Mosby's *Drug Guide for Health Professions*, the *Physician's Desk Reference (PDR)*, the *Nurse's Drug Reference (NDR)*, and *Drug Facts and Comparisons* (updated monthly) provide current information.

Know if You Have Understood a Section Before Moving Ahead.

Read a section, then work the corresponding exercise to reinforce your learning. Working the exercises throughout the chapter lets you "chunk" the material into manageable pieces.

Measure How You Are Doing in the End-of-Chapter Review Before the Test.

Complete the end-of-chapter review and check your answers in Appendix VI to ensure you understand each chapter's material. Additional practice questions are provided on the CD.

Real Life Practice Opportunities!

Imagine yourself working in your chosen health care field. The case studies and health reports you read in this book are just like the ones you will be reading when you are a health care professional! You will be fully prepared to understand the day-to-day medical terminology you will encounter.

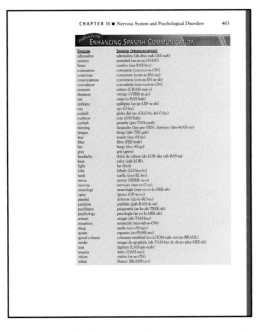

Spanish Translations Make Your Education More Valuable!

Spanish translations of selected medical terms are presented at the end of each chapter. Even if you do not speak Spanish, knowing some medical terminology in Spanish will help you put Spanish-speaking patients more at ease.

Have Fun With the Practice CD.

Additional visuals and practice exercises on the CD will help you measure how much you learned. You can work in "study mode" until you feel ready to try the "test mode" for each chapter. Your scores in the test mode are recorded and can also be printed.

The CD is also valuable in learning pronunciations. The listing of medical terms at the end of each chapter is the same as the audio chapter glossary on the CD, so you can look at the terms as you practice pronouncing them. After listening to pronunciations, review the list and be sure that you know the meanings of each term.

Preparing for a Midterm or Final Exam?

Use the Index/Glossary to review terms for the big exams. It has the definitions and the pages they were introduced so you know where to find terms as you review.

You are about to learn an entirely new language, but you have discovered a fun and easy way to do it! After the first chapter, medical terms that seem difficult now will be easy. Some terms will be easier to remember than others, but challenge yourself to understand every term in every chapter.

TABLE OF CONTENTS

CHAPTER 1

Tools for Building Medical Terms

LEARNING GOALS

In this chapter, you will learn to do the following:
1. Use the programmed learning format to learn medical terminology.
2. Identify the roles of word roots, prefixes, suffixes, and combining forms.
3. Identify examples of combining forms, prefixes, and suffixes.
4. Demonstrate correct usage of the combining vowel by correctly joining word parts to write medical terms.
5. Use the rules learned in this chapter to write the singular or plural forms of medical terms.
6. Demonstrate understanding of the use of the reference material.

THESE ARE THE MAJOR SECTIONS IN THIS CHAPTER:

- **Learning by the Programmed Method**
- **Foundations of Word Building**
- **Word Roots, Combining Forms, Prefixes, and Suffixes**
- **Combining Word Parts**
- **Pronunciation of Medical Terms**
- **Plurals of Medical Terms**
- **Enhancing Spanish Communication**
- **Pharmacology**

FUNCTION FIRST

The material in this chapter is important because it is the beginning foundation on which you will build a medical vocabulary. It explains word building and teaches you how to break down a word into its parts.

Each chapter introduces new terms and uses those you learned in previous chapters. You will gradually build a strong medical vocabulary foundation that will enable you to recognize and write thousands of medical words. It is important to study material in the order that it is presented within a chapter. It is also important to study Chapters 1 through 7 in sequential order. These early chapters form the foundation for learning material about the body systems presented in Chapters 8 through 17.

Learning by the Programmed Method

1-1 It is important to study the first seven chapters in the sequence presented in this book, because these chapters are the foundation for learning terms presented in all other chapters.

Programmed learning consists of blocks of information, often containing blanks in which you will write answers. After writing an answer, you will check to see if it is correct by comparing your answer with that in the left column, called the answer column.

1-2 A frame is a block of information preceded by a number. Each frame is given a separate number, and most frames contain at least one blank in which you will write an answer. After writing your answer in a blank, you will check to see if it is correct.

The answer column should be covered while you are filling in the blanks. To do this, position the bookmark so that it covers only the answer column. After writing your answer in a blank, check it by sliding down the bookmark just enough to see the answer. When you are not using the bookmark to cover the answer column, use it to mark your place in the book.

1-3 You have just read two frames. Information contained in frames throughout this book will help you learn medical terms. A block of information with a number is called a

frame

_____.

Write the answer in the preceding blank and check it immediately. Some students prefer to write their answers on a separate sheet of paper so that they can rework the material later. It is important to *write your answer because writing it will help you to remember it better* than if you just think of the answer. Always check your answer immediately and say it aloud if possible. This is especially helpful when you are not familiar with the term. Saying an answer aloud helps you remember it. If you make an error, look back at previous frames to see where you went wrong. Otherwise, you may repeat the error without realizing why it is incorrect.

1-4 This text provides frequent exercises to reinforce what you are learning. Answers to the reviews are in Appendix VI, Solutions to Review Exercises. The end-of-the-chapter reviews help integrate what you have learned in a chapter.

Exercise 1

Write answers in the blanks.

1. In programmed learning, a block of information preceded by a number is called a _____.

2. Position the bookmark so that it covers only the _____ column.

3. It is important to _____ your answer because this will help you remember better than just thinking of the answer.

4. After writing the answer in the blank, always _____ it using the information in the answer column.
   (Use Appendix VI to check your answers.)

Foundations of Word Building

1-5 Word building is a system of learning the meaning of various word parts to understand and write new words. Because it is impractical to memorize the medical dictionary, you will use a system of word _____ to learn medical terms.

building

1-6 Pay close attention to spelling. When writing a term, an error of only one letter can result in a different term. For example, the ilium is a pelvic bone, and the ileum is part of the small intestine. In addition to checking your answer each time, you will also check the

spelling _____.

WORD ROOTS, COMBINING FORMS, PREFIXES, AND SUFFIXES

1-7 Most medical terms are composed of word parts that have their origins in Greek or Latin. Although familiarity with either of the two languages would facilitate learning medical terms, it is not necessary. We will be learning the English translation of many Greek or Latin word parts used in medical terminology.

Word roots, combining forms, prefixes, and suffixes are word parts. Learning the meaning of these word parts eliminates the necessity of memorizing each new term you encounter. In this chapter, it is important to learn to recognize word roots, prefixes, and suffixes in terms and how to combine them parts to write terms. Word roots, prefixes, and suffixes are called word _____.

1-8 Most words have a word root, even ordinary words. The word root is the main body of the word. It is usually accompanied by a prefix or suffix or both. Word roots are the building blocks for many terms related to anatomy, diagnosis, and medical procedures. You see by reading this informa-root tion that most words have a word _____.

Look at the Greek words and their associated word roots in Table 1-1. By adding prefixes and suffixes, you will soon begin writing medical terms.

1-9 Some compound words are composed of two word roots, or words, as in *collarbone* (collar and bone). Form a compound word using eye and lid: _____.

Many words would be difficult to pronounce if they were written without a vowel to join the word roots. A vowel (usually *o*) is often inserted between word roots to make the word easier to pronounce, as in speedometer. A combining form is recognized as a word part that ends in an enclosed vowel. In this example, the combining form, *speed(o)*, is joined with another part of the word, *meter*. The parentheses are not included when the combining form joins other word parts.

The term *cephalometer* is composed of two word roots, *cephal* and *meter*. Write the combining cephal(o) form for cephal: _____.

The origins of several combining forms and their use in medical terms are shown in Table 1-2.

1-10 You will sometimes learn two word roots that have the same meaning. Table 1-1 shows the Greek word root *nephr* for kidney, whereas Table 1-2 shows the Latin word root *ren* for kidney. Both *nephric* and *renal* mean pertaining to the kidney. Likewise, both *dermal* and *cutaneous* mean pertaining to the skin (Figure 1-1). However, as a general rule, Latin roots are used to write words naming and describing structures of the body, whereas Greek roots are used to write words naming and describing diseases, conditions, diagnosis, and treatment. As with most rules, there are exceptions.

TABLE 1-1 Examples of Word Roots

Greek Word	Word Root
karkinos (crab, cancer)	carcin
lithos (stone)	lith
nephros (kidney)	nephr
stomatos (mouth)	stomat

TABLE 1-2 Examples of Word Roots and Combining Forms

Latin Word	Word Root	Combining Form	Use in a Word
articulus (joint)	articul	articul(o)	articulation
cauda (tail)	caud	caud(o)	caudal
fungi (fungus)	fung	fung(i)	fungicide
oris (mouth)	or	or(o)	oral
renes (kidney)	ren	ren(o)	renal

When two medical terms have the same meaning but look very different, it is probably because the origins of the word roots are from two different languages, Greek and

<u>   Latin   </u>.

1-11 A prefix is a word part that is placed before a word root to modify its meaning. When written alone, a prefix is usually followed by a hyphen (example: *peri-*). In *anhydrous*, *an-* is a prefix that means without. *Hydrous* means related to water. What type of word part is *an-*?

<u>   prefix   </u>.

1-12 In *anhydrous*, *hydrous* refers to water. Combining the two meanings, *anhydrous* means without

<u>   water   </u>.

1-13 In *subnormal*, *sub-* means below. In *subnormal*, which part of the word is the prefix?

<u>   sub-   </u>

Normal is a familiar word that we use to mean agreeing with the regular and established type. Its meaning is changed when a prefix is added. *Subnormal* means <u>   below   </u> normal.

1-14 A suffix is attached to the end of a word or word part to modify its meaning. Suffixes are joined to combining forms to write nouns (names; the subject of the sentence), adjectives (descriptive words), and verbs (action words). A suffix written alone is usually preceded by a hyphen, indicating that another word part precedes it.

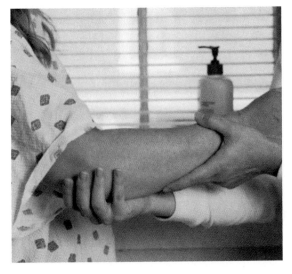

Figure 1-1 Examination of the skin. A patient's skin, the body's largest and most visible organ, can produce valuable information about his or her health. The scientific name of the skin is dermis, so named after the Greek term *derma. Cutis* (Latin) also means skin. Both *dermal* and *cutaneous* mean pertaining to the skin.

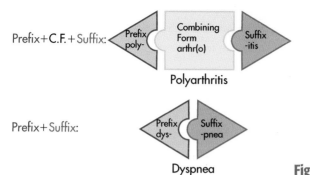

Prefix+C.F.+Suffix:

Polyarthritis

Prefix+Suffix:

Dyspnea

Figure 1-2   The relationship of prefixes, combining forms, and suffixes.

suffix

Carditis means inflammation of the heart. The word part *card* refers to the heart and is the word root. The word part *-itis* means inflammation and is being used as what part of the word?

_____

1-15 Occasionally a word is composed of only a prefix and a suffix. Join *dys-* and *-pnea* to write a new word: _____. The prefix *dys-* means bad, painful, or difficult, and *-pnea* means breathing. *Dyspnea* means difficult breathing.

dyspnea

Visualize the relationship of prefixes, combining forms, and suffixes as you study Figure 1-2.

1-16 You will be learning the combining form for word roots because word roots are often combined with other word parts. Combining forms act as the foundation for most terms (Figure 1-3). In *thermometer, therm(o)* is the combining form. Which is a combining form, *cyst* or *cyst(o)*?

cyst(o)

_____

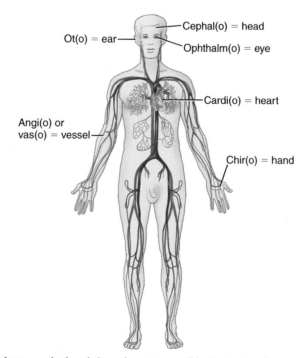

Figure 1-3   Combining forms are the foundations of most terms. All body structures have corresponding combining forms.

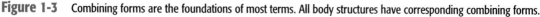

Exercise 2

Write CF (for combining form) or WR (for word root) after each of the following word parts:

1. aden(o) _____   4. derm(a) _____   7. gloss(o) _____

2. bil(i) _____   5. duoden _____   8. hemat _____

3. cyan _____   6. electr _____   9. ren _____

Exercise 3

Write CF (for combining form), P (for prefix), or S (for suffix) for each of the following word parts:

1. brady- _____   4. -graphy _____   7. mal- _____

2. -cele _____   5. hydr(o) _____   8. phon(o) _____

3. eu- _____   6. -iasis _____   9. -pathy _____

Exercise 4

A prefix or suffix is underlined in each of the following terms. Write P (for prefix) or S (for suffix) after each term:

1. adhesion _____   4. dermal _____   7. hypoglossal _____

2. adenopathy _____   5. endocardial _____   8. microscope _____

3. biliary _____   6. hematology _____   9. prenatal _____
   (Use Appendix VI to check your answers.)

Combining Word Parts

1-17 You have learned that medical terms are composed of word roots, combining forms, prefixes, and suffixes. You will now learn to combine these word parts to write medical terms.

One does not always use the vowel that is at the end of a combining form. A rule that will help you in writing medical terms is this:

The combining vowel is used before suffixes that begin with a *consonant* and before another word root.

Observe the use of the rule in building terms with these suffixes:

Combining Form	Suffixes	Term and Meaning
	+ -itis	= otitis, inflammation of the ear
	+ -logy	= otology, study of the ear
ot(o) = ear	+ -plasty	= otoplasty, plastic surgery of the ear
	+ -rrhea	= otorrhea, discharge from the ear
	+ -tomy	= ototomy, incision of the ear

(There are exceptions to the rule, and you will learn the exceptions as you progress through the material. For now, remember to drop the vowel before a suffix that begins with a vowel.) The rule for using the combining vowel shows us that the combining vowel is used in two cases. In one case,

consonant   the combining vowel is used before a suffix that begins with a _____.

1-18 The combining vowel is also used to join two combining forms. When combining *gastr(o)*, meaning stomach, and *enter(o)*, meaning intestine, *gastroentero* results. (Of course, this is not a complete word because it needs a suffix.) Combine *gastr(o)* + *enter(o)* + *-logy* to write a term that means

gastroenterology   the study of the stomach, intestines, and related structures: _____.

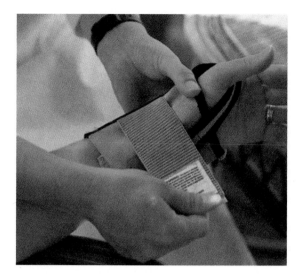

Figure 1-4 A carpal support. Maintaining the wrist in a resting position is important to prevent further irritation of the inflamed nerve in carpal tunnel syndrome, a painful disorder of the wrist and hand. It may develop spontaneously without a known cause or may result from disease or injury. A common cause is repetitive movements of the hands and wrists, such as factory work or typing. Surgery may be required to relieve severe symptoms of long duration.

carpal

aortitis

cardioaortitis

tonsillitis

uremia
urogenital

periappendicitis

enteritis
enterocyst
unilateral

combining

anti-, tri-,

suffix

1-19 The wrist is also called the carpus. Write a word that means pertaining to the wrist by combining *carp(o)*, meaning wrist, and *-al*, meaning pertaining to: _____.
A carpal support holds the wrist in a given position (Figure 1-4).

1-20 The combining form *aort(o)* means aorta, and *-itis* means inflammation. Join the two word parts to write a term that means inflammation of the aorta: _____.
(Check your spelling carefully.)
Join *cardi(o)*, meaning heart, and *aortitis*: _____.

1-21 Join the combining form *tonsill(o)* with *-itis*: _____.
Imagine how cumbersome the pronunciation would be if you did not drop the vowel.
Combine *ur(o)* with *-emia* to form a new word: _____.
Combine *ur(o)* with *genital* to form a new word: _____.
To summarize, one usually drops the combining vowel if the combining form is joined to a suffix that begins with a vowel.

1-22 The word-building rules are summarized in Box 1-1.
Notice that prefixes are not included in the rule concerning use of the combining vowel. That is because most prefixes require no change before they are joined with other word parts. (A few exceptions will be noted later.) Join *peri-* and *appendicitis*: _____.
Let us be certain that you can apply this rule. Join *enter(o)* with *-itis*: _____.

Join *enter(o)* with *cyst*: _____.
Join *uni-* and *lateral*: _____.

1-23 If you were correct on the last few blanks, you have learned the rule for using word parts to write medical terms. In this program, you will be using combining forms, prefixes, and suffixes to build many new words.
A combining form will be recognized as a word part that has a vowel enclosed in parentheses as its ending. For example, you may not know the meaning of *thorac(o)*, but you recognize that *thorac(o)* is which type of word part? _____ form

1-24 Prefixes will be designated by placing a hyphen after the word part, such as *pre-*. The hyphen indicates that something follows this word part. Which of the following word parts are prefixes: *metr(o)*, *anti-*, *tri-*, *-scope*? _____ and _____
Remember that the hyphen follows the prefix when the prefix is shown alone. If the hyphen comes before the word part, the word part is a suffix. This tells us that *-scope* is which type of word part? _____

Box 1-1 Word-Building Rules

Joining Combining Forms
The combining vowel is usually retained between two combining forms.
Example: gastr(o) + enterology = gastroenterology

Joining Combining Forms and Suffixes
The combining vowel is usually retained when a combining form is joined with a suffix that begins with a consonant.
Example: enter(o) + -logy = enterology
The combining vowel is usually omitted when a combining form is joined with a suffix that begins with a vowel.
Example: enter(o) + -ic = enteric

Joining Other Word Parts to Prefixes
Most prefixes require no change when they are joined with other word parts.
Examples: peri- + appendicitis = periappendicitis; dys- + -pnea = dyspnea

1-25 You will also learn to recognize word parts as components of other words. To help you distinguish the component parts of medical terms, the words will often be divided by a diagonal between the component parts.

For example, how many component parts are there in the word *aden/oma*?

two

three

How many component parts does *peri/ophthalm/itis* have? _____

To interpret a new word, begin by looking at the suffix. You will know the meaning of many suffixes after studying Chapters 3 and 4. Recognizing suffixes will help you identify the word as a noun, a verb, or an adjective. After deciding the meaning of the suffix, go to the beginning of the word and read across from left to right, interpreting the remaining elements to develop the full sense of the term. Using the suggested method, the interpretation of word parts in *peri/ophthalm/itis* is "inflammation, around, eye." The full sense of the term is "inflammation of tissues around the eye." See Figure 1-5 to summarize what you have learned about writing and interpreting medical terms.

1-26 Now that you have learned about word parts and how to analyze terms, you need to be aware that some terms do not follow the rules you have learned. In other cases, two spellings are accepted. Whenever you are in doubt, check a medical dictionary. Two spellings of the same term usually come about through popular use. (For example, both *thoracentesis* and *thoracocentesis* mean surgical puncture of the chest wall.) As we progress through the material, such exceptions are noted.

1-27 Eponyms are names for diseases, organs, procedures, or body functions that are derived from the name of a person. A cesarean section, a surgical procedure in which the abdomen and uterus are incised to deliver the infant, is an eponym, and is named after the manner in which Julius Caesar was supposedly born. Parkinson's disease and Alzheimer's disease are also eponyms.

Word building will not be as helpful when analyzing eponyms. Nevertheless, it is important to remember these terms also.

1-28 Abbreviations are shortened forms of words or phrases. Abbreviations include the following:
- Letters (The abbreviation for complete blood cell count is cbc.)
- Shortened words (The abbreviation stat. is short for *statim*, Latin meaning at once or immediately.)
- Acronyms, pronounceable words formed from initial letters (CABG, pronounced like the *vegetable*, means coronary artery bypass graft.)

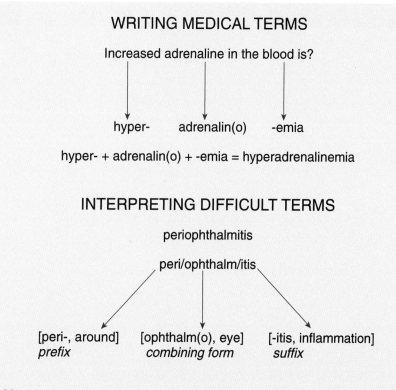

WRITING MEDICAL TERMS

Increased adrenaline in the blood is?

hyper-   adrenalin(o)   -emia

hyper- + adrenalin(o) + -emia = hyperadrenalinemia

INTERPRETING DIFFICULT TERMS

periophthalmitis

peri/ophthalm/itis

[peri-, around]   [ophthalm(o), eye]   [-itis, inflammation]
prefix   *combining form*   *suffix*

Meaning of periophthalmitis is "inflammation of tissues around the eye."

Figure 1-5   Examples of using prefixes, suffixes, and combining forms to write and interpret medical terms.

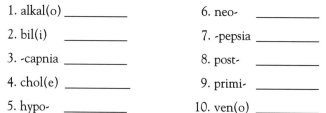

Abbreviations and symbols save time but can be confusing because some have more than one meaning. The abbreviation C means canine tooth, carbon, and Celsius among others. Also some uppercase abbreviations have different meanings than the lowercase equivalents (CC means chief complaint, and *cc* means cubic centimeter.)

abbreviations
Shortened words or phrases are called _____.

Exercise 5

Use CF (for combining form), P (for prefix), or S (for suffix) to designate each of the following word parts as a combining form, a prefix, or a suffix.

1. alkal(o) _____   6. neo- _____

2. bil(i) _____   7. -pepsia _____

3. -capnia _____   8. post- _____

4. chol(e) _____   9. primi- _____

5. hypo- _____   10. ven(o) _____

Combine the following word parts to write terms.

1. acid(o) + -osis   _____

2. acr(o) + -megaly   _____

3. anti- + -emesis   _____

4. bronch(o) + -scopy   _____

5. dys- + -phagia   _____

6. hypo- + thyroid(o) + -ism   _____

7. leuk(o) + cyt(o) + -osis   _____

8. mal- + absorption   _____

9. my(o) + metr(o) + -ium   _____

10. thromb(o) + phleb(o) + -itis _____

(Use Appendix VI to check your answers.)

Pronunciation of Medical Terms

dren
i
an
short
 	
lo
short
	1-29 A medical term is easier to remember when you know how to pronounce it. *If you have not already done so, study the rules for pronunciation that are found on the front inside cover of this book. Do this before proceeding to the remaining frames of this chapter.*
	    In the term *adrenaline* (ə-dren′ə-lin), which syllable has the primary accent? _____
	    In *adrenalitis* (ə-dre″nəl-i′tis), which syllable has the primary accent? _____
	    Which syllable receives secondary emphasis in *angiectomy* (an″je-ek′tə-me)? _____
	    Is the *a* in *angiectomy* pronounced as a long or short *a*? _____
	
	1-30 In *ankylosis* (ang″kə-lo′sis), which is the primary accented syllable? _____
	    Is the vowel in the *sis* syllable pronounced as a long or short *i*? _____
	
	1-31 Be aware that there are different ways to pronounce some medical terms. Pronunciation will be shown as new terms are introduced in later chapters. In addition, an alphabetical list of terms is presented in the Index/Glossary. The list includes the pronunciations and definitions for most medical terms presented in this book.

Write answers in the blanks to review your understanding of the rules of pronunciation used in this book.

1. How many syllables does the term *hypercalcemia* (hi″pər-kal-se′me-ə) have? _____
2. Using the pronunciation of *hypercalcemia* shown in number 1, which syllable receives the primary accent?

_____

3. Using the pronunciation of *hypercalcemia* shown in number 1, which syllable receives a secondary accent?

_____

4. Using the pronunciation of *hypercalcemia* shown in number 1, list all vowels that are pronounced as long vowels:

_____

(Use Appendix VI to check your answers.)

TABLE 1-3 Forming Plurals of Nouns with Special Endings

If the Singular Ending is	The Plural Ending is	Examples (Singular)	Examples (Plural)
is	*es*	diagnosis, prognosis, psychosis	diagnoses, prognoses, psychoses

(Some words ending in *is* form plurals by dropping the *is* and adding *ides,* as in *epididymis* and *epididymides.*)

um	*a*	atrium, ileum, septum, bacterium	atria, ilea, septa, bacteria
us	*i*	alveolus, bacillus, bronchus	alveoli, bacilli, bronchi

(Some singular forms ending in *us* form plurals by dropping the *us* and adding either *era* or *ora,* such as *viscus* and *viscera* and *corpus* and *corpora.* Others form plurals by simply adding *es,* as in *virus* and *viruses.*)

a	*ae*	vertebra, patella, petechia	vertebrae, petallae, petechiae
ix	*ices*	appendix, varix, cervix	appendices, varices, cervices

(Through common use, *appendixes* and *cervixes* have become acceptable plural forms.)

ex	*ices*	cortex	cortices
ax	*aces*	thorax	thoraces (thoraxes is also acceptable)
ma	*s* or *mata*	carcinoma, sarcoma	carcinomas or carcinomata, sarcomas or sarcomata
on	*a*	protozoon, spermatozoon	protozoa, spermatozoa

(Some singular forms ending in *on* form plurals by adding *s,* as in *chorion* and *chorions.*)

nx	*nges*	phalanx, larynx	phalanges, larynges

Plurals of Medical Terms

1-32 Although plurals of many medical terms are formed using rules you may already know, it is important to learn rules that apply when terms have special endings. When you see a noun in its singular form, you will learn to write a plural for that term, but be aware that sometimes more than one plural is acceptable.

Many plurals are formed by simply adding an *s* to the singular term. Write plurals by adding an *s* to these singular terms:

abrasions
lacerations

abrasion _____

laceration _____

1-33 Many nouns that end in *s, ch,* or *sh* form their plurals by adding *es.* The plural of abscess is abscesses. Write plurals by adding *es* to these terms:

branches
brushes
sinuses

branch _____

brush _____

sinus _____

1-34 Singular nouns that end in *y* preceded by a consonant form their plurals by changing the *y* to *i* and adding *es.* For example, the plural of allergy is allergies. Change the *y* to *i* and add *es* to write plurals of these nouns:

capillaries
extremities
ovaries

capillary _____

extremity _____

ovary _____

1-35 Use Table 1-3 to learn the rules for forming other plurals of medical terms, but be aware that there are a few exceptions and that only major rules are included. Many dictionaries show the plural forms of nouns and can be used as references. Also notice that some terms have more than one acceptable plural.

Exercise 8

Write the plural form for each of the following singular nouns.

1. capsule _____
2. cataract _____
3. calculus _____
4. cortex _____

5. diagnosis _____
6. neurosis _____
7. protozoon _____
8. virus _____

Write the singular form of each plural noun.

9. appendices _____
10. fungi _____
11. larynges _____
    (Use Appendix VI to check your answers.)

12. prognoses _____
13. sarcomata _____
14. spermatozoa _____

español ENHANCING SPANISH COMMUNICATION

Spanish translation of selected terms is presented at the end of each chapter. Appendices III and IV of *Building a Medical Vocabulary* have comprehensive lists of both English-Spanish and Spanish-English translations for easy reference. The sounds of Spanish vowels do not vary and must be fully and distinctly pronounced. This does not apply to double vowels. Use these rules to pronounce vowels:

Spanish vowel	Pronounce as	Spanish vowel	Pronounce as
a	a in mama	u	u in rule or the sound of oo in spool
e	a in day		(The u is generally silent in these syllables:
i	i in police		que, gue, and gui.)
o	o in so	y	e in see, but sounds like j if it follows n

Some consonants have similar sounds in English and Spanish. Some significant differences are noted here.

Spanish	Pronunciation	Spanish	Pronunciation
c	k or s, except ch pronounced like church	ñ	blending of n and y as in canyon
		q	k
d	sometimes as th		
		r	trilled r
g	similar to g in go, except pronounced as h before e or i	rr	strongly trilled r
h	not pronounced	z	s
j	h		
ll	blending of l and y, or simply y as in yet		

Phonetic pronunciation is presented with the stressed syllable in uppercase letters, as in the example BO-cah. In this term, the first syllable is stressed. *Boca* is the Spanish word for mouth.

Pharmacology

Pharmacology is the study of the preparation, properties, uses, and actions of drugs. Drugs are used in medicine to prevent, diagnose, and treat disease and to relieve pain. Another term for medicines is *pharmaceuticals*. Beginning with Chapter 2, additional information about medications is presented for each chapter in Appendix I.

CHAPTER 1 REVIEW

Work the following review section. The review helps you know whether you learned the material. After completing all sections of the review, check your answers with the solutions found in Appendix VI. (Don't be concerned about learning the meaning of the word parts for Chapter 1, because all of them will be included in subsequent chapters.)

Use the practice CD for additional questions and a fun way to review. However, the CD does not replace the comprehensive written reviews at the end of each chapter.

Describing
I. Describe the role of each of the following word parts:

1. combining form _____

2. prefix _____

3. suffix _____

4. word root _____

Identifying Word Parts
II. Use CF (for combining form), P (for prefix), or S (for suffix) to designate each of the following word parts as a combining form, a prefix, or a suffix.

1. bil(i) _____	6. intra- _____
2. crani(o) _____	7. multi- _____
3. -ectomy _____	8. -oid _____
4. gigant(o) _____	9. -plegia _____
5. -iatrics _____	10. spher(o) _____

Combining Word Parts
III. Using the rules you have learned in Chapter 1, combine the word parts to write terms.

1. hypo- + derm(o) + -ic _____

2. leuk(o) + -emia   _____

3. melan(o) + -oid   _____

4. my(o) + cardi(o) + -al _____

5. thromb(o) + -osis   _____

Writing Plurals

IV. *Write the plural of each term that is given.*

1. calculus   _____

2. diagnosis   _____

3. septum   _____

4. vertebra   _____

5. protozoon   _____

Checking Spelling

V. *Use the Index/Glossary to check the spelling of these terms. Circle all incorrectly spelled terms and write their correct spellings:*

canser   cerebrotomy   colorrhaphy   neurolysis   ofthalmoplasty

Pronunciation

VI. *Use the Index/Glossary to check the pronunciations of the following terms. Complete the table by indicating the syllable that has the primary accent, all syllables containing a long vowel, and all syllables containing a short vowel. The first term is done as an example:*

	SYLLABLE WITH PRIMARY ACCENT	SYLLABLE(S) WITH LONG VOWEL	SYLLABLE(S) WITH SHORT VOWEL
1. adipose	ad_____	pos_____	ad, i_____
2. aerosol	_____	_____	_____
3. cortisone	_____	_____	_____
4. lactose	_____	_____	_____
5. nephroscope	_____	_____	_____

(Check your answers with the solutions in Appendix VI. Pay particular attention to spelling. If most of your answers are correct, you are ready to move on to Chapter 2.)

CHAPTER 2

Medicine and Its Specialties

In this chapter, you will learn to do the following:

Basic Understanding
1. Recognize prefixes, suffixes, combining forms, and word roots in medical words.
2. Write the meanings of the word parts and use them to build and analyze terms.
3. Match medical specialists with the areas in which they specialize.
4. Identify the specialty associated with various medical conditions.
5. Match health professions presented in this chapter with their descriptions.

Greater Comprehension
6. Spell medical terms accurately.
7. Write the meanings of the abbreviations.
8. Pronounce medical terms correctly using the phonetic system that is presented in this book.

THESE ARE THE MAJOR SECTIONS IN THIS CHAPTER:

❏ **Medicine and Its Specialties**
❏ **Other Health Professions**

15

Medicine and Its Specialties

prefix	**2-1** You have learned that prefixes, suffixes, and combining forms are word parts that are used to write medical terms. Which word part is placed before a word root to modify its meaning? _____ You will learn many word parts as you study each chapter. Beginning now, you are expected to remember the meanings of word parts and terms that are introduced. Pronunciations will also be shown the first time a medical term is introduced.
combining	**2-2** Some word parts end in an enclosed vowel—for example, *psych(o)*. You recognize this type of word part as a _____ form. This chapter introduces several combining forms associated with the medical specialties. You will also learn a few prefixes and suffixes that are used in naming the specialties and the specialists.
suffix	**2-3** Which word part is attached to the end of a word or word part to modify its meaning? _____ Suffixes are added to other word parts (mainly combining forms) to write terms. Study the following suffixes and remember their meanings.

Suffixes Used to Write Medical Specialists and Their Specialties

SUFFIX Terms about Specialists	MEANING	SUFFIX Terms about Specialties	MEANING
-er, -ist	one who	-ac, -al, -ic, -logic, -logical	pertaining to
-iatrician	practitioner	-iatrics, -iatry	medical profession or treatment
-logist	one who studies; specialist	-logy	study or science of

one	**2-4** The suffixes *-er* and *-ist* mean _____ who. You know many terms that contain these suffixes—for example, *practitioner*, one who practices, and *specialist*, one who is devoted to a special field or occupation. In medicine, a specialist is a person who has advanced education and training in one area of practice, such as internal medicine, dermato/logy (dər″mə-tol′o-je) or cardio/logy (kahr″de-ol′ə-je).
study	**2-5** The suffix *-logy* means the _____ or science of, and the suffix *-logist* means one who studies or a specialist. Also notice that several suffixes in the list, including *-logic* and *-logical*, mean pertaining to.
profession	**2-6** The suffixes that are mentioned in the last two frames are not used exclusively in writing medical terms. You will be able to think of many words that use these word parts. The suffixes *-iatrics* and *-iatry* are more specific for medicine and mean the medical _____ or a medical treatment.

Exercise 1

Match terms in the left column with their meaning in the right column. Some choices will be used more than once.

_____ 1. -ac
_____ 2. -er
_____ 3. -iatrician
_____ 4. -iatry
_____ 5. -ic
_____ 6. -ist
_____ 7. -logist
_____ 8. -logy

A. medical profession or treatment
B. one who
C. one who studies; specialist
D. practitioner
E. pertaining to
F. study or science of

(Use Appendix VI to check your answers.)

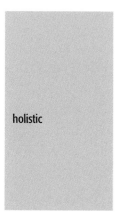

holistic

2-7 The term *medicine* has several meanings, including a drug or a remedy for illness. A second meaning of medicine is the art and science of diagnosis, treatment, and prevention of disease. Medicine recognizes that a person is a composite of physical, social, spiritual, emotional, and intellectual needs (Figure 2-1).

The holistic **(ho-lis′tik)*** viewpoint considers the human as a functioning whole. In illness, the components interact and influence one another. Recognizing that a person is a composite of physical, social, emotional, and intellectual needs is a _____ viewpoint.

2-8 Family practice is a medical specialty that encompasses several branches of medicine and coordinates health care for all members of a family. A family practice physician often acts as the primary health care provider, referring complex disorders to other specialists. The family practice physician has largely replaced the concept of a general practitioner (GP).

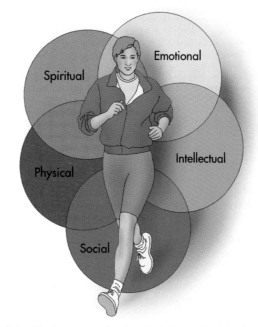

Figure 2-1   Holistic health, the concept that the physical, emotional, intellectual, social, and spiritual aspects of a person's life must be viewed as an integrated whole.

---

*Holistic (Greek: *holos*, whole).

internist

2-9 Internal medicine is a nonsurgical specialty of medicine that deals specifically with the diagnosis and treatment of diseases of the internal structures of the body. The specialist is called an internist (**in-ter′nist**). It is important not to confuse *internist* with the term *intern*. An intern in many clinical programs is any immediate postgraduate trainee. A physician intern is in postgraduate training, learning medical practice under supervision before being licensed as a physician. An internist, however, is a licensed medical specialist.

A physician who specializes in internal medicine is an _____.

Study the following combining forms associated with the medical specialties. Also remember the names of the medical specialties.

Combining Forms for Selected Medical Specialties

COMBINING FORM(S)	MEANING	MEDICAL SPECIALTY	MEDICAL SPECIALIST
cardi(o)	heart	cardiology	cardiologist
crin(o)	to secrete	endocrinology	endocrinologist
dermat(o)	skin	dermatology	dermatologist
esthesi(o)	feeling or sensation	anesthesiology	anesthesiologist
gastr(o), enter(o)	stomach, intestines*	gastroenterology	gastroenterologist
ger(a), ger(o), geront(o)	elderly	geriatrics	geriatrician
gynec(o)	female	gynecology	gynecologist
immun(o)	immune	immunology	immunologist
ne(o), nat(o)	new, birth	neonatology	neonatologist
neur(o)	nerve	neurology	neurologist
obstetr(o)	midwife	obstetrics	obstetrician
onc(o)	tumor	oncology	oncologist
ophthalm(o)	eye	ophthalmology	ophthalmologist
orth(o), ped(o)	orth(o) means straight; ped(o) means child (sometimes, foot)	orthopedics	orthopedist (orthopedic (surgeon)
ot(o), laryng(o)	ear, larynx	otolaryngology	otolaryngologist
path(o)	disease	pathology	pathologist
ped(o)	child (sometimes, foot)	pediatrics	pediatrician
psych(o)	mind	psychiatry	psychiatrist
rheumat(o)	rheumatism	rheumatology	rheumatologist
radi(o)	radiant energy (sometimes, radius)	radiology	radiologist
rhin(o)	nose	rhinology	rhinologist
ur(o)	urinary tract (sometimes, urine)	urology	urologist

*Enter(o) sometimes refers specifically to the small intestine.

skin

2-10 You may already know some of the terms that are associated with the medical specialties. If you do not recognize the combining forms used in the following frames, look back at the listing that you just studied. For example, dermato/logy is the medical specialty concerned with the diagnosis and treatment of diseases of the _____.

A person with acne problems or skin allergies would be treated by a dermatologist (**dər″mə-tol′o-jist**).

dermal (der′məl)

2-11 Combine derm(o) and -al to write a term that means pertaining to the skin:

_____.

Dermato/logic (**dər″mə-to-loj′ik**) and *dermato/logical* (**dər″mə-to-loj′ĭ-kəl**) also refer to the skin. Whether one chooses to say dermatologic or dermatological depends on one's preference. Remember that both -ic and -al mean pertaining to. The ending -ical makes use of both suffixes. Many adjectives accept either ending.

cardiologist
(kahr″de-ol′ə-jist)
cardiac (kahr′de-ak)

cardiac

eye

ophthalmologist
(of″thəl-mol′ə-jist)
eye

pathologist

disease

endocrinologist
(en″do-krĭ-nol′ə-jist)

anesthesiologist
(an″es-the″ze-ol′ə-jist)

gastroenterology

gastroenterologist
(gas″tro-en″tər-ol′ə-jist)

geriatrician
(jer″e-ə-trish′ən)

2-12 The study of the heart and its function is cardio/logy. A physician who specializes in diseases of the heart is a _____.

Combine *cardi(o)* and *-ac* to write a term that means pertaining to the heart: _____.

In a cardi/ac arrest, the heart has stopped beating. In the term *cardiac*, *cardi(o)* means heart and *-ac* means pertaining to. If the heart stops beating, the patient has had a _____ arrest.

2-13 Ophthalmo/logy (of″thəl-mol′ə-je) is the branch of medicine that specializes in the study, diagnosis, and treatment of disorders of the _____.

Write the name of the specialist in ophthalmology by combining *ophthalm(o)* and *-logist*: _____.

Ophthalmic (of-thal′mik), ophthalmologic (of″thəl-mə-loj′ik), and ophthalmological (of″thəl-mə-loj′ĭ-kəl) mean pertaining to the _____.

2-14 Pathology (pə-thol′ə-je) is the general study of the characteristics, causes, and effects of disease. Cellular pathology is the study of cellular changes in disease. Clinical pathology is the study of disease by the use of laboratory tests and methods. A medical pathologist usually specializes in either clinical or surgical pathology. A clinical pathologist (pə-thol′ə-jist) is especially concerned with the use of laboratory methods in clinical diagnosis.

Tissues and organs that are removed in surgery are sent to the surgical pathology laboratory. The physician who studies those tissues and organs to determine the cause of disease is a surgical _____.

The terms *patho/logic* (path-o-loj′ik) and *patho/logical* (path-o-loj′ĭ-kəl) mean morbid or pertaining to pathology or caused by _____.

2-15 The endo/crine (en′do-krīn, en′do-krin) glands secrete hormones (hor′mōnz) into the bloodstream. These hormones play an important role in regulating the body's metabolism. The prefix *endo-* means inside. The suffix *-crine*, from the combining form *crin(o)*, means to secrete. Glands that secrete hormones into the bloodstream are endocrine glands. One example of an endocrine gland is the adrenal (ə-dre′nəl) gland, which secretes adrenaline (epinephrine) into the bloodstream.

The science of the endocrine glands and the hormones they produce is endocrinology (en″do-krĭ-nol′ə-je). A specialist in endocrinology is called an _____.

2-16 An/esthesio/logy (an″es-the″ze-ol′ə-je) is the branch of medicine concerned with the administration of anesthetics (an″es-thet′iks) and with their effects. The physician who administers anesthetics during surgery is an _____. An anesthetic is a drug or agent that is capable of producing a complete or total loss of feeling. The prefix *an-* means no, not, or without. The literal interpretation of anesthesiology is "the study of no feeling," but you need to remember that it is the branch of medicine concerned with the administration of drugs that produce a loss of feeling.

An an/esthetist (ə-nes′thə-tist) is not a physician but is trained in administering anesthetics.

2-17 Gastro/entero/logy (gas″tro-en″tər-ol′ə-je) is the study of diseases affecting the gastrointestinal tract, including the stomach and intestines. Write the name of this specialty that deals with the stomach and intestines: _____.

Gastr/ic (gas′trik) means pertaining to the stomach. A physician who specializes in gastric disorders is a _____.

2-18 Three combining forms—*ger(a)*, *ger(o)*, and *geront(o)*—mean old age or the aged. The scientific study of all aspects of the aging process and issues encountered by older persons is geronto/logy (jer″on-tol′ə-je). The branch of medicine that deals with the problems of aging and the diseases of the elderly is geriatrics (jer″e-at′riks). A physician who specializes in gerontology is a _____.

The selection of the correct combining form may be confusing. Common usage determines which term is proper. Practice will help you to remember.

2-19 Gyneco/logy (gǐ″nə-, jin″ə-kol′ə-je) is devoted to treating diseases of the female reproductive organs, including the breasts. A physician who specializes in the treatment of females is a

_____.

Gyn is an abbreviation for gynecology. It refers to the _____

genital (jen′ĭ-təl) tract.

2-20 Many gynecologists also specialize in obstetrics (ob-stet′riks). Obstetrics (OB) deals with pregnancy, labor, delivery, and immediate care after childbirth; however, *obstetr(o)* means midwife. Midwives assisted women during childbirth before obstetrics developed as a medical specialty. Physicians who specialize in obstetrics are obstetricians (ob″stə-trĭ-′shənz). Two adjectives that mean pertaining to obstetrics are *obstetric* and *obstetrical*.

Write the name of the physician who specializes in obstetrics: _____.

2-21 Neo/nato/logy (ne″o-na-tol′ə-je) is the branch of medicine that specializes in the care of newborns, infants from birth to 28 days of age. A physician who specializes in neonatology is a

_____.

Newborns are given a physical examination (PE) soon after birth. In general, weight triples and height increases by 50 percent in the first year of a healthy infant's life. Head circumference is also measured (Figure 2-2), and subsequent measurements are taken for the first years. A rapidly rising head circumference suggests increased pressure inside the skull, and an unusually small head may indicate underdevelopment of the brain.

2-22 The word root for child is *ped(o)*. Pediatric (pe″de-at′rik) means pertaining to children. Ped/iatrics (pe″de-at′riks) is devoted to the study of children's diseases. Because diseases of children are often quite different from diseases encountered later in life, most parents prefer to take their children to a physician who specializes in _____.

The suffix *-iatrician,* which means practitioner, is used to write the name of the physician who specializes in pediatrics. A ped/iatrician (pe″de-ə-trĭ′shən) specializes in the development and care of infants and children and in the treatment of their diseases.

2-23 Onco/logy (ong-kol′ə-je), a rapidly changing specialty, is concerned with the study of malignancy. The combining form *onc(o)* means tumor. Oncology is particularly concerned with malignant (mə-lig′nənt) tumors and their treatment. *Malignant** means tending to become worse, spread, and cause death.

A specialist who practices oncology is an _____.

gynecologist (gǐ″nə-, jin-ə-kol′ə-jist)
female

obstetrician

neonatologist (ne″o-na-tol′ə-jist)

pediatrics

oncologist (ong-kol′ə-jist)

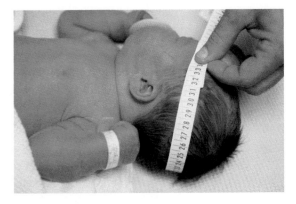

Figure 2-2 Measuring the head of a newborn. This is the appropriate placement of the measuring tape to obtain the head circumference of a newborn.

*Malignant (Latin: *malignus*, bad disposition).

2-24 *Cancer* refers to any of a large group of diseases that are characterized by the presence of malignant tumor. These tumors are called carcinomas. Invasive carcinoma is a malignant tumor that infiltrates and destroys surrounding tissues and may continue spreading. Remission, whether spontaneous or the result of therapy, is the disappearance of the characteristics of a malignant tissue.

malignant

Tumors that do not invade surrounding tissue or spread to distant sites are referred to as benign (bə-nīn′) tumors. In other words, benign tumors are not _____.

2-25 An oto/logist (o-tol′ə-jist) specializes in otology (o-tol′ə-je), the study of the ear, including the diagnosis and treatment of its diseases and disorders. Physicians who specialize in ear, nose, and throat disorders are ear, nose, and throat (ENT) specialists. The combining form *ot(o)* means ear and *laryng(o)* means larynx, or the voice box. *Oto/laryngo/logy* (o″to-lar″ing-gol′ə-je) commonly refers to the branch of medicine dealing with diseases and disorders of the ears, nose, throat, and nearby structures. An otolaryngologist (o″to-lar″ing-gol′ə-jist) is a physician who practices

otolaryngology

_____. *O/tic* (o′tik) means pertaining to the ear.

rhinologist
(ri″nol′ə-jist)

Rhino/logy (ri″nol′ə-je) focuses on the diagnosis and treatment of disorders involving the nose. Write the name of the physician who specializes in rhinology: _____.

2-26 Psych/iatry (si-ki′ə-tre) is a medical specialty that deals with the causes, treatment, and prevention of mental, emotional, and behavioral disorders. A physician who specializes in psychiatry is

psychiatrist
(si-ki′ə-trist)

a _____.

Clinical psycho/logy (si-kol′ə-je) is concerned with the diagnosis, treatment, and prevention of a wide range of personality and behavioral disorders. One who is trained in this area is a clinical

psychologist
(si-kol′ə-jist)

_____. Clinical psychology is not a branch of medicine but a branch of psychology.

2-27 Immuno/logy (im″u-nol′o-je) represents one of the most rapidly expanding areas of science, and *immun(o)* is the combining form for immune. This branch of science involves assessment of the patient's immune defense mechanism against disease, hypersensitivity, and many diseases now thought to be associated with the immune mechanism. This mechanism is the natural defenses that protect the body from pathogenic organisms and malignancies, but it is also involved in allergies, excessive reactions to common and often harmless substances in the environment.

immunologist
(im″u-nol′o-jist)

The specialist in immunology is an _____. Sometimes immunology is combined with the identification and treatment of allergies.

2-28 A physician may choose to specialize in immunology and rheumato/logy (roo″mə-tol′ə-je). A specialist in rheumatology is a _____.

rheumatologist
(roo″mə-tol′ə-jist)

Almost all words that contain the combining form *rheumat(o)* pertain to rheumatism (roo′mə-tiz-əm). Rheumato/logy is the branch of medicine that deals with rheumat/ic disorders. One may think of rheumatism as just one disease, but it is any of a variety of disorders marked by inflammation, degeneration, or other problems of the connective tissues of the body, especially the joints and related structures. This medical specialty is called _____.

rheumatology

Ancient Greeks believed that one's health was determined by the mixture of humors, certain fluids within the body. The word *rheum* meant a watery discharge; rheumatism was thought to be caused by a flowing of humors in the body and was thus named.

2-29 The combining form *radi(o)* means radiant energy. (Sometimes *radi[o]* is used to mean radius, a bone of the forearm, but usually it refers to radiant energy.) Radio/logy (ra″de-ol′ə-je) is the use of various forms of radiant energy (such as x-ray) in the diagnosis and treatment of disease. Radiology is an important part of cancer treatment. The physician who studies and interprets radiographs (x-ray examinations) is a _____. Two terms that mean pertaining to

radiologist
(ra″de-ol′ə-jist)

radiology are *radiologic* (ra″de-o-loj′ik) and *radiological* (ra″de-o-loj′ĭ-kəl).

Sometimes radiology is called roentgeno/logy (rent″gən-ol′ə-je) after the discoverer of x-rays, Wilhelm Conrad Röntgen. Roentgenology is really one branch of radiology dealing with the use of roentgen rays (x-rays). Radiology includes the use of other forms of radiant energy for diagnostic and therapeutic purposes. The combining form *therapeut(o)* means treatment, because therapy means treatment.

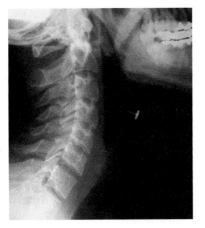

Figure 2-3   Radiograph of an aspirated thumbtack. The lodged tack appears white because it absorbs the x-rays and prevents them from reaching the film or image receptor. Also note the different appearances of air, soft tissue, bone, and teeth.

2-30 X-rays that pass through the patient expose the radiographic film or digital image receptor to create the image. X-radiation passes through different substances in the body to varying degrees. Where there is greater penetration, the image is black or darker; where the x-rays are absorbed by the subject, the image is white or light gray. Thus air appears black, fat appears dark gray, muscle tissue appears light gray, and bone appears very light or white. Heavy substances, such as lead or steel, appear white because they absorb the rays and prevent them from reaching the image receptor (see thumbtack in Figure 2-3).

Substances that do not permit the passage of x-rays are described as radiopaque (**ra″de-o-pāk′**). When *radi(o)* is joined with the word *opaque*,* one *o* is omitted to facilitate pronunciation. The combining form *radi(o)* is also joined with *lucent†* to form the term *radiolucent* (**ra″de-o-loo′sənt**), which describes substances that readily permit the passage of x-rays.

Write the term that means not permitting the passage of x-rays or other radiant energy:

radiopaque _____.

2-31 The combining form *ur(o)* means urine or urinary tract. Urology (**u-rol′ə-je**) is concerned with the urinary tract in both genders, and also the male genital tract. A specialist in urology is a

urologist
(u-rol′ə-jist) _____.

Urologic (**u″ro-loj′ik**), *urological* (**u″ro-loj′ĭ-kəl**), and *urinary* (**u′rĭ-nar″e**) mean pertaining to the urine or the urinary system. A uro/logic examination is an examination of the urinary tract.

2-32 A neuro/logist (**noo-rol′ə-jist**) is a physician who specializes in

neurology _____, the field of medicine that deals with the nervous system and its disorders.

The combining form *neur(o)* means nerve. A nerve cell is called a neuron (**noor′on**) (Figure 2-4). In many words, *neur(o)* refers to the nervous system, which comprises the brain, spinal cord, and nerves.

2-33 Neurosurgery (**noor′o-sər″jər-e**) is surgery involving the brain, spinal cord, or peripheral nerves. Build a word combining *neur(o)* with surgeon that means a surgeon who specializes in surgery of the nervous system: _____.

neurosurgeon
(noor″o-sur′jən)

*Opaque (Latin: *opacus*, dark, obscure).
†Lucent (Latin: *lux*, light).

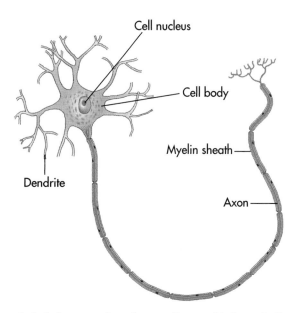

Cell nucleus

Cell body

Myelin sheath

Dendrite

Axon

Figure 2-4   The structure of a typical neuron, a type of nerve cell responsible for conducting nervous impulses. This neuron has a cell body and cytoplasmic projections, one axon, and several dendrites that are sometimes called nerve fibers. Unlike most cells in the body, the neuron cannot replicate.

The term *surgery* is derived from a Greek word that means handwork. Surgery includes several branches of medicine that treat disease, injuries, and deformities by manual or operative procedures. The term *surgery* also refers to the work performed by a surgeon or the place where surgery is performed (Figure 2-5). General surgery deals with operations of all kinds. There are many other surgical specialties, such as those dealing exclusively with the head and neck, hand, and urinary system. OR is the abbreviation for operating room, the place where surgeries are performed.

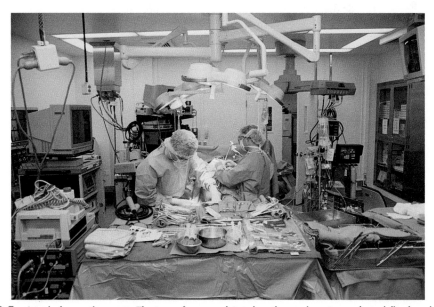

Figure 2-5   A typical operating room. The type of surgery determines the precise setup and specialized equipment that is needed. All persons in the operating room must wear surgical attire.

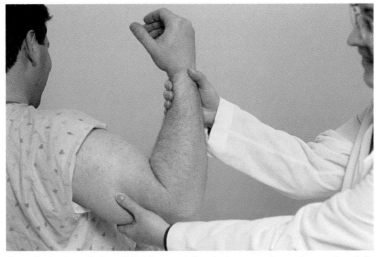

Figure 2-6   Orthopedics is a branch of medicine that specializes in the prevention and correction of disorders of the muscular and skeletal systems of the body.

plastic

2-34 Plastic surgery is the repair or reconstruction of tissue or organs by means of surgery. The combining form *plast(o)* means repair. Reconstructive surgery is an aspect of plastic surgery. It includes procedures such as resetting broken facial bones, restoring parts of the body destroyed by cancer, and correcting birth defects.

Aesthetic plastic surgery has greatly increased in the last few years, particularly that involving the face and breasts. Another notable trend is the increasing number of men who are having cosmetic surgery, with hair replacement leading the list. The medical specialist who performs plastic surgery is called a _____ surgeon.

orthopedics

2-35 Ortho/pedics (or″tho-pe′diks) is a branch of surgery that deals with the preservation and restoration of the bones and associated structures. The specialist is called an orthoped/ist (or″tho-pe′dist) or an orthopedic surgeon (Figure 2-6).

The combining form *orth(o)* means straight, and *ped(o)* refers to child or foot (*pes-,* * *pod[o]*, and *-pod* also refer to foot). The orthopedist originally straightened children's bones and corrected deformities. Today an orthopedist specializes in disorders of the bones and associated structures in people of all ages. The specialty that is concerned with diseases and disorders of the bones and associated structures is _____.

epidemiologist (ep″ĭ-de″me-ol′o-jist)

2-36 An epidemic attacks several people in a region at the same time. The field of medicine that studies the factors that determine the frequency and distribution of diseases is epidemiology (ep″ĭ-de″me-ol′o-je). The specialist is an _____. A physician with this specialty may be assigned the responsibility of directing infection control programs within a hospital. An epidemiologist nurse also has special training and experience in the control of infections.

triage

2-37 There are many other areas in which physicians specialize. Preventive medicine is concerned with preventing the occurrence of both mental and physical illness and disease. Emergency room (ER) medicine deals with acutely (ə-kūt′le) ill or injured patients who require immediate medical treatment. *Acute* (ə-kūt′) means having a short and relatively severe course. The opposite of acute is *chronic* (kron′ik), existing over a long period. In the emergency room, patients are often prioritized according to their need for treatment. This method of sorting according to the patients' needs for care is called triage (tre-ahzh′, tre′ahzh). Write the term that means the sorting and prioritizing of patients for treatment: _____.

Emergency department (ED) more accurately describes the place in a hospital where emergencies are handled, and the terminology is evolving to reflect this fact.

*Latin: *pes,* foot.

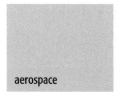

aerospace

2-38 Some physicians specialize in sports medicine, which is concerned with prevention, diagnosis, and treatment of sports injuries. A specialist in forensic (fə-ren′zik) medicine deals with the legal aspects of health care. Aerospace medicine is concerned with the effects of living and working in an artificial environment beyond Earth's atmosphere and forces of gravity. The effect of zero gravity on an astronaut's health would be an aspect of _____ medicine.

Exercise 2

Match the medical specialists with the areas in which they specialize.

_____ 1. anesthesiologist
_____ 2. dermatologist
_____ 3. geriatrician
_____ 4. gynecologist
_____ 5. neonatologist
_____ 6. neurologist
_____ 7. oncologist
_____ 8. otolaryngologist
_____ 9. pathologist
_____ 10. pediatrician

A. children
B. disease in general
C. ear, nose, and throat
D. feeling or sensation
E. females
F. nervous system
G. newborns
H. older persons
I. skin
J. tumors

Exercise 3

Write the specialty associated with the following conditions or situations.

1. heart attack   _____
2. interpreting a radiograph   _____
3. deficiency of the immune system _____
4. hormonal deficiency   _____
5. nosebleed   _____
6. miscarriage   _____
7. irritable bowel disease   _____
8. urinary infection   _____
9. broken wrist   _____
10. rheumatoid arthritis   _____
   (*Use Appendix VI to check your answers.*)

Other Health Professions

2-39 Sophisticated medical care would not be possible without a great variety of health professionals. Physicians rely on the competence of co-workers, those trained in medical specialties, as well as nurses and other allied health workers, who have completed a course of study in a field of health and whose specialized knowledge is vitally important in the diagnosis and treatment of disease.

A physician assistant (PA) is a person certified by the American Academy of Physician Assistants. Depending on their skill, their experience, and legal regulations, physician assistants can deliver pri-

assistant

mary patient care much like a licensed physician. Sometimes they work under the supervision of a licensed physician. PA is an abbreviation for physician _____.

Study the meanings of the word parts in the following list.

Word Parts Used to Write Terms About Medicine and Allied Health Professions

Combining Forms	Meanings	Prefixes	Meanings
bi(o)	life or living	an-	no, not, or without
dent(i), dent(o), odont(o)	tooth	endo-	inside
opt(o), optic(o)	vision		
or(o)	mouth	**Suffix**	**Meaning**
pharmac(o)	drugs or medicine	-crine	secrete
therapeut(o)	treatment		

drugs

2-40 The combining form *pharmac(o)* refers to drugs or medicine. Pharmaco/logy (**fahr″mə-kol′ə-je**) is the study of _____, including their origin, nature, properties, and effects. A pharmacy is a place for the preparation and dispensing of drugs and medicinal supplies by pharmacists and their assistants. The science of formulating, dispensing, and providing information on drugs is also called pharmacy.

RN

practical

2-41 Nursing is one of the oldest and most familiar fields of medicine (Figure 2-7). The registered nurse (RN) is licensed to practice by a state board of nurse examiners or other state authority. The abbreviation for registered nurse is _____.

A licensed practical nurse (LPN) is educated in basic nursing techniques and works under the supervision of a registered nurse. The LPN is a graduate of a school of practical nursing. LPN means a licensed _____ nurse. (LVN is licensed vocational nurse.)

As health care has become more complex, many nursing specialties, such as the nurse practitioner, nurse educator, nurse anesthetist, and nurse midwife, have developed.

laboratory

2-42 Medical laboratory personnel are skilled in the performance of clinical laboratory procedures used in diagnosis and the evaluation of patient progress. In descending order of responsibility and education, laboratory personnel include medical technologists, medical technicians, and laboratory assistants. The place in which these individuals work is a medical _____.

life

2-43 The combining form *bi(o)* means _____ or living. Bio/hazards (**bi′o-haz″ərds**) are objects or substances that are harmful or potentially harmful to humans, other organisms, or the environment. Laboratories that work with disease-causing organisms that require special conditions for containment post signs bearing a special biohazard symbol. This symbol is recognized internationally and warns of harmful or potentially harmful agents.

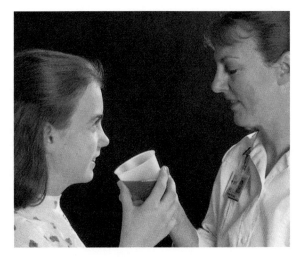

Figure 2-7 Nurse with young patient. The complexity of delivering excellent nursing care provides an even greater challenge as nursing is influenced by increased knowledge about disease, rapid changes in technology and health care, and greater promotion of wellness.

2-44 A radio/logic technologist operates diagnostic imaging equipment and assists radiologists. A radiologic technologist works under the supervision of a physician who specializes in radiology, a

radiologist

_____.

2-45 A physical therapist is specially trained to provide physical therapy to patients (Figure 2-8). A professional who is skilled in physical therapy is called a physical

therapist

_____.

Rehabilitation medicine is concerned with restoring the ability to live and work as normally as possible after an injury or illness. Physical therapy, which is often part of rehabilitation, is the treatment of body ailments by nonmedicinal means. It uses natural agents such as water, heat, massage, and exercise in the treatment of disease. This type of treatment is often written "PT," which is a

physical

way of abbreviating _____ therapy.

2-46 Respiratory therapy is the treatment of disorders in which breathing may be impaired. Any disease in which breathing is affected would be a concern of those who work in

respiratory

_____ therapy. A respiratory therapist is a specialist who holds a degree in respiratory therapy.

Medical records, medical transcription, cytotechnology (**si″to-tek-nol′ə-je**), and dietetics (**di″ə-tet′iks**) are only a few of the many other fields that are associated with health care.

2-47 The combining forms *dent(i)*, *dent(o)*, and *odont(o)* mean _____.

tooth

Dent/istry (**den′tis-tre**) is concerned with the teeth, the oral cavity, and associated structures, as well as the prevention, diagnosis, and treatment of disease and the restoration of defective or missing tissue. This includes the prevention of tooth and gum disease.

Or/al means pertaining to the mouth. The science of operative procedures on the mouth is oral surgery. If someone were having wisdom teeth pulled, it would probably be done by a specialist

surgeon

called an oral _____.

2-48 The combining forms *opt(o)* and *optic(o)* mean vision. A person who deals with optic/al (**op′tĭ-kəl**) glasses and other devices used to correct vision is an optician (**op-tish′ən**). An optic/ian

vision

specializes in correcting _____.

vision

Opto/metry (**op-tom′ə-tre**) is the measurement of _____. In optometry, the irregularities of vision are diagnosed. Corrective lenses are often prescribed. An opto/metr/ist (**op-tom′ə-trist**) is not a physician but a specialist concerned with vision.

2-49 Medical care is fast changing and influenced by increased knowledge about diseases, increased public awareness, and rapid advances in science and technology. Many new professions in

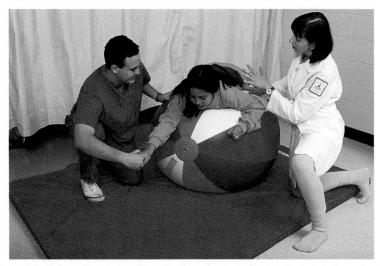

Figure 2-8   Physical therapists with young patient. The therapists are using exercise to help the patient strengthen and coordinate body movements.

the medical field have evolved in recent years, and no doubt more will continue to evolve as increasing emphasis is placed on promotion of wellness, as well as the treatment of disease.

Congratulations! You are well on your way to learning medical terminology.

SELECTED ABBREVIATIONS

Abbreviations are shortened forms of written words or phrases that are used in place of the whole. For example, MD means doctor of medicine. However, MD has other meanings, including medical department.

The Institute for Safe Medications publishes lists of what are considered dangerous abbreviations and recommends that certain terms are written in full because they are easily mistaken for another meaning (for example, qn, meaning nightly or at bedtime, is misinterpreted as qh, which means every hour). Abbreviations are presented in this book because many are still commonly used, but particular caution must be taken in both using and reading abbreviations. If a common abbreviation is missing, you may wish to check to see if its use is discouraged by the Institute for Safe Medications. The Institute's website address is www.ismp.org.

ED	emergency department		**LPN**	licensed practical nurse
ENT	ear, nose, and throat		**OB**	obstetrics
ER	emergency room		**OR**	operating room
GP	general practitioner		**PA**	physician assistant
Gyn	gynecology		**PE**	physical examination
ICU	intensive care unit		**PT**	physical therapy (also prothrombin time)
LVN	licensed vocational nurse			

PREPARING FOR A TEST OF THIS CHAPTER

Study the Word Lists

Review all lists of word parts and their meanings. If you have problems remembering certain word parts, use index cards to prepare flash cards with a word part on one side and its meaning on the reverse side. Review the cards several times before the test.

Be Careful With These!

-ist (one who) vs. -iatry (medical profession or treatment)
-logy (study of) vs. -logist (one who studies; specialist)
ne(o) (new) vs. neur(o) (nerve)
or(o) (mouth) vs. ur(o) (urinary tract or urine) vs. ot(o) (ear)
intern (one in postgraduate training) vs. internist (a physician)

Work the Review Section

Work the following review section. The review helps you know if you have learned the material. The written exercises are divided into Basic Understanding (I through VI) and Greater Comprehension (VII through IX). Your instructor will advise you concerning parts of the review you are to work. After completing all sections of the review, check your answers with the solutions found in Appendix VI.

Use the List of Medical Terms

Review each term in the Listing of Medical Terms at the end of the chapter. Look at the spelling of each term and be sure that you know its meaning. If you cannot recall its meaning, look up the term in the glossary and reread the frames that pertain to the term. It is also helpful to click on the Chapter 2 pronunciations included on the CD. Listen as the terms are pronounced. Additional questions are also included on the CD.

CHAPTER 2 REVIEW

■ Basic Understanding

Identifying Word Parts

I. Use slashes to divide the following terms into their component parts and identify the parts as CF (for combining form), P (for prefix), or S (for suffix). Example: neonatologist = neo/nato/logist <u>neo is CF; nato is CF; logist is S</u>.

1. cardiac   _____

2. gynecologist   _____

3. ophthalmological   _____

4. pathology   _____

5. psychiatry   _____

Writing the Meanings

II. Write the meanings of these word parts.

1. bi(o)   _____

2. -crine   _____

3. dent(o)   _____

4. endo-   _____

5. optic(o)   _____

6. opt(o)   _____

7. or(o)   _____

8. pharmac(o)   _____

9. rhin(o)   _____

10. ur(o)   _____

Matching

III. Match the medical specialists with the areas in which they specialize.

_____ 1. anesthesiologist	A. children	
_____ 2. dermatologist	B. drugs that produce loss of feeling or sensation	
	C. ear, nose, and throat	
_____ 3. endocrinologist	D. eyes	
_____ 4. geriatrician	E. females	
	F. hormones and the glands that secrete them	
_____ 5. gynecologist	G. mental, emotional, and behavioral disorders	
_____ 6. neurologist	H. nervous system	
	I. nose	
_____ 7. oncologist	J. older persons	
_____ 8. ophthalmologist	K. skin	
	L. tumors	
_____ 9. otolaryngologist		
_____ 10. pediatrician		
_____ 11. psychiatrist		
_____ 12. rhinologist		

IV. Match health professions in the left column with their descriptions in the right column.

_____ 1. pharmacists

_____ 2. physical therapists

_____ 3. radiologic technologists

_____ 4. rehabilitation therapists

_____ 5. respiratory therapists

A. dispense and provide information about drugs
B. operate diagnostic imaging equipment
C. restore one's ability to live and work as normally as possible after an injury
D. treat body ailments by nonmedicinal means
E. treat disorders in which breathing is impaired

Multiple Choice

V. Circle the correct answer to complete each of these sentences.

1. A 65-year-old man has a history of heart problems. Which type of specialist should he see for care of his heart condition? (cardiologist, endocrinologist, laryngologist, orthopedist)

2. Cynthia is pregnant. Which type of specialist should she see to care for her during her pregnancy, labor, and delivery? (gerontologist, obstetrician, orthopedist, otologist)

3. Which term means a person who is not a physician but is trained in administering drugs that cause a loss of feeling? (anesthesiologist, anesthesist, anesthetics, anesthetist)

4. Which of the following physicians specializes in the diagnosis and treatment of newborns through the age of 28 days? (geriatrician, gynecologist, neonatologist, urologist)

5. John suffers from persistent digestive problems. Which specialist in disorders of the stomach and intestine is John referred to? (gastroenterologist, immunologist, rheumatologist, toxicologist)

6. Sally injures her arm while ice skating. The emergency room physician orders an x-ray. Which type of physician is a specialist in interpreting x-rays? (gynecologist, ophthalmologist, plastic surgeon, radiologist)

7. Sally's x-ray reveals a fractured radius, one of the bones of her forearm. Dr. Bonelly, a bone specialist, puts a cast on Sally's arm. Which type of specialist is Dr. Bonelly? (dermatologist, orthopedist, otologist, rhinologist)

8. What does the word neuron mean? (medical specialty that deals with the nervous system, nerve cell, neurosurgery, specialist in diseases of the nervous system)

9. Which physician specializes in diagnosis of disease using clinical laboratory results? (clinical pathologist, gastroenterologist, internist, surgical pathologist)

10. Which term describes a substance that does not permit the passage of x-rays? (radiopaque, roentgen, roentgenology, x-radiation)

Writing Terms

VI. *Write a term for each of the following descriptions.*

1. a specialist in internal medicine   _____

2. existing over a long period   _____

3. having a severe and relatively short duration   _____

4. method of prioritizing patients according to their need   _____

5. permitting the passage of radiant energy   _____

6. pertaining to the heart   _____

7. study of the characteristics, causes, and effects of disease   _____

8. surgery of the nervous system   _____

9. tending to become worse, spread, and cause death   _____

10. the secretions of endocrine glands   _____

Greater Comprehension

Spelling

VII. *Circle all incorrectly spelled terms and write their correct spellings:*

cardiak   dermatologic   obstetrics   optometry   sychiatry

Interpreting Abbreviations

VIII. *Write the meaning of each of these abbreviations:*

1. ED   _____

2. ENT   _____

3. ICU   _____

4. OB   _____

5. PA   _____

Pronunciation

IX. *The pronunciation is shown for several medical words. Indicate which syllable has the primary accent by marking it with an ':*

1. anesthesiology (an es the ze ol ə je)

2. forensic (fə ren zik)

3. gastroenterology (gas tro en tər ol ə je)

4. orthopedics (or tho pe diks)

5. radiologic (ra de o loj ik)

   (Use Appendix VI to check your answers.)

LISTING OF MEDICAL TERMS

This listing of terms from Chapter 2 matches Chapter 2 Glossary on the CD. Use the practice CD to review the terms. Look closely at the spelling of each term as it is pronounced, pronounce it aloud, and be sure you know the meaning of each term.

acute
adrenal
adrenaline
anesthesiologist
anesthesiology
anesthetic
anesthetist
benign
biohazard
cardiac
cardiac arrest
cardiologist
cardiology
cellular pathology
chronic
clinical pathologist
clinical pathology
clinical psychologist
clinical psychology
dental
dentist
dentistry
dermal
dermatologic
dermatological
dermatologist
dermatology
dietetics
endocrine
endocrinologist
endocrinology
epidemic
epidemiologist
epidemiology
family practice
forensic medicine

gastric
gastroenterologist
gastroenterology
general anesthesia
geriatrician
geriatrics
gerontology
gland
gynecologist
gynecology
holistic
hormone
immunologist
immunology
internal medicine
internist
larynx
licensed practical nurse
licensed vocational nurse
malignant
medical pathologist
medical technician
medical technologist
neonatologist
neonatology
neurologist
neurology
neuron
neurosurgeon
neurosurgery
nurse anesthetist
nurse midwife
nurse practitioner
obstetric
obstetrical
obstetrician

obstetrics
oncologist
oncology
ophthalmic
ophthalmologist
ophthalmology
optical
optician
optometrist
optometry
oral
oral surgeon
orthopedic
orthopedic surgeon
orthopedics
orthopedist
otic
otolaryngologist
otolaryngology
pathogen
pathologic
pathological
pathologist
pathology
pediatric
pediatrician
pediatrics
pharmacist
pharmacology
pharmacy
physical therapist
physical therapy
physician assistant
plastic surgery
preventive medicine

primary health care
   provider
psychiatrist
psychiatry
psychologist
psychology
radiologic
radiologic technologist
radiological
radiologist
radiology
radiolucent
radiopaque
reconstructive surgery
registered nurse
rehabilitation medicine
remission
respiratory therapist
respiratory therapy
rheumatism
rheumatologist
rheumatology
rhinologist
rhinology
roentgenology
surgery
surgical pathologist
surgical pathology
therapy
triage
tumor
urinary
urologic
urological
urologist
urology

español ENHANCING SPANISH COMMUNICATION

ENGLISH	SPANISH (PRONUNCIATION)
acute	*agudo* (ah-GOO-do)
aged	*envejecido* (en-vay-hay-SEE-do)
anesthetic	*anestésico* (ah-nes-TAY-se-co)
benign	*benigno* (bay-NEEG-no)
breast	*seno* (SAY-no)
cancer	*cáncer* (CAHN-ser)
child	*niña* (NEE-nya), *niño* (NEE-nyo)
chronic	*crónico* (CRO-ne-co)
disease	*enfermedad* (en-fer-may-DAHD)
ear	*oreja* (o-RAY-hah)
eye	*ojo* (O-ho)
gland	*glándula* (GLAN-doo-lah)
gynecology	*ginecología* (he-nay-co-lo-HEE-ah)
heart	*corazón* (co-rah-SON)
hormone	*hormona* (or-MOH-nah)
intestine	*intestino* (in-tes-TEE-no)
life	*vida* (VEE-dah)
malignant	*maligno* (mah-LEEG-no)
mind	*mente* (MEN-te)
mouth	*boca* (BO-cah)
muscle	*músculo* (MOOS-coo-lo)
nerve	*nervio* (NERR-ve-o)
neurology	*neurología* (nay-oo-ro-lo-HEE-ah)
nose	*nariz* (nah-REES)
pathology	*patología* (pah-to-lo-HEE-ah)
physical examination	*examen físico* (ek-SAH-men FEE-se-co)
pregnancy	*embarazo* (em-bah-RAH-so)
psychiatry	*psiquiatría* (se-ke-ah-TREE-ah)
psychology	*psicología* (se-co-lo-HEE-ah)
radiation	*radiación* (rah-de-ah-se-ON)
stomach	*estómago* (es-TOH-mah-go)
surgeon	*cirujano(a)* (se-roo-HAH-no) (na)
surgery	*cirugía* (se-roo-HEE-ah)
therapy	*tratamiento* (trah-tah-me-EN-to)
throat	*garganta* (gar-GAHN-tah)
urinary system	*sistema urinario* (sis-TAY-mah oo-re-NAH-re-o)
urine	*orina* (o-REE-nah)
urology	*urología* (oo-ro-lo-HEE-ah)
x-ray	*radiografía* (rah-de-o-grah-FEE-ah)

CHAPTER 3

Building Surgical and Diagnostic Terms

LEARNING GOALS

In this chapter, you will learn to do the following:

Basic Understanding
1. Match suffixes with their meanings.
2. Recognize combining forms for selected body structures in terms.
3. Write the meanings of the word parts and use them to build and analyze terms.
4. Recognize several types of diagnostic imaging procedures.

Greater Comprehension
5. Spell medical terms accurately.
6. Write the meaning of the abbreviations.
7. Pronounce medical terms correctly.

THESE ARE THE MAJOR SECTIONS IN THIS CHAPTER:

- Building Terms with Suffixes
- Suffixes Pertaining to Surgical Procedures
- Combining Forms for Selected Body Structures
- Suffixes Pertaining to Diagnosis
- Diagnostic Radiology

Building Terms with Suffixes

end	**3-1** Certain terms and their related suffixes have the same meaning. For example, both *-scope* and a *scope* mean an instrument for viewing. Most suffixes are not words in themselves and are attached to the _____ of a word or word part. You will learn several suffixes in this chapter and use them to write new terms. To make the suffixes easier to remember, they are presented in groups.
noun	**3-2** The suffix that is added to a word part (mainly a combining form) generally determines its category. Some students find it helpful to know what types of words are formed by the use of various suffixes. It is for these students that information about parts of speech is provided. It is logical that a suffix coincides with how its meaning is used in speech. For example, *removal* is a noun, so *appendectomy* (ap″en-dek′tə-me), surgical removal of the appendix, is a _____.

Suffixes Pertaining to Surgical Procedures

operative	**3-3** You learned earlier that surgery is a medical specialty that is concerned with operative procedures; therefore, suffixes that pertain to surgical procedures are used to write words about _____ means of treating injury or disease.
	3-4 All the suffixes in the following list are used to name various surgical procedures, and all form nouns when combined with other word parts. It is necessary to take time to study each suffix and its meaning. It is also helpful to think of words you may know that can help you to remember the meaning. Throughout this chapter, make flashcards for word parts and their meanings. Review with the flashcards several times before the test.

Suffixes That Pertain to Surgical Procedures

SUFFIX	MEANING
-centesis	surgical puncture to aspirate or remove fluid
-ectomy	excision (surgical removal or cutting out)
-lysis	process of loosening, freeing, or destroying
-pexy	surgical fixation (fastening in a fixed position)
-plasty	surgical repair
-rrhaphy	suture (uniting a wound by stitches)
-scope	instrument used for viewing (also used in diagnostic procedures)
-scopy	visual examination with a lighted instrument (not always a surgical procedure)
-stomy	formation of an opening
-tome	an instrument used for cutting
-tomy	incision (cutting into tissue)
-tripsy	surgical crushing

puncture	**3-5** The suffix *-centesis* means surgical puncture. Amnio/centesis (am″ne-o-sen-te′sis) is surgical _____ of the amnion (am′ne-on), the thin membrane that surrounds the fetus during pregnancy. A small amount of amniotic (am″ne-ot″ik) fluid is removed for analysis to aid in the diagnosis of fetal abnormalities.
nerve	**3-6** You learned in the last chapter that *neur(o)* means _____. Neur/ectomy (noo-rek′to-me) is partial or total excision of a nerve. (Notice that partial or total is implied. Literal translation does not always indicate the full meaning.)

neurotripsy
(nŏo″o-trip′se)

-pexy

ophthalmoplasty
(of-thal′mo-plas″te)
incision

-tome

-scopy

ear

-rrhaphy

-stomy

3-7 *Neuro/lysis* (nŏo-rol′ĭ-sis) means destruction of nerve tissue or loosening of adhesions (ad-he′zhənz) surrounding a nerve. Fibrous structures called adhesions form when two structures abnormally attach to each other.

Change the suffix of neurolysis to form a word that specifically means surgical crushing of a nerve: _____.

3-8 The suffix that means surgical fixation or fastening in a fixed position is

_____.

3-9 You learned earlier that *ophthalm(o)* means eye. Combine *ophthalm(o)* and *-plasty* to write a new term: _____. The term you just wrote means surgical repair of the eye.

Ophthalmo/tomy (of″thəl-mot′ə-me) is _____ of the eye (in this case, the eyeball).

3-10 Be sure you understand the difference between incision and excision. Incision is cutting into. Excision is cutting out or removal. Write the suffix that means an instrument used for cutting: _____.

3-11 The suffix that means a visual examination with a lighted instrument is _____, and the instrument used is a scope, which can also be a suffix.

3-12 Oto/plasty (o′to-plas″te) is surgical repair of the _____.

3-13 To suture is to stitch together cut or torn edges of tissue with silk, catgut, wire, or synthetic material. Write the suffix that means suture: _____.

3-14 Perhaps you have heard of a stoma, which is a small opening, either natural or artificially created. The suffix that means formation of an opening is _____ and is derived from the same root as stoma.

Exercise 1

Match the suffixes in the left column with their meanings in the right column.

_____ 1. -centesis
_____ 2. -ectomy
_____ 3. -pexy
_____ 4. -plasty
_____ 5. -rrhaphy
_____ 6. -scopy
_____ 7. -stomy
_____ 8. -tome
_____ 9. -tomy
_____ 10. -tripsy

A. excision
B. formation of an opening
C. incision
D. instrument used for cutting
E. surgical crushing
F. surgical fixation
G. surgical puncture
H. surgical repair
I. suture
J. visual examination

Combining Forms for Selected Body Structures

3-15 Combining forms for several body structures are presented in this section. This list is not intended to be complete. You learned several combining forms in the previous chapter, and many more will be presented in later chapters. Adding various suffixes to the combining forms will determine how the resulting term is used in a sentence. Practice learning the combining forms in the same manner that you learned the list of suffixes pertaining to surgical procedures.

Combining Forms for Selected Body Structures

COMBINING FORM(S)	MEANING	COMBINING FORM(S)	MEANING
aden(o)	gland	cutane(o), derm(a), dermat(o)	skin
angi(o)	vessel		
append(o), appendic(o)	appendix	mamm(o), mast(o)	breast
blephar(o)	eyelid	nephr(o), ren(o)	kidney
cerebr(o), encephal(o)	brain; cerebr(o) sometimes means cerebrum, the main portion of the brain	oste(o)	bone
		tonsill(o)	tonsil
		vas(o)	vessel; ductus deferens (also called vas deferens, excretory duct of the testicle)
chir(o)	hand		
col(o), colon(o)	colon or large intestine		

colonoscope
(ko-lon′-o-skōp)

3-16 Both colono/scopy (ko″lən-os′kə-pe) and colo/scopy (ko-los′ko-pe) mean an examination of the lining of the colon with a special instrument. The instrument is a _____, also called a coloscope (kol′o-skōp).

suture

3-17 Colectomy (ko-lek′tə-me) is excision of the colon (or a portion of it). Colo/pexy (ko′lo-pek″se) is surgical fixation of the colon, and colo/rrhaphy (ko-lor′ə-fe) is _____ of the colon.

blepharoplasty
(blef′ə-ro-plas″te)

3-18 Write a term that means surgical repair of the eyelid: _____.

hand

3-19 Chiro/plasty (ki′ro-plas″te) is plastic surgery on the _____.

suture

3-20 Angio/plasty (an′je-o-plas″te) means plastic surgery on vessels (in this case, blood vessels). Angio/rrhaphy (an″je-or′ə-fe) means repair of a vessel by _____.

bone
osteotome
(os′te-o-tōm″)

3-21 Osteo/tomy (os″te-ot′ə-me) is cutting of a _____. Write a word that means the instrument used in osteotomy: _____.

incision

3-22 Tracheo/tomy (tra″ke-ot′ə-me) is an _____ made into the trachea (tra′ke-ə) through the neck. This procedure may be performed as an emergency measure to gain access to the airway below a blockage. Use -stomy to build a word that means the opening into the trachea through which a tube may be inserted: _____.

tracheostomy
(tra″ke-os′tə-me)
adenectomy
(ad″ə-nek′tə-me)

3-23 Combine aden(o) and -ectomy: _____. This new term means surgical removal of a gland. A gland is an organ with specialized cells that secrete or excrete materials not related to their ordinary metabolism.

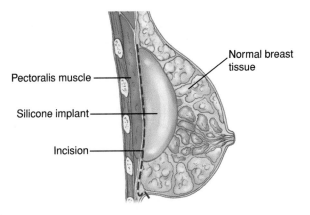

Pectoralis muscle

Silicone implant

Incision

Normal breast tissue

Figure 3-1 Augmentation mammoplasty is achieved by inserting envelopes filled with silicone gel *(shown here)* or saline beneath normal breast tissue or beneath the muscle of the chest. An incision below the breast causes the least obvious scarring.

appendectomy
(ap″en-dek′tə-me)

3-24 Use *append/o* to write a word that means surgical removal of the appendix:
_____.

mastectomy
(mas-tek′tə-me)

3-25 Use *mast(o)* to write a term that means excision of a breast:
_____.

breast

Mammo/plasty (**mam′o-plas″te**) is surgical repair of the _____.
Plastic surgery of the breasts is performed to reduce or lift large or sagging breasts, to enlarge small breasts, or to reconstruct a breast after removal of a tumor. Enlarging the breasts is called augmentation mammoplasty (Figure 3-1).

incision

3-26 *Encephalo/tomy* (**en-sef″ə-lot′ə-me**) and *cerebro/tomy* (**ser″ə-brot′ə-me**) mean _____ of the brain. Not all word parts that have the same meaning are interchangeable. You will learn which to use as you study them.
Write a word that means the instrument used in encephalotomy:
_____.

encephalotome
(en-sef′ə-lə-tōm)

Exercise 2

Write the meaning of the underlined word part in each of the following words.

1. neuro<u>lysis</u>   _____

2. <u>ophthalmo</u>plasty   _____

3. colo<u>rrhaphy</u>   _____

4. <u>oto</u>plasty   _____

5. <u>encephalo</u>tomy   _____

6. mammo<u>plasty</u>   _____

7. <u>angio</u>rrhaphy   _____

8. <u>aden</u>ectomy   _____

9. cerebro<u>tomy</u>   _____

10. <u>blepharo</u>plasty   _____

Suffixes Pertaining to Diagnosis

sign
symptom

3-27 Diagnosis (di″əg-no′sis), abbreviated Dx, is the identification of a disease or condition by a scientific evaluation of physical signs, symptoms (Sx), history, tests, and procedures. Compare *diagnosis* with *prognosis* (prog-no′sis), which means the predicted outcome of a disease.

Signs are objective, or definitive, evidence of an illness or disordered function. Symptoms are subjective evidence as perceived by the patient, such as pain. Indisputable evidence, such as a rash, is which—a sign or a symptom? _____

Is itching of the skin a sign or a symptom? _____ *Itching* and *rash* are both diagnostic terms.

3-28 Diagnostic (di″əg-nos′tik) terms are used to describe the signs and symptoms of disease (such as rash and itching), as well as the tests used to establish a diagnosis. The tests include clinical studies (measuring blood pressure), laboratory tests (determination of blood gases), and radio/logic (ra″de-o-loj′ik) studies, those that relate to the use of radiant energy (such as a chest x-ray [radiograph]).

Laboratory (lab) tests, ranging from simple to sophisticated studies, identify and quantify substances to evaluate organ functions or establish a diagnosis. The abbreviation WNL, meaning within normal limits, is sometimes used by physicians to describe the results of a laboratory test.

diagnostic

Both lab and radiologic tests that are used to establish a diagnosis are _____ terms.

softening

3-29 Suffixes that pertain to diagnosis are used to describe signs and symptoms, as well as tests and procedures that are used to diagnose disease. Some diseases are named for the diagnostic term. For example, -malacia means soft or softening and can be used to describe a sign, but some diseases are named for that particular sign (for example, ophthalmo/malacia [of-thal″mo-mə-la′shə] means an abnormal _____ of the eye).

All the suffixes in the following list form nouns unless otherwise noted. Read each suffix and its meaning.

Suffixes That Pertain to Diagnosis

Signs and Symptoms

-algia, -dynia	pain
-ectasia, -ectasis	dilatation (dilation, enlargement) or stretching of a structure or part
-edema	swelling
-emesis	to vomit, vomiting
-malacia	soft, softening
-megaly	enlargement
-oid (forms adjectives and nouns)	resembling
-penia	deficiency
-rrhage, -rrhagia	excessive bleeding or hemorrhage

-rrhea	flow or discharge
-rrhexis	rupture
-spasm	twitching, cramp
-stasis	stopping, controlling

Procedures

-gram	a record
-graph	an instrument used to record
-graphy	the process of recording
-scope	instrument used for viewing
-scopy	visual examination

ear

3-30 Both oto/dynia (o″to-din′e-ə) and ot/algia (o-tal′je-ə) mean a pain in the _____, or earache.

eye

3-31 Ophthalmo/dynia (of-thal″mo-din′e-ə) means pain in the _____.

Use -algia to write another term that means pain in the eye: _____.

ophthalmalgia
(of″thəl-mal′jə)

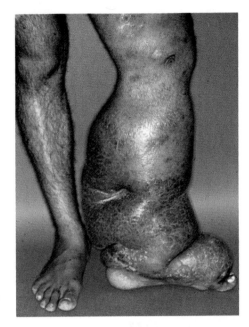

Figure 3-2 Extensive swelling, caused by chronic obstruction of the lymphatic vessels, occurs in the late stages of elephantiasis.

deficiency	**3-32** The suffix *-penia* means _____. *Calci/penia* (**kal″sĭ-pe′ne-ə**) means a deficiency of calcium.
enlargement	**3-33** You may be more familiar with the prefix *mega-*, but *-megaly* also means enlarged or enlargement. *Cardio/megaly* (**kahr″de-o-meg′ə-le**) means _____ of the heart.
discharge	**3-34** Several suffixes in the list begin with *rr*. *Oto/rrhea* (**o″to-re′ə**) means a _____ from the ear.
-rrhexis hemorrhage	**3-35** Write a suffix that means rupture: _____. Both *-rrhage* and *-rrhagia* mean excessive bleeding or _____.
swelling	**3-36** Several suffixes are also terms that can stand alone. *Emesis* (**em′ə-sis**) means the material expelled in vomiting, and *edema* (**ə-de′mə**) is the presence of abnormally large amounts of fluid in the tissues, resulting in swelling. The suffix *-edema* means swelling.\
Blephar/edema (**blef″ə-rĭ-de′mə**) is _____ of the eyelid.\
An outstanding example of edema is seen in the late stages of elephantiasis (**el″ə-fən-ti′ə-sis**), a parasitic disease generally seen in the tropics (Figure 3-2). The excessive swelling is caused by obstruction of the lymphatic vessels by the parasites.
softening ophthalmomalacia	**3-37** *Malacia* (**mə-la′shə**) means _____. Write a word that means abnormal softening of the eye: _____.
controlling	**3-38** *Stasis* (**sta′sis**), the term, means the same as the suffix *-stasis*, which means stopping or _____.
twitching	**3-39** *Spasm* means cramp or twitching. *Blepharo/spasm* (**blef′ə-ro-spaz″em**) means _____ of the eyelid.
bone	**3-40** You learned that *oste(o)* means _____. If something is described as *oste/oid* (**os′te-oid**), it resembles bone.

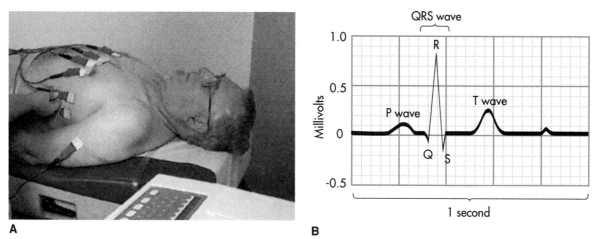

A   **B**

Figure 3-3 **A,** A patient undergoing electrocardiography, the making of graphic records produced by electrical activity of the heart muscle. The instrument, an electrocardiograph, is shown. The electrical impulses that are given off by the heart are picked up by electrodes (sensors) and conducted into the electrocardiograph through wires. **B,** An enlarged section of an ECG, a tracing that represents the heart's electrical impulses, which are picked up and conducted to the electrocardiograph by electrodes or leads connected to the body. The pattern of the graphic recording indicates the heart's rhythm and other actions. The normal ECG is composed of the labeled parts shown in the drawing. Each labeled segment represents a different part of the heartbeat. Electrocardiography is a valuable diagnostic tool.

recording

record

electrocardiograph
(e-lek″tro-kahr′de-
o-graf″)

otoscope (o′to-skōp)

ophthalmoscopy
(of″thəl-mos′kə-pe)

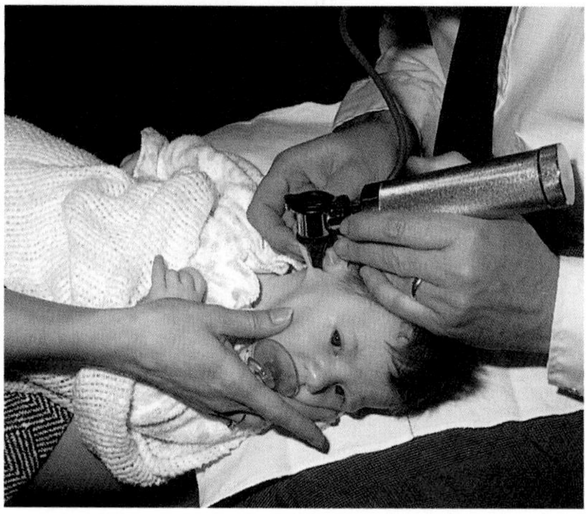

3-41 Electro/cardio/graphy (**e-lek″tro-kahr″de-og′rə-fe**), the process of recording the electrical impulses of the heart, is one example of a diagnostic procedure. The suffix *-graphy* means the process of _____. An electro/cardio/gram (**e-lek″tro-kahr′de-o-gram″**) is a record or tracing of the electrical impulses of the heart, because *-gram* means the _____ that is produced in this procedure. This is abbreviated as ECG or EKG. The suffix *-graph* means an instrument used for recording. Use *electr(o)* + *cardi(o)* + *-graph* to write the name of the instrument used in electrocardiography: _____ (Figure 3-3).

3-42 *Oto/scopy* (**o-tos′kə-pe**) means an examination of the outer ear, including the eardrum (Figure 3-4). Write a word that means the lighted instrument used in otoscopy: _____.

3-43 Using *otoscopy* as a model, write a term that means examination of the interior of the eye with an ophthalmoscope (**of-thal′mə-skōp**): _____.

Figure 3-4 Otoscopy is visual examination of the ear, including the eardrum, with a lighted instrument, an otoscope.

Exercise 3

Match the suffixes in the left column with their meanings in the right column.

_____1. -algia

_____2. -ectasis

_____3. -edema

_____4. -emesis

_____5. -malacia

_____6. -megaly

_____7. -rrhagia

_____8. -stasis

A. controlling
B. dilatation
C. enlargement
D. excessive bleeding
E. pain
F. softening
G. swelling
H. vomiting

Exercise 4

Write the suffix that means the following:

1. deficiency   _____

2. flow or discharge _____

3. resembling   _____

4. rupture   _____

5. spasm or twitching _____

Diagnostic Radiology

3-44 Radiology is the branch of medicine concerned with x-rays and radioactive substances and with the diagnosis and treatment of disease using any of the various sources of radiant energy. Diagnostic radiology is used to establish or confirm a diagnosis. Learn the following word parts and their meanings.

Word Parts Associated with Radiology

COMBINING FORM	MEANING	PREFIX	MEANING
ech(o), son(o)	sound	ultra-	excessive
electr(o)	electricity		
fluor(o)	emitting or reflecting light		
radi(o)*	radiant energy		
tom(o)	to cut		

*radi(o) sometimes means radius, a bone of the forearm.

3-45 Radio/graphy was the predominant means of diagnostic imaging for many years, using x-rays to provide film images of internal structures. Almost everyone is familiar with a chest x-ray (CXR). There are additional diagnostic imaging modalities today, including the following:

- Contrast imaging
- Computed tomography (CT), formerly known as computed axial tomography (CAT)
- Nuclear medicine (placing radioactive materials into body organs for the purpose of imaging)

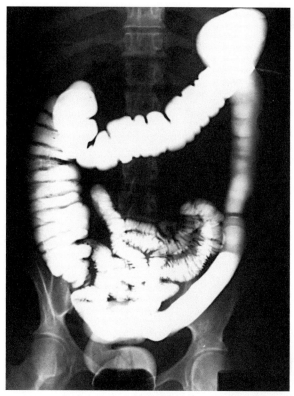

Figure 3-5 Contrast imaging. In this example of a barium enema, radiopaque barium sulfate is used to make the large intestine clearly visible.

- Magnetic resonance imaging (MRI)
- Sono/graphy (also called ultra/sono/graphy, echo/graphy, or ultra/sound)

3-46 Contrast imaging is the use of radiopaque (**ra″de-o-pāk′**) materials to make internal organs visible on x-ray images. A contrast medium may be injected into the body or swallowed, resulting in greater visibility of internal organs or cavities outlined by the contrast material. This type of imaging is called _____ imaging. One example is a barium enema, the introduction of barium sulfate, a radiopaque contrast medium, into the rectum. A barium enema increases visibility of the inner contours of the lower intestinal tract (Figure 3-5).

3-47 Fluoro/scopy (**floo-ros′kə-pe**) is a method of viewing the x-ray image directly in real time so that motion can be seen, and radiography provides a permanent record of the image at a particular point in time. Fluoroscopy and radiography are both used to follow the movement of the barium sulfate through the upper and lower portions of the gastro/intestinal (GI) tract. The studies are called upper GI series (or barium swallow) and lower GI series (barium enema), respectively.

Write the name of the instrument used in fluoroscopy: _____.
This device projects an x-ray image on a screen. Barium enemas and barium meals are done for diagnosis of certain types of obstruction, ulcers, tumors, or other abnormalities.

3-48 CT is the abbreviation for computed _____. This technique produces an image of a detailed cross section of tissue similar to what one would see if the body or body part were actually cut into sections. The *tom(o)* in tomo/graphy means to _____. The procedure, however, is painless and non/invasive, meaning it does not require the skin to be broken or a cavity or organ of the body to be entered. A CT scanner and a computed tomogram (**to′mo-gram**) of the brain are shown in Figure 3-6.

3-49 Nuclear medicine involves administering radio/pharmaceuticals (**ra″de-o-fahr″mə-soo′tĭ-kəlz**) to a patient orally, into the vein, or by having the patient breathe the material in vapor

contrast

fluoroscope
(**floor′o-skōp**)

tomography
(**to-mog′rə-fe**)

cut

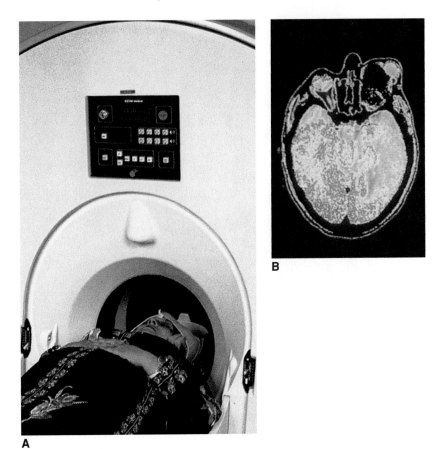

Figure 3-6   Computed tomography of the brain. **A**, Positioning of patient for computed tomography. **B**, Computed tomographic scan of the brain.

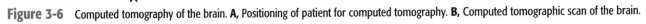

mouth

form. Computerized scanners called gamma cameras detect the radioactivity emitted by the patient and map its location to form an image of the organ or system (Figure 3-7). You remember that oral administration is by _____. Pharmaceuticals (**fahr″mə-soo′tĭ-kəlz**) are medicinal drugs, and radiopharmaceuticals are those that are radioactive.

magnetic

3-50 MRI is the abbreviation for _____ resonance (**rez′o-nəns**) imaging. It is a noninvasive technique for visualizing internal structures and creates images based on the magnetic properties of chemical elements within the body, rather than using ionizing radiation such as x-rays. In addition, it produces superior soft-tissue resolution (Figure 3-8). Soft-tissue resolution distinguishes adjacent structures. Patients must remain motionless for a time and may experience anxiety because of being somewhat enclosed inside the scanner. The newer open MRI scanners have eliminated much of the anxiety and can accommodate larger patients.

excessive

3-51 Sono/graphy (**sə-nog′rə-fe**) is known by many names, including ultrasonography (**ul″trə-sə-nog′rə-fe**) and diagnostic ultrasound (**ul′trə-sound**). The prefix *ultra-* means _____. Most of these names use the combining form *son(o)*, which means sound. Sonography is the process of imaging deep structures of the body by sending and receiving high-frequency sound waves that are reflected back as echoes from tissue interfaces. Conventional sonography provides two-dimensional images, but the more recent scanners are capable of showing a three-dimensional perspective. Sonography is very safe because it is not invasive and does not use ionizing radiation. It has many medical applications, including imaging of the fetus (Figure 3-9).

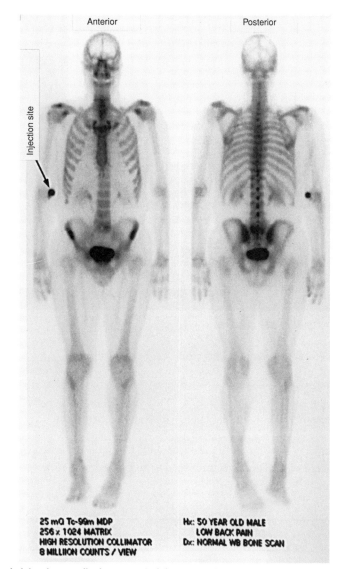

Figure 3-7 Nuclear medicine: administering a radiopharmaceutical that accumulates in a specific organ or structure to provide information about its function, and to some degree, its structure.

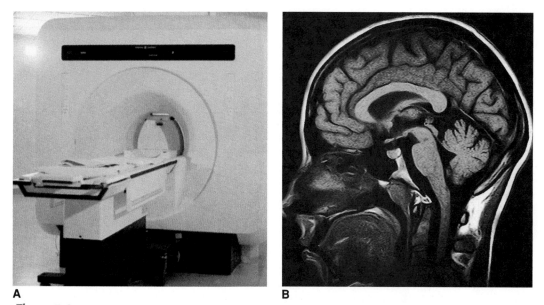

Figure 3-8 Magnetic resonance imaging. **A,** Clinical setting for magnetic resonance imaging. **B,** Image of the head.

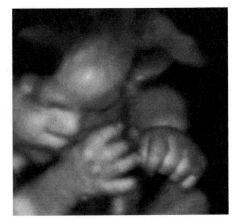

Figure 3-9 Ultrasound of fetus. Using sound waves at high frequency, ultrasound imaging provides two- and three-dimensional images of internal organs, including images of a developing fetus.

Exercise 5

Write a word in each blank to complete these sentences.

1. The use of radiopaque materials to make internal organs visible on x-ray is called _____ imaging.

2. CT means computed _____.

3. Nuclear medicine involves placing _____ materials into body organs for the purpose of imaging.

4. Creating images based on the magnetic properties of chemical elements within the body is *MRI*, which means magnetic _____ imaging.

5. Ultrasonography provides imaging of internal structures by measuring and recording _____ waves.

SELECTED ABBREVIATIONS

CT, CAT	computed tomography, computed axial tomography	**GI**	gastrointestinal
CXR	chest x-ray	**lab**	laboratory
Dx	diagnosis	**MRI**	magnetic resonance imaging
ECG, EKG	electrocardiogram	**Sx**	symptoms
		WNL	within normal limits

PREPARING FOR A TEST OF THIS CHAPTER

Review as you were instructed in the previous chapter and work the end-of-chapter review.

Be Careful With These!

-gram (a record) vs. *-graph* (an instrument) vs. *-graphy* (a process)
-rrhage (excessive bleeding) vs. *-rrhea* (discharge) vs. *-rrhexis* (rupture)
-tome (cutting instrument) vs. *-tomy* (cutting into)
-tomy (cutting into) vs. *-stomy* (formation of an opening)
incision (cutting into) vs. excision (cutting out, removal)
diagnosis (identification of disease) vs. prognosis (predicted outcome)
sign (objective) vs. symptom (subjective)

CHAPTER 3 REVIEW

■ Basic Understanding

Matching
I. Match the following surgical suffixes with their meanings.

_____ 1. -centesis   A. excision
                          B. formation of an opening
_____ 2. -ectomy   C. surgical crushing
_____ 3. -pexy   D. surgical fixation
                          E. surgical puncture
_____ 4. -plasty   F. surgical repair
_____ 5. -rrhaphy   G. suture
                          H. visual examination
_____ 6. -scopy

_____ 7. -stomy

_____ 8. -tripsy

Matching
II. Match the following diagnostic suffixes with their meanings.

_____ 1. -algia   A. dilatation
                          B. enlargement
_____ 2. -ectasia   C. excessive bleeding
_____ 3. -edema   D. flow or discharge
                          E. pain
_____ 4. -emesis   F. resembling
_____ 5. -malacia   G. rupture
                          H. softening
_____ 6. -megaly   I. swelling
                          J. vomiting
_____ 7. -oid

_____ 8. -rrhagia

_____ 9. -rrhea

_____ 10. -rrhexis

Writing the Meanings
III. Write the meaning of the following terms.

1. amniocentesis   _____

2. blepharoplasty   _____

3. calcipenia   _____

4. echography   _____

5. electrocardiograph   _____

6. fluoroscope   _____

7. osteoid   _____

8. tomogram   _____

Multiple Choice
IV. *Circle one answer for each of the following questions.*

1. Susie tells the doctor that she has a sore throat. Which term describes the sore throat? (diagnosis, prognosis, sign, symptom)

2. Mr. Jones has plastic surgery on his hand. What is the name of this procedure? (carpectomy, chiroplasty, ophthalmoplasty, otoplasty)

3. Which word means stopping or controlling? (phobia, ptosis, spasm, stasis)

4. An elderly man is told he has an enlarged heart. Which term describes his condition? (cardiomegaly, carditis, coronary artery disease, megalomania)

5. Which term means pertaining to a record of the electrical impulses of the heart? (echography, electrocardiogram, electrocardiograph, electrocardiography)

6. Which term specifically means an opening into the trachea? (tracheoplasty, tracheostomy, tracheotome, tracheotomy)

7. Which term means removal of a gland? (adenectomy, adenotomy, appendotomy, appendectomy)

8. Which term means abnormal softening of the eye? (ophthalmalgia, ophthalmomalacia, ophthalmoscopy, opthalmotomy)

9. Which term means an earache? (otodynia, otology, otoscope, otoscopy)

10. Which diagnostic procedure produces an image of a detailed cross section of tissue similar to what one would see if the organ were actually cut into sections? (computed tomography, contrast imaging, electrocardiography, nuclear medicine imaging)

Writing Terms
V. *Write a term for each clue that is given.*

1. excessive bleeding   _____

2. excision of the colon   _____

3. incision of the eye   _____

4. instrument used in encephalotomy _____

5. plastic surgery of the ear _____

6. surgical crushing of a nerve _____

7. surgical fixation of the colon _____

8. suture of a vessel   _____

9. swelling of the eyelid   _____

10. visual examination of the ear _____

Spelling
VI. *Circle all incorrectly spelled terms and write their correct spellings.*

cerebrotomy   colorrhaphy   nurotripsy   ofthalmoplasty   simptom

Interpreting Abbreviations

VII. *Write the meaning of each of these abbreviations.*

1. CT   _____

2. CXR   _____

3. ECG   _____

4. MRI   _____

5. WNL   _____

Pronunciation

VIII. *Indicate the primary-accented syllable in each of the following terms by marking it with an ´.*

1. appendectomy (ap en dek tə me)

2. calcipenia (kal sĭ pe ne ə)

3. encephalotomy (en sef ə lot ə me)

4. neurolysis (noo rol ĭ sis)

5. sonography (sə nog rə fe)
(*Use Appendix VI to check your answers*)

LISTING OF MEDICAL TERMS

Use the practice CD to review the terms that have been presented. Look closely at the spelling of each term as it is pronounced and be sure you know the meaning of each term.

adenectomy
adhesion
amniocentesis
amnion
amniotic
angioplasty
angiorrhaphy
appendectomy
blepharedema
blepharoplasty
blepharospasm
calcipenia
cardiomegaly
cerebrotomy
chiroplasty
colectomy
colonoscope
colonoscopy
colopexy
colorrhaphy
coloscope

coloscopy
computed axial
    tomography
computed tomography
diagnosis
dilatation
echography
edema
electrocardiogram
electrocardiograph
electrocardiography
elephantiasis
emesis
encephalotome
encephalotomy
excision
gland
incision
magnetic resonance
    imaging
malacia

mammoplasty
mastectomy
neurectomy
neurolysis
neurotripsy
ophthalmalgia
ophthalmodynia
ophthalmomalacia
ophthalmoplasty
ophthalmoscope
ophthalmoscopy
ophthalmotomy
osteoid
osteotome
osteotomy
otalgia
otodynia
otoplasty
otorrhea
otoscope
otoscopy

prognosis
radioactive
radiology
radiopaque
radiopharmaceuticals
sonography
spasm
stasis
stoma
suture
symptom
therapeutic
tomogram
trachea
tracheostomy
tracheotomy
ultrasonography
ultrasound

español ENHANCING SPANISH COMMUNICATION

ENGLISH	SPANISH (PRONUNCIATION)
appendix	*apéndice* (ah-PEN-de-say)
brain	*cerebro* (say-RAY-bro)
calculus	*cálculo* (CAHL-coo-lo)
diagnosis	*diagnóstico* (de-ag-NOS-te-co)
dilatation	*dilatación* (de-lah-tah-se-ON)
edema	*hidropesía* (e-dro-pay-SEE-ah)
enlargement	*aumento* (ah-oo-MEN-to)
eyelid	*párpado* (PAR-pah-do)
hand	*mano* (MAH-no)
hemorrhage	hemorragia (ay-mor-RAH-he-ah)
instrument	instrumento (ins-troo-MEN-to)
pain	dolor (do-LOR)
rupture	ruptura (roop-TOO-rah)
spasm	espasmo (es-PAHS-mo)
suture	sutura (soo-TOO-rah)
swelling	hinchar (in-CHAR)
symptom	síntoma (SEEN-to-mah)
trachea	tráquea (TRAH-kay-ah)
vessel	vaso (VAH-so)
vomiting	vómito (VO-me-to)

CHAPTER 4

Building Terms about Diseases and Disorders

LEARNING GOALS

In this chapter, you will learn to do the following:

Basic Understanding

1. Match suffixes pertaining to pathologies with their meanings.
2. Match the combining forms that describe color with their meanings.
3. Write the meanings of the word parts and use them to build and analyze terms.
4. Recognize several terms associated with treatment of diseases and disorders.

Greater Comprehension

5. Spell medical terms accurately.
6. Write the meanings of the abbreviations.
7. Pronounce medical terms correctly.

THESE ARE THE MAJOR SECTIONS IN THIS CHAPTER:

- ❏ **Word Parts Pertaining to Pathologies**
- ❏ **Miscellaneous Suffixes**
- ❏ **Combining Forms and Related Suffixes**
- ❏ **Additional Combining Forms**
- ❏ **Therapeutic Interventions**

Word Parts Pertaining to Pathologies

diseases

4-1 Suffixes joined to combining forms are used to write the names of many diseases or disorders. Patho/logies are terms that represent the names of _____ or disorders. All the suffixes in the following list are used to write nouns.

Word Parts Pertaining to Pathologies

COMBINING FORM	MEANING	SUFFIX	MEANING
cancer(o), carcin(o)	cancer	-mania	excessive preoccupation
onc(o)	tumor	-maniac	a person who shows excessive preoccupation
path(o)	disease	-oma	tumor
		-osis	condition (often an abnormal condition; sometimes an increase)
SUFFIX	**MEANING**		
-cele	hernia (protrusion of all or part of an organ through the wall of the cavity that contains it)	-pathy	disease
		-phobia	abnormal fear
-emia	condition of the blood	-ptosis	prolapse (sagging)
-ia-, -iasis	condition		
-itis	inflammation		
-lith	stone or calculus		

tumor

4-2 Carcin/oma (**kahr″sǐ-no′mə**) is cancer or a cancer/ous tumor, because *carcin(o)* means cancer and *-oma* means _____.
    You also know a combining form that means tumor, which is

onc(o)

_____.

4-3 Many tumors are benign. For example, an angi/oma (**an″je-o′mə**) is a benign tumor made up of blood vessels or lymph vessels (Figure 4-1).

4-4 The suffix that means inflammation is *-itis*. Ophthalm/itis (**of″thəl-mi′tis**) is inflammation of

eye
appendix
otitis (**o-ti′tis**)

the _____.
    Appendic/itis (**ə-pen″dǐ-si′tis**) is inflammation of the _____.
    Write a term that means inflammation of the ear: _____.
    Tonsillitis (**ton″sǐ-li′tis**) means inflammation of the tonsils, and mast/itis (**mas-ti′tis**) is inflammation of the _____.

breast

nerve

    Oste/itis (**os″te-i′tis**) is inflammation of a bone, and neuritis (**noo-ri′tis**) is inflammation of a _____.

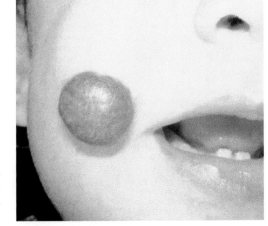

Figure 4-1   This type of angioma is filled with blood vessels. It is often called a birthmark because it is commonly found during infancy. It grows at first but may spontaneously disappear in early childhood. It can be surgically removed if bleeding or injury is a problem or later for cosmetic reasons.

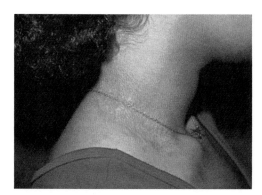

Figure 4-2 This example of allergic dermatitis is caused by nickel in the necklace. Allergic dermatitis usually results from contact with jewelry, metal clasps, or coins. Other types of allergic dermatitis may be caused by contact with poison ivy, other metals, or chemicals, including latex, dyes, and perfumes.

adenitis (ad″ə-ni′tis)
skin

Write a term that means inflammation of a gland: _____.
Dermat/itis (der″mə-ti′tis) is inflammation of the _____. One type of dermatitis is caused by an allergic reaction (Figure 4-2).

4-5 The list of suffixes that pertain to pathologies contains a word that means protrusion of all or part of an organ through an abnormal opening. That word is

hernia (hər′ne-ə)
herniation

_____. This is also called herniation (hər″ne-a′shən).
An encephalo/cele (en-sef′ə-lo-sēl″) is _____ of part of the brain through an opening in the skull, also called cerebral (sə-re′brəl, ser′ə-brəl) hernia.

fear

4-6 Phobia (fo′be-ə) means any persistent and irrational fear of something. The suffix -phobia means abnormal _____.

sagging

4-7 As a suffix, -ptosis (to′sis) means prolapse or _____. As a term, ptosis has two meanings: it can mean the same as the suffix, and also it is sometimes used to mean prolapse of one or both eyelids (Figure 4-3).

-mania

4-8 A suffix that means excessive preoccupation is _____. In klepto/mania (klep″to-ma′ne-ə), there is an excessive preoccupation that leads to an uncontrollable and recurrent urge to steal.

pyromaniac
(pi″ro-ma′ne-ak)

4-9 Pyro/mania (pi″ro-ma′ne-ə) is a disorder characterized by excessive preoccupation with seeing or setting fires. A person having characteristics of pyromania is a
_____.

condition

4-10 Several suffixes mean condition. Hyster/ia is a condition so named because long ago hysterical women were thought to suffer from a disturbed condition of the uterus (hyster/o means uterus). Neur/osis (noo-ro′sis) is a nervous _____ or disorder that is not caused by a demonstrable structural change. The suffix -iasis also means condition.

disease

4-11 The suffix -pathy means _____. Literal interpretation of adeno/pathy (ad″ə-nop′ə-the) is any disease of a gland; however, it means enlargement of a gland, especially a gland of the lymphatic (lim-fat′ik) system.

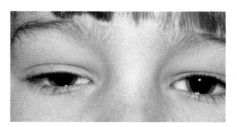

Figure 4-3 Blepharoptosis. Note the drooping of the right upper eyelid.

otopathy (o-top′ə-the) blood	**4-12** *Ophthalmopathy* (of″thəl-mop′ə-the) means any disease of the eye. Write a word that means any disease of the ear: _____.
	4-13 The suffix *-emia* means a condition of the _____. Bacter/emia (bak″tər-e′me-ə) is the presence of bacteria in the blood.
-lith	**4-14** A calculus is a stone. Write a suffix that means a calculus: _____.

Exercise 1

Circle the correct answer to complete each sentence.

1. The suffix *-iasis* means (condition, dilitation, disease, excessive).
2. The suffix *-itis* means (deficiency, inflammation, sagging, soft).
3. The suffix *-phobia* means abnormal (bleeding, deficiency, fear, preoccupation).
4. The suffix *-ptosis* means (decreased, disease, fear, prolapse).
5. The suffix that means excessive preoccupation is (-mania, -maniac, -phobia, -ptosis).
6. The suffix that means tumor is (-oid, -oma, -osis, -rrhagia).
7. The suffix that means disease is (-pathy, -penia, -phobia, -ptosis).
8. The suffix that means hernia is (-cele, -megaly, -rrhea, -stasis).
9. The suffix that means blood is (-algia, -dynia, -emia, -emesis).
10. The suffix that means a stone or calculus is (-cele, -lith, -malacia, -megaly).

Miscellaneous Suffixes

4-15 Read through this list of suffixes and their meanings. Thinking of familiar words that contain these suffixes will help you remember their meanings.

Miscellaneous Suffixes

-able, -ible	capable of, able to		-iac	one who suffers
-an, -ary, -eal, -ive, -tic	pertaining to		-opia	vision
-ase	enzyme		-ose	sugar
-eum, -ium	membrane		-ous	pertaining to or characterized by
-ia, -ism	condition or theory		-y	state or condition

otologist (o-tol′ə-jist)	Write a term that means a physician who specializes in diseases of the ear: _____.
nerve	**4-16** Several suffixes mean pertaining to. You may be wondering how you know which suffix to use, and practice will help you remember. *Neur/al* (noor′əl) means pertaining to a _____ or the nerves.
breast	**4-17** *Mamm/ary* (mam′ər-e) means pertaining to the _____.
cerebral	**4-18** Combine *cerebr(o)* and *-al* to write a word that means pertaining to the brain: _____.

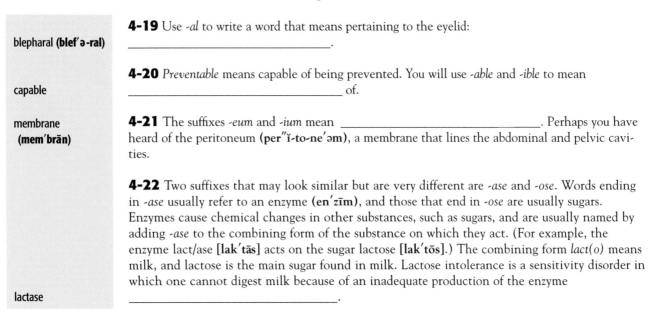

blepharal (blef′ə-ral)

4-19 Use *-al* to write a word that means pertaining to the eyelid:
_____.

capable

4-20 *Preventable* means capable of being prevented. You will use *-able* and *-ible* to mean
_____ of.

membrane (mem′brān)

4-21 The suffixes *-eum* and *-ium* mean _____. Perhaps you have heard of the peritoneum (per″ĭ-to-ne′əm), a membrane that lines the abdominal and pelvic cavities.

4-22 Two suffixes that may look similar but are very different are *-ase* and *-ose*. Words ending in *-ase* usually refer to an enzyme (en′zīm), and those that end in *-ose* are usually sugars. Enzymes cause chemical changes in other substances, such as sugars, and are usually named by adding *-ase* to the combining form of the substance on which they act. (For example, the enzyme lact/ase [lak′tās] acts on the sugar lactose [lak′tōs].) The combining form *lact(o)* means milk, and lactose is the main sugar found in milk. Lactose intolerance is a sensitivity disorder in which one cannot digest milk because of an inadequate production of the enzyme

lactase

_____.

Exercise 2

Match suffixes in the left column with their meanings in the right column.

_____ 1. -able
_____ 2. -ase
_____ 3. -eum
_____ 4. -iac
_____ 5. -ism
_____ 6. -opia
_____ 7. -ose
_____ 8. -ous
_____ 9. -tic
_____ 10. -y

A. capable of
B. condition or theory
C. enzyme
D. membrane
E. one who suffers
F. pertaining to
G. pertaining to or characterized by
H. state or condition
I. sugar
J. vision

Combining Forms and Related Suffixes

specialist

4-23 A few combining forms and suffixes are so often combined that they remain fixed and easily recognized. For example, *log(o)* means knowledge or words. The suffix *-logist*, meaning one who studies or a specialist, results when *log(o)* is combined with *-ist*. You have already learned that the suffix *-logist* means one who studies or a _____.

In analyzing the component parts of a word, begin by looking at the suffix. This identifies it as a noun, a verb, or an adjective. After deciding the meaning of the suffix, go to the beginning of the word and read across from left to right, interpreting the remaining elements to develop the full sense of the term. Practice this technique with a word that you learned in the previous

ophthalmo/logist

chapter. Use slashes to divide ophthalmologist: _____. Literal interpretation yields specialist, eye. The full meaning is a physician who treats disorders of the eye.

4-24 Study the following list of word parts and their meanings. All the suffixes are used to form nouns, with the exception of those ending in *-ic* and *-tic*. The suffixes *-genic*, *-lytic*, *-phagic*, and *-trophic* are used to form adjectives, words that modify or describe nouns. The suffix *-ic* can also be used to form words with several of the combining forms presented.

Selected Combining Forms and Related Suffixes

COMBINING FORMS AND MEANINGS	SUFFIXES AND MEANINGS (IF DIFFERENT THAN THE COMBINING FORM)
cyt(o) means cell	-cyte
gen(o) means beginning, origin	-genic (produced by or in); -genesis (producing or forming)
kinesi(o) means movement	-kinesia, -kinesis (movement, motion)
leps(o) means seizure	-lepsy
log(o) means knowledge or words	-logy (study or science of); -logist (one who studies)
lys(o) means destruction, dissolving	-lysin (that which destroys); -lysis (process of destroying); -lytic (capable of destroying; *note the change in spelling*)
megal(o) means large, enlarged	-megaly (enlargement)
metr(o) means measure; uterine tissue	-meter (instrument used to measure); -metry (process of measuring)
path(o) means disease	-pathy
phag(o) means eat, ingest	-phagia, -phagic, -phagy (eating, swallowing)
phas(o) means speech	-phasia
plas(o) means formation, development	-plasia
plast(o) means repair	-plasty (surgical repair)
pleg(o) means paralysis	-plegia
schis(o), schiz(o), schist(o) mean split, cleft	-schisis
scler(o) means hard	-sclerosis (hardening)
scop(o) means to examine, to view	-scope (instrument used for viewing); -scopy (process of visually examining)
troph(o) means nutrition	-trophic, -trophy

4-25 A micro/scope (**mi'kro-skōp**) is an instrument for viewing small objects that must be magnified so they can be studied. The process of viewing things with a microscope is _____ .

microscopy
(mi-kros'kə-pe)

4-26 Hemo/lysis (**he-mol'ə-sis**) is the destruction of red blood cells that results in the liberation of hemoglobin (**he'mo-glo"bin**), a red pigment. A substance that causes hemolysis is a _____ . This is also called a hemolytic (**he"mo-lit'ik**) substance. Hemolyze (**he'mo-līz**) is a verb that means to destroy red blood cells and cause them to release hemoglobin.

hemolysin
(he-mol'ə-sin)

4-27 Ophthalmo/pathy (**of"thəl-mop'ə-the**) is any _____ of the eye.

disease

4-28 A patho/gen (**path'o-jən**) is any agent or microorganism (**mi"kro-or'gən-iz-əm**) that produces disease. *Patho/genic* (**path-o-jen'ik**) means capable of causing _____ .

disease

4-29 A carcino/gen (**kahr-sin'ə-jen**) is a carcinogenic substance, one that produces cancer. The production or origin of cancer is called _____ .

carcinogenesis
(kahr"sĭ-no-jen'ə-sis)

4-30 Cephalo/metry (**sef"ə-lom'ə-tre**) (*cephal[o]* means head) is measurement of the dimensions of the head. A device or instrument for measuring the head is a _____ .

cephalometer
(sef"ə-lom'ə-tər)

4-31 A phago/cyte (**fag'o-sīt**) is a cell that can ingest and destroy particulate substances such as bacteria. *Ingest* means to _____ .

eat

epilepsy

4-32 *Epi/lepsy* (ep′ĭ-lep″se) refers to a group of neurologic (noor″o-loj′ik) disorders characterized by seizures. Literal translation of this term does not give the full meaning. Write this term that refers to a group of neurologic disorders characterized by seizures:

_____.

dystrophy (dis′trə-fe)

4-33 *Dys/trophic* (dis-trof′ik) muscle deteriorates because of defective nutrition or metabolism. Any disorder caused by defective nutrition or metabolism is called a

_____.

Exercise 3

Match the following suffixes in the left column with their meanings in the right column.

_____ 1. -cyte
_____ 2. -genic
_____ 3. -kinesia
_____ 4. -lepsy
_____ 5. -lysin
_____ 6. -lysis
_____ 7. -lytic
_____ 8. -plasty
_____ 9. -scope
_____ 10. -scopy

A. capable of destroying
B. cell
C. instrument used for viewing
D. movement
E. process of destroying
F. process of examining visually
G. produced by or in
H. surgical repair
I. seizure
J. that which destroys

Exercise 4

Match the following suffixes in the left column with their meanings in the right column.

_____ 1. -megaly
_____ 2. -meter
_____ 3. -metry
_____ 4. -pathy
_____ 5. -phagia
_____ 6. -phasia
_____ 7. -plegia
_____ 8. -schisis
_____ 9. -sclerosis
_____ 10. -trophy

A. disease
B. eating or swallowing
C. enlargement
D. hardening
E. instrument used to measure
F. nutrition
G. paralysis
H. process of measuring
I. speech
J. split or cleft

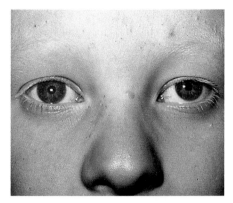

Figure 4-4   The white hair and pale skin of albinism. This condition is characterized by partial or total lack of melanin pigment in the body.

Additional Combining Forms

4-34 Most medical terms have one or more combining forms as their foundation. You will learn many new combining forms as you study later chapters pertaining to the body systems or the body in general. Some common combining forms will be introduced in this section. It is sometimes easier to learn them in groups, such as combining forms that describe color and commonly used combining forms.

Study the combining forms for several colors and their meanings. Again, try to think of words that you know that will help you remember the combining forms. For example, it will be easy to remember that *chlor(o)* means green if you think of chlorophyll.

Combining Forms That Describe Color

COMBINING FORM	MEANING	COMBINING FORM	MEANING
alb(o), albin(o), leuk(o), occasionally leuc(o)	white	erythr(o)	red
		melan(o)	black
chlor(o)	green	xanth(o)	yellow
cyan(o)	blue		

white

4-35 An albino (**al-bi′no**) is an individual with congenital (**kən-jen′ĭ--təl**) absence of pigment in the skin, hair, and eyes. The skin and hair appear _____ because of the lack of pigment. An albino has a hereditary condition known as albinism (**al′bĭ-niz-əm**). Congenital conditions are those that exist at, or before, birth.

black

Albinism is characterized by partial or total lack of the pigment called melanin (**mel′ə-nin**). Melan/in is a _____ or dark brown pigment that naturally occurs in the hair, skin, and eyes but is partially or totally lacking in albinos (Figure 4-4).

cyan(o)

4-36 Cyan/osis (**si″ə-no′sis**) is a bluish discoloration of the skin and mucous (**mu′kəs**) membranes caused by a deficiency of oxygen in the blood (Figure 4-5). The part of the term *cyanosis* that means blue is _____. Mucous membranes are thin sheets of tissue that cover or line various cavities or parts of the body that open to the outside, such as the lining of the mouth. They are named mucous membranes because they secrete mucus (**mu′kəs**).

red

4-37 Erythro/cytes (**ə-rith′ro-sītz**) are _____ blood cells. (Erythrocytes are not actually red but are so named because they contain a red-pigmented protein.)

yellow

4-38 Xantho/derma (**zan″tho-der′mə**) is a _____ coloration of the skin, as in jaundice (**jawn′dis**). Jaundice is characterized by the yellow discoloration of the skin, mucous membranes, and sclera (**sklēr′ə**) (white outer part of the eyeball) and is caused by an increased amount of bilirubin in the blood (Figure 4-6).

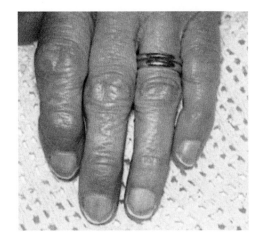

Figure 4-5   Cyanosis. The bluish discoloration is generally not as obvious as the extremely cyanotic skin of this patient.

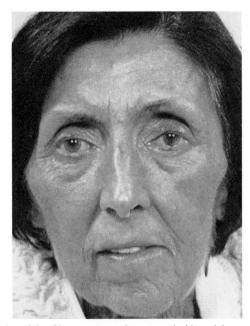

Figure 4-6   Jaundice. This yellow discoloration of the skin, mucus membranes, and whites of the eyes is caused by greater than normal amounts of bilirubin in the blood. Jaundice accompanies many diseases, including liver disorders.

Exercise 5

Write the color associated with each of the following combining forms.

1. alb(o)   _____

2. chlor(o)   _____

3. cyan(o)   _____

4. erythr(o)   _____

5. leuk(o)   _____

6. melan(o)   _____

7. xanth(o)   _____

4-39 Study the following list of commonly used combining forms. Again, try to think of words that you know that will help you remember the combining forms.

Commonly Used Combining Forms

COMBINING FORM	MEANING	COMBINING FORM	MEANING
bi(o)	life or living	nas(o), rhin(o)	nose
cephal(o)	head	ne(o)	new
electr(o)	electricity	pod(o)	foot
hist(o)	tissue	pyr(o)	fire
muscul(o), my(o)	muscle	therm(o)	heat

study

living

4-40 Bio/logy (**bi-ol´ə-je**) is the _____ of life and living things.

Bi/opsy (**bi´op-se**) is the examination of tissue from the _____ body. The suffix -opsy means to view. In a biopsy (Bx), tissue is removed, sectioned, and viewed through a microscope. A biopsy is performed to establish a precise diagnosis. You may have already heard of a post/mortem examination. This may be written *postmortem* or as two words, *post mortem*. This is an examination of the organs and tissues of a body to determine the cause of death or pathological conditions. Another name for postmortem examination is *autopsy* (**aw´top-se**).

4-41 Histo/logy (**his-tol´ə-je**) is the study of the structure, composition, and functions of tissues. A microscope is used to study the minute cells that make up tissue. Stated simply, *histo/logy* means the study of tissue. One who specializes in histology is a _____.

histologist
(**his-tol´ə-jist**)

4-42 A thermo/meter is an instrument for measuring temperature. Body temperature is the level of heat produced and sustained by the body processes. Variations and changes in body temperature may indicate disease. Normal adult body temperature as measured orally is 98.6°F or 37°C. (F and C are abbreviations for Fahrenheit and Celsius.)

mouth

An oral (**or´əl**) thermometer is placed in the _____. A rectal (**rek´təl**) thermometer is inserted in the rectum (**rek´təm**). Rectal temperatures are generally slightly higher than oral temperatures. Most hospitals use electronic thermometers that record temperatures rapidly and accurately. Newer instruments are capable of measuring body temperature on the skin surface.

head

4-43 *Cephal/ic* (**sə-fal´ik**) means pertaining to the _____.

4-44 You have leaned that *rhin(o)* means nose. Another combining form that means nose is *nas(o)*. Combine *nas(o)* and *-al* to write word that means pertaining to the nose: _____.

nasal (**na´zəl**)

4-45 You learned that *chir(o)* means hand. Write the combining form from the list that means foot: _____.

pod(o)

electrical

4-46 An electro/cardio/gram is a record or tracing of the _____ impulses of the heart.

4-47 *Muscul/ar* (**mus´ku-lər**) means pertaining to muscle. Write the second combining form that means muscle: _____.

my(o)

Now write a term that means muscular pain by combining *my(o)* and *-algia*: _____.

myalgia (**mi-al´jə**)

Exercise 6

Match each combining form in the left column with its meaning in the right column.

_____ 1. bi(o)

_____ 2. cephal(o)

_____ 3. electr(o)

_____ 4. hist(o)

_____ 5. my(o)

_____ 6. pod(o)

_____ 7. therm(o)

A. foot
B. electric
C. head
D. heat
E. living
F. muscle
G. tissue

Therapeutic Interventions

treatment

4-48 *Therapeutic* (**ther″ə-pu′tik**) means pertaining to therapy, or _____. The abbreviation for treatment is Tx. Learn the following word parts and their meanings.

Word Parts Pertaining to Treatment

COMBINING FORM	MEANING	COMBINING FORM	MEANING
algesi(o)	sensitivity to pain	therapeut(o)	treatment
chem(o)	chemical	tox(o), toxic(o)	poison
esthesi(o)	feeling or sensation		
narc(o)	stupor	**SUFFIX**	**MEANING**
pharmac(o), pharmaceut(i)	drugs or medicine	-therapy	treatment

treat

4-49 Therapeutic radiology uses radiation to _____ cancer. Radiation therapy, also called radiation onco/logy (**ong-kol′ə-je**), is the treatment of cancer using ionizing radiation, such as x-ray. The literal translation of onco/logy is the study of

tumors

_____, but radiation oncology is treatment of tumors with ionizing radiation.

The source of radiation can be external or internally implanted radioactive substances. The goal of this type of therapy is to deliver a maximum dose of radiation to the cancerous tissue and a minimal dose to the surrounding healthy tissue. A natural consequence of this type of therapy is at least some damage to normal cells. Radiation oncology is used to treat

cancer

_____.

4-50 In addition to radiation, several approaches are used to treat cancer, including surgery to remove the cancer and chemo/therapy (**ke″mo-ther′ə-pe**), which is treatment of disease by chemical agents. The combining form *chem(o)* means chemical. Cyto/toxic (**si″to-tok′sik**) agents are used

cells

in cancer treatment to kill cancer _____.

new

4-51 A neo/plasm (**ne′o-plaz-əm**) is a _____ growth of tissue, a tumor, either benign or malignant. Anti/neo/plastics (**an″te-, an″ti-ne″o-plas′tiks**) are medications that are used to treat neoplasms. (The prefix *anti-* means against. You will study it in the next chapter.) Many malignant tumors are curable if detected and treated in the early stage.

You will also learn how medications are administered in the next chapter.

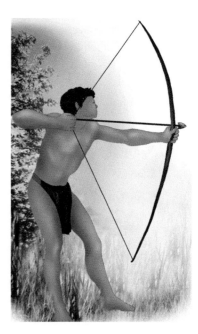

Figure 4-7 Curare is a deadly poison used by South American Indians to coat the tips of arrows used to kill animals. Wounded monkeys tend to grab hold of branches or tree trunks, but the curare relaxes their muscles and the monkeys fall to the ground. Curare was the forerunner of neuromuscular blocking agents that are used today to prevent contraction of muscle during general surgery.

4-52 You have heard of the word *esthetic,* also spelled *aesthetic,* which pertains to the sense of beauty or to sensation (feeling). The prefix *an-* means not or without; *esthesi(o)* refers to feeling (nervous sensation). *An/esthetic* (**an″əs-thet′ik**) means characterized by or producing anesthesia, and the same term is applied to a drug that brings about this numbing effect. Literal translation of

without

an/esthesia (**an″es-the′zhə**) is _____ feeling. The term *anesthesia* is formed by combining *an-* + *esthesi(o)* + *-ia.* (An *i* is dropped to avoid double *i* and to facilitate pronunciation.)

4-53 Anesthesia is partial or complete loss of sensation, with, or without loss of consciousness. Anesthesia may be local, regional, or general. Local anesthesia is confined to one area of the body. Brief surgical or dental procedures can be performed when anesthesia is administered to a localized area; thus it is called local anesthesia. When an anesthetic blocks a group of nerve fibers, regional anesthesia occurs. In this case, loss of feeling occurs in a certain region of the body. For this reason, it is called regional anesthesia.

general

General anesthesia produces a state of unconsciousness with absence of sensation over the entire body. The drugs producing this state are called _____ anesthetics.

4-54 Certain drugs called neuromuscular (**noor″o-mus′ku-lər**) blocking agents may be used to stop muscle contraction during surgery. *Neuro/muscul/ar* means pertaining to the

nerves

_____ and muscles. Later you will study how the nerves and muscles interact to bring about movement. Curare, a poison, was one of the first neuromuscular blocking agents to be studied (Figure 4-7).

4-55 An an/alges/ic (**an″əl-je′zik**) is a drug that relieves pain. The term results from combining *an-* + *algesi(o)* + *-ic,* but notice that one *i* is omitted to facilitate pronunciation. The combining form

pain

algesi(o) means sensitivity to _____.

An analgesic such as aspirin is a type of pharmaceutical (**fahr″mə-soo′tĭ-kəl**). The term *pharmaceutical* means pertaining to pharmacy or drugs, but it also means a medicinal drug. Some drugs require a doctor's prescription and others, such as aspirin, are over-the-counter (OTC) drugs, in other words, not requiring a prescription.

4-56 Pharmaco/therapy (**fahr″mə-ko-ther′ə-pe**) is the treatment of diseases with

medicine (drugs)

_____. The combining form therapeut(o) means treatment. Write an adjective that means pertaining to treatment by combining therapeut(o) and -ic:

therapeutic

_____. A second meaning of the term you just wrote is curative.

poison

4-57 You already have an idea of the meaning of *toxic* (**tok´sik**), which is another word for poisonous. The use of *tox(o)* and *toxic(o)* originates with a Greek word that means archery or the archer's bow. Ancient Greeks smeared poison on arrowheads that were used in hunting. In a regular dictionary, you will find the word *toxophilite*, one fond of archery. But in medical words, *tox(o)* almost always means _____. A tox/in (**tok´sin**) is a poison. If a substance is poisonous, it is said to be a toxic (**tok´sik**) substance.

Combine *toxic(o)* and *-logy* to write a word that means the science or study of poisons: _____.

**toxicology
(tok″sĭ-kol´ə-je)**

**toxicologist
(tok″sĭ-kol´ə-jist)**

A specialist in toxicology is a _____.

stupor

4-58 A narcotic (**nahr-kot´ik**) is a substance that produces insensibility or _____. The term also means a narcotic drug. Narcotic analgesics alter perception of pain, induce a feeling of euphoria, and may induce sleep. Repeated use of narcotics may result in physical and psychological dependence. In large amounts (for example, in an overdose [OD]), narcotics can depress respiration.

Exercise 7

Write a word in each blank to complete these sentences.

1. A drug that relieves pain is an _____.

2. Partial or complete loss of sensation is _____.

3. Drugs that are used to stop muscle contraction are _____ blocking agents.

4. A word that means pertaining to treatment is _____.

5. A _____ is a substance that produces insensibility or stupor.

6. Treatment of cancer using ionizing radiation is called _____ oncology.

4-59 The list of abbreviations that follows has several common abbreviations that physicians use when writing prescriptions. A prescription drug (Rx) can be dispensed to the public only with an order given by a properly authorized person.

SELECTED ABBREVIATIONS

Bx	biopsy	**OTC**	over the counter (drug that can be obtained without a prescription)
C	Celsius, centigrade		
F	Fahrenheit	**Rx**	prescription
OD	overdose; right eye (*oculus dexter*)	**Tx**	treatment

PREPARING FOR A TEST OF THIS CHAPTER

Review as you were instructed in Chapter 2 and work the end-of-chapter review.

Be Careful With These!

-ase (enzyme) vs. *-ose* (sugar)
-ia (condition) vs. *-iac* (one who suffers)
-lysin (that which destroys) vs. *-lytic* (capable of destroying)
-phagia (eating, swallowing) vs. *-phasia* (speech)
-plasia (formation, development) vs. *-plasty* (surgical repair)
-rrhage (hemorrhage) vs. *-rrhea* (discharge) vs. *-rrhexis* (rupture)
analgesic (relieves pain) vs. anesthetic (causes loss of feeling or sensation)
diagnosis (identifying disease/condition) vs. prognosis (probable outcome)

CHAPTER 4 REVIEW

■ Basic Understanding

Matching

I. Match suffixes in the left column with their meanings in the right column.

_____ 1. -cele

_____ 2. -emia

_____ 3. -iasis

_____ 4. -lith

_____ 5. -mania

_____ 6. -oma

_____ 7. -phobia

_____ 8. -ptosis

    A. abnormal fear
    B. calculus
    C. condition
    D. condition of the blood
    E. excessive preoccupation
    F. hernia
    G. prolapse
    H. tumor

II. Match combining forms for colors and their meanings:

_____ 1. alb(o)

_____ 2. chlor(o)

_____ 3. cyan(o)

_____ 4. erythr(o)

_____ 5. melan(o)

_____ 6. xanth(o)

    A. black
    B. blue
    C. green
    D. red
    E. white
    F. yellow

Multiple Choice

III. Circle the correct answer to complete each sentence.

1. Julie experiences redness of the skin around her recently acquired earrings. What is Julie's condition called? (dermatitis, malacia, mastitis, ptosis)

2. When James and Cynthia's baby is born, it has a yellow discoloration of the skin and mucous membranes. Which condition is most likely? (albinism, cyanosis, jaundice, myalgia)

3. Johnny, a college student, sees the physician and is told that his appendix is inflamed. What is the name of his condition? (appendectomy, appendicitis, appendorrhexis, appendotomy)

4. Karen sustains a severe head injury in which there is herniation of the brain through an opening in the skull. What is the name of this pathology? (cerebritis, cerebrotomy, encephalocele, encephaloplasty)

5. Ken suffers an abnormal fear of heights. What type of pathology does he have? (dilatation, mania, phobia, ptosis)

6. What is the term for examination of tissue from a living body? (autopsy, biopsy, postmortem, ptosis)

7. A 70-year-old man is undergoing therapeutic radiology for cancer. What is this type of therapy called? (chemotherapy, neuromuscular blocking, radiation oncology, toxicology)

8. *Histology* means the study of which of the following? (disease, function, structure, tissue)

9. Which of the following produces insensibility or stupor? (analgesic, anesthetics, narcotic, pharmaceutic)

10. Which of the following is a medication that is used to treat neoplasms? (analgesic, antineoplastic, local anesthesia, regional anesthesia)

Writing Terms
IV. *Write a term for each clue that is given.*

1. a red (blood) cell   _____

2. a substance that causes hemolysis   _____

3. a substance that produces cancer   _____

4. any disease of the eye   _____

5. excessive preoccupation with fires   _____

6. inflammation of a bone   _____

7. muscular pain   _____

8. pertaining to the nose   _____

9. treatment of disease with medicines   _____

10. viewing things with a microscope   _____

■ Greater Comprehension

Spelling
V. *Circle all incorrectly spelled terms and write their correct spellings:*

anasthetic   angioma   cefalic   epilepsy   serebral

Interpreting Abbreviations
VI. *Write the meanings of these abbreviations.*

1. Bx   _____

2. OD   _____

3. OTC   _____

4. Rx   _____

5. Tx   _____

Pronunciation
VII. *Indicate the primary-accented syllable in each term by marking it with an ′.*

1. adenopathy (ad ə nop ə the)

2. cephalometry (sef ə lom ə tre)

3. cytotoxic (si to tok sik)

4. hemolytic (he mo lit ik)

5. lactose (lak tōs)
(Check your answers with the solutions in Appendix VI.)

LISTING OF MEDICAL TERMS

Use the practice CD to review the terms that have been presented. Look closely at the spelling of each term as it is pronounced and be sure you know the meaning of each term.

adenitis	dermatitis	mammary	otoplasty
adenopathy	dystrophic	mania	pathogen
albinism	dystrophy	mastitis	pathogenic
albino	electrocardiogram	melanin	pathology
analgesic	encephalocele	microscope	peritoneum
anesthesia	enzyme	microscopy	phagocyte
anesthetics	epilepsy	mucous membrane	pharmaceuticals
angioma	erythrocyte	muscular	pharmacotherapy
antineoplastics	general anesthesia	myalgia	phobia
appendicitis	hemolysin	narcotic	postmortem
autopsy	hemolysis	nasal	ptosis
bacteremia	hemolytic	neoplasm	pyromania
biopsy	hemolyze	neuritis	pyromaniac
blepharal	hernia	neurologic	rectal thermometer
carcinogen	herniation	neuromuscular blocking	rectum
carcinogenesis	histologist	agent	regional anesthesia
carcinoma	histology	neurosis	therapeutic
cephalic	hysteria	oncology	tonsillitis
cephalometer	ingest	ophthalmitis	toxicologist
cephalometry	jaundice	ophthalmopathy	toxicology
cerebral	kleptomania	oral thermometer	toxin
chemotherapy	lactase	osteitis	xanthoderma
cyanosis	lactose	otitis	
cytotoxic	local anesthesia	otopathy	

español ENHANCING SPANISH COMMUNICATION

ENGLISH	SPANISH (PRONUNCIATION)
anesthesia	*anestesia* (ah-nes-TAY-se-ah)
biopsy	*biopsia* (be-OP-see-ah)
blood	*sangre* (SAHN-gray)
bone	*hueso* (oo-AY-so)
electricity	*electricidad* (ay-lec-tre-se-DAHD)
enlargement	*aumento* (ah-oo-MEN-to)
enzyme	*enzima* (en-SEE-mah)
fear	*miedo* (me-AY-do)
fire	*fuego* (foo-AY-go)
foot (pl., feet)	*pie* (PE-ay), *pies* (PE-ays)
head	*cabeza* (cah-BAY-sah)
heat	*calor* (cah-LOR)
hernia	*hernia* (AYR-ne-ah), *quebradura* (kay-brah-DOO-rah)
membrane	*membrana* (mem-BRAH-nah)
movement	*movimiento* (mo-ve-me-EN-to)
narcotic	*narcótico* (nar-CO-te-co)
nutrition	*nutrición* (noo-tre-se-ON)
seizure	*ataque* (ah-TAH-kay)
skin	*piel* (pe-EL)
speech	*habla* (AH-blah), *lenguaje* (len-goo-AH-hay)
sugar	*azúcar* (ah-SOO-car)

COLORS	LOS COLORES
black	*negro* (NAY-gro)
blue	*azul* (ah-SOOL)
green	*verde* (VERR-day)
red	*rojo* (ROH-ho)
white	*blanco* (BLAHN-co)
yellow	*amarillo* (ah-mah-REEL-lyo)

CHAPTER 5

Building Medical Terms with Prefixes

In this chapter, you will learn to do the following:

Basic Understanding
1. Match prefixes with their meanings.
2. Recognize prefixes in terms and write their meanings.
3. Use prefixes to build and analyze terms.
4. Use *a-* or *an-* correctly to write terms of negation.

Greater Comprehension
5. Spell medical terms accurately.
6. Write the meanings of the abbreviations.
7. Pronounce medical terms correctly.

THESE ARE THE MAJOR SECTIONS IN THIS CHAPTER:

- ❑ **Using Prefixes in Medical Terms**
- ❑ **Prefixes That Pertain to Numbers or Quantity**
- ❑ **Prefixes That Pertain to Position or Direction**
- ❑ **Prefixes Related to Negation**
- ❑ **Using Other Prefixes to Build Terms**

Using Prefixes in Medical Terms

prefix	**5-1** You have learned that prefixes, suffixes, and combining forms are word parts that are used to write medical terms. Which word part is placed before a word to modify its meaning? _____ Most prefixes, including those ending with a vowel, can be added to the remainder of the word without change. You will encounter some exceptions, however. Prefixes in this chapter will be grouped as those pertaining to numbers or quantity, to position or direction, and to negation, plus some miscellaneous prefixes.

Prefixes That Pertain to Numbers or Quantity

5-2 Study the following prefixes that pertain to numbers or quantity. Many of the prefixes in the list are used in everyday language, so think of words you may know that can help you remember their meanings.

Prefixes That Pertain to Numbers or Quantity

Specific Numbers		Quantities	
PREFIX	**MEANING**	**PREFIX**	**MEANING**
mono-, uni-	one	diplo-	double
bi-, di-	two	hemi-, semi-	half, partly
tri-	three	hyper-	excessive, more than normal
quad-, quadri-, tetra-	four	hypo-	beneath or below normal
centi-	one hundred or one-hundredth	multi-, poly-	many
milli-	one-thousandth (1/1000)	nulli-	none
		pan-	all
		primi-	first
		super-, ultra-	excessive

one	**5-3** The terms *monorail* and *unicorn* contain prefixes that mean one. Both a mono/rail and a uni/corn have _____ rail and horn, respectively.
two	**5-4** A bi/cycle has _____ wheels and carbon di/oxide (CO_2) contains two atoms of oxygen.
three	**5-5** A tri/cycle has _____ wheels.
four	**5-6** Quad/ruplets (**kwod″roop′letz**) are four offspring born at one birth, and carbon tetra/chloride has _____ chloride atoms.
centi-	**5-7** When trying to remember the meaning of centi/grade, it is helpful to remember that centigrade is a temperature scale in which 0° is the freezing point and 100° is the boiling point of water at sea level. Centigrade is the same as Celsius, named after the Swedish scientist, Anders Celsius. Write the prefix used to write the term *centigrade* that means 100: _____.
milli-	**5-8** A milli/meter is one-thousandth of a meter. Write the prefix that means one-thousandth: _____.
two	**5-9** *Dipl/opia* (**dĭ-plo′pe-ə**) means double vision. How many images of a single object are seen in diplopia? _____ (Note that one *o* is dropped when *diplo-* is joined with *-opia* to facilitate pronunciation.)

half	**5-10** In *hemi/sphere* and *semi/circle*, the prefixes mean _____ .
super-	**5-11** *Hyper/active* means excessively active. In addition to *hyper-*, two more prefixes mean excessive: *ultra-* and _____ .
below	**5-12** A prefix that means the opposite of *hyper-* is *hypo-*. In the word *hypo/derm/ic* (**hi″po-dər′mik**), *hypo-* means _____ .
many	**5-13** In the terms *multi/tude* and *poly/unsaturated*, the prefixes mean _____ .
nulli-	**5-14** *Null* is a word that means having no value, nothing, or equal to zero. Write the prefix that means none: _____ .
pan-	**5-15** *Pan/demic* (**pan-dem′ik**) means occurring throughout (in other words, affecting all) the population of a country, people, or the world. Write the prefix that means all: _____
first	**5-16** Primitive humans were some of the first people on earth. *Primary* means what position in rank or importance? _____

Exercise 1

Match the prefixes in the left column with their meanings in the right column. The choices on the right may be used more than once.

_____ 1. bi-

_____ 2. di-

_____ 3. centi-

_____ 4. milli-

_____ 5. mono-

_____ 6. quad-

_____ 7. tri-

_____ 8. uni-

A. one
B. two
C. three
D. four
E. one-hundredth (1/100)
F. one-thousandth (1/1000)

Exercise 2

Write the meaning of these prefixes.

1. diplo- _____

2. hyper- _____

3. hypo- _____

4. nulli- _____

5. poly- _____

6. primi- _____

7. semi- _____

Prefixes That Pertain to Position or Direction

5-17 Several important prefixes pertain to position or direction. Study the following list. Again, think of familiar words to help you remember their meanings.

Prefixes That Pertain to Position or Direction

PREFIX	MEANING	PREFIX	MEANING
ab-	away from	intra-	within
ad-	toward	ipsi-	same
ante-, pre-	before in time or in place	meso-, mid-, medio-	middle
circum-, peri-	around	para-	near, beside, or abnormal
dia-	through	per-	through or by
ecto-, ex-, exo-, extra-	out, without, away from	post-	after, behind
en-, end-, endo-	inside	retro-	behind, backward
epi-	above, on	super-, supra-	above, beyond
hypo-, infra-, sub-	beneath, under	sym-, syn-	joined, together
inter-	between	trans-	across

ab-

5-18 Ab/duct (**ab-dukt′**) means to carry away by force or draw away from a given position. The prefix that means away from is _____. The prefix *ad-* is the opposite of *ab-*. In chemical addiction, a person has a compulsive need for a certain drug, or in other words, is drawn toward a habit-forming drug.

before

5-19 Both *ante-* and *pre-* mean _____ in time or place. A preview is shown before a show or performance. After is the opposite of before, and the corresponding prefix for after is *post-*. To postdate a check is to write a date after the date that the check is written. The prefix *post-* in many medical terms also means behind. *Post/nasal* (**pōst-na′zəl**) means lying or occurring behind the nose. Another prefix, *retro-*, means behind or backward, as in the term *retroactive*, which means extending back to a prior time or condition.

around

5-20 The perimeter is the outer boundary or the line that is drawn around the outside of an area. Both *peri-* and *circum-* mean _____.

dia-

5-21 The diameter passes through the center of a circle. The prefix in diameter that means through is _____. Another prefix, *per-*, means through or by. To perspire* is to excrete fluid through the pores of the skin.
   A trans/dermal (**trans-dər′məl**) drug is one that can be absorbed through unbroken skin. An example is the patch to prevent motion sickness. The literal translation of trans/dermal is

across

_____ the skin.

5-22 Several prefixes, *ecto-*, *ex-*, *exo-*, and *extra-*, mean out, without, or away from. Practice will help you know which prefix to use when writing terms.
   Enclose means to close up inside something. Both *en-* and *endo-* mean

inside

_____.

epi-

5-23 Write the prefix from the list that means above or on: _____. The prefixes *super-* and *supra-* can also mean above and sometimes mean beyond. Supernormal is beyond normal human powers. Supra/renal (**soo″prə-re′nəl**) glands are located

above

_____ the kidneys.

*Perspire (Latin: *perspirare*, to breathe through)

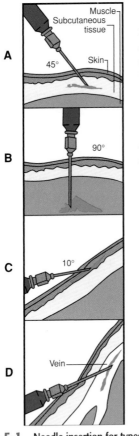

Subcutaneous
A subcutaneous injection places a small amount (0.5 to 2 ml) of medication below the skin layer into the subcutaneous tissue. The needle is inserted at a 45° angle.

Intramuscular
An intramuscular injection deposits medication into a muscular layer. As much as 3 to 5 ml may be administered in one injection, and depending on the size of the patient, a needle from 1 to 3 inches in length is used.

Intradermal
An intradermal injection places very small amounts (0.05 to 0.01 ml) of a drug into the outer layers of the skin with a very fine gauge, short needle. This type of injection is often used to test allergic reactions.

Intravenous
An intravenous injection is used to administer medications directly into the blood stream for immediate effect or to withdraw blood for testing purposes. A few milliliters of medication or much larger amounts (given over a long period of time) may be administered after venipuncture of the selected vein has been performed.

Figure 5-1   Needle insertion for types of injections. **A,** Subcutaneous; **B,** intramuscular; **C,** intradermal; **D,** intravenous.

under

5-24 The prefixes *hypo-*, *infra-*, and *sub-* mean beneath or _____. *Hypo/dermic* means beneath the skin. A hypodermic needle is used to inject a drug or medication under the skin or into blood vessels and for withdrawing a fluid, such as blood. Following are four important types of injections:

- sub/cutaneous (**sub″ku-ta′ne-əs**), beneath the skin
- intra/muscular (**in″trə-mus′ku-lər**), within a muscle
- intra/dermal (**in″trə-dər′məl**), within the dermis (**dər′mis**), the layer of skin that contains the blood vessels
- intra/venous (**in″trə-ve′nəs**), within a vein, because *venous* means pertaining to a vein

under

The literal translation of subcutaneous is _____ the skin. In a subcutaneous injection, the needle is placed into the subcutaneous tissue beneath the skin. Study the four types of injections in Figure 5-1 and be able to describe each type.

5-25 The prefix *-ipsi* means same. *Ipsi/lateral* (**ip″sĭ-lat′ər-əl**) means affecting the same side of the body. The opposite of this, *contra/lateral* (**kon″trə-lat′ər-əl**), means affecting the opposite side of the body. The prefix *contra-* means against, but here it is used to mean opposite or opposed to a particular side of the body.

middle

5-26 The prefix *mid-* means _____. Two other prefixes that mean middle are *meso-* and *medio-*.

5-27 Parallel lines run beside each other. This may help you remember that *para-* means

beside

_____.

inter-	**5-28** An interval is a space of time between events. Write the prefix that means *between*: _____.
intra-	**5-29** Intracollegiate activities occur within a college or are engaged in by members of a college. The prefix that means *within* is _____.
together	**5-30** Both *sym-* and *syn-* mean *joined* or _____. A syn/drome (**sin'drōm**) is a set of symptoms that occur together and collectively characterize a particular disease or condition.

Exercise 3

Write answers in the blank lines to complete the sentences. (Although an answer may require more than one word, it is represented by a blank line.)

1. The prefix *ab-* means _____, but *ad-* means _____.

2. *Postnasal* pertains to the region _____ the nose.

3. Two prefixes that have opposite meanings are *endo-* and *ecto-*. An abbreviated meaning of *ecto-* is *outside*, and *endo-* means _____.

4. *Inter-* means between, and *intra-* means _____.

5. Suprarenal glands are located _____ each kidney.

Prefixes Related to Negation

5-31 When a prefix of negation is placed before a term, it forms a new word with the opposite meaning. For example, *symptomatic* (**simp″to-mat′ik**) means having symptoms, and *asymptomatic* (**a″simp-to-mat′ik**) means without (not having) symptoms.

Prefixes Related to Negation

PREFIX	MEANING
a-, an-	no, not, without
in-	not or inside (in)

	5-32 *Hydrous* (**hi′drəs**) means containing water. *Anhydrous* (**an-hi′drəs**) means absence of water. An important rule for using *a-* or *an-* is: • Use *a-* before a consonant. • Use *an-* before a vowel or the letter *h*.
trauma (injury)	**5-33** *Trauma* (**traw′mə, trou′mə**) means a wound or injury, whether physical or emotional. *Traumatic* (**trə-mat′ik**) means pertaining to or occurring as the result of _____. Write a word that means not inflicting or causing damage or injury: _____.
atraumatic (a″traw-mat′ik)	
in-	**5-34** Another prefix that means not, as in the term *inconsistent*, is _____. Sometimes *in-* means inside, as in the terms *include* and *inhale* (to breathe in).

Use either a- or an- to write words that have the opposite meanings of these terms.

1. The opposite of esthesia is _____.

2. The opposite of hydrous is _____.

3. The opposite of plastic is _____.

4. The opposite of traumatic is _____.

Using Other Prefixes to Build Terms

5-35 There are additional prefixes that one needs to know to write medical terms. Their meanings should be easy to remember, because many of them are used in everyday language. Note that some prefixes have more than one meaning and may pertain to two classifications, such as position and time. An example is *post-*, which means "after" to describe time or "behind" to describe position. Study the list of miscellaneous prefixes, using word association to help you remember their meanings.

Miscellaneous Prefixes

PREFIX	MEANING	PREFIX	MEANING
Related to Size		**Related to Description**	
macro-, mega-, megalo-	large or great	anti-, contra-	against
micro-	small	brady-	slow
		dys-	bad, difficult
Related to Time		eu-	good, normal
ante-, pre-, pro-	before	mal-	bad
post-	after or behind	pro-	favoring, supporting
		tachy-	fast

post-

5-36 The prefixes *ante-*, *pre-*, and *pro-* mean before in time. *Pre/cancerous* (**pre-kan′sər-əs**) is a term that is used to describe an abnormal growth that is likely to become cancerous. The prefix that means after in time is _____. *Post/anesthetic* (**pōst″an-əs-thet′ik**) describes the time after anesthetic is administered.

microscopic (mi″kro-skop′ik)

5-37 When referring to size, macro/scopic (**mak″ro-skop′ik**) structures are large enough to be seen by the naked eye. If the structures are so small that they can only be seen with a microscope, they are called _____ structures.

small

5-38 Micr/ot/ia (**mi-kro′shə**) is an unusually small size of the external ear (one o is omitted to facilitate pronunciation). Literal translation of microtia is _____ ear (Figure 5-2).

against

5-39 Both *anti-* and *contra-* mean _____, as in the terms *anti/perspirant* (**an″te-, an″ti-pər′spər-ant″**) and *contra/ceptive* (**kon″trə-sep′tiv**). An antiperspirant inhibits or prevents perspiration (sweating). A contraceptive prevents conception or diminishes the likelihood of conception.

The prefix that means the opposite of against is *pro-*, which means favoring or supporting (in other words, for).

fast
slow

5-40 The prefixes *brady-* and *tachy-* have opposite meanings, slow and _____, respectively. You learned that *-phasia* means speech. *Brady/phasia* (**brad″ĭ-fa′zhə**) means an abnormally _____ manner of speech, often associated with mental illness. The opposite of bradyphasia is tachy/phasia (**tak″e-fa′zhə**), rapid speech, as may be present in the manic phase of bipolar disorder.

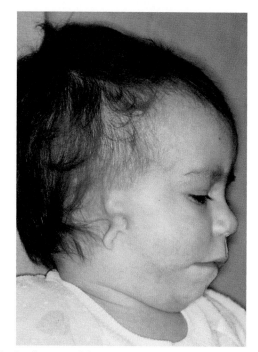

Figure 5-2 An example of microtia, underdevelopment of the external ear. Otoplasty, reconstructive surgery of the ear, is generally performed before the child reaches school age.

5-41 Both *dys-* and *mal-* mean bad, but *dys-* can also mean difficult, as in the term *dys/lexia* (**dis-lek′se-ə**), which means difficulty in reading, often reversing letters or distinguishing letter sequences.

The prefix *eu-* means good or normal. *Eu/phoria* (**u-for′e-ə**) is a feeling or state of well-being, and *dys/phoria* (**dis-for′e-ə**) is characterized by depression and anguish.

Exercise 5

Match the prefixes in the left column with their meaning(s) in the right column. The choices on the right may be used more than once.

_____ 1. anti-

_____ 2. brady-

_____ 3. contra-

_____ 4. dys-

_____ 5. eu-

_____ 6. mal-

_____ 7. micro-

_____ 8. macro-

_____ 9. megalo-

_____ 10. tachy-

A. against
B. bad
C. fast
D. good or normal
E. large
F. slow
G. small

5-42 Prescriptions contain a number of terms and abbreviations that are a combination of English and Latin, sometimes called a type of "medical shorthand." Common abbreviations that are used in writing prescriptions are included in the following list, with their Latin origins in parentheses.

SELECTED ABBREVIATIONS

a.c.	before meals (*ante cibum*)		**PO**	by mouth (*per os*)
ad lib.	freely as needed, at pleasure (*ad libitum*)		**p.r.n.**	as the occasion arises, as needed (*pro re nata*)
Aq.	water (*aqua*)		**q.**	every (*quaque*)
b.i.d.	twice a day (*bis in die*)		**q.i.d.**	four times a day (*quater in die*)
b.i.n.	twice a night (*bis in noctis*)		**stat.**	immediately (*statim*)
Noct.	night (*nocte*)		**t.i.d.**	three times a day (*ter in die*)
NPO	nothing by mouth (*nil per os*)			

PREPARING FOR THE TEST

Review as you were instructed in Chapter 2 and work the end-of-chapter review.

Be Careful With These!

in- (not) vs. *in-* (inside)
infra- (under) vs. *intra-* (within)
Opposites:
ab- (away from) vs. *ad-* (toward)
ante-, *pre-* (before) vs. *post-* (after)
en-, *end-*, *endo-* (inside) vs. *ecto-*, *exo-*, *extra-* (outside)
hyper- (more than normal) vs. *hypo-* (less than normal)
macro- (large) vs. *micro-* (small)
nulli- (none) vs. *pan-* (all)
super-, *supra-* (above) vs. *hypo-*, *infra-*, *sub-* (below)

CHAPTER 5 REVIEW

■ Basic Understanding

Matching
I. Match the suffixes on the left with their meanings on the right.

_____ 1. di-   A. all
                          B. below normal
_____ 2. diplo-   C. double
_____ 3. hyper-   D. four
                          E. many
_____ 4. hypo-   F. more than normal
_____ 5. nulli-   G. none
                          H. one
_____ 6. pan-   I. three
_____ 7. poly-   J. two
_____ 8. quad-
_____ 9. tri-
_____ 10. uni-

Multiple Choice
II. Circle the correct answer in each of the following questions.

1. What does *primi-* mean? (above, beneath, excessive, first)

2. What does *tachy-* mean? (bad, good, fast, slow)

3. What does *dys-* mean? (difficult, good, normal, slow)

4. What does *hypo-* mean? (above, after, before, beneath)

5. Which term describes a structure that can be seen with the naked eye? (macroscopic, microscopic, ophthalmoscopic, ophthalmoscopy)

6. What does the prefix in *antibiotic* mean? (against, before, effective, supporting)

7. What does the prefix in *hemisphere* mean? (all, double, favoring, half)

8. What is the meaning of the prefix in *bilateral*? (one, two, three, four)

9. In which type of injection is the needle placed in the subcutaneous tissue? (intradermal, intramuscular, intravenous, subcutaneous)

10. Which term means a set of symptoms that occur together and characterize a particular disease or condition? (dysphoria, symptomatic, syndrome, tachyphasia)

Writing Terms
III. Use a- or an- to write terms that have the opposite meanings of these words.

1. esthesia vs. _____.

2. hydrous vs. _____.

3. plastic vs. _____.

4. symptomatic vs. _____.

5. traumatic vs. _____.

IV. Write a term for each of the following:

1. abnormally slow speech   _____

2. absence of an external ear   _____

3. behind the nose   _____

4. double vision   _____

5. occurring on the opposite side   _____

■ Greater Comprehension

Spelling
V. Circle all incorrectly spelled words and write their correct spellings.

adiction   antiperspirant   ipselateral   postanethetic   suprarenal

Interpreting Abbreviations
VI. Write the instructions for dosage of the medications after reading the following prescription.

John Butler, M.D.
220 Hospital Drive
Any City, USA 22222

PATIENT: *Jerry McGinnis*   DATE: *1/12/04*
ADDRESS: <u>*15022 9ᵗʰ ST.*</u>
          <u>CITY, STATE</u>

Zocor 40 mg daily
Mirapex 1 mg t.i.d.
Zoladex q. three months
Imdur 120 mg b.i.d.
NitroQuick p.r.n.

- Dispense as written
- Generic equivalent OK

Refill <u>2</u> times

John Butler, M.D.

---

1. Zocor   _____

2. Mirapex   _____

3. Zoladex   _____

4. Imdur   _____

5. NitroQuick   _____

Pronunciation

VII. Indicate the primary accented syllable by marking it with an ′.

1. abduct (ab dukt)

2. contraceptive (kon trə sep tiv)

3. hypodermic (hi po dər mik)

4. syndrome (sin drōm)

5. transdermal (trans dər məl)

 # LISTING OF MEDICAL TERMS

Use the practice CD to review the terms that have been presented. Look closely at the spelling of each term as it is pronounced, and be sure you know the meaning of each term.

abduct	contralateral	intravenous injection	subcutaneous injection
addiction	diplopia	ipsilateral	suprarenal
anhydrous	dyslexia	macroscopic	symptomatic
anotia	dysphoria	microscopic	syndrome
antiperspirant	euphoria	microtia	tachyphasia
asymptomatic	hydrous	pandemic	transdermal
atraumatic	hyperactive	postanesthetic	trauma
bradyphasia	hypodermic	postnasal	traumatic
Celsius	intradermal injection	precancerous	
centigrade	intramuscular injection	quadruplets	

español ENHANCING SPANISH COMMUNICATION

ENGLISH	SPANISH (PRONUNCIATION)
hypodermic	hipodérmico (e-po-DER-me-co)
microscope	microscopio (me-cros-CO-pe-o)
trauma	daño (DAH-nyo), herida (ay-REE-dah)
treatment	tratamiento (trah-tah-me-EN-to)

CHAPTER 6

Organization of the Body

The Body's Organizational Scheme

6-1 Order and organization are outstanding features of the human body. All its parts, from tiny atoms to visible structures, work together as a functioning whole. The organizational structure has several levels. These are illustrated in Figure 6-1. From simplest to complex, the levels are as follows:

- atoms or ions (carbon, oxygen, hydrogen, nitrogen)
- molecules (proteins, sugars, water)
- organelles (specialized structures within cells—for example, the nucleus)
- cells (fundamental units of life)
- tissues (similar cells acting together to perform a function)
- organs (tissue types working together to perform one or more functions)
- body systems (several organs working together to accomplish a set of functions)
- total organism (a human capable of carrying on life functions)

chemical

The simplest level is the _____ level.

6-2 Every individual begins life as a single cell, a fertilized egg. This single cell divides into two cells, then four, eight, and so on, until maturity. During development, cells become specialized. Cells that have the ability to divide without limit and give rise to specialized cells are called stem cells. They are abundant in a fetus and in cord blood of a newborn. Stem cells are being used in bone marrow transplants, but controversy surrounds the use of stem cells in research for organ or tissue regeneration. These undifferentiated cells that can give rise to other types of cells are called

stem

_____ cells.

6-3 There are a number of different types of body cells (blood cells, bone cells, liver cells, and many others), but all share certain characteristics such as metabolism, building up substances, and breaking down substances for the body's use. Chromosomes, threadlike structures within the nucleus of a cell, contain deoxyribonucleic acid (DNA), which functions in the transmission of genetic information. Write the abbreviation for the material in cells that contains genetic information:

DNA

_____.

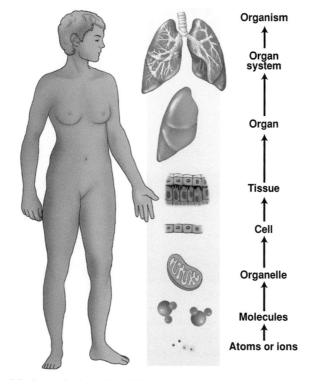

Figure 6-1 Organizational scheme of the body. The formation of the human organism progresses from different levels of complexity. All its parts, from tiny atoms to visible structures, work together to make a functioning whole.

body

6-4 In humans, each somatic cell has 23 pairs of chromosomes. The combining forms *somat(o)* and *som(a)* mean body. Somatic **(so-mat′ik)** cells are all the cells of the body except the sex cells, sperm and ova (singular: ovum). *Somat/ic* means pertaining to the _____.

An abnormality in the chromosomes themselves, or too many chromosomes, usually results in defects. Down syndrome **(sin′drōm)**, the most common chromosomal abnormality of a generalized syndrome, is a congenital **(kən-jen′ĭ-təl)** condition characterized by varying degrees of mental retardation and multiple defects (see Figure 13-7). The incidence is generally associated with advanced age of the mother. *Congenital* (Latin: *congenitus*, born together) means existing at, and usually before, birth. This example of a congenital defect, usually caused by an extra chromosome 21, is

Down

_____ syndrome.

6-5 A tissue is a group of cells that have similar structure and function as a unit. Using the following information, label the four types of tissues in Figure 6-2.

Figure 6-2, A Epithelial **(ep″ĭ-the′le-əl)** tissue forms the covering of body surfaces, both inside and on the surface of the body; an example is the outer layer of the skin.

Figure 6-2, B Connective tissue supports and binds other body tissues and parts; examples are bone and cartilage.

Figure 6-2, C Nervous tissue coordinates and controls many body activities; it is found in the brain, spinal cord, and nerves.

Figure 6-2, D Muscle tissue produces movement; an example is skeletal muscle that makes bending of the arm possible.

A group of cells that have similar structure and function as a unit are called a

tissue

_____.

6-6 Organs are made up of two or more tissue types that work together to perform one or more functions and form a more complex structure. You are familiar with many organs, such as the liver, the lungs, and the reproductive organs.

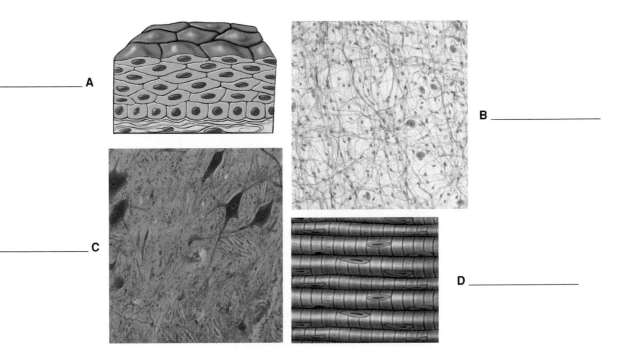

_____ A

B _____

_____ C

D _____

Figure 6-2 Label the four types of tissue. **A,** Epithelial tissue of the type that comprises several cellular layers; **B,** connective tissue of elastic fibers; **C,** nervous tissue; **D,** muscle tissue of the striated type.

TABLE 6-1 Major Body Systems

Body System	Major Functions
Cardiovascular system	Delivers oxygen, nutrients, and vital substances throughout the body; transports cellular waste products to the lungs and kidneys for excretion
Lymphatic system	Helps maintain the internal fluid environment; produces some types of blood cells; regulates immunity
Respiratory system	Brings oxygen into the body and removes carbon dioxide and some water waste
Digestive system	Provides the body with water, nutrients, and minerals; removes solid wastes
Urinary system	Filters blood to remove wastes of cellular metabolism; maintains the electrolyte and fluid balance
Reproductive system	Procreation (producing offspring)
Muscular system	Makes movement possible
Skeletal system	Provides protection, form, and shape for the body; stores minerals and forms some blood cells
Nervous system	Coordinates the reception of stimuli; transmits messages to stimulate movement
Integumentary system	Provides external covering for protection; regulates the body temperature and water content
Endocrine system	Secretes hormones and helps regulate body activities

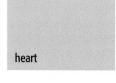

heart

A body system consists of several organs that work together to accomplish a set of functions. See Table 6-1 for a listing of the major body systems and their functions. Body systems will be covered in Chapters 8 through 17 of this book. Some systems will be combined in the same chapter; for example, the cardiovascular and lymphatic systems are presented in Chapter 8. You have already learned that *cardi(o)* means the _____.

Exercise 1

Write a word in each of the blanks to complete these sentences.

1. Every individual begins life as a single _____.

2. Similar cells acting together to perform a function is called a/an _____.

3. Tissue types working together to perform a function is called a/an _____.

4. The type of tissue that supports and binds other body tissues and parts is called _____ tissue.

5. The tissue type that forms the covering of body surfaces is _____ tissue.

6. The type of tissue that produces movement is _____ tissue.

7. The tissue type that coordinates and controls many body activities is _____ tissue.

8. All cells of the body except the sex cells are called _____ cells.

9. Undifferentiated cells that give rise to specialized cells are called _____ cells.

10. The term that means existing at or before birth is _____.

Anatomic Position and Directional Terms

6-7 Anatomy (ə-nat′ə-me) is the study, description, and classification of structures and organs of the body. Anatomists use directional terms and planes to describe the position and direction of the body. Locations and positions are always described relative to the body in the anatomic (an″ə-tom′ik) position—that is, the position that a person has while standing erect with the arms at the sides and the palms forward, as shown in Figure 6-3.

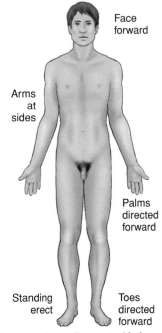

Face
forward

Arms
at
sides

Palms
directed
forward

Standing
erect

Toes
directed
forward

Figure 6-3   Anatomic position. The person is standing erect with the arms at the sides and the palms forward.

palm

plantar

In the anatomic position, the palms are forward. The palm* is the hollow of the hand. *Palm/ar* (**pahl′mər**) pertains to the _____.

Plantar (**plan′tər**)† pertains to the sole. Write the word that means pertaining to the sole:

_____.

chest (thorax)

6-8 In the anatomic position, the chest faces forward. The combining form *thorac(o)* means chest. The scientific name of the chest is the thorax (**thor′aks**). Thoraco/tomy (**thor″ə-kot′ə-me**) is incision into the _____. *Thoracotomy* refers to any incision of the chest wall.

The thorac/ic (**thə-ras′ik**) region is the area of the chest.

chest

thoracodynia

6-9 Thoraco/dynia (**thor″ə-ko-din′e-ə**) is a type of pain in the _____. (It differs from angina pectoris (**an-ji′nə, an′jə-nə pek′to-ris**), a heart disease in which the chest pain results from interference with the supply of oxygen to the heart muscle.) A term for pain in the chest is

_____.

suprathoracic
(**soo″prə-thə-ras′ik**)
across

Two directional terms that pertain to the chest are written by combining the prefixes *supra-* and *trans-*. Write a term that means pertaining to a location above the chest:

_____

Trans/thorac/ic (**trans″thə-ras′ik**) means through the chest cavity or _____ the chest wall.

frontal (**frun′təl**)

6-10 Body planes, imaginary flat surfaces, are used to identify the position of the body (Figure 6-4). Locations and positions are described relative to the body in the anatomic position. Complete these sentences while studying Figure 6-4:

The _____ plane divides the body into front and back portions. This plane is also called the coronal (**kor′ə-nəl**) plane.

transverse
(**trans-vərs′**)
midsagittal
(**mid-saj′ĭ-təl**)

A _____ plane divides the body into upper and lower portions. A sagittal (**saj′ĭ-təl**) plane divides the body into right and left sides. A _____ plane divides the body into equal right and left halves.

*Palm (Latin: *palma*).
†Plantar (Latin: *planta*, sole).

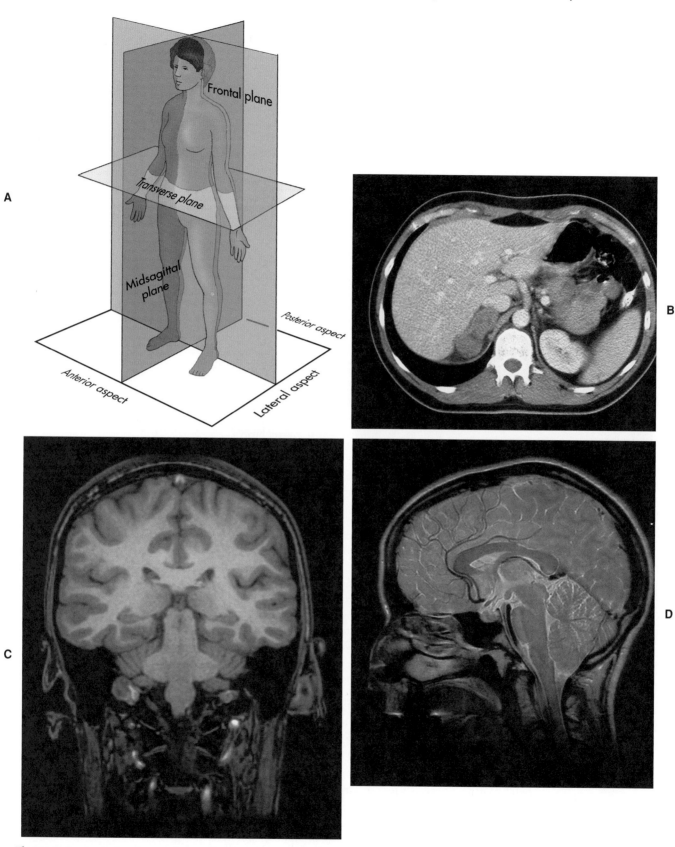

Figure 6-4   Anatomic reference planes and aspects. **A,** The frontal, transverse, and midsagittal planes are shown. The anterior, posterior, and lateral aspects are used to describe locations of various structures or parts. **B,** CT of the abdomen, transverse image. **C,** MRI of a frontal/coronal scan through the head, showing the brain. Note the ears on the sides of the head. **D,** MRI of a sagittal scan through the head.

anterior
  (an-tēr´e-ər)
posterior
  (pos-tēr´e-or)
lateral (lat´ər-əl)

6-11 *Aspects* refer to the surface of the figure when seen from various perspectives. The aspects shown in Figure 6-4 are used to describe locations of various structures or parts. The front is called the _____ aspect.

The back of the figure is the _____ aspect.

The side of the figure is the _____ aspect.

Study the following combining forms used in directional terms. Associate the combining forms with words you already know. For example, it is easier to remember that *tel(e)* means far or distant if you think of a telephone, which allows you to talk with someone distant from you.

Combining Forms Used in Directional Terms

COMBINING FORM	TERM	MEANING
anter(o)	anterior	nearer to or toward the front
poster(o)	posterior	nearer to or toward the back
ventr(o)	ventral	belly side
dors(o)	dorsal	directed toward or situated on the back side
medi(o)	medial, median	middle or nearer the middle
later(o)	lateral	farther from the midline of the body or from a structure
super(o)	superior	uppermost or above
infer(o)	inferior	lowermost or below
proxim(o)	proximal	nearer the origin or point of attachment
dist(o), tel(e)	distal	far or distant from the origin or point of attachment
caud(o)	caudad or caudal	in an inferior position
cephal(o)	cephalad	toward the head

front

6-12 *Anterior* means nearer to or toward the front. *Antero/medial* (an″tər-o-me´de-əl) indicates the aspect that is toward the _____ and toward the middle.

6-13 In humans, the anterior or front side is also the ventral (ven´tral) surface. *Ventral* refers to the belly side. *Ventro/median* (ven″tro-me´de-ən) is another way of saying anteromedial, but the latter is more common.

ventral

In humans, the anterior or front side is the same as the _____ surface. In dogs, for example, the ventral surface is not the front side.

behind

within (inside)

front

6-14 The opposite of anterior is posterior (pos-tēr´e-or). *Posterior* means directed toward or situated at the back. *Postero/external* (pos″tər-o-ek-ster´nəl) indicates that something is situated on the outside of a posterior part. Thus posteroexternal is situated _____ and outside. *Postero/internal* (pos″tər-o-in-tər´nəl) is situated behind and _____.

Antero/posterior (an″tər-o-pos-tēr´e-ər) pertains to both the _____ and the back sides. *Anteroposterior* means from the front to the back of the body.

front

back

6-15 In radiology, directional terms are used to specify the direction of the x-ray beam from its source to its exit surface before striking the film. In an anteroposterior projection, the x-ray beam strikes the anterior aspect of the body first. In other words, the beam passes from _____ to back. *Postero/anterior* (pos″tər-o-an-tēr´e-or) means from the posterior to the anterior surface, or, in other words, from _____ to front.

Positions for some common radiographic projections of the chest are shown in Figure 6-5.

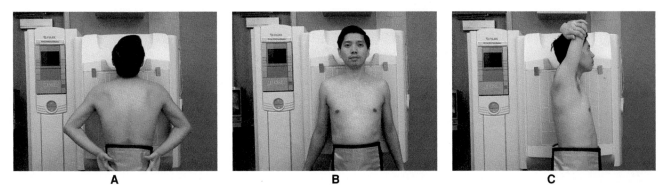

Figure 6-5   Patient positioning for a chest x-ray. **A,** In a posteroanterior (PA) projection, the anterior aspect of the chest is closest to the image receptor. **B,** In an anteroposterior (AP) projection, the posterior aspect of the chest is closest to the image receptor. **C,** In a left lateral chest projection, the left side of the patient is placed against the image receptor.

belly (front)	**6-16** Both *dorsal* (dor´səl) and *posterior* mean directed toward or situated on the back side. *Dorso/ventral* (dor″so-ven´trəl) pertains to the back and _____ surfaces. (Notice the order in which the two word parts are presented. The importance of the order becomes obvious when one is describing the path of a bullet, for example. *Dorsoventral* sometimes means passing from the back to the belly surface.)
	Lateral means side, so *dorso/lateral* (dor″so-lat´ər-əl) means behind and to one side of the body. Use the other word part that you learned that means behind to write another term that means
posterolateral (pos″tər-o-lat´ər-əl) side	behind and to one side: _____. *Medio/lateral* (me″de-o-lat´ər-əl) means from the middle to one _____. This term also denotes the direction of a line, as in the path of a bullet or the passage of an x-ray beam.
anter(o) anterolateral (an″tər-o-lat´ər-əl) side	**6-17** *Lateral* means side and denotes a position away from the midline of the body. Write the combining form for anterior: _____. Write a new word using *lateral* that means situated in front and to one side: _____.
sides back	**6-18** *Uni/lateral* (u″nĭ-lat´ər-əl) means affecting only one _____. *Bi/lateral* (bi-lat´ər-əl) pertains to two _____. In other words, *bilateral* refers to both sides of the body. *Postero/medial* (post″tər-o-me´de-əl) means situated in the middle of the_____ side of an organism.
front	**6-19** Anatomists use the term *superior* (soo-pe´re-or) to indicate uppermost or situated above. *Antero/superior* (an″tər-o-soo-pēr´e-ər) indicates a position in _____ and above. Using the combining form for posterior, build a word that means behind and above:
posterosuperior (pos″tər-o-soo-pēr´e-or)	_____. *Super/ficial* (soo″pər-fish´əl) means situated on or near the surface. Superficial radiation therapy is sometimes used for surface lesions such as skin tumors. *Superficial* comes from a similar-appearing Latin word that contains *super(o)*, the combining form that means uppermost or situated
above	_____.
	6-20 *Inferior* (in-fēr´e-ər) is the opposite of superior. There may be certain products that you consider inferior to your favorite brand. When you consider something inferior, you believe that product is lower in value than something else. *Inferior* means lower or below. In anatomy, *inferior* means

below	situated _____. It is often used in reference to the lower surface of a structure or the lower of two or more similar structures.
middle	*Infero/median* (**in″fәr-o-me′de-әn**) means situated in the _____ of the underside.
	Only a few medical words use the combining form *infer(o)*. The prefix *sub-* is more often used in medicine.
tail	**6-21** The combining form *caud(o)* means toward the tail or the end of the body away from the head. *Caudad* (**kaw′dad**) or *caudal* (**kaw′dәl**) pertains to a _____ or tail-like structure. In human anatomy, it also means inferior.
caudal	Another word in human anatomy that means the same as inferior is _____, which also refers to the tail.
proximal	**6-22** The combining form *proxim(o)* means near. *Proxim/al* (**prok′sĭ-mәl**) refers to something that is near. *Proximal* describes the position of structures that are nearest their origin or point of attachment. The end of the thigh bone that joins with the hip bone is the _____ end.
distal	**6-23** Distal (**dis′tәl**) is the opposite of proximal. If the upper end of the thigh bone is proximal, the lower end of the thigh bone is _____ to the hip bone.
proximal	Which is nearer its origin, a structure that is proximal or one that is distal? _____
distant	Another combining form, *tel(e)*, also means distant. A *tele/cardio/gram* (**tel″ә-kahr′de-o-gram**) registers the heart impulses of patients in _____ places. With a telecardiogram, the cardiologist and the patient may be in different cities, and the heart tracing is sent by phone.
	6-24 The combining form *cephal(o)* means head, and the suffix *-ad* means toward. *Cephalad* (**sef′ә-lad**) means toward the head. *Dorso/cephalad* (**dor″so-sef′ә-lad**) means situated toward the back of the head. Write another word using *-ic* that means pertaining to the head:
cephalic (**sә-fal′ik**)	_____.
	6-25 Locations and directions are generally described relative to the body in the anatomic position. Physicians rely on additional positions for examination or surgery. *Prone** (**prōn**) and *supine*† (**soo-pīn′**) are terms used to describe the position of a person who is lying face downward and lying on the back, respectively (Figure 6-6, *A* and *B*). If a person is prone, is the face turned up or down?
down	_____
	Pronation (**pro-na′shәn**) and *supination* (**soo″pĭ-na′shәn**) are generally used to indicate positioning of the hands and feet, but their complete meanings include the act of lying prone or face downward and assumption of a supine position. Pronation of the arm is the rotation of the forearm so that the palm faces downward.
up	Supination is the rotation of a joint that allows the hand or foot to turn upward. Supination of the wrist allows the palm to turn _____. Compare pronation and supination of the wrist in Figure 6-6, *C*.
	Recumbent (**re-kum′bәnt**) means lying down. The lateral recumbent position is assumed by the patient lying on the side, because *lateral* means pertaining to the
side	_____.

*Prone (Latin: *pronus*, inclined forward).
†Supine (Latin: *supinus*, lying on the back, face upward).

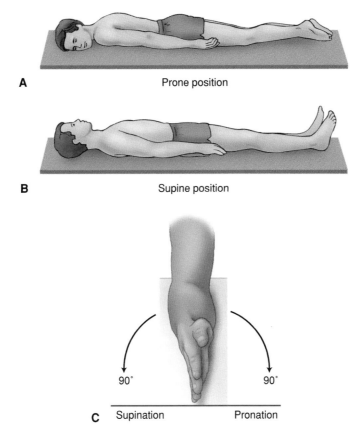

A   Prone position

B   Supine position

90°   90°

C   Supination   Pronation

Figure 6-6 Comparison of pronation and supination. **A,** Prone, lying face downward. **B,** Supine, lying on the back. **C,** Supination and pronation of the elbow and wrist joints, which permit the palm of the hand to turn upward or downward.

Exercise 2

Complete the table by writing the meaning of each word part that is listed. Also write the corresponding anatomic term for 1 through 12. (Numbers 2 and 8 have two anatomic terms each.) The first one is done as an example.

COMBINING FORM	MEANING	ANATOMIC TERM
1. anter(o)	*front*	*anterior*
2. caud(o)		
3. cephal(o)		
4. dist(o)		
5. dors(o)		
6. infer(o)		
7. later(o)		
8. medi(o)		
9. poster(o)		
10. proxim(o)		
11. super(o)		
12. ventr(o)		

Body Regions and Body Cavities

6-26 The body is made up of two major regions:

- head, neck, and trunk (chest, abdomen, and pelvis)
- extremities (arms and legs)

The chest, abdomen (**ab′də-mən, ab-do′mən**), and pelvis make up the body's

trunk

_____. The trunk has two major cavities that contain internal
organs.
    Learn the following combining forms that are used to describe the body.

Selected Combining Forms Used to Describe the Body

COMBINING FORM	MEANING	COMBINING FORM	MEANING
abdomin(o)	abdomen	pelv(i)	pelvis
acr(o)	extremities (arms and legs)	periton(o)	peritoneum
cephal(o)	head	pod(o)	foot
crani(o)	cranium (skull)	som(a), somat(o)	body
dactyl(o)	finger or toe	spin(o)	spine
encephal(o)	brain	thorac(o)	thorax (chest)
herni(o)	hernia	viscer(o)	viscera (large abdominal organs)
omphal(o), umbilic(o)	umbilicus (navel)		

abdominothoracic
(ab-dom″ĭ-no-thə-
ras′ik)

6-27 The abdomen is that part of the body lying between the thorax and the pelvis. Write a word
that means pertaining to the abdomen and thorax by combining *abdomin(o)* + *thorac(o)* + *-ic*:
_____.

6-28 Because of its large area and numerous internal organs, the abdomen is frequently subdivided
using imaginary lines to indicate points of reference. There are two methods of using imaginary
lines to divide the abdomen into regions. Dividing the abdomen into four quadrants (**kwod′rəntz**)
is a convenient way to designate areas in the abdominal (**ab-dom′ĭ-nəl**) cavity (Figure 6-7, A).
Refer to the diagram to answer the following:
Quadrant is a term that means any one of four corresponding parts. *RUQ* and *LUQ* refer to the right

upper
lower

and left _____ quadrants, respectively. *RLQ* and *LLQ* refer to
the right and left _____ quadrants.
    Abdominal quadrants are used to describe the location of pain or of body structures. The system
of naming four abdominal areas that are determined by drawing two imaginary lines through the

quadrant

umbilicus is the four- _____ system. Principal organs contained
in the four abdominal quadrants are shown in Table 6-2.

6-29 Anatomists describe the abdomen as having nine regions, shown in Figure 6-7, B. The nine-
region system is also used in clinical and surgical settings. Some of the terms may be unfamiliar, but
try to remember the divisions. When the terms are studied in more detail in later chapters, they will
acquire more meaning. Look at Figure 6-7, B while working this frame.
    The upper lateral regions beneath the ribs are the right and left

hypochondriac
(hi″po-kon′dre-ak)

_____ regions.

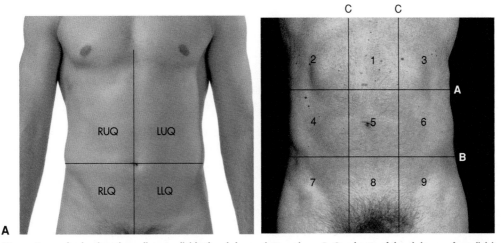

Figure 6-7   Two systems of using imaginary lines to divide the abdomen into regions. **A,** Quadrants of the abdomen, four divisions of the abdomen determined by drawing a vertical line and a horizontal line through the umbilicus. *RUQ, LUQ, RLQ,* and *LLQ* are abbreviations for right upper quadrant, left upper quadrant, right lower quadrant, and left lower quadrant, respectively. **B,** The nine anatomic regions of the abdomen, determined by four imaginary lines: A, B, C, and D. The regions are: *1,* epigastric; *2,* right hypochondriac; *3,* left hypochondriac; *4,* right lumbar; *5,* umbilical; *6,* left lumbar; *7,* right inguinal (or iliac); *8,* hypogastric; *9,* left inguinal (or iliac).

epigastric (ep″ĭ-gas′trik)	Between the hypochondriac regions lies the _____ region. The stomach is in this region.
umbilical (əm-bil′ĭ-kəl)	The _____ region lies just below the epigastric region. The umbilical region is that of the navel, or umbilicus.
lumbar (lum′bahr)	The right and left _____ regions lie on each side of the umbilical region.
hypogastric (hi″po-gas′trik)	The lower middle region is called the _____ region.
iliac (il′e-ak) inguinal (ing′gwĭ-nəl)	Finally, the two lower lateral regions are the right and left _____ or _____ regions.

TABLE 6-2 Abdominal Quadrants and Their Contents

Right upper quadrant (RUQ)	Contains the right lobe of the liver, gallbladder, right kidney, and parts of the large and small intestines
Left upper quadrant (LUQ)	Contains the left lobe of the liver, stomach, pancreas, left kidney, spleen, and parts of the large and small intestines
Right lower quadrant (RLQ)	Contains the right ureter, right ovary and uterine tube, appendix, and parts of the large and small intestines
Left lower quadrant (LLQ)	Contains the left ureter, left ovary and uterine tube, and parts of the large and small intestines

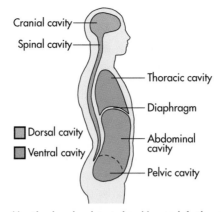

Cranial cavity
Spinal cavity
Thoracic cavity
Diaphragm
Abdominal cavity
Pelvic cavity
☐ Dorsal cavity
☐ Ventral cavity

Figure 6-8   The body has two principal body cavities, the dorsal and ventral cavities, each further subdivided. The dorsal cavity is divided into the cranial cavity and the spinal cavity. The ventral cavity is divided into the thoracic cavity and the abdominopelvic cavity, which is subdivided into the abdominal cavity and the pelvic cavity.

---

abdomen

6-30 The first region that you named in the preceding frame was the hypochondriac region. (You have probably also heard the term *hypochondriac* applied to a person who has a false belief of suffering from some disease. Ancient Greeks believed that organs in the hypochondriac region of the abdomen were the cause of melancholy and imaginary diseases, hence the term *hypochondriac*.) The hypochondriac region is just one of nine abdominal divisions. *Abdomin/al* means pertaining to the _____.

back (posterior)
front (belly)

6-31 The body has two major cavities, spaces that contain internal organs. The two principal body cavities are the dorsal cavity and the ventral cavity. We learned previously that *dorsal* means situated toward the _____ surface of the body. *Ventral* means situated toward the _____ surface.

cranial
spinal

dorsal

6-32 The dorsal and ventral cavities are subdivided as shown in Figure 6-8. The dorsal cavity is divided into the _____ cavity and the _____ cavity.
    The cranial (kra′ne-əl) cavity contains the brain, and the spinal (spi′nəl) cavity contains the spinal cord and the beginnings of the spinal nerves. The cranial and spinal cavities are divisions of the _____ body cavity.

thorax (chest)

6-33 The ventral cavity is the anterior body cavity. It is subdivided into the thoracic, abdominal, and pelvic (pel′vik) cavities. You have learned that *thoracic* means pertaining to the _____. The thoracic cavity contains several divisions, which you will learn in a later chapter. The abdominal and pelvic cavities are not separated by a muscular partition, and together they are often called the abdominopelvic (ab-dom″ĭ-no-pel′vik) cavity. The muscular diaphragm (di′ə-fram) separates the thoracic cavity from the abdominopelvic cavity.

pelvic

abdominal

6-34 The pelvis is the lower portion of the trunk of the body. You learned that *pelv(i)* is the combining form for pelvis. The cavity formed by the pelvis is the _____ cavity.
    The pelvic cavity contains the urinary bladder, the lower portion of the large intestine, the rectum, and the male or female reproductive organs. However, organs such as the stomach, spleen, and liver are contained in the _____ cavity.

peritoneum

6-35 The abdominopelvic cavity is lined with a membrane called the peritoneum (per″ĭ-to-ne′əm). This membrane also invests the internal organs (Figure 6-9). Write the name of the membrane that lines the abdominopelvic cavity and is reflected over the internal organs: _____.

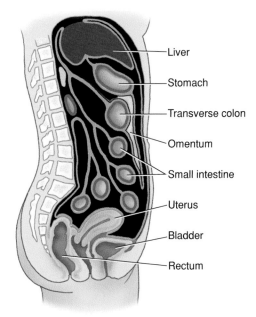

Figure 6-9   The peritoneum. This extensive membrane lines the entire abdominal wall and is reflected over the viscera. The free surface of the peritoneum is smooth and lubricated by a fluid that permits the viscera to glide easily against the abdominal wall and against one another.

There are two types of peritoneum:

• The parietal (pǝ-ri′ǝ-tǝl) peritoneum lines the abdominal and pelvic walls.
• The visceral (vis′er-ǝl) peritoneum contains large folds that weave in between the organs, binding them to one another and to the walls of the cavity.

parietal

The peritoneum that lines the abdominopelvic cavity is _____ peritoneum.

Organs within the ventral body cavity, especially the abdominal organs, are called *viscera* (vis′ǝr-ǝ). Peritoneum that invests the viscera is called _____ peritoneum.

visceral

peritoneal
(per″ĭ-to-ne′ǝl)

6-36 Build a word that means pertaining to the peritoneum using the suffix *-eal*:
_____.

Serous membranes such as the peritoneum secrete a lubricating fluid that allows the organs to slide against one another or against the cavity wall. The peritoneal cavity is the space between the parietal peritoneum and the visceral peritoneum.

abdominoplasty
(ab-dom″ĭ-no-
plas′te)

6-37 Write a word using *-plasty* that means surgical repair of the abdomen:
_____. (This type of plastic surgery, when done for aesthetic reasons to tighten the abdominal muscles, is commonly called a tummy tuck.)

abdomen

6-38 Abdomino/centesis (ab-dom″ĭ-no-sen-te′sis) is surgical puncture of the
_____. Abdominal paracentesis (par″ǝ-sǝn-te′sis) is another name for abdominocentesis. This procedure is performed to remove fluids or to inject a therapeutic agent. It is most often done to remove excess fluid, ascites (ǝ-si′tēz), from the peritoneal cavity (Figure 6-10).

Ascites is abnormal accumulation of serous fluid in the peritoneal cavity, sometimes resulting in considerable distension (enlargement, stretching) of the abdomen. The removal of the excess fluid in the peritoneal cavity is called abdominal _____.

paracentesis

6-39 The body's extremities are the four limbs. Each arm, elbow, forearm, wrist, hand, and associated fingers make up one of the body's upper extremities. Each thigh, knee, leg, ankle, foot, and associated toes make up one of the lower extremities. Fingers and toes are digits. When referring to the bones

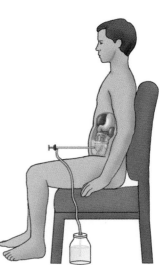

Figure 6-10   Paracentesis, a procedure in which fluid is withdrawn from a body cavity. It is performed to remove excess fluid from the abdomen.

of the digits, *phalanges* is the proper term. When referring to a digit in its entirety (multiple phalanges plus surrounding soft tissues), *digit*, *finger*, or *toe* should be used. Many medical terms use combining forms for the body extremities—hands, feet, and phalanges (bones of the fingers and toes). The combining form for extremities is _____. In acro/paralysis (**ak″ro-pə-ral′ĭ-sis**), movement of the _____ is impaired.

    Build a word by combining *acr(o)*, *cyan(o)*, and *-osis*: _____.

Literal translation of this new word is a blue condition of the
_____. This is an intermittent cyanosis of the extremities, caused by exposure to cold or emotional stimuli. Acrocyanosis is also called Raynaud's (**ra-nōz′**) sign or phenomenon.

6-40 Acro/megaly (**ak″ro-meg′ə-le**) is a disorder in which there is enlargement of the
_____. In acromegaly, there is enlargement of many parts of the skeleton, particularly the distal portions such as the nose, ears, jaws, fingers, and toes (see Figure 17-11). It is caused by increased secretion of growth hormone by the pituitary (**pǐ-too′ĭ-tar″e**) gland.

6-41 The suffix *-osis* means condition but sometimes implies a disease or abnormal increase. It usually indicates an abnormal noninflammatory condition. Inflammation is tissue reaction to injury and is recognized by pain, heat, redness, and swelling.
    Literal translation of *dermat/osis* (**der″mə-to′sis**) is a _____
condition. Its true meaning is any disease of the skin in which inflammation is not present. Inflammation of the skin is called dermatitis. Acro/dermat/itis (**ak″ro-dər″mə-ti′tis**) is inflammation of the skin of the _____, especially the hands and feet.
    Write another word that, translated literally, means surgical repair of the skin:
_____. In this surgery, skin grafts are used to cover destroyed or lost skin.

6-42 The combining form *dactyl(o)* usually refers to a finger but sometimes to a toe. Fingers and toes are also called digits (**dij′its**). Whenever you see *dactyl(o)* or *digit*, immediately think of a finger or toe. A dactylo/gram (**dak-til′o-gram**) is a mark or record of a fingerprint. The part of the word that refers to the finger is *dactyl(o)*. The process of taking fingerprints is _____.

    Dactyl/itis (**dak″tə-li′tis**) is inflammation of a finger or toe.
    Dactylo/spasm (**dak′tə-lo-spaz-əm**) is a cramping or twitching of a digit. Write this word that means cramping of a finger or toe: _____.

6-43 The combining form for hand is *chir(o)*. Use *chir(o)* and *-spasm* to form a new word:
_____. Writer's cramp is a form of chirospasm.

---

acr(o)
extremities
acrocyanosis
(ak″ro-si″ə-no′sis)
extremities

extremities

skin

extremities

dermatoplasty
(dər′mə-to-plas″te)

dactylography
(dak″tə-log′rə-fe)

dactylospasm

chirospasm
(ki′ro-spaz-əm)

hand
hands
feet
podiatry
podogram

Chiro/plasty (**ki′ro-plas″te**) is surgical repair of the _____.
Chiro/pod/y (**ki-rop′ə-de**) literally refers to the _____ and feet and was once a term for podiatry (**po-di′ə-tre**). A pod/iatrist (**po-di′ə-trist**) specializes in the care of _____. The specialized field dealing with the foot, including its anatomy, pathology, and medical and surgical treatment, is _____.

6-44 A podo/gram (**pod′o-gram**) is a print or record of the foot. The term *footprint* is more commonly used than _____.

Exercise 3

Write combining forms for the following terms:

1. abdomen _____

2. chest _____

3. extremities _____

4. finger or toe _____

5. pelvis _____

6. peritoneum _____

7. spine _____

8. skull _____

Terms Related to the Body as a Whole

fever
without
fever
hyperpyrexia
against

6-45 A disease or a disorder in one structure can affect the functioning of the body as a whole. In the next chapter, you will learn how an infectious disease such as influenza can spread from one person to someone else. Infections occur when the body is invaded by pathogenic microorganisms. Infection is just one of several causes of an abnormal elevation of the body temperature, which is called fever or pyr/exia (**pi-rek′se-ə**). The latter term is written using a combining form *pyr(o)*, which means fire; however, *pyrexia* means a _____ or a febrile condition.
   Febrile (**feb′ril**) pertains to fever. *A/febrile* (**a-feb′ril**) means _____ fever.
   An anti/pyretic (**an″te-, an″ti-pi-ret′ik**) is an agent that is effective against _____. *Anti/febrile* (**an″te-, an″ti-feb′ril**) and *anti/pyretic* both mean effective against fever. Aspirin is a well-known antipyretic.

6-46 A pyro/gen (**pi′ro-jən**) is a substance or agent that produces fever, such as some bacterial toxins. *Hyper/pyrexia* (**hi″pər-pi-rek′se-ə**) denotes a highly elevated body temperature, because *hyper-* means excessive or more than normal. This can be produced by physical agents such as hot baths or hot air, or by reaction to infection. A body temperature that is much greater than normal is called _____. An abnormally high temperature is considered to be hyperpyrexial (**hi″pər-pi-rek″se-al**).

6-47 *Anti/infective* (**an″te-in-fek′tiv**) means capable of killing infectious micro/organisms or of preventing them from spreading. Agents that are capable of this action are called antiinfectives. The literal translation of *antiinfective* is acting _____ infection. Anti/microb/ial (**an″te-, an″ti-mi-kro′be-əl**) agents act against microbes (**mi′krōbz**). Antimicrobial means the same as antiinfective.

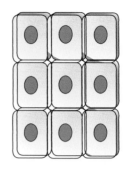
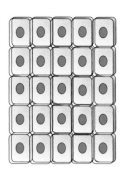
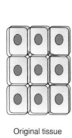

Figure 6-11 A representation of tissue enlargement by hypertrophy and hyperplasia.

Original tissue   Increase in tissue size by hypertrophy   Increase in tissue size by hyperplasia

living

There are many types of antiinfectives. Because the term *anti/bio/tic* (**an″te-, an″ti-bi-ot′ik**) contains the combining form *bi(o)*, we know that antibiotics act against _____ microscopic organisms. Antibiotics are derived from microorganisms or they are produced semi-synthetically and are used to treat infections, largely bacterial infections. Read more about other types of antiinfectives in the Chapter Pharmacology section, Appendix I, pages 531-547.

against

6-48 Inflammation is the body's protective response to irritation or injury. You are familiar with some of the signs of inflammation, such as heat and redness. *Antiinflammatory* (**an″te-in-flam′ə-to″re**) means acting _____ inflammation. In other words, it means counteracting or reducing inflammation.

6-49 Earlier in this chapter, you studied how tissue is a collection of similar cells acting together to perform a particular function. The suffix *-plasia* means formation. Several terms that contain *-plasia* are used to describe abnormal tissue formation. *Dys/plasia* (**dis-pla′zhə**) is the abnormal development of tissues or organs. *A/plasia* (**ə-pla′zhə**) is the lack of development of an organ or tissue.

without

Translated literally, *aplasia* means _____ development. *An/otia* (**an-o′shə**), congenital absence of one or both ears, is an example of aplasia.

Hypo/plasia (**hi″po-pla′zhə**) is less severe than aplasia; it is the underdevelopment of an organ or tissue and usually results from fewer than the normal number of cells.

hyperplasia (hi″pər-pla′zhə)

6-50 Write a new term by combining *hyper-* and *-plasia*: _____. Literal translation of the word parts yields "increased development," but you will need to remember that *hyperplasia* means an abnormal increase in the number of normal cells in tissue. *Hyperplasia* contrasts with another term, *hyper/trophy* (*hyper-*, increased, *-trophy*, nutrition), which means an increase in the size of an organ caused by an increase in the size of the cells rather than the number of cells. Figure 6-11 will help you understand the difference between hyperplasia and hypertrophy. It may be helpful to note that, despite the technical difference between hyperplasia and hypertrophy, these terms are sometimes used interchangeably to indicate increased size of a body part.

Cells of the heart are particularly prone to hypertrophy (**hi-pər′tro-fe**). In other words, the heart increases in size by enlarging individual cells. An enlargement of the adult heart may be caused by an increased workload. This differs from hyperplasia, in which the number of cells increases. The new cells may be either benign or malignant, so hyperplasia does not necessarily mean that the new cells are cancerous.

6-51 However, a change in the structure and orientation of cells, characterized by a loss of differentiation and reversal to a more primitive form, is characteristic of malignancy. This change in cell structure is call *ana/plasia* (**an″ə-pla′zə**). The prefix *ana-* means upward, excessive, or again. The important thing to remember about anaplasia is that it is especially characteristic of

malignancy

_____.

6-52 You have learned that both *som(a)* and *somat(o)* refer to the body in general. The death of a person, somatic (**so-mat′ik**) death, is usually defined as absence of electrical activity of the brain for a specified period under rigidly defined circumstances. Practice will help you learn which word part to use in writing terms about the body.

body somat(o)	*Somato/genic* (so″mə-to-jen′ik) means originating in the _____. The part of *somatogenic* that means body is _____.
head	**6-53** You have already learned that *cephal(o)* refers to the head and that *cephal/ad* means toward the _____. The combining form *encephal(o)* means the brain and is so called because it is located inside the head. Electro/encephalo/graphy (e-lek″tro-ən-sef″ə-log′rə-fe) is the process of recording electrical activity of the brain and can be used to determine somatic death.
brain inflammation disease	**6-54** An electro/encephalo/gram (e-lek″tro-en-sef′ə-lo-gram) is a record produced by the electrical impulses of the _____. (You see why the abbreviation EEG is commonly used!) The instrument used to record electrical impulses of the brain is an electroencephalograph (e-lek″tro-ən-sef′ə-lo-graf″). Encephal/itis (en-sef″ə-li′tis) is _____ of the brain. There are many types of encephalitis, but a large percentage of cases are caused by viruses. The symptoms include mild to severe convulsions, coma, and even death in some cases. Encephalo/pathy (en-sef″ə-lop′ə-the) is any _____ of the brain.
body	**6-55** *Som/esthetic* (so″mes-thet′ik) pertains to _____ feeling. The *a* is dropped from *som(a)* to facilitate pronunciation. A particular part of the brain is the somesthetic area and is responsible for receiving and pinpointing where and what sensations occur in the body. A lesion in this part of the brain could affect one's ability to read, write, or speak and also one's ability to recognize objects by touch. A lesion is a wound or other pathologic change in body tissue.
mind	**6-56** *Somato/psych/ic* (so″mə-to-si′kik) pertains to both body and _____. Somatopsychic disorders are physical disorders that influence mental activity. A brain lesion (physical disorder) often produces significant intellectual difficulties and memory loss (mental activities). Physiology is the study of the function of the body. Psycho/physio/logic (si″ko-fiz-e-o-loj′ik), also called psycho/somatic (si″ko-so-mat′ik), disorders are the opposite of somatopsychic. Extreme or prolonged emotional states that influence the physical body's functioning are psychophysiologic disorders. Emotional factors may precipitate conditions such as high blood pressure. You learned that *physi(o)* means nature. In psychophysiologic disorders, the natural functioning of the body is influenced by emotional factors.
mind	**6-57** *Psychosomatic* is also the commonly used term that refers to the interaction of the mind, or psyche, and the body. You have learned that *psych(o)* means _____. *Psych/ic* (si′kik) has two meanings: A person said to be endowed with the ability to read the minds of others is called a psychic. *Psychic* also means pertaining to the mind.
umbilicus umbilicus omphalocele	**6-58** *Omphalus* (om′fə-ləs) is another name for the umbilicus (əm-bil′ĭ-kəs) or navel. *Omphalic* (om-fal′ik) means pertaining to the _____ . An omphalo/cele (om′fə-lo-sēl″) is a congenital hernia of the _____. Babies are sometimes born with an omphalocele, protrusion of part of the intestine through a defect in the abdominal wall at the umbilicus. Write the formal name for an umbilical (əm-bil′ĭ-kəl) hernia: _____. Hernio/plasty (hər′ne-o-plas″te), surgical repair of a hernia, is sometimes used specifically to denote repair using a mesh patch or plug to reinforce the area of the defect.
incisional	**6-59** A hernia can occur through any weakness or defect in the peritoneum that lines the abdominal or pelvic cavities. In addition to the umbilicus, frequent sites of such weaknesses are old surgical scars and the inguinal (ing′gwĭ-nəl) (groin) and femoral (fem′or-əl) (thigh) canals (Figure 6-12). Read the information that accompanies the illustration and write answers in the blanks. A hernia that occurs through inadequately healed surgery is an _____ hernia.

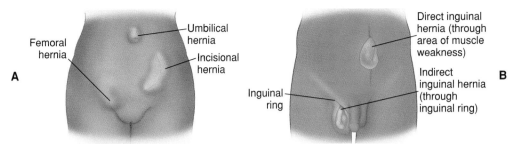

Figure 6-12   Common types of abdominal hernias. **A,** Umbilical hernias result from a weakness in the abdominal wall around the umbilicus. An incisional hernia is herniation through inadequately healed surgery. In a femoral hernia, a loop of intestine descends through the femoral canal into the groin. **B,** Inguinal hernias are of two types. A direct hernia occurs through an area of weakness in the abdominal wall. In an indirect hernia, a loop of intestine descends through the inguinal canal, an opening in the abdominal wall for passage of the spermatic cord in males and a ligament of the uterus in females.

femoral	The type of hernia that occurs if a loop of intestine descends through the femoral canal into the groin is a _____ hernia.
inguinal	A direct or indirect hernia that occurs in the groin is an _____ hernia.
umbilicus	**6-60** Omphal/oma (om″fə-lo′mə) is a tumor of the _____.
inflammation	Omphal/itis (om″fə-li′tis) is _____ of the umbilicus.
	Write a term that means hemorrhage from the umbilicus by combining *omphal(o)* and *-rrhagia*:
omphalorrhagia (om″fə-lo-ra′jə)	_____.
rupture	*Omphalorrhexis* (om″fə-lo-rek′sis) means _____ of the umbilicus.

Exercise 4

Write a word in each blank to complete the sentence.

1. A term that means a fever is _____.

2. An agent that causes fever is a/an _____.

3. Abnormal development of tissue or organs is called _____.

4. Lack of development of an organ or tissue is _____.

5. Underdevelopment of an organ or tissue is _____.

6. Abnormal increase in the number of normal cells in tissue is _____.

7. A change in the structure and orientation of cells that is characteristic of malignancy is _____.

8. *Omphalus* is another name for the navel, also called the _____.

9. The death of a person is called _____ death.

10. Electroencephalography is the process of recording electrical activity of the _____.

11. Congenital herniation of the navel is called _____.

12. A term that means pertaining to the body and the mind is psychosomatic or _____.

The Physical Examination

walk	**6-61** *Ambulation* (am″bu-la′shən) means the act of walking. *Ambulant* (am′bu-lənt) describes a person who is able to _____. It is also accurate to say that the person is ambulatory (am′bu-lə-tor″e).

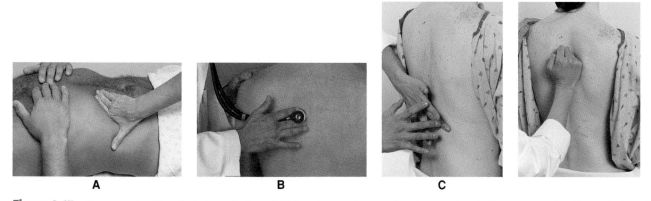

Figure 6-13   Three aspects of the physical examination, which help in assessing the internal organs. **A,** palpation; **B,** percussion; **C,** auscultation with a stethoscope.

Vital signs (VS) are the measurements of pulse, respiration, and body temperature. Blood pressure is also customarily included. The vital signs are often considered the base indicator of a patient's health status. You will learn more about the vital signs in later chapters.

6-62 A physical examination (PE) is an investigation of the body to determine its state of health, using any of several techniques, which include the following:

- inspection (The examiner uses the eyes to observe the patient.)
- palpation (**pal-pa′shən**) (The examiner feels the texture, size, consistency and location of certain body parts with the hands; Figure 6-13, A.)
- percussion (**pər-ku′shən**) (The examiner taps the body with the fingertips or fist to evaluate the size, borders, and consistency of internal organs and to determine the amount of fluid in a body cavity; Figure 6-13, B).
- auscultation (**aws″kəl-ta′shən**) (The examiner listens for sounds within the body to evaluate the heart, blood vessels, lungs, intestines, or other organs or to detect the fetal heart sound. Auscultation is performed most commonly with a stethoscope; Figure 6-13, C.)

Using the hands to feel the location or size of the liver is an example of
_____. Tapping the chest with the fingertips is an example of
_____. Listening to the heart with a stethoscope is an example of
_____.

palpation
percussion
auscultation

Exercise 5

Write answers to these questions.

1. What is the name of the procedure in which the physician listens with a stethoscope for sounds within the body?
_____

2. What is the name of the procedure in which the physician taps the patient's body with the fingertips to evaluate an internal organ? _____

3. What is the name of the procedure in which the physician feels the texture, size, consistency, and location of body parts with the hands? _____

4. What is the term for the act of walking? _____

SELECTED ABBREVIATIONS

abd	abdomen, abdominal	**LUQ**	left upper quadrant
AP	anteroposterior	**PA**	posteroanterior
BSA	body surface area	**PE**	physical examination
DNA	deoxyribonucleic acid	**RLQ**	right lower quadrant
EEG	electroencephalogram	**RUQ**	right upper quadrant
lat.	lateral	**VS, v.s.**	vital signs
LLQ	left lower quadrant		

PREPARING FOR THE TEST

Review as you were instructed in Chapter 2 and work the end-of-chapter review.

Be Careful With These Opposites!

anter(o) vs. poster(o)
ventr(o) vs. dors(o)
proxim(o) = proximal vs. dist(o) or tel(e) = distal
medial vs. lateral
prone vs. supine

CHAPTER 6 REVIEW

■ Basic Understanding

Labeling

I. *Label the body cavities that are indicated on the diagram.*

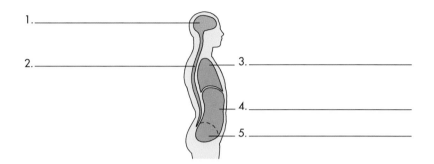

1. _____

2. _____   3. _____

4. _____

5. _____

II. *Write the names or the abbreviations of the abdominal quadrants that are indicated on the diagram.*

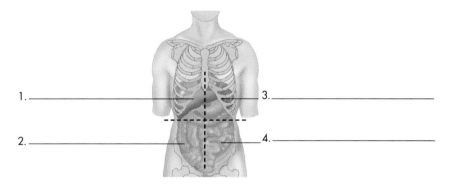

1. _____   3. _____

2. _____   4. _____

III. *Label the body planes and aspects that are indicated on the illustration.*

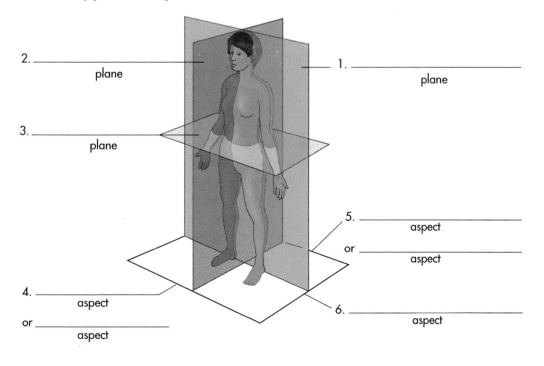

2. _____
    plane

1. _____
    plane

3. _____
    plane

5. _____
    aspect

or _____
    aspect

4. _____
    aspect

or _____
    aspect

6. _____
    aspect

Matching

IV. Using the diagram, identify the following abdominal regions with the correct letter (A-I). The first region is done as an example.

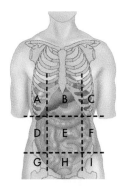

1. epigastric   _B_   4. left iliac   _____   7. right iliac   _____

2. hypogastric   _____   5. left lumbar   _____   8. right lumbar   _____

3. left hypochondriac _____   6. right hypochondriac _____   9. umbilical   _____

V. Match each directional term with its meaning, A through H. (Selections may be used more than once.)

_____ 1. anterior   A. above
                              B. back
_____ 2. distal   C. below
_____ 3. dorsal   D. far
_____ 4. inferior   E. front
                              F. middle
_____ 5. lateral   G. near
_____ 6. medial   H. side
_____ 7. posterior
_____ 8. proximal
_____ 9. superior
_____ 10. ventral

Listing

VI. List four main types of tissue.

1. _____

2. _____

3. _____

4. _____

Sequencing

VII. *Four levels of human organization are listed. Label each level with a number (1, 2, 3, or 4) to indicate simple levels to more complex levels.*

1. body systems _____

2. cells _____

3. organs _____

4. tissues _____

Multiple Choice

VIII. *Circle the correct answer for each of the following.*

1. Similar cells acting together to perform a function defines a/an (body system, organ, organism, tissue).

2. Pete is trying to explain the two methods of drawing imaginary lines to designate abdominal areas. He explains that dividing the abdomen into (bilateral areas, eight regions, six regions, four quadrants) is a convenient way to describe the location of pain or of body structures.

3. A term that means from the middle to one side is (anteromedian, anterolateral, mediolateral, posteromedial).

4. Dr. Ray explains in a radiology report that a fracture has occurred in the distal portion of the thigh bone. *Distal* means (farther from the origin, in the middle of the bone, nearer the origin, on the side of the bone).

5. Which plane divides the body into anterior and posterior portions? (frontal, midsagittal, sagittal, transverse)

6. Which term means inflammation of the brain? (cephaloitis, craniitis, encephalitis, sephalitis)

7. What is the term that means lying face downward? (ambulatory, prone, proximation, supine)

8. Shelley has a noninflammatory skin condition. What is the skin condition called? (dermatitis, dermatosis, pyosis, pyrexia)

9. What is another name for the navel? (angina, ascites, omphalocele, umbilicus)

10. Which of these terms means a muscular partition that separates the thoracic and abdominopelvic cavities? (diaphragm, paracentesis, peritoneum, pyrogen)

Writing Terms

IX. *Write words for the following:*

1. pertaining to above the chest _____

2. affecting only one side _____

3. lying flat on the back _____

4. pertaining to the peritoneum _____

5. pertaining to the sole _____

6. inflammation of the skin _____

7. pertaining to the abdomen and pelvis _____

8. cramping of the hand _____

9. abnormal development of tissue _____

10. a record of electrical impulses of the brain _____

■ Greater Comprehension

Spelling

X. *Circle all incorrectly spelled terms and write their correct spelling:*

abdomin   acrosyanosis   hyperpyrexia   palmar   superficial

Interpreting Abbreviations

XI. *Write the meaning of each of these abbreviations:*

1. abd _____

2. AP _____

3. lat. _____

4. PE _____

5. VS _____

Pronunciation

XII. *The pronunciation is shown for several medical words. Indicate the primary accented syllable in each term with a ʹ.*

1. bilateral (bi lat ər əl)

2. cephalic (sə fal ik)

3. omphalic (om fal ik)

4. posterosuperior (pos tər o soo pēr e or)

5. visceral (vis ər əl)
(Check your answers with the solutions in Appendix VI.)

LISTING OF MEDICAL TERMS

Use the practice CD to review the terms that have been presented. Look closely at the spelling of each term as it is pronounced and be sure you know the meaning of each term.

abdomen	chiropody	iliac	posteromedial
abdominal	chirospasm	inferior	posterosuperior
abdominal cavity	chromosomes	inferomedian	pronation
abdominal paracentesis	congenital	inflammation	prone
abdominal quadrant	connective tissue	inguinal	proximal
abdominocentesis	coronal plane	lateral	psychic
abdominopelvic cavity	cranial cavity	lesion	psychophysiologic
abdominoplasty	cranium	lumbar	psychosomatic
abdominothoracic	dactylitis	medial	pulse
acrocyanosis	dactylogram	median	pyrexia
acrodermatitis	dactylography	mediolateral	pyrogen
acromegaly	dactylospasm	melancholy	Raynaud's phenomenon
acroparalysis	dermatitis	microorganism	recumbent
afebrile	dermatoplasty	midsagittal plane	respiration
ambulant	dermatosis	noninflammatory	sagittal plane
ambulation	diaphragm	omphalic	serous membrane
ambulatory	digit	omphalitis	somatic cell
anaplasia	distal	omphalocele	somatic death
anatomic position	dorsal	omphaloma	somatogenic
anatomic plane	dorsal cavity	omphalorrhagia	somatopsychic
anatomy	dorsocephalad	omphalorrhexis	somesthetic
angina pectoris	dorsolateral	omphalus	sperm
anotia	dorsoventral	organ	spinal cavity
anterior	Down syndrome	organism	stem cells
anterolateral	dysplasia	ova	superficial
anteromedial	electroencephalogram	ovum	superior
anteroposterior	electroencephalograph	palmar	supination
anterosuperior	electroencephalography	palpation	supine
antibiotic	encephalitis	paracentesis	suprathoracic
antifebrile	encephalopathy	parietal peritoneum	telecardiogram
antiinfective	epigastric	pelvic cavity	thoracic
antiinflammatory	epithelial cells	pelvis	thoracic cavity
antimicrobial	epithelial tissue	percussion	thoracodynia
antipyretic	extremities	peritoneal	thoracotomy
aplasia	facial	peritoneal cavity	thorax
ascites	febrile	peritoneum	tissue
auscultation	femoral	phalanges	transthoracic
bilateral	frontal plane	pituitary gland	transverse plane
blood pressure	hernia	plantar	umbilical
body plane	hernioplasty	podiatrist	umbilicus
body system	hyperplasia	podiatry	unilateral
caudad	hyperpyrexia	podogram	ventral
caudal	hyperpyrexial	posterior	ventral cavity
cellular	hypertrophy	posteroanterior	ventromedian
cephalad	hypochondriac	posteroexternal	viscera
cephalic	hypogastric	posterointernal	visceral peritoneum
chiroplasty	hypoplasia	posterolateral	vital signs

español ENHANCING SPANISH COMMUNICATION

ENGLISH	SPANISH (PRONUNCIATION)
abdomen	abdomen (ab-DOH-men), vientre (ve-EN-tray)
anatomy	anatomía (ah-nah-to-MEE-ah)
antibiotic	antibiótico (an-te-be-O-te-co)
arm	brazo (BRAH-so)
aspirate	aspirar (as-pe-RAR)
belly	barriga (bar-REE-gah)
bladder	vejiga (vah-HEE-gah)
blood	sangre (SAHN-gray)
body	cuerpo (coo-ERR-po)
breathing	respiración (res-pe-rah-se-ON)
chest	pecho (PAY-cho)
face	cara (CAH-rah)
fever	fiebre (fe-AY-bray)
finger	dedo (DAY-do)
fingerprint	impresión digital (im-pray-se-ON de-he-TAHL)
hip	cadera (cah-DAY-rah)
kidney	riñon (ree-NYOHN)
leg	pierna (pe-ERR-nah)
liver	hígado (EE-ga-do)
navel	ombligo (om-BLEE-go)
palm	palma (PAHL-mah)
rib	costilla (cos-TEEL-lyah)
skull	cráneo (CRAH-nay-o)
sole	planta (PLAHN-tah)
thigh	muslo (MOOS-lo)
toe	dedo del pie (DAY-do del PE-ay)
uterus	útero (OO-tay-ro)
wrist	muñeca (moo-NYAY-cah)

CHAPTER **7**

Body Fluids and Immunity

LEARNING GOALS

In this chapter, you will learn to do the following:

Basic Understanding
1. Recognize general facts about body fluids.
2. Recognize the meaning of word parts pertaining to body fluids and immunity and use them to write terms.
3. Identify the functions and principal conditions that affect erythrocytes, leukocytes, and blood platelets.
4. List several body defense mechanisms.
5. List four general types of microorganisms.
6. Recognize the four classifications of bacteria.
7. Define active versus passive immunity and natural versus artificial immunity.
8. Name several nonspecific body defense mechanisms and describe the two aspects of specific immune response.

Greater Comprehension
9. Define terms that are presented in health care reports.
10. Recognize the meaning of several signs and symptoms of anemia.
11. Spell medical terms accurately.
12. Pronounce medical terms correctly.
13. Write the meanings of the abbreviations.
14. Categorize terms as anatomy, diagnostic test or procedure, pathology, surgery, or therapy.

THESE ARE THE MAJOR SECTIONS IN THIS CHAPTER:

- ❏ **Cellular Needs and Body Fluids**
- ❏ **Composition of Blood**
- ❏ **Anemias and Abnormal Hemoglobins**
- ❏ **Blood Coagulation**
- ❏ **Classification of Disease**
- ❏ **Bioterrorism**
- ❏ **Immunity**
- ❏ **Medical Records**
- ❏ **Categories of Medical Terms**

Cellular Needs and Body Fluids

7-1 Fluids constitute more than half of an adult's weight under normal conditions, and they are vital in the transport of oxygen and nutrients to all cells and removal of wastes from the body. Water is the most important component of body fluids. Body fluids are not distributed evenly throughout the body, and they move back and forth between compartments that are separated by cell membranes. The most important component of body fluids is

water

_____.

Several body fluids are associated with specific body systems. For example, spinal fluid bathes the brain and spinal cord and is associated with the nervous system. Urine is formed and excreted by the urinary system. Other fluids include saliva, mucus, perspiration, and gastric juices. Chemical and microscopic studies are performed on various body fluids to determine the body's internal status. Laboratory tests are commonly used to detect, identify, and quantify substances; evaluate organ functions; help establish or confirm a diagnosis; and aid in the management of disease.

7-2 Blood and lymph are the fluids that we generally associate with the cardio/vascul/ar (**kahr″de-o-vas′ku-lər**) (_cardi[o]_, heart; _vascul[o]_, vessel; _-ar_, pertaining to) and lymphatic (**lim-fat′ik**) systems, but these fluids circulate throughout the body, providing nutrients for cells and transporting wastes for removal. As blood circulates, needed substances move across the vessel walls into the fluid that surrounds the body cells and fluid accumulates in the tissue spaces. This excess fluid is normally transported away from the tissues by the lymphatic system, another vascular network that helps maintain the internal fluid environment. Lymph (**limf**) is the fluid that circulates through the lymphatic vessels. Cyan/osis (**si″ə-no′sis**) is caused by a deficiency of oxygen and an excess of carbon dioxide in the blood, as in severe conditions that interfere with normal breathing or circulation (see Figure 4-5). The color of the person's skin appears bluish in cyanosis, so named because _cyan(o)_ means

blue

_____.

Study the word parts and their meanings in the following list.

Word Parts for Selected Body Fluids

Word Part	Meaning	Word Part	Meaning
hem(a), hem(o), hemat(o), -emia	blood	muc(o)	mucus
		py(o)	pus
hidr(o)	sweat, perspiration	sial(o)	saliva; salivary glands
hydr(o)	water	ur(o)	urine; urinary tract

7-3 More than a million tiny structures called sweat glands are found in the skin. Sweat, or perspiration (**per″spĭ-ra′shən**), contains water, salts, and other waste products. These substances are excreted through pores in the skin when one perspires, and this serves as a means of ridding the body of wastes and regulating the body temperature. Another name for sweat is

perspiration
hidr(o)

_____.

The combining form for sweat is _____. Do not confuse this combining form with _hydr(o)_, which has the same pronunciation.

7-4 It is easy to confuse the terms _excrete_ and _secrete_. Secretion (**se-kre′shən**) is the process of discharging a substance into a cavity. For example, saliva (**sə-li′və**) is secreted into the mouth to keep the mouth moist, along with other functions. Excretion (eks-kre′shən) is the body's way of elimi-nating waste substances. Perspiration is excreted through pores in the skin. Substances that are secreted or excreted are called secretions or excretions, respectively.

Saliva is the clear fluid secreted by the salivary (sal′ĭ-var-e) glands in the mouth. It serves to mois-ten the oral cavity, to aid in chewing and swallowing, and contains an enzyme that initiates digestion of starch. The combining form that means saliva is _____. This combining form also means the salivary glands.

sial(o)

7-5 Mucus (mu′kəs) is the slippery secretion of glands within mucous membranes. *Muc/ous* means composed of or secreting _____. As you learned in Chapter 4, mucous membranes line cavities or canals of the body that open to the outside, such as the digestive tract. Notice the difference in spelling and meaning of the terms *mucus* and *mucous*.

mucus

7-6 Pus (pus) is the liquid product of infection and is composed of protein substances, fluid, bacteria, and white blood cells (or their remains). It is generally yellow; if it is red, this suggests blood from the rupture of small vessels. The combining form that means pus is _____. Discharges from infected tissue are described as purulent (pu′roo-lənt) or suppurative (sup′u-ra″tiv). Both terms mean pertaining to, consisting of, or producing pus. *Sanguinous* (sang′gwi-nəs) means containing blood.

py(o)

Several factors that slow the process of healing are listed below:

- infection, presence of foreign material, or necrotic tissue
- movement (lack of immobilization) of the wound
- poor blood circulation in the area of the abscess, or in the individual in general
- decreased number of white blood cells in the blood
- deficiency of antibodies in the blood
- malnutrition in the individual

A localized collection of pus in a cavity surrounded by inflamed tissue is called an abscess (ab′ses). The inflamed tissue may disintegrate and become necrotic (nə-krot′ik), increasing the difficulty of delivering medication to the site of infection and slowing the healing process. The combining form *necr(o)* means death. In necrosis (nə-kro′sis), there is localized tissue death in response to either injury or disease. Abscesses may need to be excised or surgically drained for healing to occur.

7-7 A hemat/oma (he″mə-to′mə) is a localized collection of blood, usually clotted, in an organ, space, or tissue, resulting from a break in the wall of a blood vessel. The term *hematoma* (hemat[o], blood + -oma, tumor) is derived from the old meaning of tumor, a swelling, because there is a raised area wherever a hematoma exists. Hematomas can occur almost anywhere in the body. They are especially dangerous when they occur inside the skull, but most hematomas are not serious. Bruises are familiar forms of hematomas.

You will use the suffix *-oma* to write words for tumors of many kinds, but you'll also need to remember that a localized collection of blood in an organ, tissue, or space is called a _____.

hematoma

7-8 Translated literally, *hyper/emia* (hi″pər-e′me-ə) means excessive _____. You need to know that hyperemia is an excess of blood in part of the body caused by increased blood flow, as one often sees in inflammation. In hyperemia, the overlying skin usually becomes reddened and warm.

blood

cell

Several combining forms will be used in this chapter to describe cells and body fluids. You already know that *cyt(o)* and *-cyte* mean _____. Learn the meanings of the word parts in the following list.

Word Parts Used to Describe Aspects of Cells and Body Fluids

WORD PART	MEANING	WORD PART	MEANING
Word Parts Commonly Used to Describe Cells		**Combining Forms for Blood Clotting**	
cellul(o)	little cell or compartment	coagul(o)	coagulation
chrom(o)	color	fibrin(o)	fibrin
cyt(o), -cyte	cell	thromb(o)	thrombus; clot
hemoglobin(o)	hemoglobin		
kary(o), nucle(o)	nucleus	**Miscellaneous Word Parts**	
morph(o)	shape; form	aer(o)	air or gas
necr(o)	death	angi(o), vascul(o)	vessel
norm(o)	normal	home(o)	sameness; constant
phil(o)	attraction	is(o)	equal
poikil(o)	irregular	lith(o)	stone; calculus
spher(o)	round	necr(o)	death
		-ant	that which causes
Combining Forms for Selected Electrolytes		-ate	to cause an action or the result of an action
calc(i)	calcium	-cidal	killing
kal(i)	potassium	-poiesis	production
natr(o)	sodium	-poietin	that which causes production

7-9 Body fluids are found either within the cells, intra/cellul/ar (in″trə-sel′u-lər), or outside the cells, extra/cellul/ar (eks″trə-sel′u-lər) (Figure 7-1).

The prefix *intra-* means within, the combining form *cellul(o)* means little cell or compartment, and the suffix *-ar* means pertaining to. Extra/cellul/ar fluid is not contained inside the cells. The prefix *extra-* means outside.

Only about one fourth of the extracellular fluid is plasma, the liquid portion of the blood. Blood remains inside blood vessels in humans, so it is an intra/vascular fluid. Write this term that means within a vessel by combining *intra-*, *vascul(o)*, and *-ar*: _____.

intravascular

Plasma (plaz′mə) is the fluid part of the blood. Another type of extracellular fluid fills the spaces between most of the cells of the body. This type of fluid is called interstitial* (in″tər-stish′əl) fluid. Knowing that *inter-* means between should be helpful.

7-10 Look again at Figure 7-1. Review these new terms that are used to describe body fluids by choosing one of these terms (*extracellular, intracellular, intravascular,* or *interstitial*) to complete these sentences:

More than half of all body fluid is contained within cells and is called

intracellular
extracellular
interstitial

_____ fluid. Body fluid is classified as either intracellular or _____ fluid. There are two types of extracellular fluid: plasma and _____ fluid.

7-11 The regulation of the amount of water in the body is called fluid balance. This balance is maintained through intake and output of water. Water is obtained by drinking fluids and eating foods. Water leaves the body via urine, feces, sweat, tears, and other fluid discharges. This balance depends on the proper intake of water and the elimination (output) of body wastes, including excess water (Figure 7-2). Note that most of the water gained by the body is through drinking water, and most water is excreted in the urine.

---

*Interstitial (Latin: *interstitium,* space or gap in a tissue or structure).

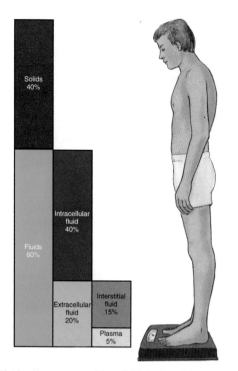

Figure 7-1   The body's fluid compartments. Fluid makes up 60% of the adult's body weight, and most of that is intracellular fluid. Two types of extracellular fluid are interstitial fluid and plasma. Accumulation of fluid in the interstitial compartment results in a condition called edema.

fluid

The fluid balance depends on proper functioning of several body systems, particularly the urinary system. Dehydration (de″hi-dra′shən) (excessive loss of water from body tissue) or generalized edema (ə-de′mə) (swelling caused by excessive accumulation of fluid in the body tissues) can occur if the body cannot maintain fluid balance. This regulation of the amount of water in the body is called _____ balance.

7-12 Fluid balance is one aspect of homeo/stasis (ho″me-o-sta′sis) (home[o], constant + -stasis, controlling), a relative constancy in the internal environment of the body. When the body is healthy, the tissue fluid that bathes and maintains the cells remains fairly constant within very limited normal ranges. Homeostasis is naturally maintained by sensing and control mechanisms that promote healthy survival. The combining form *home(o)* means

constant

_____ or sameness, and -*stasis*, in this case, means controlling.

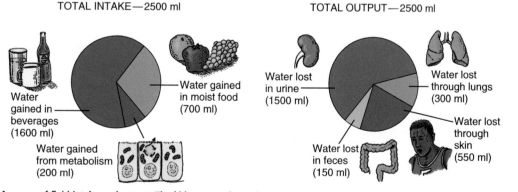

Figure 7-2   Avenues of fluid intake and output. The kidneys are the main regulators of fluid loss. Generally, fluid intake equals fluid output so that the total amount of fluid in the body remains constant. Water is the most important constituent of the body and is essential to every body process. Depriving the body of needed water eventually leads to dehydration.

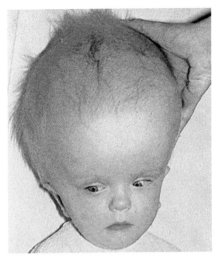

Figure 7-3   Four-month-old child with hydrocephalus. Hydrocephalus is usually caused by obstruction of the flow of cerebrospinal fluid. If hydrocephalus occurs in an infant, the soft bones of the skull push apart as the head increases in size.

7-13 The nervous system and endocrine system work together to bring about homeostasis by affecting various functions, including the heartbeat, respiration, blood pressure, body temperature, and the concentration of electrolytes (**e-lek′tro-līts**) in the body fluids. Electrolytes are molecules that conduct an electrical charge. Some examples of electrolytes in body fluids are calcium, potassium, and sodium. Certain diseases, conditions, and medications may lead to an imbalance of the electrolytes. Hypo/calc/emia (**hi″po-kal-se′me-ə**) is a deficiency of

calcium
_____ in the blood. Hypo/kal/emia (**hi″po-kə-le′me-ə**) is a
potassium
deficiency of _____ in the blood. Write a word that means a defi-
hyponatremia
ciency of sodium in the blood: _____. Hyper/calcemia,
   (**hi″po-nə-tre′me-ə**)
hyper/kalemia, and hyper/natremia are greater than normal blood levels of calcium, potassium, and sodium, respectively. Proper quantities of electrolytes are critical to normal metabolism and function.

7-14 The combining form *hydr(o)* means water. In chemistry, *hydr(o)* refers to hydrogen, but more commonly *hydr(o)* means water. Hydro/cephaly (**hi″dro-sef′ə-le**) appears to mean

water; head
_____ in the _____. In medical terms, some interpretation is needed in dividing words into their components. Hydrocephaly is more commonly called hydrocephalus (**hi″dro-sef′ə-ləs**). *Hydrocephalus* means a condition characterized by abnormal accumulation of cerebrospinal (**ser″ə-bro-spi′nəl**) fluid (see Chapter 15) within the skull, causing enlargement of the head, mental retardation, and convulsions (Figure 7-3).

Treatment of hydrocephalus generally consists of surgical intervention to correct the cause or to shunt the excess fluid away from the skull. *Shunt* (**shunt**) means to redirect the flow of a body fluid from one cavity or vessel to another. The device that is implanted in the body to redirect the fluid is also called a shunt. Write this new term for what is often used in treating hydrocephalus:

shunt
_____.

7-15 A calculus or stone is formed in body tissues by an accumulation of mineral salts in body tissues—for example, calcium carbonate. Calculi may occur in many organs, but they are more common in the kidney and gallbladder. Nephro/lith/iasis (**nef′ro-lǐ-thi′ə-sis**) is the presence of kidney stones. Litho/tomy (**lǐ-thot′ə-me**) is the incision of an organ or duct for removal of a calculus, especially one from the urinary tract. The suffix *-tomy* means incision, so the meaning of lithotomy is implied. Write this term that means an incision of an organ or duct for removal

lithotomy
of a calculus: _____. Be aware that the term *lithotomy* is also used to mean the lithotomy position, often used in obstetrics and gynecology. In the lithotomy position, the patient lies on the back with the hips and the knees flexed and the thighs rotated outward.

stone
Litho/tripsy (**lith′o-trip″se**) is the crushing of a _____ within the body, followed by the washing out of the fragments. This was originally done by surgical removal, but noninvasive methods such as high-energy shock waves or laser are now available and often eliminate the need for surgery.

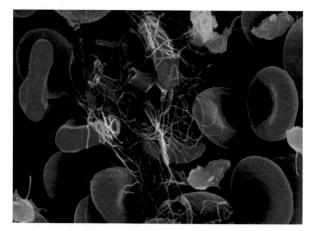

Figure 7-4   Blood coagulation. This scanning electron micrograph has been colored to emphasize the different structures. Red blood cells *(red)* are entangled with the fibrin *(yellow)*. Note the thin center and the thick edges that give red blood cells a concave appearance. The platelets *(blue)*, which initiate clotting, are also visible.

Exercise 1

Write a word in each blank to complete these sentences.

1. A relative constancy in the internal environment of the body is called _____.

2. Fluid that is contained within cells is _____ fluid.

3. Fluid found outside cells is called _____ fluid.

4. Fluid that is located between cells and in tissue spaces is called _____ fluid.

5. Regulation of the amount of water in the body is called fluid _____.

6. A term for a deficiency of potassium in the blood is _____.

7. A term for a deficiency of calcium in the blood is _____.

8. A term for excessive sodium in the blood is _____.

9. A concretion that is formed in body tissues by an accumulation of mineral salts is called a stone or

_____.

10. Excision of a stone is commonly called _____.

Composition of Blood

study

7-16 Blood, the most studied of all body fluids, is composed of a liquid portion, plasma, and several formed elements (cells or cell fragments). The study of blood and blood-forming tissues is called hematology (he″mə-tol′ə-je). You have learned that *-logy* means

_____ of.

The combining form *hemat(o)* means blood, but in the word *hematology*, the definition includes the blood-forming tissues. The blood-forming tissues are bone marrow and lymphoid tissue (spleen, thymus, tonsils, and lymph nodes).

blood
hematologist
   (he″mə-tol′ə-jist)

Hemato/logic (he″mə-to-loj′ik) means pertaining to hematology or the study of the _____. Change the ending of hematology to create a word that means one who studies blood: _____.

hematopoeisis

7-17 The suffix *-poiesis* means production. Hemato/poiesis (he″mə, hem″ə-to-poi-e′sis) is the production of blood, specifically the formation and development of its cells. Write this new word that means the formation and development of blood cells: _____.

7-18 Blood clots when it is removed from the body. Coagulation (ko-ag″u-la′shən) is the formation of a clot (Figure 7-4). Blood coagulation is a series of chemical reactions in which special fibers (fibrin) entrap blood cells, resulting in a blood clot.

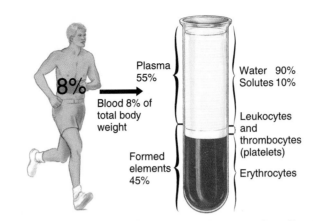

Figure 7-5   The blood in this test tube has been treated with anticoagulant to prevent clotting and centrifuged to separate its components. Red blood cells, the heaviest of the three components, make up the bottom layer. The middle layer of white blood cells and platelets is often called the buffy coat. The liquid part of treated blood, plasma, constitutes the upper layer. Any of these blood components can be given in a transfusion.

Blood transfusions and many hematologic studies require blood that has not coagulated. An anti/coagulant (**an″te-, an″ti-ko-ag′u-lənt**) is used to prevent blood from clotting. You have learned that *anti-* is a prefix that means against. An anti/coagulant acts

against coagulation   _____ coagulation. In other words, it prevents blood from clotting. Another word for blood clotting is _____.

A coagul/ant (**ko-ag′u-lənt**) promotes or accelerates coagulation, because *-ant* means that which causes. A substance that prevents coagulation is called an _____.

anticoagulant   Another suffix, *-ate*, means to cause an action or the result of an action. Thus *coagulate* (**ko-ag′u-lāt**) has two meanings, either to cause to clot or to become clotted. When you read that blood coagulates when removed from the body, it means that the blood clots.

7-19 Write a word that means any disease (disorder) of coagulation:

coagulopathy (ko-ag″u-lop′ə-the)   _____.

Exposure to air is not the reason that blood coagulates when removed from the body. A circulating anticoagulant normally prevents blood from clotting within the body. An anticoagulant can also be placed in blood as soon as it is removed from the body to prevent

coagulation   _____.

7-20 *In vitro** (**in ve′tro**) means occurring in a laboratory test tube (or glass) or occurring in an artificial environment. Because the anticoagulant is placed in the blood in an artificial environment (outside the body), this is in vitro use of an anticoagulant. A Latin term meaning in an artificial

in vitro   environment or outside the body is _____.

Some patients tend to form clots within blood vessels, a serious condition that can result in death. For these patients, a physician prescribes in vivo (**in ve′vo**) anticoagulants to prevent

clotting (coagulation)   _____. *In vivo* is a Latin term that means occurring in a living organism.

7-21 Laboratory tests often require treating blood with an anticoagulant to prevent clotting. The blood in the tube in Figure 7-5 has been treated with an anticoagulant. The formed elements are erythrocytes (**ə-rith′ro-sīts**), leukocytes (**loo′ko-sīts**), and thrombocytes. *Thrombo/cyte* (**throm′bo-sīt**) is another name for a blood platelet. The layer that is made up of leukocytes and platelets is sometimes called the buffy coat.

An erythro/cyte is a red blood cell (RBC), often simply called red cell or red corpuscle (**kor′pəs-əl**). A corpuscle is defined as any small mass or cell. Many structures, including red blood cells, are corpuscles. Normally, erythrocytes are biconcave disks that have no nucleus when seen in circulating

---

*In vitro (Latin: *in*, within; *vitreus*, glassware).

blood. Look again at the shape of the red blood cells in Figure 7-4. Their major function is transportation of oxygen and carbon dioxide.

The hemato/crit (**he-mat′ə-krit**) measures the percentage of red blood cells in a volume of blood. The part of *hematocrit* that means blood is _____. (Hematocrit is often abbreviated HCT.) The hematocrit is not a difficult concept. It simply tells us what percentage of the blood is made up of red blood cells. Normal values are based on packed red cell volume, which is determined by centrifuging the blood. Exact normal values vary among children, men, and women, but they usually range between 37% and 54%. (The hematocrit can also be calculated based on the size and number of red cells in a minute sample of blood.)

hemato-

7-22 The suffix in the term *thrombocyte* implies that it is a cell; however, thrombocytes are not typical cells but simply cell fragments without a nucleus (see Figure 7-4). Thrombocyte is another name for a blood _____.

platelet

7-23 *Erythro/cyt/ic* (**ə-rith″ro-sit′ik**) means pertaining to erythrocytes. Erythro/poiesis (**ə-rith″ro-poi-e′sis**) is the production of _____.

Erythro/poietin (**ə-rith″ro-poi′ə-tin**) is a hormone that stimulates erythropoiesis. (Notice the slight change in the suffix *-poiesis*. The suffix *-poietin* means a substance that causes production.) Erythropoietin acts on stem cells of the bone marrow to produce erythrocytes.

erythrocytes

7-24 A leukocyte is a white blood cell (WBC), often simply called a white cell or white corpuscle. The primary function of leukocytes is to protect the body against pathogenic organisms. You remember from Chapter 4 that *patho/genic* means capable of causing _____.

disease

7-25 The blood of healthy persons has normal numbers of erythrocytes and leukocytes. This number is determined by blood counts. A leukocyte count is a determination of the number of _____ blood cells. An erythrocyte count is the evaluation of the number of _____ blood cells.

white
red

7-26 Erythrocytes, leukocytes, and thrombocytes (more commonly called blood platelets) are the formed elements of the blood. The combining form *thromb(o)* means thrombus (**throm′bəs**), a blood clot that is attached to a vessel wall and tends to obstruct a blood vessel or a cavity of the heart. You should be aware that some specialists differentiate between a blood clot (occurring outside the body) and a thrombus (occurring internally).

A thrombo/cyte is not a cell that has clotted. It is a cell fragment that initiates the formation of the clot and is commonly called a blood platelet. Another name for a blood platelet is a _____.

thrombocyte

7-27 A stained blood smear, as shown in Figure 7-6, A allows examination of the erythrocytes, leukocytes, and blood platelets. The cells and platelets are stained for microscopic examination. A normal red cell in circulating blood has matured and lost its nucleus; however, a white blood cell still has a nucleus. There are five major types of leukocytes that can be classified by the presence or absence of granules in the cytoplasm and their staining characteristics:

- neutrophil (**noo′tro-fil**)
- eosinophil (**e″o-sin′o-fil**)
- basophil (**ba′so-fil**)
- lymphocyte (**lim′fo-sīt**)
- monocyte (**mon′o-sīt**)

The leukocyte in Figure 7-6, A is a neutrophil. Neutrophils, eosinophils, and basophils have granules and are called granulo/cytes (**gran′u-lo-sītz″**). The combining form *phil(o)* in these terms means attraction. Neutro/phils are so named because they are easily stained with (attracted to) neutral dyes. The granules of eosino/phils appear orange because they stain with eosin, an acid dye (Figure 7-6, B). On the other hand, the granules of baso/phils are stained dark by basic dyes (Figure 7-6, C). Lymphocytes and monocytes are a/granulo/cytes (**a-gran′u-lo-sītz**), meaning _____ that lack granules (Figure 7-6, D and E).

cells

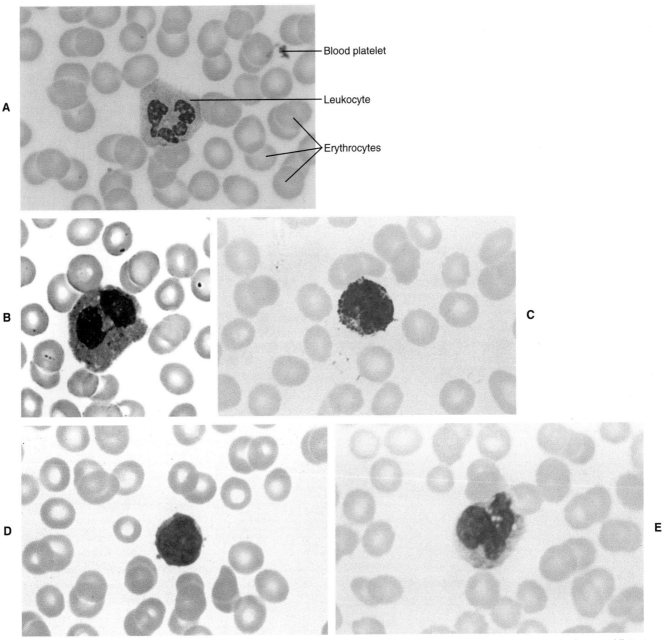

Figure 7-6 Human blood, stained. **A,** A leukocyte, a blood platelet, and erythrocytes are labeled. The leukocyte is a segmented neutrophil. **B,** An eosinophil; **C,** a basophil; **D,** a lymphocyte; **E,** a monocyte.

A differential white cell count is an examination and enumeration of the distribution of leukocytes in a stained blood smear. This laboratory test provides information related to infections and various diseases and is included in a complete blood cell count (CBC).

7-28 *Poly/morpho/nuclear* **(pol″e-mor″fo-noo′kle-ər),** a word often encountered when one is reading about leukocytes, is often shortened to *polymorph* **(pol′e-morf),** and is abbreviated PMN. *Polymorphonuclear* means having a nucleus that is divided in such a way that the cell may appear to have several nuclei, such as in the neutrophil in Figure 7-6, A. The combining form *morph(o)* means form or shape. In the term *polymorphonuclear, poly-* means _____, *morph(o)* means shape, and *nuclear* pertains to a nucleus. A leukocyte with a nucleus that is divided in such a way that it appears multiple is polymorphonuclear.

many

nucleus	**7-29** The word part for nucleus is *nucle(o)* or *kary(o)*. A nucleo/protein (**noo″kle-o-pro′tēn**) is a protein found in the _____. Karyomegaly (**kar″e-o-meg′ə-le**) is abnormal enlargement of a cell nucleus.
nucleus	*Nucle/oid* (**noo′kle-oid**) means resembling a _____.
clot	**7-30** Thrombo/genesis (**throm″bo-jen′ə-sis**) is the formation of a blood _____. When a clot forms inside a blood vessel or the heart, the clot itself is called a thromb/us (**throm′bəs**) (plural: thrombi [**throm′bi**]).
	Thrombo/lysis (**throm-bol′ĭ-sis**) is dissolution or destruction of a clot that has formed in a blood vessel. In other words, thrombolysis is destruction of a _____.
thrombus	Thromb/osis (**throm-bo′sis**) is the presence of a _____. If a thrombus does not dissolve spontaneously, or if a thrombolytic agent cannot be used, the clot may need to be surgically removed, a procedure known as a thromb/ectomy (**throm-bek′tə-me**). *Thrombo/lytic* (**throm″bo-lit′ik**) means capable of dissolving a thrombus.
thrombus	
blood	**7-31** Literal translation of *hemo/lysis* (**he-mol′ə-sis**) is destruction of _____. Hemolysis is destruction of the red blood cell membrane, resulting in the release of hemoglobin (**he′mo-glo″bin**), the red pigment of blood. Because you have learned three combining forms that mean blood, you may be wondering how one knows which form to use. Common usage determines the proper form. Even though *hemato/lysis* (**he″mə-tol′ə-sis**) is a word, *hemolysis* is much better known.
destruction (hemolysis)	A hemo/lysin (**he-mol′ə-sin**) is a substance that causes _____ of red blood cells. When blood is placed in water or another substance that hemolyzes it, the destruction refers to the dissolving of the erythrocytes, which burst and release their red pigment.
	7-32 Infectious mononucleosis (**mon″o-noo″kle-o′sis**) is an acute infection caused by the Epstein-Barr virus. It is characterized by fever, sore throat, swollen lymph glands, leukocytosis with atypical lymphocytes, abnormal liver function, and enlargement of the spleen. *Leukocytosis* means an
increase; white	_____ in the number of _____ blood cells.
	Young people are most often affected. Treatment is primarily symptomatic, with analgesics to control pain and enforced bed rest to prevent serious complications of the liver or spleen.
blood	**7-33** Literal translation of *leuk/emia* (**loo-ke′me-ə**) is white _____ and is so called because of the large number of white cells in the blood of patients with this disease. Leukemia is a progressive, malignant disease of the hemato/poietic (**he″mə-to-, hem″ə-to-poi-et′ik**) (blood-forming) organs, characterized by a sharp increase in the number of leukocytes, as well as the presence of immature forms of leukocytes in the blood and bone marrow. A malignancy in which there is a sharp increase in the number of leukocytes is _____.
leukemia	Write a word using *leuk(o)*, *cyt(o)*, and *-penia*: _____. This is often shortened to *leukopenia* (**loo″ko-pe′ne-ə**). Either word means a decrease or deficiency in the number of leukocytes.
leukocytopenia (loo″ko-si″to-pe′-ne-ə)	
blood	**7-34** An/emia (**ə-ne′me-ə**) literally means without _____. Because no one can live without blood, the name *anemia* is an exaggeration of the condition.
deficiency	Erythro/cyto/penia (**ə-rith″ro-si″to-pe′ne-ə**) is a _____ of erythrocytes. *Erythrocytopenia* can be shortened to *erythropenia* (**ə-rith″ro-pe′ne-ə**). Either word means a deficiency in the number of red blood cells. Anemia, however, is a deficiency in the number of red blood cells or a deficiency in hemoglobin, or sometimes, a reduction in both red cells and hemoglobin.
	7-35 Anemia is not a disease but a sign of various diseases. The severity of signs and symptoms depends on the severity of the anemia. Table 7-1 lists classic signs and symptoms of anemia.
	Several new terms are included in the table. *Tachycardia* (**tak″ĭ-kahr′de-ə**) means an increased pulse rate; it will be studied in the next chapter. Analyzing its word parts, *tachy-* means
fast	_____, *cardi(o)* means heart, and *-ia* means condition. One *i* is omitted to facilitate pronunciation.

TABLE 7-1 Classic Signs and Symptoms of Anemia

- Pallor (color of nail beds, palms, and mucous membranes of the mouth and conjunctivae are more reliable than skin color for assessing paleness)
- Tachycardia (increased pulse rate)
- Heart murmur
- Angina (chest pain)
- Severe anemia
- Congestive heart failure
- Dyspnea (difficult breathing)
- Shortness of breath
- Fatigue on exertion
- Headache
- Dizziness
- Syncope (fainting)
- Tinnitus (ringing in the ears)
- Gastrointestinal symptoms (anorexia, nausea, sore tongue and mouth)
- Constipation or diarrhea

Dys/pnea (**disp′ne-ə**) means difficult breathing because the suffix, *-pnea*, means breathing. You will learn more about dyspnea in Chapter 9. Note that *pallor* (**pal′ər**), named after the Latin term, refers to an unnatural paleness or absence of color. The table defines *syncope** (**sing′kə-pe**) as _____ and *tinnitus†* (**tin′ĭ-təs, tĭ-ni′təs**) as _____ in the ears.

fainting
ringing

7-36 Iron deficiency anemia results when there is a greater demand for iron than the body can supply. It can be caused by blood loss or insufficient intake or absorption of iron from the intestinal tract. Iron deficiency anemia is often treated successfully with iron tablets and a well-balanced diet.

Ancient Greeks drank water in which iron swords had been allowed to rust, thinking that they derived strength from the sword. The French steeped iron filings in wine and then drank it! Like the French wine with added iron, some modern products contain iron and vitamins with substantial alcohol. It is said that long ago, Ozark mountain people stuck nails in apples and let the nails rust. They removed the nails and fed the apples to their children. If the children's anemia improved after eating the apples, it is possible that they had _____ deficiency anemia.

iron

7-37 Thrombo/cyto/penia (**throm″bo-si″to-pe′ne-ə**) is a decrease in the number of _____. This is also called thrombopenia (**throm″bo-pe′ne-ə**). Because thrombo/cytes are important in the process of blood coagulation, thrombocytopenia, if severe, results in a bleeding disorder.

thrombocytes

Thrombo/cyt/osis (**throm″bo-si-to′sis**) means an increase in the number of thrombocytes in the circulating blood. You learned that *-osis* means condition, but sometimes it implies an increased condition.

7-38 Because coagulation involves several factors, a bleeding disorder can result from any number of deficiencies, including a deficiency of vitamin K. Classic hemo/philia (**he″mo-fil′e-ə**) is a hereditary bleeding disorder in which there is deficiency of one coagulation factor called antihemophilic (**an″te-, an″ti-he″mo-fil′ik**) factor VIII. Other types of hemophilia may result from the deficiencies of other coagulation or clotting factors. In hemophilia, there is spontaneous bleeding or prolonged

*Syncope (Greek: *synkoptein*, to cut short).
†Tinnitus (Latin: *tinnire*, to tinkle).

bleeding after a minor injury. Perhaps the naming of hemophilia came about because of excessive and prolonged bleeding that occurs in the disorder, thus leading to an inaccurate conclusion that affected individuals had an affinity or attraction to blood.

anemia

Prolonged bleeding leads to a deficiency of both red blood cells and hemoglobin. This condition is called _____.

7-39 Erythro/cyt/osis (ə-rith″ro-si-to′sis) means an increase in the number of

erythrocytes
leukocytosis
(loo″ko-si-to′sis)

_____.

An increase in the number of leukocytes is _____. You learned earlier that leukemia is characterized by leukocytosis. But there is a major difference between leukemia and most conditions that cause leukocytosis. In leukemia, the production of leukocytes is uncontrolled, and many of the leukocytes produced are immature and nonfunctional.

leukocytes

Leukocytosis may be transitory and often accompanies a bacterial, but not usually a viral, infection. Because the main function of leukocytes is protection against harmful invading microorganisms such as bacteria, this should help you remember which type of cell is likely to increase during a bacterial infection: _____.

7-40 Infection is sometimes confused with inflammation. Inflammation is a protective response of body tissues to irritation or injury, often resulting in elimination of offending agents and establishment of conditions necessary for repair. Infection (the presence of living microorganisms within the tissue) is but one cause of inflammation. Which of these two words is part of the body's natural

inflammation

defense? _____. The cardinal signs of inflammation are redness, heat, swelling, and pain, sometimes accompanied by loss of function.

Inflammation may be acute or chronic, lasting for months or even years. In chronic inflammation, the injurious agent persists or repeatedly injures tissue and can be debilitating to the individual.

7-41 Anemia and polycythemia represent abnormalities in the number of erythrocytes. Leukemia, leukocytosis, and leukopenia are abnormalities in the number of leukocytes. An increase or a decrease in blood platelets is also abnormal.

There is an increase in the number of erythrocytes in polycythemia. There are two forms of this condition, primary polycythemia (also called polycythemia vera [pol″e-si-the′me-ə ve′rə]) and secondary polycythemia. In both there is an increase in the number of

erythrocytes

_____.

Primary polycythemia is a serious disorder in which the bone marrow overproduces many types of cells and is associated with a chromosomal defect. Secondary polycythemia occurs as a physiologic response to prolonged exposure to high altitude or to lung or heart disease. In the described situations, insufficient oxygen in the tissue brings about the response. Sometimes the cause of secondary polycythemia is not known.

There is also an increase in the number of leukocytes in this disease, as well as the more marked erythrocytosis. This increased cell mass results in a sluggish flow of blood through the blood vessels. The increased red cell mass leads to several secondary alterations, such as elevated blood pressure, increased viscosity, and thrombotic tendencies. Viscosity is the ability or inability of a fluid to flow well. A solution with high viscosity is thick and flows more slowly than one of lower viscosity.

thrombi

Thrombotic tendencies favor formation of _____.

7-42 Principal conditions that are associated with abnormalities in the blood cells and platelets are listed in Table 7-2. The table lists a few terms that you have not yet studied. A/granulo/cyt/osis

granulocyte

means absence of what type of blood cell? _____.

Disseminated (meaning scattered or distributed over a considerable area; that is, an organ or the body) intra/vascul/ar coagulation (DIC) is a grave coagulopathy (ko-ag″u-lop′ə-the) in which there is generalized intravascular clotting.

TABLE 7-2 Principal Conditions Affecting Blood Cells and Platelets

Conditions Involving Erythrocytes	Conditions Involving Leukocytes	Conditions Involving Blood Platelets
Anemia	Leukocytosis	Disseminated intravascular coagulation
Bone marrow failure	Leukopenia	Thrombocytopenia
Hemolysis	Agranulocytosis	Thrombocytosis
Polycythemia	Leukemia (acute or chronic)	

Exercise 2

Write a word in each blank to complete these sentences.

1. The liquid portion of blood is _____.

2. A term that means production of blood is _____.

3. The formation of a clot is _____.

4. A term for a substance that prevents blood from clotting is _____.

5. A determination of the number of white blood cells is a _____ count.

Exercise 3

Write a word in each blank to complete these sentences.

1. Another name for a blood platelet is _____.

2. *Polymorphonuclear* is used to describe cells that appear to have several _____.

3. Thrombogenesis is the formation of a blood _____.

4. Destruction of a thrombus is _____.

5. Destruction of red blood cells, resulting in the release of hemoglobin, is called _____.

6. A progressive, malignant disease of the hematopoietic organs, characterized by a sharp increase in the number of leukocytes, is called _____.

7. *Leukopenia* means a deficiency of _____.

8. An increase in the number of thrombocytes is called _____.

9. A term for a deficiency in the number of red blood cells, a deficiency in hemoglobin, or sometimes a reduction in both red cells and hemoglobin is _____.

10. The meaning of syncope is _____.

Anemias and Abnormal Hemoglobins

7-43 Hemoglobin, the iron-containing pigment of erythrocytes, carries oxygen from the lungs to tissues throughout the body. Microscopic variations in the erythrocytes are often observed in anemias and can be seen on a stained blood smear. A microscope is used to view cells and other objects too small to be seen with the naked eye. A micro/cyte (**mi′kro-sīt**) is a _____ cell. Microcytes are undersized red blood cells sometimes seen in anemia. A condition in which there is an increase in the number of undersized red blood cells can be named by combining *micr(o)* + *cyto/(o)* + *-osis*: _____.

small

microcytosis
(**mi″kro-si-to′sis**)

7-44 Macro/cyte (**mak′ro-sīt**) usually refers to a large erythrocyte. Macrocytes are seen in certain types of anemia. An increase in the number of larger-than-normal erythrocytes is called

macrocytosis (mak″ro-si-to′sis)	
small	
large	
anisocytosis (an-i″so-si-to′sis)	
equal	
isotonic	
round	
round	
spherocytosis (sfēr″o-si-to′sis)	
poikilocyte poikilocytosis (poi″kĭ-lo-si-to′sis)	
below	
hyperchromic (hi″pər-kro′mik)	
blood	
smaller larger size shape	
hemoglobinopathy (he″mo-glo″bin-op′ə-the)	

_____. *Macrocyte* and *megalo/cyte* (**meg′ə-lo-sīt**) both mean large cell (usually an erythrocyte).

Micro/scopy (**mi-kros′kə-pe**) is examining something _____. *Macro/scopy* (**mə-kros′kə-pe**), as opposed to micro/scopy, is examining something _____. We can see a macro/scopic (**mak″ro-skop′ik**) object with the naked eye. The term *macroscopic examination* is used more commonly than macroscopy.

Using a microscope, erythro/cytes can be studied to determine if they appear normal. If erythrocytes appear to be of normal size, we refer to them as normocytes (**nor′mo-sīts**) or we describe them as normocytic (**nor″mo-sit′ik**).

7-45 Combine *an-* + *is(o)* + *cyt(o)* + *-osis* to write a word that means that cells are not of equal size: _____. Anisocytosis is common in the blood of people who are anemic.

Iso/tonic (**i″so-ton′ik**) means _____ tension. *Isotonic* also denotes a solution in which body cells can be bathed without damage to the cells through diffusion of water into or out of the cells, because the concentration of electrolytes in the solution is equal to that in the cell. A solution in which cells can be placed without damage to the cells or change in their general appearance is an _____ solution.

7-46 A sphere is round. A *sphero/cyte* (**sfēr′o-sīt**) is a _____ cell. A normal red blood cell is biconcave, resembling a disk indented on opposite sides. A sphero/cyte is a red blood cell that is less concave than normal and appears _____.

Using *spherocyte* and *-osis*, write a term that means the presence of spherocytes in the blood: _____.

7-47 *Poikilo/cytes* (**poi′kĭ-lo-sītz**) are red blood cells that have an abnormal shape. The combining form *poikil(o)* means irregular. If a red blood cell has an irregular shape, we call it a _____. The presence of poikilocytes in the blood is _____.

Poikilocytes are seen in several disorders, including sickle (**sik′əl**) cell anemia. People with sickle cell anemia, a hereditary anemia that mainly afflicts blacks, inherit an abnormal type of hemoglobin. Their red blood cells appear elongated and sickled and are highly fragile. In vivo hemolysis occurs, resulting in hemolytic anemia. Sickle cells are irregularly shaped erythrocytes, so they are also poikilocytes.

7-48 *Hypo/chrom/ia* (**hi″po-kro′me-ə**) is a condition in which the red blood cells have a _____ normal amount of color. These are called hypochromic (**hi″po-kro′mik**) cells. Cells that have more than the normal amount of color—in other words, excessive pigmentation—are called _____ cells.

Hemo/globin is the red pigment found inside erythrocytes that gives blood its red color. Globins (**glo′binz**) or globulins (**glob′u-linz**) are types of proteins; therefore, hemo/globin is a type of protein found in _____. Hemoglobin is often abbreviated Hb or Hgb.

7-49 Figure 7-7 shows several abnormal types of erythrocytes. You can see that microcytes are _____ than normal, macrocytes are _____ than normal, anisocytes are erythrocytes that vary in _____, and poikilocytes are erythrocytes that have an unusual _____. In anemia, erythrocytes usually do not have a normal appearance. Table 7-3 shows two ways in which anemias are classified, one on the basis of appearance of red cells and the other on the basis of cause.

7-50 Some anemias are hereditary and are caused by abnormal hemoglobins. Use *hemoglobin(o)* to write a word that literally is any disease of the hemoglobins: _____.

The hemoglobinopathies are a group of diseases caused by or associated with the presence of abnormal hemoglobin in the blood.

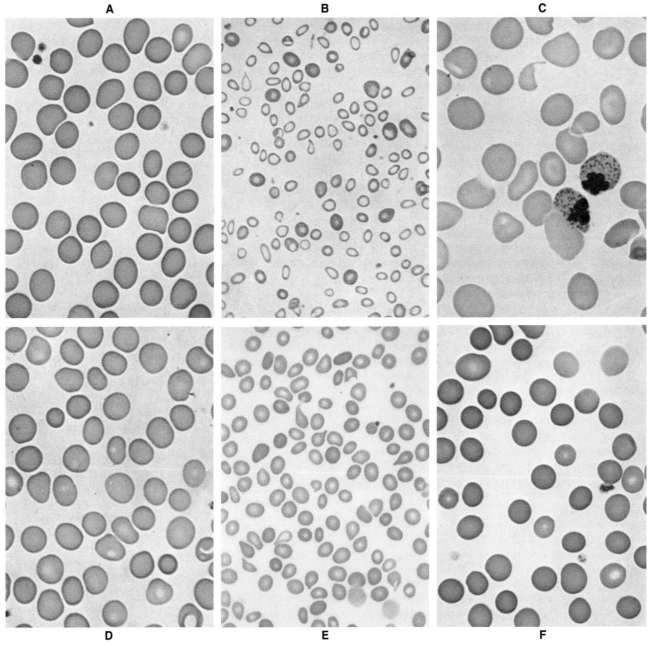

Figure 7–7　Morphologic variations of red blood cells in a stained blood smear. **A,** Normal erythrocytes. **B,** Hypochromic microcytes. A few cells are normal, but most have central paleness and small diameter. **C,** Macrocytes in pernicious anemia. In addition to erythrocytes of a larger size than normal, two immature ones still have a nucleus. These cells also show anisocytosis and poikilocytosis. **D,** Anisocytosis. Note the varying sizes of erythrocytes. **E,** Poikilocytes. Several erythrocytes have abnormal shapes. **F,** Spherocytes. About half the cells show dense staining and a small diameter.

TABLE 7-3　Two Classifications of Anemia

Morphologic Classification (Based on the Appearance of Red Cells in Stained Smear)
1. Normocytic normochromic (from sudden blood loss, hemolytic anemias, kidney disorders, and certain chronic diseases)
2. Macrocytic normochromic (deficiency of vitamin B_{12} or folic acid is a leading cause of certain chronic diseases)
3. Microcytic hypochromic (insufficient iron or hemoglobin production, chronic blood loss)

Etiologic Classification (Based on Cause)
1. Increased loss or destruction of red cells (bleeding or hemolysis owing to heredity or change in the red cell environment)
2. Decreased or defective production of red cells (deficiencies in diet; defective absorption; bone marrow interference, such as malignancies, toxic drugs, or irradiation)

7-51 Because hemoglobins are proteins, they move at various speeds across paper or starch gel, based on their electrical charge, their size, and their mobility. Hemoglobin electrophoresis (e-lek″tro-fə-re′sis) is used to identify abnormal hemoglobin.

Hemoglobins are generally identified by letters or sometimes by their place of occurrence and discovery. Normal adult hemoglobin is designated hemoglobin A. There are many abnormal types. One type of abnormal hemoglobin, S, is found in sickle cell anemia. Abnormal hemoglobins such as Hb S generally result in distortion and fragility of the erythrocytes, causing them to hemolyze more readily. *Hemo/lyze* means that the erythrocytes _____.

dissolve

7-52 Hemo/lytic anemia is a disorder characterized by premature destruction of the erythrocytes. This type of anemia may be an inherited disorder, may be associated with some infectious diseases, or may occur as a response to drugs, various toxic agents, or certain incompatibilities in blood or tissue types. The disorder in which erythrocytes are destroyed prematurely is called _____ anemia.

hemolytic

Hemolytic disease of the newborn (HDN) is also called erythro/blast/osis fetalis (e-rith″ro-blas-to′sis fe-tă′ləs). The blood of infants who are born with this type of hemolytic anemia contains erythro/blasts (e-rith′ro-blasts) (immature erythrocytes), and it is for this reason the condition was named *erythroblastosis fetalis*. It results from an incompatibility of the blood groups of the mother and fetus, such as the Rh factor, ABO blood groups, or other blood incompatibilities. Diagnosis of the disease is confirmed during pregnancy by amnio/centesis and analysis of the amniotic fluid. Treatment may consist of an intrauterine (in″trə-u′tər-in) (within the uterus) transfusion or immediate exchange transfusions after birth. In Rh factor incompatibility, sensitization to the Rh factor can be prevented by injection of the mother with a preparation such as RhoGAM. Hemolytic reactions involving the ABO blood groups are generally less severe than those involving the Rh factor.

7-53 Write a word that means the opposite of plastic by using either *a-* or *an-*: _____. You previously learned that *plast(o)* means repair. *Aplastic* means having no tendency to develop new tissue. In aplastic anemia, the bone marrow is diseased and produces few cells.

aplastic (a-plas′tik)

Irregularities in the blood often indicate abnormal conditions of various body systems; however, certain diseases or disorders are associated mainly with the blood or bone marrow and are called dyscrasias (dis-kra′zhəz).* Some examples of the latter, such as leukemia and aplastic anemia, have already been discussed.

Exercise 4

Write words for the following meanings.

1. an undersized erythrocyte   _____

2. an increase in the number of oversized erythrocytes _____

3. presence of cells of unequal size   _____

4. a red blood cell that appears round   _____

5. an irregularly shaped erythrocyte   _____

6. excessive pigmentation of erythrocytes   _____

7. decreased pigmentation of erythrocytes   _____

8. a disease associated with abnormal hemoglobin   _____

9. having no tendency to develop new tissue   _____

10. red pigment found in erythrocytes   _____

---

*Dyscrasia (Greek: *dys*, bad; *krasis*, mingling).

Blood Coagulation

fibrin

fibrinolysin
(fi″bri-nol′ə-sin)

thrombus

7-54 Coagulation of the blood is a series of chemical reactions that results in a blood clot. Fibrin (fi′brin) is formed when blood clots. Fibrino/gen (fi-brin′o-jən) is a precursor of _____. Fibrinogen is a protein that is changed into fibrin in the process of coagulation.

Fibrino/lysis (fi″bri-nol′ə-sis) is the destruction of fibrin. Write a word that means a substance that can dissolve fibrin: _____.

A fibrinolysin can dissolve a blood clot, which is another name for a _____. Heparin and warfarin (Coumadin) are in vivo anticoagulants that are used to prevent blood clots. The blood of persons taking anticoagulants is tested regularly using laboratory tests such as PT and PTT (abbreviations for prothrombin [pro-throm′bin] time and partial thromboplastin [throm″bo-plas′tin] time). Prothrombin and thromboplastin are factors involved in different parts of the coagulation process, and the tests provide information about various stages of the coagulation process. The importance of accurate and reliable prothrombin time measurements has resulted in a standardized reporting system for prothrombin times called the International Normalized Ratio (INR).

platelets

7-55 Blood coagulation saves lives when it occurs in response to injury but can result in death if it occurs in the circulating blood. An internal blood clot, a thrombus, usually starts with tissue damage and is particularly life-threatening if the clot occurs in the heart or if it breaks off and is taken by the bloodstream to the brain or heart. Thrombocyt/osis, an increase in the number of blood _____, can also cause thrombosis. Blood coagulation brings about hemo/stasis (he″mo-sta′sis, he″mos′tə-sis). *Stasis* means stoppage or flow. Hemo/stasis can also mean interruption of blood flow through a vessel or to any part of the body.

The most common cause of bleeding disorders is thrombocyto/penia, an insufficiency of blood platelets, resulting from either decreased production/survival or increased destruction. In addition, malfunction or absence of any of the coagulation factors causes at least some degree of bleeding tendency. Hemostasis may be delayed in these cases, resulting in the loss of large amounts of blood. A transfusion may be necessary to replace the lost blood.

across

agglutination

7-56 The prefix *trans-* means through or across. The introduction of whole blood or blood components into the bloodstream of a person is called a blood transfusion. In the earliest transfusions, blood was passed directly _____ from one person to another. When blood is used for transfusion, grouping or typing of the blood is necessary. Blood typing determines the blood group of a person. There are four main blood groups (A, B, O, and AB). Rh factors are also always considered. Tests determine a person's blood type by mixing blood with commercially prepared sera (and blood cells, for reverse type) and observing for agglutination (ə-gloo″ti-na′shən). In this type of agglutination, aggregates or small clumps of erythrocytes form, which may be visible macro/scopically or perhaps only micro/scopically.

Write the term that is another name for blood clumping: _____.

destruction

7-57 A transfusion reaction is an adverse reaction to the blood a person receives in a transfusion. Among the most common reactions are those that result from blood group incompatibilities. In other words, something in the donor's blood is not compatible with the blood of the recipient. Symptoms of transfusion reactions vary in degree from mild to severe. Some are manifested immediately, whereas others may not occur for several days. Blood group incompatibilities often result in agglutination or hemolysis of the erythrocytes. Hemo/lysis is _____ of the erythrocytes.

Certain diseases can be transmitted to the recipient through blood transfusion, so various screening tests are performed to avoid using infected blood. Screening generally includes testing for several types of hepatitis (hep″ə-ti′tis)—hepatitis A, B, C, and D; human immunodeficiency (im″u-no-də-fish′ən-se) virus (the agent that causes acquired immunodeficiency syndrome [AIDS]); cytomegalovirus (CMV); and syphilis (rapid plasma reagin test [RPR], is commonly used). Certain areas of the United States are beginning to also test for the West Nile virus (WNV), which causes West Nile encephalitis.

autologous

7-58 *Autologous** (**aw-tol′ə-gəs**) and *homologous*† (**ho-mol′o-gəs**) are terms that are often associated with blood transfusions or skin grafts. In an autologous transfusion, blood is removed from a donor and stored for a variable period before it is returned to the donor's circulation. In an _____ graft, tissue is transferred from one site to another on the same body.

In contrast, a homologous graft is a tissue removed from a donor for transplantation to a recipient of the same species. This is also called an allograft (**al′o-graft**). A transplant from one's identical twin is an iso/graft, but a transplantation from all other individuals of one's species is an allo/graft. Best results occur with an isograft or when the donor is closely related to the recipient. Transplantation of certain organs, such as kidneys, have a high degree of success.

7-59 Bone marrow transplants are used in treating patients with leukemia or aplastic anemia. Allo/gene/ic (**al″o-jə-ne′ik**), also called allo/genic (**al″o-jen′ik**), bone marrow transplants have a lower success rate than many organ transplants, such as the kidneys. For this reason, autologous transplants are preferred, using marrow previously obtained from the patient and stored, then reinfused when needed.

In allogeneic bone marrow transplants, a donor with a close human leukocyte antigen (HLA) type is selected. The recipient is given chemotherapy or irradiation to destroy the diseased cells and much of the normal bone marrow. Bone marrow cells are aspirated from the donor's hip, repeating many times to obtain sufficient marrow. The cells are treated with anticoagulant and prepared for intravenous transfusion into the patient. Subsequent problems may include infection and graft versus host disease (immune response due to histo/incompatibility of the donor cells and recipient tissues).

Exercise 5

Write words in the blanks to complete these sentences.

1. A series of chemical reactions that result in a blood clot is blood _____.

2. Macroscopic clumps or masses of erythrocytes are blood _____.

3. A substance that can dissolve a thrombus is called a _____.

4. Stoppage of the flow of blood is _____.

5. A _____ reaction is an adverse reaction to the blood a person receives.

6. The term for the transfusion of a person's own blood after it is collected and stored is called an _____ transfusion.

7. A _____ graft is tissue removed from a donor for transplantation to a recipient of the same species.

Classification of Disease

7-60 Diseases are specific illnesses or disorders characterized by recognizable sets of signs and symptoms, caused by heredity, infection, diet, or the environment. There are several ways to classify diseases. A classification based on structure/function would be as follows:

- organic diseases, which are associated with a demonstrable physical change in an organ or tissues; for example, a tumor
- functional disorders, which are marked by signs or symptoms but no physical changes; for example, most psychological disorders

*Autologous (Greek: *autos*, self)
†Homologous (Greek: *homos*, same).

physical

It is important to remember that organic diseases, unlike functional disorders, are associated with a demonstrable _____ change.

Classification of diseases according to cause includes infectious (caused by pathogenic organisms; for example, bacterial infections), hereditary, degenerative (deterioration of structure or function), traumatic, auto/immune (**aw″to-ĭ-mūn′**) (altered function of the immune system resulting in the production of antibodies against one's own cells), and nutritional deficiencies. The combining form *aut(o)* means self.

7-61 Other terms that are applied to various circumstances when disease occurs are *idio/pathic* (**id″e-o-path′ik**) (*idi[o]* means individual) diseases; *iatro/genic* (**i-at″ro-jen′ik**) (*iatr[o]* means physician or treatment) disorders; and *nosocomial,** (**nos″o-ko′me-əl**) infections. An idiopathic disease develops without an apparent or known cause (for example, high blood pressure for which there is no known cause). An iatrogenic disorder is an unfavorable response to medical treatment (for example, a transfusion reaction). Nosocomial infections are hospital-acquired infections (for example, infection of a surgical wound). More specifically, this type of infection was not present or incubating prior to the patient's admission to the hospital and is acquired 72 hours or longer after admission.

A disease that develops without an apparent or known cause is an

idiopathic
iatrogenic
nosocomial

_____ disease.

An unfavorable response to medical treatment is an _____ disorder, and a hospital-acquired infection is a _____ infection.

7-62 Infectious diseases are caused by pathogenic organisms. *Contagious* means capable of being transmitted from one individual to another. When contagious diseases are passed from one person to another, there is transmission of the disease. A communicable disease, also called a contagious disease, is transmitted from one person or animal to another by one of these means:

- directly by contact with discharges or airborne droplets from an infected person
- indirectly via substances (for example, bloodborne transmission through contact with blood or body fluids that are contaminated with blood) or inanimate objects (such as a contaminated spoon)
- via vectors (for example, mosquitoes, which transmit malaria)

communicable

A contagious disease is also called a _____ disease. Study the word parts that pertain to disease and immunity in the following list.

Word Parts Related to Disease

Word Part	Meaning		Word Part	Meaning
			Word Parts Associated with Immunity	
iatr(o)	physician or treatment			
idi(o)	individual		aut(o)	self
immun(o)	immunity		immun(o)	immune
nos(o), path(o)	disease			
seps(o)	infection		**Suffix**	
sept(i), sept(o)†	infection		-phylaxis	protection

Combining Forms for Microorganisms
bacter(i), bacteri(o)	bacteria
staphyl(o)	grapelike cluster; uvula
strept(o)	twisted
fung(i), myc(o)	fungus
vir(o), virus(o)	virus

---

*Nosocomial (Greek: *nosokomeian*, hospital).
†Also means septum.

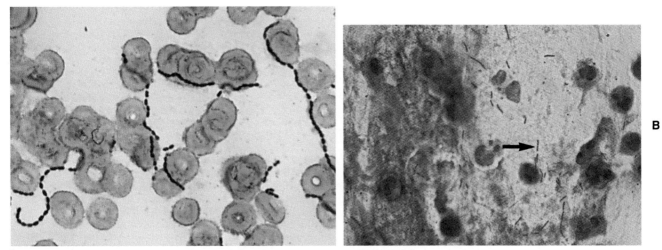

A   B

Figure 7-8   Gram stains of direct smears—body fluids collected, stained, and examined for the presence of leukocytes, bacteria, or other significant findings. **A,** Gram-positive cocci. The cocci are arranged in chains. Cells are also present on the smear. **B,** Gram-negative bacilli *(arrow)* are shown in the presence of numerous leukocytes.

7-63 Pathogenic microorganisms generally include various types of bacteria, fungi, viruses, and protozoa. Bacteria are unicellular micro/organisms that are classified according to their shape as spheric (cocci), rod-shaped (bacilli), spiral (spirochetes and spirilla), and comma-shaped (vibrios). Most bacteria are helpful rather than harmful. They are responsible for decay and are used extensively in food production, as in vinegar, sour cream, and cheese. Bacteria are also beneficial in the intestinal tract, where they are responsible for production of vitamin K. Normal bacterial flora of the skin help prevent the establishment of pathogenic bacteria. Only a few of the total number of species of bacteria are pathogenic.

Micro/bio/logy (**mi″kro-bi-ol′ə-je**) is a special branch of biology. Micro/bio/logists study bacteria, fungi, viruses, and other small organisms. Very small or microscopic organisms are called

microorganisms _____. *Virulence* (**vir′u-ləns**) means the degree of disease-causing capability of a microorganism.

7-64 Gram stain is a special staining technique that serves as a primary means of identifying and classifying bacteria. Gram-positive bacteria appear violet (purple) by this method and gram-negative bacteria appear pinkish. Observe the cocci (**kok′si**) and bacilli (**bə-sil′i**) in Figure 7-8, and then write answers in these blanks.

The bacteria in Figure 7-8, A, are gram-positive cocci. This is noted by their shape, which is

spherical _____, and their color, which is
violet or purple _____. The bacteria in Figure 7-8, B, are gram-
elongated (rod- negative bacilli. This is noted by their shape, which is _____, and
** shaped); pinkish** their color, which is _____.

7-65 Summarizing information in the previous frame, spherical-shaped bacteria are called
cocci _____.
bacilli Rod-shaped bacteria are called _____.
Bacteria that stain pink or red after undergoing Gram staining are called gram-
negative _____, whereas bacteria that stain violet or purple are gram-
positive _____.

7-66 Cocci are often seen in particular arrangements when viewed with the microscope. For this reason, cocci are further classified according to their arrangement. Although there are others, three commonly seen arrangements are shown in Figure 7-9.

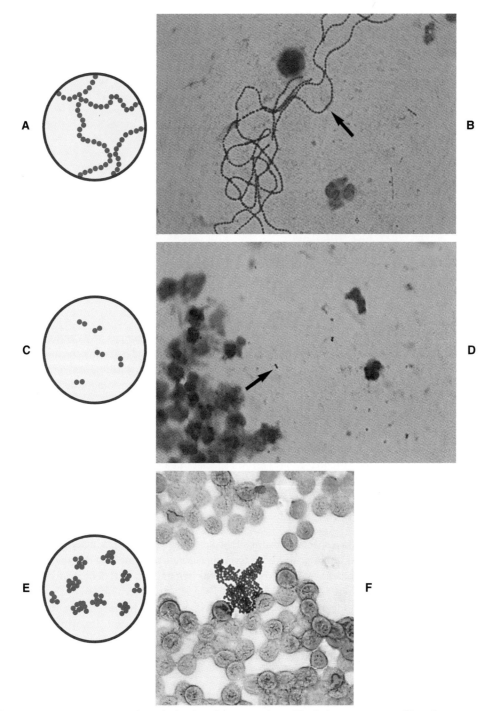

Figure 7-9   Three coccal arrangements. **A,** Schematic drawing of streptococci, cocci in chains. **B,** Streptococci in a direct smear. **C,** Schematic drawing of diplococci, cocci in pairs. **D,** Diplococci in a direct smear. **E,** Schematic drawing of staphylococci, cocci arranged in grapelike clusters. **F,** Staphylococci in a direct smear.

Learning these arrangements will give more meaning when you hear words such as *streptococcal* (**strep″to-kok′əl**) (often shortened to *strep*) and *staphylococcal* (**staf″ə-lo-kok′əl**) (often shortened to *staph*) infections. Although the combining form *strept(o)* means

twisted

_____, strepto/cocci (**strep″to-kok′si**) appear to grow in a chain that does not necessarily appear twisted.

7-67 *Strep throat* is a common way of saying strepto/coccal pharyng/itis (**far″in-ji′tis**). The combining form *pharyng(o)* means pharynx or throat. In strep throat, inflammation of the throat is caused

streptococci

by what type of bacteria? _____. There are many types of streptococci, and not all streptococci cause pharyngitis.

7-68 The combining form *staphyl(o)* means a grapelike cluster. Cocci that are arranged like a cluster of grapes are called _____.

The combining form *staphyl(o)* is also used to mean uvula (u′vu-lə), a structure that hangs like a bunch of grapes from the soft palate in the back of the mouth. When *staphyl(o)* is joined to *cocci*, it refers to a type of bacteria. When it is not joined to *cocci*, you will have to decide which meaning is intended. Staphylo/cocc/emia (staf″ə-lo-kok-se′me-ə) is _____ in the blood.

7-69 When cocci occur in pairs, they are called diplococci (dip″lo-kok′si). The reason they remain in pairs is incomplete separation after cell division. Cocci in pairs (double cocci) are called _____. A well-known diplococcus is the bacteria that causes gonorrhea.

7-70 The blood is normally free of microorganisms. Bacter/emia (bak″tər-e′me-ə) is the presence of _____ in the blood. Streptococc/emia (strep″to-kok-se′me-ə), a type of bacter/emia, is the presence of _____ in the blood. A blood culture is helpful in detecting and identifying many types of bacteria that cause bacteremia. A sensitivity test provides information about which antibiotic is likely to be most effective for treatment.

Systemic (sis-tem′ik) means pertaining to the whole body rather than to a specific area of the body. Septic/emia (*sept[i]*, infection + *-emia*, blood) (sep″tĭ-se′me-ə) is a systemic infection in which pathogens have spread from some part of the body and are not only present in the circulating blood but are multiplying and causing blood infection. This is also called sepsis, and the patient is described as septic.

The presence of microbial toxins in the blood is tox/emia (tok-se′me-ə), a serious condition. A unique type of toxemia is seen in toxic shock syndrome (TSS). The severity of the disease is caused by toxins of a pathogenic strain of *Staphylococcus* and can become life-threatening unless it is recognized and treated. It is most common in menstruating females using high-absorbency tampons but has been seen in other persons. Although *toxemia* is generally reserved to describe the presence of toxins in the blood, it is sometimes used to mean severe and progressive (for example, toxemia of pregnancy).

7-71 The need for oxygen varies with each species of bacteria, but most are aerobic. The combining form *aer(o)* means air or gas, but sometimes the usage is extended to mean oxygen. Two meanings of aerobic (ār-o′bik) are requiring oxygen (air) to maintain life and growing or occurring in the presence of oxygen. Use the prefix *an-* to write a term that means the opposite of aerobic: _____. Anaerobic bacteria (for example, the bacteria that cause tetanus) grow in complete or almost complete absence of oxygen. Tetanus (tet′ə-nəs) is an acute, potentially fatal infection of the central nervous system caused by an anaerobic bacillus, *Clostridium tetani*. The bacteria can infect wounds and produce a lethal neurotoxin. Tetanus injections or booster shots are generally recommended for persons who have a wound and have not been immunized within the past 5 years.

7-72 An anti/septic (an″tĭ-sep′tik) is a substance that inhibits the growth of microorganisms without necessarily killing them. *Bacterio/static* (bak-tēr″e-o-stat′ik) means inhibiting the growth of bacteria. However, *bacteri/cidal* (bak-tēr″ĭ-si′dəl) means killing _____. Both these terms can be written using either *bacter(i)* or *bacteri(o)*, but note the more commonly used terms.

7-73 Bacterial food poisoning results from eating food that is contaminated by certain types of bacteria. One type is caused by various species of *Salmonella* and is characterized by fever and digestive symptoms that include nausea, vomiting, and diarrhea beginning 8 to 48 hours after eating contaminated food. Similar symptoms caused by another type of bacteria, *Staphylococcus*, usually appear much sooner and usually last only a few hours. Botulism (boch′u-liz-əm), an often fatal form of food poisoning, is caused by a toxin produced by the anaerobic bacteria *Clostridium botulinum*. Most botulism occurs after eating improperly canned or improperly cooked foods. Of the types of bacterial food poisoning described, the one that is caused by a toxin and can be fatal is called _____.

Margin answers:

staphylococci
(staf″ə-lo-kok′si)

staphylococci

diplococci

bacteria
streptococci

anaerobic
(an″ə-ro′bik)

bacteria

botulism

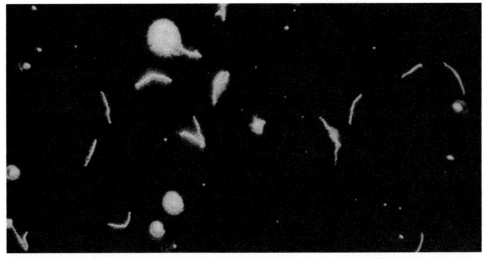

Figure 7-10   Dark-field preparation demonstrating the spirochete of syphilis. In the early stages of syphilis, the organism *Treponema pallidum,* can be observed in material from a chancre using a special dark-field preparation. The organisms are long, tightly coiled spirals that are motile.

spiral

7-74 Viruses and some bacteria do not grow in commonly used culture media. They require living cells and in some cases are difficult or impossible to grow outside a host.

Spirochetes (**spi′ro-kētz**) are _____-shaped bacteria. Observe the spiral shape of the spirochete in Figure 7-10. The special technique called dark-field preparation is used to search for spirochetes that cause syphilis (**sif′ĭ-lis**). The slide is examined microscopically using high-power magnification of 400×. The organism can often be observed in material from a chancre, the painless skin lesion that begins at the infection site in the early stages of syphilis. Syphilis is a sexually transmitted disease (STD), formerly called venereal disease. STDs are usually acquired by sexual intercourse or genital contact.

Vibrios are comma-shaped bacteria. Cholera (**kol′ər-ə**) and several other epidemic forms of gastro/enter/itis (**gas″tro-en″tər-i′tis**), inflammation of the stomach and intestines, are caused by various types of pathogenic vibrios.

7-75 Fungi are microorganisms that feed by absorbing organic molecules from their surroundings. They may be parasitic and may invade living organic substances. Yeasts and molds are included in this group. Only a few of the known fungi are pathogenic to humans. *Candida albicans*, a microscopic fungus, is normally present in the mouth, intestinal tract, and vagina of healthy individuals. Infections may occur under certain circumstances, particularly when immunity is deficient (Figure 7-11). Athlete's foot and ringworm are other diseases caused by fungi. Ringworm is so named because of the

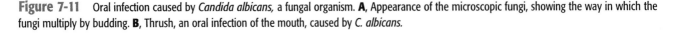

Figure 7-11   Oral infection caused by *Candida albicans,* a fungal organism. **A,** Appearance of the microscopic fungi, showing the way in which the fungi multiply by budding. **B,** Thrush, an oral infection of the mouth, caused by *C. albicans.*

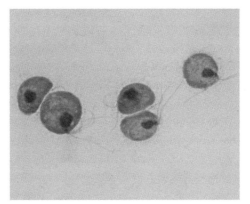

Figure 7-12 *Trichomonas* in a stained smear. *Trichomonas* is a sexually transmitted protozoon that is pathogenic to humans. Five protozoa are shown. The flagella, the hairlike projections that the protozoa use for movement, are visible.

fungus

shape of the lesion on the skin. Ringworm is not caused by a worm but by a

_____.

Only a few species of protozoa are pathogenic to humans, including the protozoa that cause malaria. Malaria is transmitted by the bite of an insect vector, the female *Anopheles* mosquito. In its acute form, the disease is characterized by anemia, enlarged spleen, chills, and fever. Trichomoniasis (**trik″o-mo-ni′ə-sis**) is another human protozoal infection and is also a sexually transmitted disease. A stained preparation of this protozoa is shown in Figure 7-12.

7-76 Microscopy laboratory reports often cite the number of organisms per microscopic high-power field (HPF), not just in reporting bacteria but also in other areas such as the study of urine or in hematology. Sometimes the number of organisms or cells per low-power field (LPF) is reported.

low-

HPF and LPF are abbreviations for microscopic high- and _____ power field, respectively.

Exercise 6

Match the types of diseases/disorders in the left column with their descriptions in the right column.

_____ 1. functional disorder

_____ 2. infectious disease

_____ 3. organic disease

A. caused by pathogenic organisms
B. demonstrable physical change
C. signs or symptoms without physical change

Exercise 7

Match word parts with their meanings.

_____ 1. iatr(o)

_____ 2. idi(o)

_____ 3. nos(o)

_____ 4. seps(o)

_____ 5. staphyl(o)

_____ 6. strept(o)

A. disease
B. grapelike cluster
C. individual
D. infection
E. physician or treatment
F. twisted

Bioterrorism

7-77 Weapons of mass destruction (WMD) have been a concern for many years but have come to the forefront as acts of terrorism have increased. The Federal Emergency Management Agency (FEMA) and the Centers for Disease Control and Prevention (CDC) use the following categories to define weapons of mass destruction:

B Biological
N Nuclear
I Incendiary (incendiaries, flammable substances used to ignite fires, or explosives)
C Chemical
E Explosive

living

Health care providers must be trained to recognize and deal with these emergencies. Biological weapons of mass destruction use _____ organisms that are pathogenic to humans.

7-78 Bio/terrorism is the use of pathogenic biological agents to cause terror in a population. High-priority agents include microorganisms that pose a risk to national security largely for the following reasons:

- They can be easily disseminated (distributed over a general area) or transmitted from person to person.
- They cause high mortality and a major public health impact.
- They can cause public panic and social disruption.
- They require special action for public health preparedness.

bioterrorism

The use of pathogenic biological agents to cause terror in a population is known as _____. CDC lists the highest priority agents as those that cause the following diseases: anthrax, botulism, plague, smallpox, tularemia, and viral hemorrhagic fevers. Botulism, a type of bacterial food poisoning, was described in the previous section. It is suggested that you use a medical dictionary to learn additional facts about these diseases. CDC also provides other categories of biological agents that could be used or engineered for mass dissemination. Many hospitals are implementing emergency preparedness plans to deal with threats or acts of bioterrorism.

Exercise 8

Write words in the blanks to complete these sentences.

1. WMD is an abbreviation for _____ of mass destruction.

2. CDC is an abbreviation for Centers for _____ Control and Protection.

3. The use of pathogenic biological agents to cause terror in a population is called _____.

4. A term that means scattered or distributed over a general area is _____.

Immunity

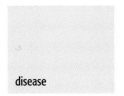

disease

7-79 Our bodies have many defenses, including immunity that usually protects us from pathogenic organisms and other foreign substances. The immune reaction that can occur in a blood transfusion is part of the same system that provides protection against disease-causing organisms. We are continually exposed to pathogens and other harmful substances. Patho/gens (**path'o-jənz**) are microorganisms that are capable of causing _____.

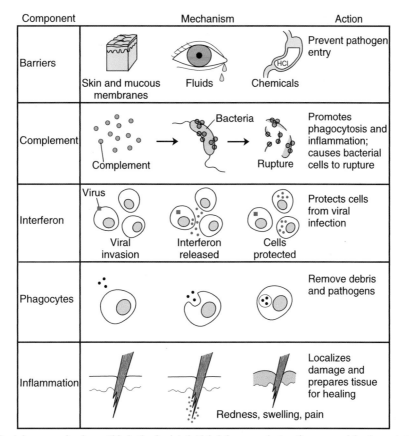

Component	Mechanism	Action
Barriers	Skin and mucous membranes — Fluids — Chemicals (HCl)	Prevent pathogen entry
Complement	Complement → Bacteria → Rupture	Promotes phagocytosis and inflammation; causes bacterial cells to rupture
Interferon	Virus — Viral invasion — Interferon released — Cells protected	Protects cells from viral infection
Phagocytes		Remove debris and pathogens
Inflammation	Redness, swelling, pain	Localizes damage and prepares tissue for healing

Figure 7-13 Nonspecific defense mechanisms. This is the body's initial defense against pathogens and foreign substances. Unlike cell-mediated immunity or antibody-mediated immunity, these defense mechanisms are nonspecific and directed against all types of invaders.

Any substance that is capable, under appropriate conditions, of inducing a specific immune response is an antigen (an′tĭ-jən). Antigens may be bacteria, tissue cells, toxins, or foreign proteins. The body's natural ability to counteract microorganisms or toxins is called resistance (re-zis′təns). Susceptibility (sə-sep″tĭ-bil′ĭ-te) is a lack of resistance. For example, when we are exposed to the influenza virus, we do not become ill if our body has sufficient

_____.

The term for lacking resistance (or being susceptible) is _____.

resistance
susceptibility

7-80 Two types of body defenses are nonspecific resistance and specific resistance. Nonspecific defensive mechanisms are directed against all pathogens and include unbroken skin, phagocytes, inflammation, and proteins such as complement (kom′plə-mənt) and interferon (in″tər-fēr′on) (Figure 7-13). Interferon is of particular importance because it is formed when cells are exposed to a virus. Additional nonspecific defenses include mucus of mucous membranes, which traps foreign particles; hairlike projections (cilia) that form the lining of the respiratory tract and transport dust and microorganisms out of the body; beneficial normal flora that prevent the overgrowth of undesirable organisms; the composition and outward flow of urine; chemicals in human tears; and acids of the stomach, vagina, and skin, which help destroy invading microorganisms.

Phagocytosis (fag″o-si-to′sis) is the ingestion and destruction of microorganisms and cellular debris by certain cells. The combining form *phag(o)* means to eat. Certain tissue cells called macrophages (mak′ro-fāj-ez) and leukocytes are the primary phago/cyt/ic cells. *Phago/cyt/ic* means pertaining to phagocytes or phagocytosis. Phagocytes (fag′o-sīts) are cells that _____ microorganisms and cellular debris.

ingest (or eat)

7-81 The second type of defense, specific defense mechanisms, is selective (specific) for particular pathogens. This specific resistance is called immunity, and it protects us from a particular disease or

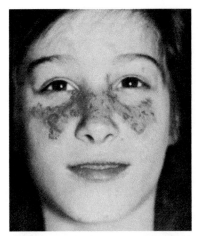

Figure 7-14   The characteristic "butterfly" rash of systemic lupus erythematosus. The word *lupus* is the Latin term for wolf. The rash is usually red, and thus the term *erythematosus,* a Latin word meaning reddened, was added in naming this disease.

immunity

condition. Both specific and nonspecific defenses occur simultaneously and work together to overcome pathogens. Resistance to a particular disease is called _____.

Specific defense incorporates cell-mediated immunity and antibody-mediated humoral (**hu′mər-əl**) immunity. A type of white blood cell, T-lymphocytes (also called T cells), is responsible for cell-mediated immunity. B-lymphocytes (also called B cells) are responsible for antibody-mediated immunity.

against

7-82 Anti/bodies (**an′tĭ-bod″ēz**) are formed _____ antigens (**an′tĭ-jənz**). People do not generally form antibodies against their own body cells; however, this happens in autoimmune diseases, a group of diseases characterized by altered function of the immune system that results in the production of antibodies against one's own cells. An example of an autoimmune disease is systemic lupus erythematosus* (**loo′pəs er″ə-them″ə-to′sis**), so named for the characteristic butterfly rash that appears across the bridge of the nose in some cases (Figure 7-14). The disease can cause major body organs and systems to fail and is potentially fatal. One forms antibodies against one's own cells in lupus erythematosus (LE), an example of an

autoimmune

_____ disease.

against

7-83 Antibodies are immuno/globulins (**im″u-no-glob′u-linz**) and are classified as IgA, IgD, IgE, IgG, or IgM. The combining form *immun(o)* means immune. An antibody interacts with the antigen that induced its synthesis. Immuno/globulins, or antibodies, are found in the blood plasma and act _____ harmful invading microorganisms.

Specific antibodies provide us with immunity against disease-causing organisms. We generally acquire antibodies either by having a disease or by receiving a vaccination (**vak″sĭ-na′shən**). A vaccination causes our bodies to produce _____.

antibodies

antibodies

7-84 Polio vaccine contains polio antigen, which causes the formation of polio _____. After receiving the polio vaccine, one is immunized against poliomyelitis (**po″le-o-mi″ə-li′tis**).

Occasionally the interaction of our defense mechanisms with an antigen results in injury. This excessive reaction to an antigen is called hyper/sensitivity (**hi″pər-sen″sĭ-tiv′ĭ-te**). Write this word that means a heightened reaction to an antigen: _____.

hypersensitivity

Anaphylaxis (**an″ə-fə-lak′sis**) or anaphylactic (**an″ə-fə-lak′tik**) reactions are exaggerated, life-threatening hypersensitivity reactions to a previously encountered antigen. The suffix *-phylaxis* means protection. With a wide range in the severity of symptoms, the reactions may include generalized itching, difficult breathing, airway obstruction, and shock. Insect stings and penicillin are two common causes of anaphylactic shock, a severe and sometimes fatal systemic hypersensitivity reaction.

*Erythematosus (Greek: *erythema,* flush upon the skin, reddish).

Natural   Artificial

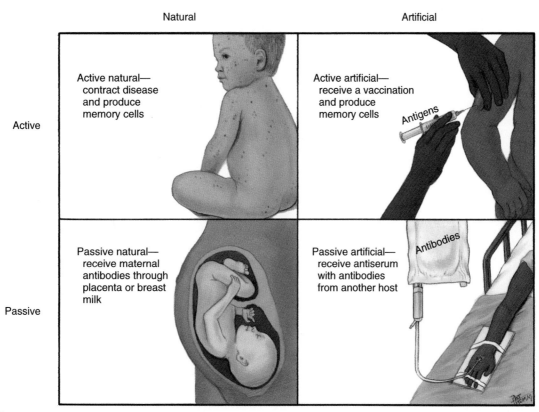

Active

Active natural—
contract disease
and produce
memory cells

Active artificial—
receive a vaccination
and produce
memory cells

Antigens

Passive

Passive natural—
receive maternal
antibodies through
placenta or breast
milk

Passive artificial—
receive antiserum
with antibodies
from another host

Antibodies

Figure 7-15   Four types of specific immunity. Active natural and passive natural immunities, as the names imply, occur through the normal activities of either an individual contracting a disease or a fetus being exposed to maternal antibodies. Both active artificial and passive artificial immunities require deliberate actions of receiving vaccinations or antibodies.

7-85 Allergies (al′ər-jēz) are conditions in which the body reacts with an exaggerated immune response to common, harmless substances, most of which are found in the environment. A substance that can produce an allergic reaction but is not otherwise harmful is called an allergen (al′ər-jen).

Some common environmental substances that may cause allergic reactions are certain foods, pollen, animal dander, feathers, and house dust. These essentially harmless substances that cause

allergens

allergies are called _____. Allergy testing is used to identify the specific allergens. The most common is skin testing, which exposes the patient to small quantities of the suspected allergens.

In an allergic reaction, injured cells release a substance called histamine (his′tə-mēn), which causes dilation of the capillaries (the smallest blood vessels), an increase in gastric secretion, and contraction of smooth muscle of several internal organs. Histamine is responsible for the symptoms of hay fever: teary eyes, sneezing, and swollen membranes of the upper respiratory tract. An anti/histamine (an″te-, an″ti-his′tə-mēn), a preparation that acts

against

_____ histamine, usually relieves the symptoms.

7-86 Immunization (im″u-nǐ-za′shən) is the process by which resistance to an infectious disease is induced or augmented. Active immunity occurs when the individual's own body produces an immune response to a harmful antigen. Passive immunity results when the immune agents develop in another person or animal and then are transferred to an individual who was not previously immune. This second type of immunity is borrowed immunity that provides immediate protection but is effective for only a short time. Immunity that an individual develops in response to a harmful

active
passive

antigen is _____ immunity. Borrowed immunity that is effective for only a short time is _____ immunity.

7-87 In both active and passive immunity, the recognition of specific antigens is called specific immunity. The terms *natural* and *artificial* refer to how the immunity is obtained (Figure 7-15).

A vaccination is any injection or ingestion of inactivated or killed microbes or their products that is administered to induce immunity. Vaccinations are available to immunize against many diseases such as typhoid, diphtheria, polio, measles, and mumps. Depending on its type, vaccine is administered orally or by injection. Vaccination is a form of prophylaxis* **(pro″fə-lak′sis)**, prevention of or protection against disease.

7-88 Toxoids **(tok′soidz)** contain toxins, which are antigens. Toxoids cause our bodies to produce _____, thus providing us with immunity. *Tox/oid*, when broken down into its components, means resembling a _____. Actually, a toxoid is simply a toxin that has been treated to eliminate its harmful properties without destroying its ability to stimulate antibody production.

A toxoid is a helpful form of toxin. However, words containing *tox(o)* usually refer to substances that have an adverse effect. For example, a cyto/toxin **(si″to-tok′sin)** has harmful effects on _____. Cyto/tox/icity **(si″to-tok-sis′ĭ-te)** is the degree to which an agent possesses a specific destructive action on cells. This term is used in referring to the lysis of cells by immune phenomena, and it is also used to describe the activity of anti/neoplas/tic drugs that selectively kill cells. *Antineoplastic* means inhibiting or preventing the development of neoplasms, malignant tumors.

Tox/icity **(tok-sis′ĭ-te)** is the degree to which something is poisonous or a condition that results from exposure to a toxin or to toxic amounts of a substance that does not cause adverse effects in smaller amounts.

7-89 *Immuno/compromised* **(im″u-no-kom′prə-mīzd)** pertains to an immune response that has been weakened by a disease or an immuno/suppressive **(im″u-no-sə-pres′iv)** agent. Radiation and certain drugs are immuno/suppressants **(im″u-no-sə-pres′ənts)**, meaning that they suppress the _____ response.

To transplant **(trans-plant′)** is to transfer tissue. The tissue that is transplanted is called a transplant **(trans′plant)**. Note that the pronunciation of the term depends on its usage as a verb or a noun. When tissue is transplanted from one person to another, rejection **(re-jek′shən)** is often a problem. Rejection is an immune reaction to the donor's tissue cells, with ultimate destruction of the transplanted tissue. Medications are used to suppress immune reactions, but the drugs have side effects. Rejection is still the most common problem encountered in transplantation of tissue from one person to another.

7-90 Immunodeficiency diseases are a group of health conditions caused by a defect in the immune system and are generally characterized by susceptibility to infections and chronic diseases. One of the most publicized immunodeficiency diseases is AIDS, a viral disease involving a defect in cell-mediated immunity that is manifested by various opportunistic infections. Infections caused by normally nonpathogenic organisms in a host whose resistance has been decreased are called opportunistic infections. There is no known cure for AIDS, and the prognosis is poor. Some persons with AIDS are susceptible to malignant neoplasms, especially Kaposi's sarcoma (see Figure 13-10).

AIDS is caused by either of two varieties of the human immunodeficiency virus, designated HIV-1 and HIV-2. AIDS is transmitted by sexual intercourse or exposure to contaminated body fluid of an infected person. It was originally found in homosexual men and intravenous (IV) drug users but now occurs increasingly among heterosexual men and women, and babies born of infected mothers. *AIDS* means acquired _____ syndrome.

Margin terms: antibodies | toxin (or poison) | cells | immune | immunodeficiency

Exercise 9

Write words in the blanks to complete these sentences.

1. A foreign substance that induces production of antibodies is called an _____.

2. Lacking resistance is being _____ to a disease.

3. Phagocytosis of pathogens is part of the body's _____ defense mechanism.

4. Antibody-mediated immunity is part of the body's _____ defense mechanism.

5. _____ immunity occurs when an individual's body produces an immune response to a harmful antigen.

6. AIDS is an abbreviation for acquired _____ syndrome.

*Prophylaxis (Greek: *prophylax*, advance guard).

Medical Records

physical

7-91 Health records are written forms of communication that document information that is relevant to the care of the patient. Medical reports communicate the patient's health status to other health professionals and to insurance companies and federal and state agencies. Inpatients are persons who have been admitted to a hospital or other health care facility for at least an overnight stay. An outpatient (OP) is one who is not admitted to a hospital and is being treated in an office, clinic, hospital, or other health care facility.

There are many types of medical records, including those for the history and physical (H & P) examination, operative (surgical) reports, consultation notes and letters, medication records, and laboratory and radiology reports. Medical reports often include statistical data (patient's legal name; date of birth [DOB]; file number, which may be the patient's social security number [SSN]; physician's name, etc.) and a signature line. H & P means history and _____.

A few representative samples will be included in this book to give you experience with understanding health care records. To apply terminology in practical situations, you will be asked to read and explain various medical terms that are in medical reports.

privacy

7-92 The Health Insurance Portability and Accountability Act (HIPAA) is a federal privacy act that went into effect in 2003. It gives the patient certain rights, including the rights to request restrictions of protected health information and to receive confidential communications concerning one's own medical condition and treatment. HIPAA is a federal _____ act concerning a patient's medical records.

Exercise 10

Write a word in each blank space to answer these questions.

1. What is the term for persons who have been admitted to a hospital or other health care facility for at least an overnight stay? _____

2. What is the term for patients who are not hospitalized and are being treated in an office, clinic, or other health care facility? _____

3. What is the abbreviation for the federal privacy act that gives the patient certain rights concerning his or her own health information? _____

CATEGORIES OF MEDICAL TERMS

7-93 As you study medical terminology, you will observe that terms are used in a variety of ways. For example, certain terms are names of structures or diseases, others represent surgical procedures, and others describe means of arriving at a diagnosis, as well as still other groupings you will begin to recognize. Here are some of the categories that will be used in this book:

- Anatomy: names of structures and related words, such as *colon* (large intestine) and *colonic* (pertaining to the colon), *erythrocyte* and *erythrocytic*.
- Diagnostic (di″əg-nos′tik) tests and procedures: terms used to describe the signs and symptoms of disease (*fever, headache*) and the tests used to establish a diagnosis. The tests include clinical studies (measuring blood pressure), laboratory tests (determination of blood gases), and radiologic studies, those that relate to the use of radiant energy (such as in a chest x-ray examination).
- Pathologies: names of diseases or disorders (*botulism, leukemia*).
- Surgeries: operative procedures (*tonsillectomy*, removal of the tonsils).
- Therapies: treatment of a disease or abnormal condition. Therapeutic terms include prescribed drugs (such as penicillin) and physical treatments (such as electric stimulation to enhance the healing process).

anatomy

The femur is commonly called the thigh bone. *Femur* is the name of a structure. The appropriate category for *femur* is _____.

Exercise 11

Categorize the terms in the left column by selecting A, B, C, D, or E.

_____ 1. antibiotics

_____ 2. erythrocyte

_____ 3. hematocrit

_____ 4. hemoglobinopathy

_____ 5. thrombectomy

A. anatomy
B. diagnostic test or procedure
C. pathology
D. surgery
E. therapy

SELECTED ABBREVIATIONS

ABO	blood groups		**hx, Hx**	history
ADL	activities of daily living		**IgA, IgD, IgG,**	immunoglobulins
AHF	antihemophilic factor		**IgM, IgE**	
AIDS	acquired immunodeficiency syndrome		**INR**	International Normalized Ratio
ALL	acute lymphoblastic leukemia		**LE**	lupus erythematosus
AML	acute myelogenous leukemia		**LPF**	low-power field
CBC, cbc	complete blood cell count		**MCH**	mean corpuscular hemoglobin (average amount of hemoglobin in each RBC)
CDC	Centers for Disease Control and Prevention			
CMV	cytomegalovirus		**MCHC**	mean corpuscular hemoglobin concentration (amount of hemoglobin per unit of blood)
diff	differential count (WBCs)			
DIC	disseminated intravascular coagulation			
DOB	date of birth		**MCV**	mean corpuscular volume (average size of individual red cells)
ELISA	enzyme-linked immunosorbent assay (commonly used in AIDS diagnosis)			
			OP	outpatient
ESR	erythrocyte sedimentation rate		**PCV**	packed cell volume
FEMA	Federal Emergency Management Agency		**PMN**	polymorphonuclear
H & P	history and physical		**PT**	prothrombin time (also physical therapy)
HAV	hepatitis A virus		**PTT**	partial thromboplastin time
Hb, Hgb	hemoglobin		**RBC**	red blood cell, red blood count
HBV	hepatitis B virus		**Rh**	rhesus factor in blood
HCT	hematocrit		**RPR**	rapid plasma reagin (blood test for syphilis)
HCV	hepatitis C virus			
HDN	hemolytic disease of the newborn		**SSN**	social security number
HDV	hepatitis D virus		**STD**	sexually transmitted disease
HIPAA	Health Insurance Portability and Accountability Act		**TSS**	toxic shock syndrome
			WBC	white blood cell, white blood cell count
HIV	human immunodeficiency virus		**WMD**	weapons of mass destruction
HLA	human leukocyte antigens		**WNV**	West Nile virus
HPF	high-power field			

PREPARING FOR THE TEST

Review as you were instructed in Chapter 2, and work the end-of-chapter review.

Be Careful with These Word Parts and Terms!

hidr(o) vs. hydr(o)
autologous vs. homologous
excretion vs. secretion
lithotomy (a surgical procedure) vs. the lithotomy position
mucus vs. mucous

CHAPTER 7 REVIEW

■ Basic Understanding

Matching
I. Match descriptions in the left column with A, B, or C.

_____ 1. body defense
_____ 2. blood platelet
_____ 3. contains hemoglobin
_____ 4. initiates coagulation
_____ 5. transports oxygen

A. leukocyte
B. erythrocyte
C. thrombocyte

II. Match each type of immunity with its description in the right column.

_____ 1. active natural
_____ 2. active artificial
_____ 3. passive artificial
_____ 4. passive natural

A. contracting a disease
B. exposure of the fetus to maternal antibodies
C. receiving a vaccination
D. receiving an injection of antibodies

III. Match the types of bacteria in the left column with clues in the right column.

_____ 1. bacilli
_____ 2. diplococci
_____ 3. spirochetes
_____ 4. staphylococci
_____ 5. streptococci
_____ 6. vibrios

A. comma-shaped bacteria
B. rod-shaped bacteria
C. spherical bacteria in grapelike clusters
D. spherical bacteria in pairs
E. spherical bacteria in twisted chains
F. spiral-shaped bacteria

True or False
IV. Mark each statement T for true or F for false:

_____ 1. Body fluids move back and forth between compartments that are separated by cell membranes.

_____ 2. Blood is an intravascular fluid.

_____ 3. Respiration is the main way that water is lost from the body.

_____ 4. Most extracellular fluid is plasma.

_____ 5. Lymph is the fluid that circulates through the lymphatic vessels.

Listing

V. *List four general types of microorganisms.*

1. _____

2. _____

3. _____

4. _____

VI. *Name five nonspecific body defenses.*

1. _____

2. _____

3. _____

4. _____

5. _____

VII. *Name two types of specific body defenses.*

1. _____

2. _____

Fill in the Blanks

VIII. *Write a word in each blank to complete these sentences.*

1. Mr. Perkins' physician tells him that he has hypokalemia, probably resulting from the use of diuretics. *Hypokalemia* means that Mr. Perkins has an inadequate amount of _____ in the blood.

2. Blood _____ is a series of chemical reactions that result in a blood clot.

3. Fluid that is located between cells and in tissue spaces is called _____ fluid.

4. Mrs. Klott forms a blood clot, called a _____, after surgery.

5. Mrs. Klott's physician prescribes an in vivo _____ after she develops a blood clot.

6. A vital function of body fluids is to transport nutrients and remove body _____.

7. A relative constancy in the internal environment of the body is called _____.

8. An examination and enumeration of the distribution of leukocytes in a stained blood smear is called a _____ white cell count.

9. Destruction of the red blood cell membrane resulting in the release of hemoglobin is called _____.

10. A term given to a group of malignant diseases characterized by abnormal numbers and forms of immature white blood cells in the blood is _____.

Multiple Choice

IX. Circle the correct answer in these sentences.

1. The name of the substance from which fibrin originates is (fibrinogen, fibrinolysis, thrombogen, thrombolysis).

2. The degree of disease-causing capability of an organism is called (resistance, sensitivity, susceptibility, virulence).

3. Transportation of oxygen to body cells is a major function of (blood platelets, erythrocytes, leukocytes, thrombocytes).

4. A term that means having no tendency to repair itself or develop into new tissue is (analytic, anisocytosis, aplastic, hemolytic).

5. The surgical procedure whereby living organs are transferred from one part of the body to another or from one individual to another is (rejection, transmission, transplant, transreaction).

6. Intracellular fluid is found (around, between, inside, outside) cells.

7. One of the specific body defense mechanisms is (cell-mediated immunity, intact skin, interferon, phagocytosis).

8. A normal defensive response of the body to a pathogen is (erythropia, infection, inflammation, xanthoderma).

9. The most abundant body fluid is (extracellular, interstitial, intracellular, plasma).

10. A decrease in the number of blood platelets is called (hemophilia, leukemia, leukocytosis, thrombopenia).

Writing Terms

X. Write a term for each of the following meanings:

1. any erythrocyte of irregular shape _____

2. below normal sodium in the blood _____

3. between cells _____

4. blood clotting _____

5. dissolving of a thrombus _____

6. a homologous graft _____

7. localized collection of pus in a cavity _____

8. neutral-staining granulocyte _____

9. production of blood _____

10. use of biological agents to cause terror _____

■ Greater Comprehension

Health Care Report

XI. Read the following consultation report and define the terms or abbreviations that follow the report. Although you may be unfamiliar with some of the terms, you should be able to determine their meanings by considering their word parts.

MID-CITY MEDICAL CENTER

222 Medical Center Drive   Main City, US 63017-1000   Phone: (555) 437-0000
                                                                        Fax (555) 437-0001

CONSULTATION REPORT

Patient Name: Thomas Byerly   **File Number:** 12361   **Date of Birth:** November 6, 1933
Examination Date: February 11, 2004
REASON FOR CONSULTATION: neutropenia/thrombocytopenia
HISTORY OF PRESENT ILLNESS: This is a 70-year-old white male with history of coronary artery disease and melanoma, who underwent a four vessel coronary artery bypass grafting on 1/10/2004. He was readmitted to the hospital on 1/22/2004 with wound dehiscence and wound infection. He was treated with vancomycin but had supratherapeutic vancomycin levels and was switched to Timentin 6 days ago, on 1/06/2004. He has had decreasing white cell counts and has been mildly neutropenic since 2/06. His WBC count today is 3.4 with an absolute neutrophil count of 1.53.
MEDICAL HISTORY:
1. Coronary artery disease
2. Remote history of melanoma
3. Deep vein thrombosis
4. Hypertension
5. Anemia
ALLERGIES: Coumadin and tape
CURRENT MEDICATIONS: Aspirin 325 mg per day; Lopressor 25 mg BID; Timentin 3.2 mg IV every 6 hours; Lisinopritl 20 mg per day
LABORATORY VALUES: WBC 3.4
                      HGB 9.3
                      Platelets 210 with absolute neutrophil count of 1.53
                      CRP 2.3
IMPRESSION: Neutropenia. This most likely is due to medications. The patient's white count was normal upon admission to the hospital. In the case of medication-related thrombocytopenia, Timentin and vancomycin could well be the cause of this hematologic abnormality.
PLAN: Discontinue Timentin and obtain hematology and infectious disease consults for recommendations on treating this *Staphylococcus* (not *aureus*) infection.

Thank you for this consultation.
JHM:amb D: 2/11/2004 T: 2/12/2004
Dictated by: Jay H. Miller, MD

Define:

1. neutropenia _____

2. thrombocytopenia _____

3. melanoma _____

4. supratherapeutic _____

5. thrombosis _____

6. anemia _____

7. BID _____

8. hematologic _____

9. staphylococcus _____

XII. Read the following physical examination report and define the terms or abbreviations that follow the report. Although you may be unfamiliar with some of the terms, you should be able to determine their meanings by considering their word parts.

MID-CITY MEDICAL CENTER

222 Medical Center Drive   **Main City, US 63017-1000**   **Phone:** (555) 437-0000
                                                                                                    Fax (555) 437-0001

PHYSICAL EXAMINATION

Name: Thomas Byerly   **Date:** 4/23/2003   **File Number:** 20511
Date of Birth: November 6, 1933
GENERAL APPEARANCE: Dyspneic with pallor
PHYSICAL EXAMINATION:
   HEENT: No jugular vein distension
   LUNGS: Decreased breath sounds bilaterally
   HEART: Regular rate and rhythm
   EXTREMITIES: No edema
   NEUROLOGIC: Alert
LABORATORY DATA: Hgb 8.8; HCT 26.5; Na 127
IMPRESSION:
1. Iron deficiency anemia secondary to chronic blood loss
2. Worsening hyponatremia
3. Exacerbation COPD
PLAN/RECOMMENDATION/DISPOSITION:
1. Anemia—has required parenteral iron in the past, secondary to inability to tolerate iron by mouth. Will transfuse.
2. Hyponatremia—some improvement after infusion of normal saline today. Recommend fluid restriction.
3. COPD to be followed by pulmonologist.

Leslie Moore, MD
Leslie Moore, M.D.

LM:aba
D: 4/23/2003
T: 4/24/2003

Define:

1. dyspneic _____

2. pallor _____

3. bilaterally _____

4. edema _____

5. Hgb _____

6. HCT _____

7. hyponatremia _____

Matching

XIII. *Match the signs and symptoms of severe anemia in the left column with the correct meaning in the right column:*

_____ 1. dyspnea

_____ 2. pallor

_____ 3. syncope

_____ 4. tinnitus

A. difficult breathing
B. fainting
C. loss of appetite
D. nausea
E. paleness
F. ringing in the ears

Spelling

XIV. *Circle all incorrectly spelled terms and write their correct spelling:*

anarobic   botulism   fibrinolisis   polymorfonuclear   toxisity

Interpreting Abbreviations

XV. *Write the meaning of these abbreviations:*

1. AIDS _____

2. CBC _____

3. HIV _____

4. PMN _____

5. RBC _____

Pronunciation

XVI. *The pronunciation is shown for several medical words. Indicate the primary accented syllable in each term with an ´.*

1. coagulopathy (ko ag u lop ə the)

2. erythropoietin (ə rith ro poi ə tin)

3. allogenic (al o jen ik)

4. microscopy (mi kros kə pe)

5. prophylaxis (pro fə lak sis)

Categorizing Terms

XVII. *Categorize the terms in the left column by selecting A, B, C, D, or E.*

_____ 1. hematocrit

_____ 2. in vivo anticoagulant

_____ 3. leukocyte

_____ 4. septicemia

_____ 5. thrombectomy

A. anatomy
B. diagnostic test or procedure
C. pathology
D. surgery
E. therapy

(Check your answers with the solutions in Appendix VI.)

LISTING OF MEDICAL TERMS

Use the practice CD to review the terms that have been presented. Look closely at the spelling of each term as it is pronounced, and be sure you know the meaning of each term.

abscess	calculus	fibrinolysis	idiopathic disease
acquired	cardiovascular	functional disorder	immunity
immunodeficiency	cerebrospinal fluid	fungal	immunization
syndrome	chancre	fungi	immunocompromised
active immunity	cholera	fungus	immunodeficiency
aerobic	*Clostridium*	gastroenteritis	immunoglobulin
agglutination	coagulant	gonorrhea	immunosuppressant
agranulocytosis	coagulate	Gram stain	immunosuppressive
allergen	coagulation	granulocyte	in vitro
allergy	coagulopathy	hematocrit	in vivo
allogeneic	cocci	hematologic	incompatibility
allogenic	complement	hematologist	infection
allograft	corpuscle	hematology	infectious disease
amniocentesis	Coumadin	hematoma	infectious mononucleosis
amniotic fluid	cyanosis	hematopoiesis	inflammation
anaerobic	cytotoxicity	hematopoietic	intercellular
analgesic	cytotoxin	hemoglobin	interferon
anaphylactic	dehydration	hemoglobinopathy	interstitial fluid
anaphylaxis	differential white cell count	hemolysin	intracellular
anemia	diphtheria	hemolysis	intrauterine
angina	diplococci	hemolytic anemia	intravascular
anisocytosis	disseminated	hemolyze	isotonic
anthrax	dissemination	hemophilia	Kaposi's sarcoma
antibiotic	dyscrasia	hemostasis	karyomegaly
antibody	dyspnea	heparin	leukemia
anticoagulant	edema	histamine	leukocyte
antigen	electrolyte	homeostasis	leukocytopenia
antihemophilic factor	electrophoresis	homologous	leukocytosis
antihistamine	eosinophil	homologous graft	leukopenia
antineoplastic drugs	Epstein-Barr virus	humoral immunity	lithotomy
antiseptic	erythroblast	hydrocephalus	lithotripsy
aplastic	erythoblastosis fetalis	hydrocephaly	lupus erythematosus
autoimmune disease	erythrocyte	hypercalcemia	lymphocyte
autologous graft	erythrocytic	hyperchromic	macrocyte
autologous transfusion	erythrocytopenia	hyperemia	macrocytosis
bacilli	erythrocytosis	hyperkalemia	macrophage
bacteremia	erythropenia	hypernatremia	macroscopic
bacterial infection	erythropoiesis	hypersensitivity	macroscopy
bactericidal	excrete	hypocalcemia	malaria
bacteriostatic	excretion	hypochromia	measles
basophil	extracellular	hypochromic	megalocyte
biological	fibrin	hypokalemia	metabolism
bioterrorism	fibrinogen	hyponatremia	microbiologist
botulism	fibrinolysin	iatrogenic disease	microbiology

microcyte
microcytosis
microorganism
microscope
microscopy
monocyte
mucoid gland
mucous
mucus
mumps
necrosis
nephrolithiasis
neurotoxin
neutrophil
normochromic
normocyte
normocytic
nosocomial infection
nucleoid
nucleoprotein
opportunistic infection
organic disease
pallor
partial thromboplastin time
passive immunity
pathogen
perspiration
phagocyte

phagocytosis
plague
plasma
poikilocyte
poikilocytosis
poliomyelitis
polycythemia
polycythemia vera
polymorph
polymorphonuclear
prophylaxis
prothrombin
protozoal
purulent
pus
rejection
resistance
salivary gland
Salmonella
sanguinous
secrete
sepsis
septic
septicemia
shunt
sickle cell anemia
skin graft
smallpox

spherocyte
spherocytosis
spinal fluid
spirochete
staphylococcal infection
staphylococcemia
staphylococci
Staphylococcus
streptococcal infection
streptococcal pharyngitis
streptococcemia
streptococci
suppurative
susceptibility
syncope
syphilis
systemic
tachycardia
tetanus
thrombectomy
thrombocyte
thrombocytopenia
thrombocytosis
thrombogenesis
thrombolysis
thrombolytic
thrombopenia
thromboplastin

thrombosis
thrombotic
thrombus
tinnitus
tissue rejection
toxemia
toxicity
toxoid
transfusion
transmission
transplant
trichomoniasis
tularemia
typhoid
urinary tract
urine
uvula
vaccination
vaccine
vibrio
viral hemorrhagic fever
viral infection
virulence
viscosity
warfarin

español ENHANCING SPANISH COMMUNICATION

ENGLISH	SPANISH (PRONUNCIATION)
allergy	alergia (ah-LEHR-he-ah)
anemia	anemia (ah-NAY-me-ah)
bacilli	bacilos (bah-SE-los)
clot	coágulo (co-AH-goo-lo)
constipation	estreñimiento (es-tray-nye-me-EN-to)
destruction	destrucción (des-trooc-se-ON)
diagnostic	diagnóstico (de-ag-NOS-te-co)
diarrhea	diarrea (de-ar-RAY-ah)
dizziness	vértigo (VERR-te-go)
excretion	excreción (ex-cray-se-ON)
fainting	languidez (lan-gee-DES), desmayo (des-MAH-yo)
fatigue	fatiga (fah-TEE-gah)
fiber	fibra (FEE-brah)
fluid	fluido (floo-EE-do)
hair	pelo (PAY-lo)
headache	dolor de cabeza (do-LOR day cah-BAY-sa)
inflammation	inflamación (in-flah-mah-se-ON)
influenza	gripe (GREE-pay)
injection	inyección (in-yec-se-ON)
injury	daño (DAH-nyo)
leukemia	leucemia (lay-oo-SAY-me-ah)
lymph	linfa (LEEN-fa)
lymphatic	linfático (lin-FAH-te-co)
mucus	moco (MO-co)
murmur	murmullo (moor-MOOL-lyo)
oxygen	oxígeno (ok-SEE-hay-no)
parasite	parásito (pah-RAH-se-to)
perspiration	sudor (soo-DOR)
ringing	zumbido (zoom-BEE-do)
saliva	saliva (sah-LEE-vah)
sweat	sudor (soo-DOR)
tears	lágrimas (LAH-gre-mahs)
tests	pruebas (proo-AY-bahs)
tongue	lengua (LEN-goo-ah)
transfusion	transfusión (trans-foo-se-ON)
water	agua (AH-goo-ah)
wound	lesión (lay-se-ON)

CHAPTER 8

Cardiovascular and Lymphatic Systems

FUNCTION FIRST

The cardiovascular system circulates blood throughout the body, delivering nutrients and other essential materials to the fluids surrounding the cells, removing waste products, and conveying the wastes to organs where they can be excreted. As blood circulates, interstitial fluid accumulates in the tissue spaces. This excess fluid is normally transported away from the tissues by another vascular network that helps maintain the internal fluid environment—the lymphatic system. The lymphatic system helps maintain the internal fluid environment of the body returning proteins and tissue fluids to the blood, aiding in the absorption of fats into the bloodstream, and helping to defend the body against microorganisms and disease.

Cardiovascular System

ANATOMY AND PHYSIOLOGY

vessel

8-1 The heart and blood vessels make up the cardio/vascul/ar (*cardi[o]*, heart + *vascul[o]*, vessel + *-ar*, pertaining to) (kahr″de-o-vas′ku-lər) system. This vast network of blood vessels delivers oxygen, nutrients, and vital substances to the interstitial (in″tər-stish′əl) fluids surrounding all the body's cells.

   Vascul/ar means pertaining to a _____, specifically a blood vessel. The heart, arteries, arterioles (ahr-tēr′e-ōlz), capillaries, venules (ven′ūlz), and veins make up the cardiovascular system (Figure 8-1). Learn these word parts that are used to describe the anatomy and physiology of the cardiovascular system.

Word Parts for Cardiovascular Anatomy and Physiology

Combining Form	Meaning	Combining Form	Meaning
Main Components of the Cardiovascular System		**Other Word Parts**	
angi(o), vas(o), vascul(o)	vessel	atri(o)	atrium
aort(o)	aorta	coron(o)	crown
arter(o), arteri(o)	artery	mediastin(o)	mediastinum
arteriol(o)	arteriole	ox(i)	oxygen
cardi(o)	heart	pulmon(o)	lung
phleb(o), ven(i), ven(o)	vein	sept(o)*	septum; partition
venul(o)	venule	sin(o)	sinus
		steth(o), thorac(o)	chest
Tissues of the Heart		valv(o), valvul(o)	valve
endocardi(o)	endocardium	ventricul(o)	ventricle
myocardi(o)	myocardium		
pericardi(o)	pericardium	**Suffix**	**Meaning**
		-ole	small

*Sept(o) sometimes means infection.

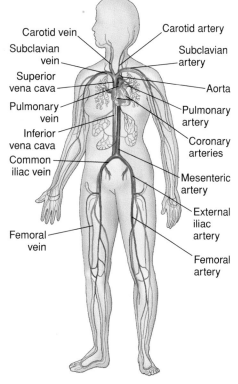

Figure 8-1   The cardiovascular system, the heart, and blood vessels. Two major components of the vascular network are shown, the arteries *(red)* and the veins *(blue)*. Only the larger or more common blood vessels are labeled.

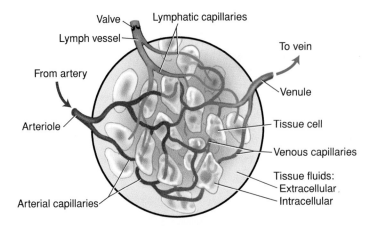

Figure 8-2   A capillary bed showing the relationship of blood vessels. Blood that is rich in oxygen is carried by the arteries that branch many times to become arterioles. Arterioles branch to become capillaries, the site of oxygen and carbon dioxide exchange. Oxygen-poor blood is returned to the heart through the venules, which flow into the veins. The veins carry the blood to the two largest veins, the superior and inferior vena cavae, which empty into the heart. Venae cavae is plural for vena cava.

8-2 The arteries are shown in red and the veins are shown in blue in Figure 8-1. This oversimplifies blood circulation, but it will help you remember that, in general, arteries carry oxygen-rich blood to body tissues and veins carry oxygen-poor blood back to the heart.

    You already know that *cardi(o)* means heart. You also need to remember that *arter(o)* and *arteri(o)* mean artery. *Arteri/al* (**ahr-tēr′e-əl**) means pertaining to one or more

_____.

arteries

8-3 *Arteri/ole* means little artery when translated literally, because *-ole* means little. The combining form for arteriole is _____. Capillaries are microscopic blood vessels that receive blood from the arterioles. Capillaries are so small that erythrocytes must pass through them in single file. Blood and tissue fluids exchange various substances across the capillary walls.

arteriol(o)

8-4 The capillaries join arterioles and venules (Figure 8-2). You will be using three combining forms that mean vein: *phleb(o)*, *ven(i)*, and *ven(o)*. *Phleb(o)* is used more often to write medical terms, but you will need to remember that *veni/puncture* (**ven′ĭ-punk″chər**) means puncture of a _____. Both *venipuncture* and *phlebo/tomy* (**flə-bot′ə-me**) mean opening of a vein to draw blood for laboratory analysis. Translated literally, *phlebotomy* means _____ of a vein. Phlebotomists (**flə-bot′ə-mists**) are persons with special training in the practice of drawing blood. *Ven/ous* means pertaining to the veins.

vein

incision

    Venules join the capillaries and veins. The combining form *venul(o)* means venule.* *Venul/ar* (**ven′u-lər**) means pertaining to, composed of, or affecting venules.

    Arterio/ven/ous (**ahr-tēr″e-o-ve′nəs**) means pertaining to both _____ and veins.

arteries

8-5 Blood circulation is the circuit of blood through the body, from the heart through the arteries, arterioles, capillaries, venules, and veins and back to the heart. *Circulation* means movement in a regular or circular fashion. If you study blood circulation more closely, you learn that it consists of many events that occur simultaneously. There are two important types of circulation that occur each time the heart beats:

- Systemic circulation: the general circulation that carries oxygenated blood from the heart to the tissues of the body and returns the blood with much of its oxygen exchanged for carbon dioxide back to the heart.

*Venule (Latin: *venula*, small vein).

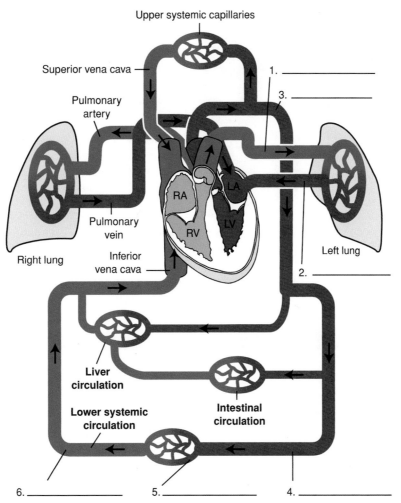

Figure 8-3 Schematic drawing of blood circulation and the relationship of blood vessels. *Arrows* indicate the direction of blood flow through the heart to the lungs and the major vessels of the cardiovascular system. *RA, RV, LA,* and *LV* are abbreviations for the four chambers of the heart. Blood circulation consists of two types of circulation: pulmonary circulation and systemic circulation. Label the diagram as indicated. **Pulmonary circulation:** Pulmonary arteries carry oxygen-deficient blood *(blue)* to the lungs, where it is oxygenated. Label the left pulmonary artery *(1)*. Oxygenated blood is returned to the heart via pulmonary veins. Label the left pulmonary vein *(2)*. **Systemic circulation:** Oxygen-rich blood *(red)* is pumped from the heart into the aorta *(3)* and is routed to arteries that branch to become arterioles, which branch to become capillaries. Label the artery *(4)* and capillary *(5)*. In the capillaries, blood is provided to the tissues of the body and the blood, with much of its oxygen exchanged for carbon dioxide, passes into the venules, then veins. Label the vein indicated by number *6*. Blood then returns to the heart via veins called the superior and inferior venae cava.

- Pulmonary circulation: the circuit that the blood makes from the heart to the lungs for the purpose of ridding the body of carbon dioxide and picking up oxygen.

The general circulation that transports oxygen to all tissues of the body is _____ circulation.

systemic

The combining form *pulmon(o)* means lung, and the suffix *-ary* means pertaining to. *Pulmon/ary* **(pool′mo-nar″e)** means pertaining to the lungs. The heart has four chambers: right atrium (RA), right ventricle (RV), left atrium (LA), and left ventricle (LV). Study and label Figure 8-3 as you read about pulmonary and systemic circulation.

8-6 All tissues of the body, including heart tissue and lung tissue, receive oxygen via the systemic circulation. However, you will need to remember that pulmonary circulation provides the means for the blood to take on oxygen from air that we take into our lungs. Oxygen-deficient blood leaves the heart via the pulmonary _____. After oxygenation that takes place in the lungs, the blood is returned to the heart via the pulmonary _____.

arteries
veins

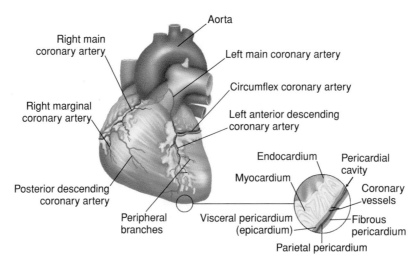

Figure 8-4   Coronary arteries and heart tissues. The two main coronary arteries are the left coronary artery (LCA) and right coronary artery (RCA). The three layers of the heart, beginning with the innermost layer, are endocardium, myocardium, and epicardium (also called the visceral pericardium).

Exercise 1

Match the combining forms in the left column with the structures in the right column. (Selections A-E may be used more than once.)

_____ 1. arter(o)

_____ 2. arteri(o)

_____ 3. arteriol(o)

_____ 4. phleb(o)

_____ 5. pulmon(o)

_____ 6 ven(i)

_____ 7. ven(o)

_____ 8. venul(o)

A. arteriole
B. artery
C. lung
D. vein
E. venule

---

chest

8-7 The muscular heart is the center of the cardiovascular system. It beats normally about 70 times per minute, or more than 100,000 times per day. In the adult, it weighs 230 grams to 340 grams (about one-half pound) and is the size of a clenched fist. The heart lies in the thorac/ic **(thə-ras′ik)** cavity. You learned earlier that the thoracic cavity is the _____ cavity.

The heart lies just left of the midline of the body, between the lungs, in a space called the medi-astinum **(me″de-əs-ti′nəm)**. The media/stinum is an area in the chest cavity between the lungs. The mediastinum contains the heart and its large vessels, the trachea, the esophagus, and nearby structures such as the lymph nodes. Write this new word, which refers to the area between the lungs: _____.

mediastinum

8-8 Special arteries supply blood to the heart itself. The combining form *coron(o)* means crown. *Coronary* **(kor′ə-nar″e)** means encircling in the manner of a crown. Blood vessels that supply oxy-gen to the heart encircle it in a crownlike fashion (Figure 8-4). Arteries that supply blood to the heart are _____ arteries.

coronary

The wall of the heart consists primarily of cardiac muscle tissue, myocardium **(mi″o-kahr′de-əm)**. You probably remember that *my(o)* means muscle. The term *myocardium* is the product of combining *my(o)* with *cardi(o)* and *-ium*, which means membrane. (One *i* is dropped to facilitate pronunciation.) *My(o)* and *cardi(o)* are often used together, so it is easier to remember that *myocardi(o)* means myocardium.

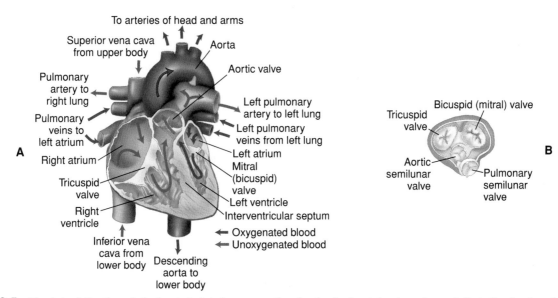

Figure 8-5   Blood circulation through the heart. **A,** Anterior cross section showing the heart chambers. *Arrows* indicate the direction of blood flow through the heart. **B,** Heart valves (viewed from above), the structures that prevent backflow of blood by opening and closing with each heartbeat.

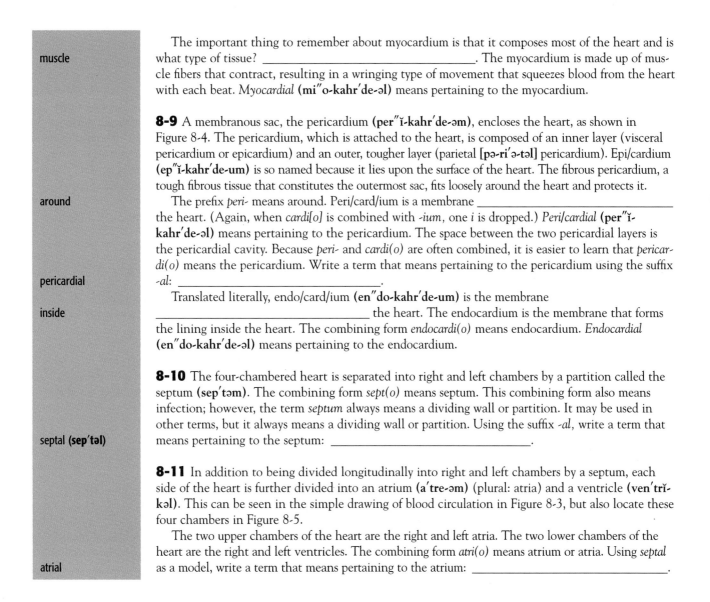

muscle

    The important thing to remember about myocardium is that it composes most of the heart and is what type of tissue? _____. The myocardium is made up of muscle fibers that contract, resulting in a wringing type of movement that squeezes blood from the heart with each beat. *Myocardial* (**mi″o-kahr′de-əl**) means pertaining to the myocardium.

    8-9 A membranous sac, the pericardium (**per″ĭ-kahr′de-əm**), encloses the heart, as shown in Figure 8-4. The pericardium, which is attached to the heart, is composed of an inner layer (visceral pericardium or epicardium) and an outer, tougher layer (parietal [**pə-ri′ə-təl**] pericardium). Epi/cardium (**ep″ĭ-kahr′de-um**) is so named because it lies upon the surface of the heart. The fibrous pericardium, a tough fibrous tissue that constitutes the outermost sac, fits loosely around the heart and protects it.

around

    The prefix *peri-* means around. Peri/card/ium is a membrane _____ the heart. (Again, when *cardi[o]* is combined with *-ium,* one *i* is dropped.) *Peri/cardial* (**per″ĭ-kahr′de-əl**) means pertaining to the pericardium. The space between the two pericardial layers is the pericardial cavity. Because *peri-* and *cardi(o)* are often combined, it is easier to learn that *pericardi(o)* means the pericardium. Write a term that means pertaining to the pericardium using the suffix

pericardial

-al: _____.

inside

    Translated literally, endo/card/ium (**en″do-kahr′de-um**) is the membrane _____ the heart. The endocardium is the membrane that forms the lining inside the heart. The combining form *endocardi(o)* means endocardium. *Endocardial* (**en″do-kahr′de-əl**) means pertaining to the endocardium.

    8-10 The four-chambered heart is separated into right and left chambers by a partition called the septum (**sep′təm**). The combining form *sept(o)* means septum. This combining form also means infection; however, the term *septum* always means a dividing wall or partition. It may be used in other terms, but it always means a dividing wall or partition. Using the suffix *-al,* write a term that

septal (**sep′təl**)

means pertaining to the septum: _____.

    8-11 In addition to being divided longitudinally into right and left chambers by a septum, each side of the heart is further divided into an atrium (**a′tre-əm**) (plural: atria) and a ventricle (**ven′trĭ-kəl**). This can be seen in the simple drawing of blood circulation in Figure 8-3, but also locate these four chambers in Figure 8-5.

    The two upper chambers of the heart are the right and left atria. The two lower chambers of the heart are the right and left ventricles. The combining form *atri(o)* means atrium or atria. Using *septal*

atrial

as a model, write a term that means pertaining to the atrium: _____.

8-12 The term *ventricle* is also applied to a chamber of the brain. Therefore *ventricul(o)* refers to a ventricle of either the heart or the brain. By analyzing other parts of the term or the sentence, one can often determine which organ is affected, the brain or the heart.

The heart has both a left ventricle and a right ventricle. *Ventricular* (**ven-trik′u-lər**) means pertaining to a ventricle. Combine *atri(o)*, *ventricul(o)*, and *-ar* to write a term that means pertaining to an atrium and a ventricle of the heart: _____.

8-13 Study the pattern of blood flow through the heart in Figure 8-5, A. Blood that has had much of its oxygen removed enters the heart on the right side of the body through its two largest veins. The large vein by which blood from the trunk and legs enters the heart is the inferior vena cava (**ve′nə ka′və**).* Blood from the head and arms enters the heart by way of the large vein, the superior vena cava. The venae bring the blood to which chamber of the heart? The right _____.

8-14 The right atrium contracts to force blood through a valve to the right ventricle. This is the tricuspid (**tri-kus′pid**) valve, and it is located between the right atrium and the right ventricle. Contraction of the right ventricle forces blood through the pulmonary artery, which branches and carries blood to the _____. As blood flows through the lungs, it picks up a fresh supply of oxygen and returns to the left side of the heart by way of the pulmonary veins. The pulmonary veins bring the blood to the left atrium.

The left atrium contracts and forces blood into the left ventricle. The flow of blood from the left atrium to the left ventricle is controlled by the mitral (**mi′trəl**) _____, also called the bicuspid valve. This richly oxygenated blood is then pumped into the aorta (**a-or′tə**) from the left ventricle. The aorta is the largest artery of the body. It branches into smaller arteries to carry blood all over the body.

8-15 In normal heart function, valves close and prevent backflow of blood when the heart contracts. Valves between the atria and ventricles are atrioventricular valves—the tricuspid valve on the right side and the bicuspid or mitral valve on the left side (Figure 8-5, B). *Cuspid* refers to the little flaps of tissue that make up the valve. Remembering that *bi-* means two, the bi/cuspid valve has _____ flaps. The left atrioventricular valve is generally called the mitral (**mi′trəl**) valve in medicine, so named because the two valve flaps are shaped somewhat like the mitered corner joints of a picture frame.

The prefix *tri-* means three. The valve that regulates the flow of blood between the right atrium and the right ventricle is the _____ valve.

8-16 Once again, look at Figure 8-5 and locate the pulmonary valve. It regulates the flow of blood from the right ventricle to the pulmonary trunk, which divides into _____ arteries that lead to the lungs. *Pulmonary* means pertaining to the lungs, and vessels that carry blood from the heart to the lungs are pulmonary arteries. Note that vessels that carry blood from the lungs back to the heart are pulmonary _____.

After flowing from the left atrium to the left ventricle, blood leaves the heart by way of the _____ valve, which regulates the flow of blood into the aorta. The pulmonary and aortic valves are also called semilunar (**sem″e-loo′nər**) valves (because of the half-moon appearance of the valve cusps).

8-17 Only a few words use this combining form *valv(o)*, but all pertain to a valve. *Valv/al* (**val′vəl**) and *valv/ar* (**val′vər**) both pertain to a _____. *Valv/ate* (**val′vāt**) means pertaining to or having valves.

Valvula means a valve, especially a small valve. The combining form *valvul(o)* is also used in words to mean valve. *Valvul/ar* (**val′vu-lər**), having valves, is a synonym for *valvate*.

8-18 It is important to remember that both atria contract simultaneously, followed by simultaneous contraction of both ventricles. The cardiac conduction system, composed of highly specialized

Margin terms:

atrioventricular (a″tre-o-ven-trik′u-lər)

atrium

lungs

valve

two

tricuspid

pulmonary

veins

aortic (a-or′tik)

valve

---

*Vena cava (Latin: *vena*, veins; *cava*, cavity).

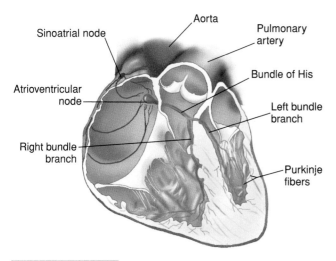

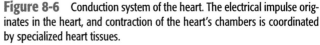

Figure 8-6   Conduction system of the heart. The electrical impulse originates in the heart, and contraction of the heart's chambers is coordinated by specialized heart tissues.

tissue that is capable of producing and conveying electrical impulses, is responsible for the coordinated contraction (Figure 8-6).

Find the sino/atrial (**si″no-a′tre-əl**) (SA) node, located at the junction of the right atrium and the superior vena cava. Electrical impulses arise spontaneously in the SA node and stimulate contraction. The SA node is the natural pacemaker of the heart. The SA node is also called the sinus node. The combining form *sin(o)* means sinus. A sinus is a cavity or channel. Perhaps you are more familiar with the sinuses near the nose (air cavities that sometimes drain or become inflamed in sinus/itis). The term *sinusitis* does not use the combining form.

Use *sin(o)* + *atrial* to write the name of the natural pacemaker of the heart, the

sinoatrial

_____ node.

8-19 The electrical impulse generated by the SA node travels through both atria to the atrio/ventricul/ar node (AV node), which in turn conducts the impulse to the atrioventricular bundle (AV bundle, called also the bundle of His) and then to the Purkinje (**pər-kin′je**) fibers and walls of the ventricles. This highly specialized system results in simultaneous contraction of the atria, followed by contraction of the ventricles.

atrioventricular

AV node means the _____ node. This special type of cardiac tissue is located near the septal wall between the left and right atria. The atria contract while the electrical impulse is briefly delayed in the AV node.

Another name for the atrioventricular bundle or AV bundle is the bundle of His, named after the Swiss physician Wilhelm His, Jr. Purkinje fibers are the termination of the bundle branches. These fibers, spread throughout the right and left ventricles, are specialized to carry the impulse at a high velocity and cause the ventricles to contract.

8-20 The heart and blood vessels work together to provide a continuous supply of oxygen and nutrients to cells throughout the body. Observe the difference in thickness of arteries, veins, and capillaries in Figure 8-7. All three types of vessels are lined with endothelium, a layer of epithelial cells, which secretes substances that prevent blood clotting and regulate the tone of the vessels. Arteries and veins have three additional layers: an inner layer, a muscular layer, and a white fibrous outer layer. Arteries are thicker than veins, and their outer layer is elastic, allowing them to expand as the heartbeat forces blood into them.

Arteries carry blood away from the heart. For this reason, blood pressure is much higher in

arteries

_____ than in veins. Veins also contain valves at various intervals to control the direction of the blood flow back to the heart.

8-21 The aorta is the main trunk of the systemic arterial system (Figure 8-8). Arteries branch out either directly or indirectly from the aorta, which arises from the left ventricle of the heart. Each artery is responsible for conveying oxygen and nutrients to specific organs and tissues, as indicated in Figure 8-9.

To identify and discuss location, anatomists divide the aorta into three major portions: the ascending aorta, the aortic arch, and descending aorta. The descending aorta is further divided into the thoracic and the abdominal aorta.

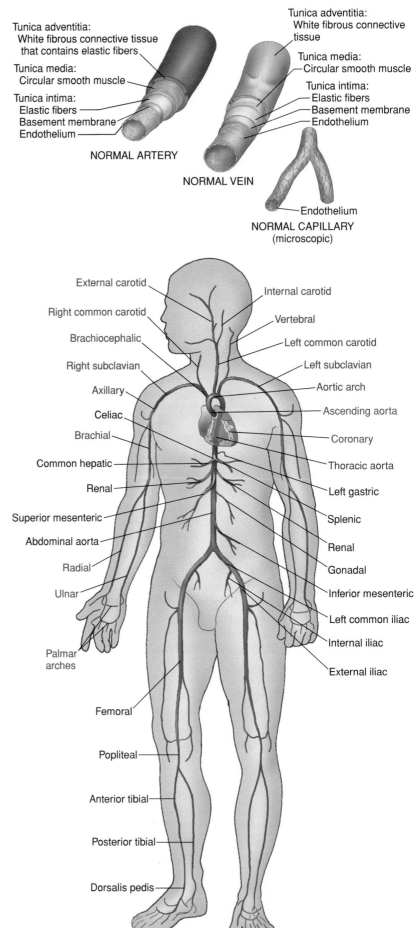

Figure 8-7 Comparison of blood vessels. Observe the difference in thickness of the walls of arteries, veins, and capillaries. A capillary wall consists of a single layer of endothelial cells. Arteries are thicker than veins, and their outer walls contain elastic fibers. The thickness of the outer wall varies with the location of the artery.

Tunica adventitia:
 White fibrous connective tissue
  that contains elastic fibers
Tunica media:
 Circular smooth muscle
Tunica intima:
 Elastic fibers
 Basement membrane
 Endothelium
NORMAL ARTERY

Tunica adventitia:
 White fibrous connective
  tissue
Tunica media:
 Circular smooth muscle
Tunica intima:
 Elastic fibers
 Basement membrane
 Endothelium
NORMAL VEIN

Endothelium
NORMAL CAPILLARY
(microscopic)

External carotid
Right common carotid
Brachiocephalic
Right subclavian
Axillary
Celiac
Brachial
Common hepatic
Renal
Superior mesenteric
Abdominal aorta
Radial
Ulnar
Palmar arches
Femoral
Popliteal
Anterior tibial
Posterior tibial
Dorsalis pedis

Internal carotid
Vertebral
Left common carotid
Left subclavian
Aortic arch
Ascending aorta
Coronary
Thoracic aorta
Left gastric
Splenic
Renal
Gonadal
Inferior mesenteric
Left common iliac
Internal iliac
External iliac

Figure 8-8 Anterior view of the aorta and its principal arterial branches. Labels for the ascending, arch, thoracic, and abdominal aorta and their corresponding arteries are shown in *red, green, purple,* and *black,* respectively.

THE AORTA AND ITS BRANCHES

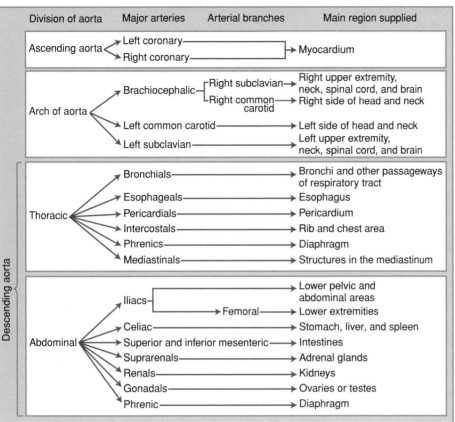

Figure 8-9 Schematic presentation of the divisions of the aorta and the corresponding regions of the body to which blood is supplied.

8-22 As the aorta emerges from the left ventricle, it stretches upward. At this point it is called the _____ aorta. It gives off two branches, the right and left coronary arteries, that transport blood to the heart. The ascending aorta then turns to the left, forming an arch that is called the arch of the aorta, or the aortic arch.

ascending

The descending aorta is a continuation of the aortic arch. The portion of the descending aorta in the thorax is called the _____ aorta. The portion of the descending aorta in the abdomen is called the _____ aorta.

thoracic
abdominal
aorta

Aort/ic (**a-or´tik**) means pertaining to the _____. *Intra/aortic* (**in″trə-a-or´tik**) means within the aorta.

Exercise 2

Complete the table by writing the meaning of each word part that is listed.

COMBINING FORM	MEANING
1. aort(o)	_____
2. atri(o)	_____
3. endocardi(o)	_____
4. mediastin(o)	_____
5. myocardi(o)	_____
6. pericardi(o)	_____
7. sept(o)	_____
8. valv(o)	_____
9. valvul(o)	_____
10. ventricul(o)	_____

EXERCISE 3

Write a word in each blank to complete these sentences that describe circulation.

Oxygen-poor blood is delivered to the right side of the heart via the two largest veins, the superior and inferior

(1) _____ _____. The blood from these two largest

veins is emptied into the chamber of the heart called the right (2) _____. When

the heart contracts, blood is forced through the tricuspid valve to the lower chamber called the

(3) _____ _____. Another contraction of the heart forces

the blood into the pulmonary artery, which branches and carries blood to the (4) _____,

where it picks up oxygen. The pulmonary veins take blood back to the heart chamber called the

(5) _____ _____. The flow of blood from the left atrium

to the left ventricle is controlled by the (6) _____ valve. Blood is then pumped into the

largest artery in the body, the (7) _____. This vessel branches many times to become

arteries, which again branch many times to become the smallest arteries, called

(8) _____, which in turn branch to become the smallest vessels, where oxygen is

delivered to body tissues. These vessels, called (9) _____, are composed of only a single

layer of cells and are continuous with venules, which in turn are continuous with larger vessels called

(10) _____. These vessels are directly or indirectly connected with the venae cavae.

DIAGNOSTIC TESTS AND PROCEDURES

arteries

8-23 The <u>heart rate</u> and <u>blood pressure</u> (BP) give a preliminary indication of how the heart is functioning. Arteries are popularly used to measure blood pressure, and the reading is a reflection of cardiac output and arterial resistance. In other words, blood pressure measures the amount of pressure on the walls of the arteries. The blood pressure reading is a reflection of the quantity of blood flow from the heart and resistance in the walls of the _____.

hypotension (hi″po-ten′shən)

8-24 Hyper/tension (hi″pər-ten′shən) is increased blood pressure. Decreased blood pressure is _____.

Blood pressure is measured using an apparatus called a <u>sphygmomanometer</u>* (sfig″mo-mə-nom′ə-ter) (Figure 8-10). A direct measurement can be obtained only by measuring pressure within a vessel or the heart itself, as in heart catheterization, which is described later in this section.

Blood pressure is at its highest point when the ventricles contract. This is known as systole (sis′to-le). Relaxation of the ventricles is diastole (di-as′to-le).† See the blood flow in the atria and ventricles during contraction and relaxation of the heart (Figure 8-11). The blood pressure measured when the ventricles contract is the <u>systolic</u> (sis-tol′ik) <u>pressure</u>. The blood pressure measured when the ventricles relax is called the _____ pressure.

diastolic (di″ə-stol′ik)

8-25 Blood pressure is usually expressed as a fraction. The standard unit of measurement is millimeters of mercury (mm Hg). For example, a healthy young person has a blood pressure of approximately 120/80 mm Hg. The higher reading is the systolic pressure, and the lower reading is the diastolic pressure. In the example of a BP reading of 120/80, the systolic pressure is 120 mm Hg and the _____ pressure is 80 mm Hg.

diastolic

Four factors that increase blood pressure are increased cardiac output, increased blood volume, increased blood viscosity, and loss of elasticity of the arterial walls.

---

*Sphygmomanometer (Greek: *sphygmos*, pulse + *manos*, thin + *metron*, measure).
†Diastole (Greek: *diastole*, expansion).

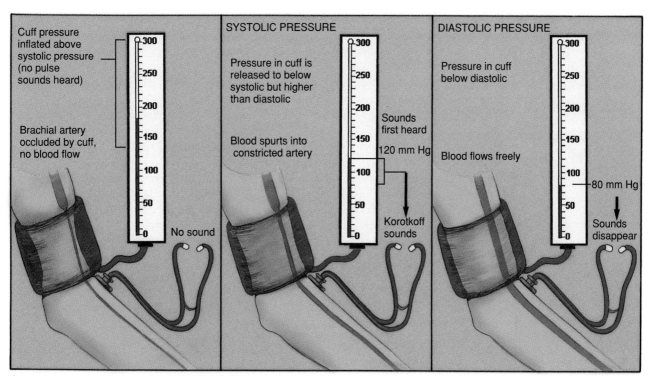

Figure 8-10 Measurement of blood pressure. Systolic pressure is due to ventricular contraction. Diastolic pressure occurs when the ventricles relax. The sounds heard through the stethoscope result from blood flow in the artery. The first sound heard represents the systolic pressure. As the pressure declines, the last sound heard represents the diastolic pressure. This example represents a normal blood pressure reading of 120/80. In arteriosclerosis the arteries lose their elasticity and cannot expand when blood is pumped into them.

---

stethoscope

8-26 Used less often than *thorac(o)*, another combining form, *steth(o)*, also means chest. The stetho/scope (steth′o-skōp) is placed on the chest to listen to heart sounds, particularly closing of the heart valves. Heart murmurs are abnormal sounds produced by improper functioning of the valves. The stethoscope is also used to hear sounds of breathing (see Figure 6-13, *B*) and intestinal action and to take blood pressure. Write the name of this instrument placed on the chest to hear heart sounds: _____.

8-27 The rhythmic expansion of an artery lying near the surface of the skin can be felt with the finger. This is known as the pulse (puls). All arteries have a pulse, but the one most often used is the radial artery on the anterolateral aspect of the wrist.

A normal pulse rate in a resting state is 60 to 100 beats per minute. An increased pulse rate (greater than 100 beats per minute) is tachy/cardia (tak″ĭ-kahr′de-ə). Using *brady-*, write a word that means a decreased pulse rate (less than 60 beats per minute):
_____.

bradycardia
(brad″e-kahr′de-ə)

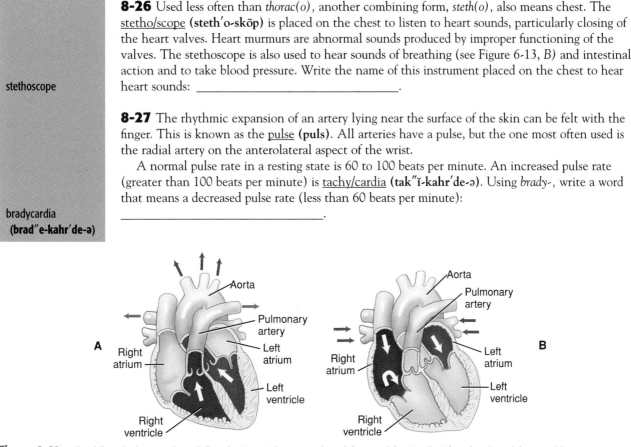

Figure 8-11 Blood flow during systole and diastole. **A,** Systole, contraction of the ventricles. **B,** Diastole, relaxation of the ventricles.

8-28 The impulses arising in the SA node and carried by the cardiac conduction system produce electrical currents that can be measured in electro/cardio/graphy (e-lek″tro-kahr″de-og′rə-fe), the process of recording the electrical currents of the heart (see Figure 3-3). Write the name of the record produced in electrocardiography: _____.The name of the instrument used in electrocardiography is an electrocardiograph (e-lek″tro-kahr′de-o-graf″). Normal heart rhythm is called sinus rhythm.

A Holter (hōl′tər) monitor is a portable electrocardiograph that a person can wear while conducting normal daily activities. This device records heart activity over time and during various activities to aid in the diagnosis of cardiac problems that occur intermittently.

8-29 Laboratory tests for cardiovascular disorders include testing for fats and cardiac enzymes in the blood. Lipids (lip′idz) are fatty substances in the body and include cholesterol (kə-les′tər-ol″) and triglycerides (tri-glis′ər-īdz). High levels of these two lipids are associated with greater risk of arteriosclerosis (ahr-tēr″e-o-sklə-ro′sis), hardening of the arteries. Two examples of lipids associated with a greater risk of cardiovascular disease are triglycerides and

_____.

Lipo/proteins (lip″o, li″po-pro′tēnz) are special proteins that transport lipids in the blood. The elevation of low-density lipoproteins (LDL) is associated with an increased risk of cardiovascular disease. High levels of high-density lipoproteins (HDL) are associated with decreased cardiac risk profiles.

8-30 Certain enzymes are released into the bloodstream by damaged heart muscle. Levels of these enzymes can be measured in blood tests called lactate dehydrogenase (lak′tāt de-hi′dro-jən″ās) test (LDH) and creatine kinase (kre′ə-tin ki′nās) test (CK), also called creatine phosphokinase (fos″fo-ki′nās) (CPK). Levels of these enzymes usually rise within a few hours after a heart attack. LDH and CPK are blood tests to assess _____ damage.

8-31 Several diagnostic procedures are used to help assess heart disease, many of which are noninvasive. Examination of a chest x-ray gives information about the size and position of the heart.

Stress tests measure the heart's response during controlled physiologic stress, usually exercise. In the treadmill exercise test (or treadmill stress test), an electrocardiogram (ECG) and other measurements are taken while the patient walks on an inclined treadmill at varying speeds and inclines. Measuring the heart's response while exercising in this manner is called a treadmill _____ test. The thallium stress test and other nuclear medicine procedures, also measure cardiovascular function, particularly coronary artery disease.

8-32 Diagnostic procedures are often able to detect abnormalities before the heart is damaged. Because each procedure has special benefits, several may be performed. Echo/cardio/graphy (ek″o-kahr″de-og′rə-fe), or ECHO, is the use of ultrasonography (ul″trə-sə-nog′rə-fe) in diagnosing heart disease. A record of the heart obtained by directing ultrasonic waves through the chest wall is an_____. Figure 8-12 is an echocardiogram that shows the chambers of the heart and a large thrombus.

Doppler echocardiography gives information about the direction and pattern of blood flow within the heart. Doppler scanning and additional specialized radiographic procedures provide additional information about heart functions.

8-33 Cardiac MRI, magnetic resonance imaging, may be done, as well as computed tomography (to-mog′rə-fe) (CT).The latter produces cross-sectional images of an organ similar to what one would see if the organ were actually cut into sections. The record produced by tomography is a _____.

Margin terms: electrocardiogram (e-lek″tro-kahr′de-o-gram″); cholesterol; heart; stress; echocardiogram (ek″o-kahr′de-o-gram″); tomogram (to′mo-gram)

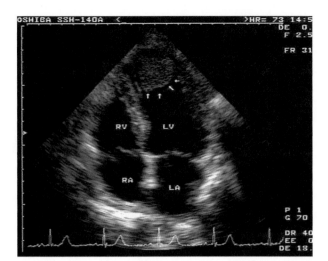

Figure 8-12   Echocardiogram. The heart is viewed from the top, and the four chambers *(RV, RA, LV, LA)* are visible, as well as a large thrombus, indicated by the *arrows.*

Positron emission tomography (PET) is used in other areas also but is especially helpful in examining blood flow in the heart and blood vessels. In this procedure, the patient is injected with a radioactive element, which becomes concentrated in the heart, and color-coded images are produced.

8-34 Arterio/graphy (ahr″tēr-e-og′rə-fe) is radiography of arteries after injection of radiopaque material into the bloodstream. Literally, this word means recording of the arteries. Build a word that means the film produced in arteriography: _____. Through common usage, arteriograph (ahr-tēr′e-o-graf) is used interchangeably with arteriogram, just as *photo/graph* is used to mean the record (picture) produced in photography. The combining form *phot(o)* means light. Coronary arteriography is a radiographic procedure used to study coronary arteries.

Digital subtraction angiography (DSA) provides computer-enhanced radiographic images of blood vessels filled with contrast material.

arteriogram
(ahr-tēr′e-o-gram)

8-35 Aorto/graphy (a″or-tog′rə-fe) is radiography of the aorta after introducing a contrast medium. The film produced by aortography is an _____. Different areas of the aorta are generally studied, rather than visualizing all of its divisions. Thoracic, abdominal, and renal aortography are examples of areas of the aorta that are studied. Radiology of the aorta in the abdominal area is called abdominal _____.

aortogram
(a-or′to-gram″)

aortography

8-36 There are also several invasive tests available to diagnose cardiovascular disease. Cardiac catheterization (kath″ə-tər-ĭ-za′shən) is a diagnostic procedure in which a catheter (kath′ə-tər) is introduced through an incision into a large blood vessel of the arm, leg, or neck and threaded through the circulatory system to the heart. Pressures and patterns of blood flow can be determined in catheterization (Figure 8-13).

The catheter enables the use of contrast media that enhance x-ray images of the heart and its vessels. A radiographic procedure that produces an angiogram (an′je-o-gram″) is called angiography (an″je-og′rə-fe). Radiography of the coronary arteries is coronary _____. Cardiac angiography, also called angiocardiography (an″je-o-kahr″de-og′rə-fe), is radiography of the heart and its vessels.

angiography

Electrophysiologic studies (EPS) use electrode catheters to pace the heart and can identify disturbances in the rhythm of the heart that would otherwise be inapparent.

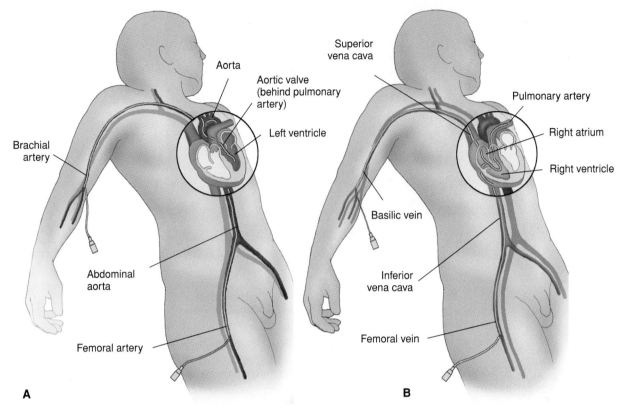

Figure 8-13   Heart catheterization. **A,** Left-sided. **B,** Right-sided. Progress of the catheter is monitored by fluoroscopy as it is threaded through blood vessels to reach the heart. Fluoroscopy gives the physician immediate images of the location of the catheter throughout the procedure. The right side of the heart may be the only side examined because left-sided heart catheterization is riskier.

Exercise 4

Write a word in each blank to complete these sentences.

1. Increased blood pressure is _____.

2. Decreased pulse is _____.

3. Relaxation of the ventricles is called _____.

4. Blood pressure that is measured when the ventricles contract is the _____ pressure.

5. A portable electrocardiograph that a person can wear is a _____ monitor.

6. Cholesterol and triglycerides are fatty substances called _____.

7. LDL and HDL are special proteins called _____.

8. Cardiac ultrasonography is called _____.

✚ PATHOLOGIES

Heart Pathologies

cardiovascular

8-37 Cardiovascular disease is any abnormal condition characterized by dysfunction of the heart and blood vessels. Diagnosis and treatment of cardiovascular disorders have improved, but cardiovascular disease remains the major cause of death in the United States.

Heart disease can be classified in many ways. One method is based on whether the cause of the heart dysfunction developed away from the heart (as in diseases of the arteries), or if the heart itself was the primary site of the dysfunction. The leading cause of death in the United States is _____ disease.

Learn the meaning of these word parts that are used to describe heart abnormalities.

Additional Word Parts for Heart Pathologies

Word Part	Meaning
rhythm(o), rrhythm(o)	rhythm
de-	down, from, or reversing
-stenosis	narrowing; stricture

atrium

8-38 <u>Primary cardiac diseases</u> include those caused by structural cardiac defects, as well as inflammation and infection that originate within the heart. Defects are sometimes present in one of the four chambers of the heart, in one of the heart valves, or in the septum that divides the two sides of the heart. If heart disease is present at birth, it is a <u>congenital heart disease</u>.

Atrio/megaly (**a″tre-o-meg′ə-le**) is abnormal enlargement of an
_____ of the heart.

atria

8-39 A <u>ventricular septal defect</u> (VSD) is an abnormal opening in the septum dividing the right and the left ventricles. Look at Figure 8-5 and be sure that you can locate where a ventricular septal defect would occur. This defect is a type of congenital heart disease. An <u>atrial septal defect</u> (ASD) is also a congenital heart disease. An atrial septal defect is an abnormal opening in the part of the septum that separates the right and the left _____.

blue (or bluish)

8-40 There are other congenital heart diseases, but atrial septal defects and ventricular septal defects account for 30% to 40% of heart diseases that are present at birth. Almost all <u>congenital heart defects</u> interrupt the normal flow of blood through the heart and vessels. Heart murmurs—abnormal heart sounds—are often heard. <u>Cyanosis</u> may also be present. Cyan/osis is a _____ discoloration of the skin and mucous membranes that results from insufficient oxygen to the tissues.

Three other congenital heart diseases are <u>patent ductus arteriosus</u> (**duk′təs ahr-tēr″e-o′səs**) (PDA), <u>coarctation of the aorta</u> (CoA), and <u>tetralogy of Fallot</u> (**tĕ-tral′ə-je ov fə-lo′**). Patent ductus arteriosus is an abnormal opening between the pulmonary artery and the aorta. There is narrowing of a part of the aorta in coarctation of the aorta. There are four congenital heart defects in tetralogy of Fallot, named for a French physician. It is difficult to remember the types of defects, but it is important to remember that these three diseases are congenital heart diseases and surgery may be indicated.

without

8-41 Normally the intervals between pulses are of equal length. Remembering that *a-* means no or without, <u>a/rrhythmia</u> (**ə-rith′me-ə**) is _____ rhythm. The combining forms *rrhythm(o)* and *rhythm(o)* mean rhythm. Arrhythmia is the same as arhythmia and is the more common spelling.

A variation in the normal rhythm of the heartbeat is an arrhythmia. Although this term is more commonly used, *dysrhythmia* (**dis-rith′me-ə**) would be more technically correct. Dysrhythmia is a disturbance of rhythm. Common usage generally determines whether one uses one or two *r*s in medical terms that pertain to rhythm. Write this new term that means an abnormal, disordered, or disturbed rhythm: _____.

dysrhythmia

Heart flutters are rapid contractions of either the atria or the ventricles and can be seen on the electrocardiogram. Heart <u>palpitations</u>,* however, are subjective sensations of a pounding or racing heart. It can be associated with heart disease, but some persons experience palpitations and yet have no evidence of heart disease. In these cases, the palpitations are believed to be normal emotional responses to stress.

fibrillation

8-42 <u>Ventricular fibrillation</u> (**fĭ-brĭ-la′shən**) is a severe cardiac arrhythmia in which ventricular contractions are too rapid and uncoordinated for effective blood circulation. A cardiac arrhythmia marked by rapid, uncoordinated contractions is called _____.

*Palpitations (Latin: *palpitare*, to move frequently and rapidly).

fibrillation

Sometimes a defibrillator is used to alleviate fibrillation. (The prefix *de-* is used to mean down, from, or reversing. It is in the latter sense that it is used here.) A defibrillator (**de-fib″rĭ-la′tər**) is an electronic apparatus that has defibrillator paddles that are used to make contact with the patient and deliver a preset voltage of electricity to shock the heart. Defibrillation (**de-fib″rĭ-la′shən**) stops_____. Ventricular fibrillation is often a cause of cardiac arrest. Another name for cardiac arrest is a/systole (**a-sis′to-le**), which means absence of heartbeat or contraction.

block

You learned earlier that the heart has a special structure, the sinoatrial node, where electrical impulses arise and stimulate contraction. Impairment in the conduction of the impulse from the SA node to other parts of the heart is known as a heart block. When the electrical impulse is not conducted throughout the heart, normal heart contraction does not occur. This condition is known as a heart _____. The condition may be asymptomatic and require no intervention, but implantation of an artificial pacemaker (described later in the surgical intervention section) may be necessary in complete heart block.

8-43 Atrial fibrillation, a cardiac arrhthymia characterized by disorganized electrical activity in the atria, results in reduced stroke volume (the amount of blood ejected by a ventricle during contraction) but is not as life threatening as ventricular fibrillation. Other arrhythmias that can be detected by electrocardiography include bradycardia, tachycardia, premature ventricular contractions (PVC), and atrio/ventricular block (AVB).

In paroxysmal (**par″ok-siz′məl**) atrial tachycardia (PAT), the patient may detect palpitations and a racing heartbeat (150-250 beats per minute) that occur and stop suddenly. *Paroxysmal* means occurring in sudden, repeated episodes.

ventricles

Atrio/ventricular block is a disorder of impulse transmission between the atria and the _____.

8-44 In many types of heart disease, the heart attempts to compensate for its deficit by working harder. Cardio/megaly (**kahr″de-o-meg″ə-le**) may result. Cardio/megaly is _____ of the heart.

enlargement

smallness

Micro/cardia (**mi-kro-kahr′de-ə**), the opposite of cardiomegaly, is abnormal _____ of the heart.

oxygen

8-45 Myocardial infarction (**in-fahrk′shən**) is necrosis of a portion of cardiac muscle caused by an obstruction or a blood clot in a coronary artery. Cells die when deprived of oxygen. The death of cells in an area of the myocardium because of oxygen deprivation is myocardial infarction. A myocardial infarction (MI) is a heart attack. An/ox/ia means an abnormal condition characterized by absence of _____. A localized area of damaged tissue resulting from anoxia is called an infarct* (**in′fahrkt**).

infarction

MI is the most common cause of death in the United States. Whether death occurs after MI largely depends on the resulting damage to the myocardium. Those who survive often suffer complications of heart function. When areas of the myocardium die because of lack of oxygen, this is called myocardial _____.

congestive

8-46 Myocardial infarction and other disorders in which there is insufficient oxygen to the heart may lead to congestive heart failure (CHF), also called congestive heart disease. CHF is an abnormal condition that reflects impaired cardiac function. The patient experiences weakness, breathlessness, and edema (**ə-de′mə**). Edema is an abnormal accumulation of fluid in the interstitial spaces of tissue. This condition is called _____ heart failure.

ischemia

8-47 Insufficient blood flow to an area is termed ischemia (**is-ke′me-əh**). If the myocardial demand for oxygen exceeds the capability of diseased coronary arteries, myocardial _____ results. The patient may experience chest pain, often called angina pectoris† (**an-ji′nə, an′ jə-nə pek′tə-ris**), or simply angina. The pain usually radiates along the neck, jaw, and shoulder and down the left arm. The pain may be relieved by rest or medication.

---

*Infarct (Latin: *infarcire*, to stuff).
†Angina pectoris (Latin: *angor*, quinsy; *pectus*, breast or chest).

If myocardial ischemia is prolonged, it often leads to myocardial infarction. Rest is an important part of recovery after a heart attack. The patient is usually left with some heart damage, often resulting in failure of the heart to function normally. This deficiency of the heart is called <u>cardiac insufficiency</u>. If the damage is too severe, surgical intervention may be necessary.

8-48 Heart valves can also be defective, resulting in the valves not opening fully, as in <u>valvul/ar</u> <u>stenosis</u>. *Stenosis* (**stə-no′sis**) means narrowing. When a valve is stenos/ed, it becomes constricted or

narrowing

narrower. Valvular stenosis is _____ of the opening created by the valve. Stenosis of any of the heart's valves can decrease blood circulation.

Valves may also become infected and inflamed. <u>Valvul/itis</u> (**val″vu-li′tis**) is inflammation of a valve, especially a heart valve. Build a new word that specifically means inflammation of the valves of the heart by using a combining form that means heart + valvulitis:

**cardiovalvulitis
(kahr″de-o-val″vu-
li′tis)**

_____.

Weakening of one or both cusps when the heart contracts is called <u>mitral valve prolapse</u> (MVP). *Prolapse* means sagging. When a valve prolapses, such as in MVP, the valve sags rather than opening fully. Symptoms vary from absent to severe, and the condition may be associated with sounds heard through a stethoscope, including a clicking sound or heart murmur.

8-49 <u>Rheumatic</u> (**roo-mat′ik**) <u>fever</u>, usually occurring in childhood, may develop as a delayed reaction to an inadequately treated infection of the upper respiratory tract by certain pathogenic streptococci (group A beta-hemolytic). The disease may affect the brain, heart, joints, or skin. <u>Rheumatic heart disease</u> is damage to heart muscle and heart valves caused by episodes of rheumatic fever. Permanent damage to the heart or the valves may occur. This type of damage is called

rheumatic

_____ heart disease.

8-50 <u>Cardio/myo/pathy</u> (**kahr″de-o-mi-op′ə-the**) is a general diagnostic term that designates primary myocardial disease. In other words, the disease originated in the myocardium. A disease of the myocardium that is not attributable to outside causes that results in insufficient oxygen, damaged

cardiomyopathy

valves, or high blood pressure is called a _____. <u>Myocarditis</u> (**mi″o-kahr-di′tis**) is an example of a cardiomyopathy.

inflammation

Myocard/itis means _____ of the myocardium. This may be caused by an infection, rheumatic fever, a chemical agent, or a complication of another disease.

8-51 Inflammation of the inner lining of the heart is _____.

**endocarditis
(en″do-kahr-di′tis)**

<u>Endocarditis</u> is caused by infectious microorganisms that invade the lining of the heart, quite often the valves.

Using *-itis*, build a word that means inflammation of the pericardium:

**pericarditis
(per″ĭ-kahr-di′tis)**

_____. In <u>pericarditis</u>, the pericardium becomes inflamed, owing to an infectious microorganism, a cancerous growth, or a variety of other causes.

8-52 <u>Hemo/pericardium</u> (**he″mo-per″ĭ-kahr′de-əm**) is an effusion (**ə-fu′zhən**)* of blood into the pericardial space. *Effusion* means the escape of fluid into a part, such as a cavity. Blood in the pericardial space is called _____. An accumulation of fluid

hemopericardium

in the pericardial space can lead to compression of the heart, which is called <u>cardiac tamponade</u> (**tam″pon-ād′**).

8-53 <u>Shock</u> is a life-threatening condition in which there is inadequate blood flow to the body's tissues. It is usually associated with inadequate cardiac output, hypotension, and tissue damage. Causes of shock include hemorrhage or dehydration resulting in hypo/vol/emia (**hi″po-vo-le′me-ə**).

low

The term *hypovolemia* means an abnormally _____ circulating blood volume.

---

*Effusion (Latin: *effusion*, pour out).

Write the names of the cardiac pathologies represented by the following definitions. The first letter of each term is given as a clue.

1. enlarged heart c_____

2. a bluish discoloration of the skin resulting from insufficient oxygen c_____

3. a disturbance in the heart rhythm d_____

4. a localized area of damaged tissue resulting from insufficient oxygen i_____

5. insufficient blood flow to an area i_____

6. inflammation of the valves of the heart c_____

7. inflammation of the pericardium p_____

8. a word that means narrowing s_____

9. inflammation of the lining of the heart e_____

10. a life-threatening condition in which blood flow is inadequate s_____

Blood Vessel Pathologies

vasodilation

8-54 Arteries, arterioles, capillaries, venules, and veins make up the network of blood vessels that carry blood. The dilation and constriction of blood vessels influence blood pressure and the distribution of blood to various parts of the body. The vaso/motor (**vas″o-, va″zo-mo′tər**) center located in the brain regulates vasoconstriction (**vas″o-, va″zo-kən-strik′shən**) and vasodilation (**vas″o-, va″zo-di-la′shən**), thus influencing the diameter of the blood vessels.

Vaso/dilation is stretching or dilation of a vessel. In the word *vasodilation*, *dilation* means expansion or stretching. An increase in the diameter of a blood vessel is _____. The opposite of vasodilation is vaso/constriction. When blood vessels constrict, they become narrow. A decrease in the diameter of blood vessels is vasoconstriction.

Learn the meaning of these word parts used to describe disorders of the blood vessels.

Additional Word Parts for Blood Vessel Pathologies

WORD PART	MEANING
aneurysm(o)	aneurysm
ather(o)	yellowish, fatty plaque
embol(o)	embolus

hardening

8-55 The coronary arteries supply blood to the heart tissue. A heart attack may be preceded by coronary artery disease (CAD), an abnormal condition of the coronary arteries that causes a reduced flow of oxygen and nutrients to the myocardium. Arterio/sclerosis (**ahr-tēr″e-o-sklə-ro′sis**) is a thickening and loss of elasticity of the walls of the arteries. Literal interpretation of *arterio/scler/osis* is _____ of the arteries.

Arterio/sclero/tic (**ahr-tēr″e-o-sklə-rot′ik**) heart disease (ASHD) is hardening and thickening of the walls of the coronary arteries. This reduces the oxygen supply to the myocardium and may lead to a heart attack.

atherosclerosis

8-56 Athero/sclerosis (**ath″ər-o-sklə-ro′sis**), a form of arteriosclerosis, is characterized by the formation of fatty deposits on the walls of arteries. Only a few words use the combining form *ather(o)*, which means yellow, fatty plaque. Write the term that means a form of arteriosclerosis characterized by the formation of fatty deposits on the walls of arteries: _____.

The yellowish plaques in atherosclerosis are cholesterol, other lipids, and cellular debris that accumulate in the inner walls of arteries. As atherosclerosis progresses, the vessel walls become fibrotic and calcified and the lumen (cavity) narrows, resulting in reduced blood flow. The plaque creates a risk for occlusion (**o-kloo′zhən**) (blockage) or thrombosis and is one of the major causes of coronary heart disease, angina pectoris, myocardial infarction, and other cardiac disorders. An occlusion is an obstruction or closure.

8-57 Formation of a blood clot in a coronary artery is <u>coronary thrombosis</u> (**throm-bo'sis**). <u>Coronary occlusion</u> is a closing off of a _____ artery. The occlusion may result from a thrombus, but it is more likely due to a narrowing of the lumen of the blood vessel.

Myocardial infarction occurs if an occlusion is complete and no blood is being supplied to an area of the myocardium.

A blood clot in a vessel in the brain is one cause of a <u>cerebro/vascular accident</u> (CVA). This abnormal condition is characterized by occlusion of a vessel of the brain by an embolus, thrombus, or cerebrovascular hemorrhage or spasm and results in ischemia of the brain tissues. CVA, also called stroke, is an abbreviation for _____ accident.

8-58 <u>Scler/osis</u> is a condition characterized by abnormal hardening of tissue. Build a word that means hardening of the aorta: _____.

<u>Stenosis</u> (**stə-no'sis**) means constriction or narrowing of a passage or orifice. <u>Stricture</u> (**strik'chər**) is also used in this sense. Two terms often have the same meaning because words are derived from both the Latin and the Greek languages. In <u>aortic stenosis</u>, narrowing of the aorta, blood cannot flow efficiently from the left ventricle into the aorta and may lead to congestive heart failure. <u>Aortic insufficiency</u> (AI), also called aortic regurgitation, is somewhat less severe, but blood flows back into the left ventricle during diastole because the aortic valve does not close completely. The heart will work harder in an attempt to deliver needed oxygen and nutrients to all the body's cells.

Build a word that means inflammation of the aorta by using the combining form for aorta plus the suffix for inflammation: _____. <u>Angio/card/itis</u> (**an"je-o-kahr-di'tis**) is inflammation of the heart and large blood vessels.

8-59 <u>Angio/stenosis</u> (**an"je-o-stə-no'sis**) is _____ of the diameter of a vessel. Any disease of the arteries is an <u>arterio/pathy</u> (**ahr-ter"e-op'ə-the**). Use *arter(o)* to write a word that means inflammation of an artery: _____.

<u>Peripheral vascular disease</u> (PVD) is blockage or narrowing of arteries that results in interference of adequate blood flow to the extremities, especially those conditions affecting the lower extremities. Atherosclerosis is one cause of PVD.

8-60 An <u>aneurysm</u> (**an'u-rizm**) is a localized dilation or ballooning out of the wall of a blood vessel. Aneurysms can occur in many blood vessels, but most aneurysms are arterial. This is because pressure is higher in the arteries, particularly the aorta. Use the combining form *aneurysm(o)* to write words about aneurysms. *Aneurysm/al* (**an"u-riz'məl**) means pertaining to an

_____.

An aneurysm may rupture, causing hemorrhage, or thrombi may form in the dilated vessel and give rise to emboli (**em'bo-li**) that may obstruct smaller vessels. An <u>embolus</u> (**em'bo-ləs**) is foreign matter (air or gas, a bit of tissue or tumor, or a piece of a thrombus) that circulates in the bloodstream until it becomes lodged in a smaller vessel. An <u>embolism</u> is an abnormal condition in which an embolus becomes lodged in a blood vessel.

8-61 Aneurysms tend to occur at specific sites, most commonly in the abdominal aorta (Figure 8-14). Most patients are asymptomatic until the aneurysm ruptures. Aneurysms may be first discovered by routine examination or during radiographic study performed for another reason. Computed tomography and ultrasound are usually helpful in establishing a diagnosis. Aortography (**a"or-tog'rə-fe**), also called aortic arteriography, is performed for all patients who are to undergo surgical repair of a thoracic aneurysm. The radiographic process in which the aorta and its branches are injected with contrast media for visualization is called

_____.

8-62 An <u>angi/oma</u> (**an"je-o'mə**) is a benign tumor of either blood or lymph vessels. Angiomas are not malignant and sometimes disappear spontaneously. An angioma is either a <u>hem/angi/oma</u> (**he-man"je-o'mə**) or a <u>lymph/angi/oma</u> (**lim-fan"je-o'mə**). A hemangioma is a tumor of

_____ vessels. (Note that the vowel is dropped from *hem[a]* and *lymph[o]* when they are joined with combining forms that begin with a vowel.) A lymph/angi/oma is a tumor composed of lymph vessels.

Margin terms (left column):

coronary

cerebrovascular

aortosclerosis
(a-or"to-sklə-ro'sis)

aortitis (a-or"ti'tis)

narrowing

arteritis (ahr"tə-ri'tis)

aneurysm

aortography

blood

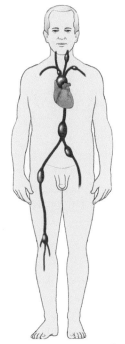

Figure 8-14   Common anatomic sites of arterial aneurysms.

varicose

phlebitis (flə-bi′tis)

8-63 <u>Varicose</u> **(var′ĭ-kōs)** <u>veins</u> are swollen and knotted and occur most often in the legs. They result from sluggish blood flow in combination with weakened walls and incompetent valves in the veins. Unlike arteries that have substantially more muscle and elastic tissue, veins have flaplike valves that prevent blood from flowing backward. Defective valves allow the blood to collect in the veins, which become swollen and knotted. This condition is called

_____ veins (Figure 8-15).

8-64 Using *phleb(o)*, build a word that means inflammation of a vein:

_____.

    <u>Thrombo/phleb/itis</u> **(throm″bo-flə-bi′tis)** is inflammation of a vein associated with a blood clot. <u>Venous thrombosis</u>, formation of a thrombus within a vein, may be a complication of phleb/itis. It may also result from an injury to the leg or prolonged bed confinement.

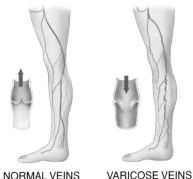

NORMAL VEINS
Functional valves aid
in flow of venous blood
back to heart

VARICOSE VEINS
Failure of valves and
pooling of blood in
superficial veins

Figure 8-15   Normal veins versus varicose veins. Sluggish blood flow, weakened walls, and incompetent valves contribute to varicose veins in the legs, a common location for these enlarged and twisted veins near the surface of the skin.

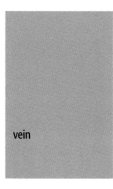

vein

Hemorrhoids (**hem′ə-roidz**) are a type of varicose veins in the lower rectum or anus (see Figure 10-18, B).

8-65 Phlebo/stasis (**flə-bos′tə-sis**) may be a spontaneous slowing down of blood flow in a vein or the result of a deliberate act in which one compresses the vein to control the flow of blood temporarily. In many words, *-stasis* will be used for either of these two meanings.

You will need to remember that *phlebostasis* means either a spontaneous venous stasis or stopping the flow of blood in a _____ by application of a tourniquet (**toor′nĭ-kət**) on an extremity. A tourniquet is a device applied around an extremity to control the circulation and prevent the flow of blood to or from the distal area.

Exercise 6

Write a word in each blank to complete these sentences.

1. A term for a localized dilation or ballooning out of the wall of a blood vessel is _____.

2. CAD is an abbreviation that means _____ artery disease.

3. A closing off of a coronary artery is called coronary _____.

4. Formation of a blood clot in a coronary artery is coronary _____.

5. Formation of fatty deposits on the walls of arteries is a form of arteriosclerosis, called _____.

6. Hardening of the aorta is _____.

7. The term for inflammation of a vein associated with a blood clot is _____.

8. Narrowing of the diameter of the aorta is called aortic _____.

SURGICAL AND THERAPEUTIC INTERVENTIONS

cardiopulmonary

8-66 Cardio/pulmonary resuscitation (**re-sus-ĭ-ta′shən**) (CPR) is a basic emergency procedure for life support, consisting of manual external cardiac massage and artificial respiration. *Pulmonary* refers to the lungs, so *cardio/pulmonary* pertains to the heart and lungs. The artificial respiration can be mouth-to-mouth breathing or a mechanical form of ventilation.

CPR is used in cases of cardiac arrest to establish effective circulation and ventilation in order to prevent irreversible cerebral damage resulting from anoxia. CPR is an abbreviation for _____ resuscitation.

pacemaker

8-67 You learned earlier that the SA node is called the pacemaker of the heart. A second meaning of pacemaker is an artificial cardiac pacemaker, a small battery-powered device that is generally used to increase the heart rate by electrically stimulating the heart muscle. Depending on the patient's need, a cardiac pacemaker may be permanent or temporary and may fire only on demand or at a constant rate (Figure 8-16). Severe bradycardia may indicate the need for an artificial cardiac _____.

Figure 8-16   Artificial cardiac pacemaker.

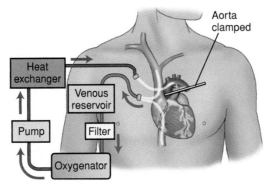

Figure 8-17 Components of a cardiopulmonary bypass system used during heart surgery.

---

cardioverter

pericardium

cardioplegic
(kahr″de-o-plej′ik)

extracorporeal

bypass

atria

artery

8-68 <u>Cardio/version</u> (kahr′de-o-ver″zhən) uses electrical shock to restore the normal rhythm of the heart with a device that delivers a direct-current shock. An <u>automatic implantable cardioverter</u> (kahr′de-o-vər″tər) is a device that detects sustained ventricular tachycardia or fibrillation and terminates it by a shock that restores the normal rhythm. This implanted device is called an automatic implantable _____.

8-69 <u>Peri/cardio/centesis</u> (per″ĭ-kahr″de-o-sən-te′sis) is surgical puncture of the _____. This procedure is performed to draw off fluid that has accumulated in the pericardial space.

8-70 If surgery is to be performed on the heart, <u>cardio/plegia</u> (kahr″de-o-ple′jə) may be necessary to stop myocardial contractions. Solutions used to stop the heart's action so that surgery may be performed on the heart are called _____ solutions.

   Surgeries involving the heart and major vessels generally require <u>cardiopulmonary</u> (kahr″de-o-pool′mə-nar-e) <u>bypass</u>, a procedure in which the heart is bypassed by providing an extra/corporeal* (eks″trə-kor-por′e-əl) (outside the body) device to pump blood. The term that means "outside the body" is _____. The blood is diverted from the heart and lungs to a <u>pump oxygenator</u> (ok′sĭ-jə-na″tor), then returned directly to the aorta and pumped to the rest of the body (Figure 8-17).

8-71 The term *bypass* (bi′pas) is also used to mean bypass surgery. A <u>coronary artery bypass</u> is an open heart surgery in which a prosthesis or a section of a blood vessel is grafted onto one of the coronary arteries, bypassing a blocked or narrowed coronary artery in coronary artery disease. If a vessel from elsewhere in the patient's body is used to provide an alternate route for the blood to circumvent the obstructed coronary artery, the surgery is called a <u>coronary artery bypass graft</u> (CABG), often referred to as "cabbage" (Figure 8-18).

   The vessels that are generally used are a segment of the saphenous (sə-fe′nəs) vein from the patient's leg or the mammary artery. A bypass is also called a <u>shunt</u> (shunt). One that circumvents a vessel that supplies blood to the heart is called a coronary artery

_____.

   Developments in cardiac surgery are heart transplantation and use of an artificial heart. Research continues to bring improvements in these two types of surgeries.

8-72 Atrial or ventricular septal defects usually require surgical closure of the abnormal opening. <u>Atrio/septo/plasty</u> (a″tre-o-sep′to-plas″te) is surgical repair of the septum in the area between the right and left _____.

8-73 There are several procedures used to remove plaque accumulation in major arteries. <u>End/arter/ectomy</u> (end-ahr″tər-ek′tə-me) is surgical excision of arteriosclerotic plaque from the inner wall of an obstructed _____. Endarterectomy does not desig-

---

*Extracorporeal (Latin: *corpus*, body).

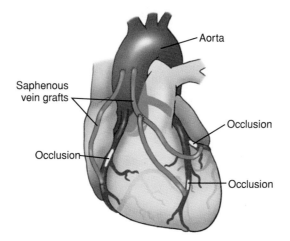

Figure 8-18 Coronary artery bypass graft using saphenous vein grafts. Sections of the patient's own saphenous veins are grafted onto the coronary arteries to bypass the blocked coronary arteries.

endarterectomy

nate a particular artery. There are several sites in the body where plaque commonly forms. One of these is the carotid artery, and this occlusion causes restricted blood flow to the brain. Removal of arteriosclerotic plaque from an obstructed carotid artery, usually done to prevent stroke, is called carotid _____.

8-74 Ather/ectomy (ath″or-ek′to-me) is surgical removal of plaque from a major artery using a rotary cutter inside a special catheter that is guided radiographically. The catheter has openings through which the plaque fragments can be aspirated (withdrawn by suction). Removal of plaque from an artery is called _____.

atherectomy

An occluded artery can sometimes be opened with laser angioplasty. In this procedure, laser energy is delivered to the site through a fiberoptic probe affixed to an arterial catheter. Laser angioplasty is used to open an occluded _____.

artery

8-75 Percutaneous (per″ku-ta′ne-əs) transluminal coronary angioplasty (PTCA) is a technique that is used in the treatment of atherosclerotic coronary heart disease. This procedure involves flattening the plaque against the arterial walls, resulting in improved circulation. It involves threading a catheter through the vessel to the plaque, then inflating and deflating a small balloon at the tip of the catheter (balloon angioplasty). Sometimes a wire cylinder or tube, called a coronary stent, is placed in the artery to keep it open.

PTCA means percutaneous transluminal coronary _____.

angioplasty

8-76 As a term written alone, angio/plasty means surgical repair of blood vessels that have become damaged by disease or injury. Angio/stomy (an″je-os′to-me) is formation of a new _____ into a blood vessel.

opening

Incision of a vessel is angiotomy (an″je-ot′o-me). Use angi(o) to write a word that means the removal (excision) of a vessel: _____.

angiectomy
(an″je-ek′to-me)
vein

8-77 Phleb/ectomy (flo-bek′to-me) is surgical removal of a _____. This procedure may involve removing only a segment of the vein. Phlebectomy may be necessary for treatment of varicose veins.

vein

Phlebo/plasty (fleb′o-plas″te) is plastic surgery of a _____.

8-78 In some cases, blood flow can be increased by using methods that do not require extensive surgery. A blood clot in a coronary artery in a patient with acute myocardial infarction may be treated with a thrombo/lytic (throm″bo-lit′ik) agent to dissolve the clot. This is called thrombolytic therapy (TT). The thrombolytic agent is administered through a catheter.

Heparin is prescribed in the treatment and prophylaxis (for example, to prevent a blood clot after surgery) of a variety of thromboembolic (throm″bo-em-bol′ik) disorders. Thrombo/embol/ic pertains to an embolus resulting from a blood _____. Embol/ectomy

clot

(em″bə-lek′tə-me), excision of the embolus, may be indicated, especially if the aorta or the common iliac artery is obstructed. In other cases, heparin is given and followed by frequent monitoring of the coagulation status of the patient's blood.

8-79 Vaso/dilators (vas″o-, va″zo-di′la-tərz) are medications that cause
_____ of blood vessels. The pain of angina pectoris is often
relieved by rest and vasodilation of the coronary arteries using nitroglycerin, a coronary vasodilator.
<u>Calcium channel blockers</u> are drugs that help diminish muscle spasms and are used primarily in treatment of spasms of the coronary artery.
Another type of drug, <u>beta blockers</u>, are often given after a myocardial infarction to allow the heart to work less.

dilation

8-80 <u>Digoxin</u> is a well-known drug that is prescribed in the treatment of congestive heart failure and certain arrhythmias. <u>Anti/arrhythmic</u> (an″te-ə-rith′mik) drugs prevent, alleviate, or correct an abnormal heart _____.

rhythm

8-81 <u>Anti/hyper/tensive</u> (an″te-, an″ti-hi″pər-ten′siv) means acting
_____ hypertension, or counteracting high blood pressure. The term also applies to agents that reduce high blood pressure.
<u>Diuretics</u> (di″u-ret′ikz) are also used in the treatment of hypertension and act to reduce the blood volume through greater excretion of water by the kidneys.

against

8-82 <u>Anti/lipid/emic</u> (an″te, an″ti-lip″ĭ-de′mik) drugs are prescribed to reduce the risk of atherosclerotic cardiovascular disease (ACVD). Combined with exercise and a low-fat diet, antilipidemic drugs lower cholesterol levels in the blood. Lower incidence of coronary heart disease and lower cholesterol levels are found in populations consuming a low-fat diet. Medications that lower cholesterol in the blood are called _____ drugs.

antilipidemic

Exercise 7

Read the surgical schedule and match the diagnoses in the left column with the surgical interventions in the right column. (All selections are used.)

SURGICAL SCHEDULE

_____ 1. arrhythmia

_____ 2. atrial septal defect

_____ 3. blocked coronary artery

_____ 4. plaque in a peripheral artery

_____ 5. severe bradycardia

_____ 6. varicose veins

A. atherectomy
B. atrioseptoplasty
C. cardiac pacemaker
D. internal cardioverter
E. phlebectomy
F. PTCA

Exercise 8

Match the drugs in the left column with their use in the right column. (All selections are used.)

_____ 1. antiarrhythmics

_____ 2. antihypertensives

_____ 3. antilipidemics

_____ 4. vasodilators

A. alleviate abnormal heart rhythm
B. dilate blood vessels
C. lower blood cholesterol levels
D. reduce blood pressure

Lymphatic System

ANATOMY AND PHYSIOLOGY

8-83 The lymphatic (**lim-fat'ik**) system, also called the lymphatics, is composed of lymphatic vessels, a fluid called lymph (**limf**), lymph nodes, and three organs: the spleen, thymus, and tonsils. The system helps protect and maintain the internal fluid environment of the body by producing, filtering, and conveying lymph; absorbing and transporting fats to the blood system; and serving as an important part of the immune system. Lymph nodes filter lymph and trap substances, helping prevent the spread of infection or cancer cells. In addition, lymph nodes contain macro/phages that can phagocytize foreign substances. Lymphocytes undergo maturation in lymphatic tissue to become B lymphocytes (B cells) or T lymphocytes (T cells). B cells and T cells are involved in antibody- and cell-mediated immunity, respectively.

lymph

The fluid transported by the lymphatic vessels is _____. Learn the meaning of the following word parts.

Word Parts Pertaining to the Lymphatic System

COMBINING FORM	MEANING	COMBINING FORM	MEANING
aden(o)	gland	lymphat(o)	lymphatics
adenoid(o)	adenoids	splen(o)	spleen
lymph(o)	lymph, lymphatics	thym(o)	thymus
lymphaden(o)	lymph node	tonsill(o)	tonsil
lymphangi(o)	lymph vessel		

lymphogenous

8-84 *Lympho/genous* (**lim-foj'ə-nəs**) means both forming lymph or derived from lymph or the lymphatics. Write this word that means originating in the lymphatics:
_____.

interstitial

8-85 Study the major parts of the lymphatic system (Figure 8-19). Only the major lymph vessels and nodes are shown. The smallest vessels of this system are lymph capillaries that are found in almost all regions of the body. Look at the detailed drawing of the proximity of the lymphatic capillaries to the cardiovascular capillaries, venules, and arterioles. The lymphatic capillaries pick up _____ fluid that has collected from the normal course of blood circulation.

Fluid enters but does not leave the lymph vessels because of valves that carry the fluid away from the tissue. The system depends on muscular contraction because there is no pump, and transport of fluid is slow. Lymph ducts eventually empty the lymph into the subclavian (**səb-kla've-ən**) veins, thus returning the fluid to the systemic circulation.

chest

8-86 Note the bean-shaped lymph nodes along the course of the lymph vessels shown in Figure 8-19. The cisterna chyli (**sis-tər'nə ki'li**) and the ducts are structures that are formed by the merging of many lymph vessels and their trunks.

As its name indicates, the thorac/ic duct is located in the _____.

lymphaden(o)

8-87 Three types of lymph nodes are shown in the drawing. The combining form that you will use to write terms about lymph nodes is _____.

neck

The cervic/al (**sər'vĭ-kəl**) lymph nodes are located in the area of the _____. In later chapters, you will study the combining forms *axill(o)* and *inguin(o)*, which mean armpit and groin, respectively. For now, remember the locations of the cervical, axillary (**ak'sĭ-lar″e**), and inguinal (**ing'gwĭ-nəl**) lymph nodes.

lymphangi(o)

8-88 Lymph is the fluid transported by the lymphatic vessels. Sometimes *lymph(o)* is used to mean lymphatics, but it is also a combining form for lymph. The combining form that you will use to write terms about lymph vessels is _____.

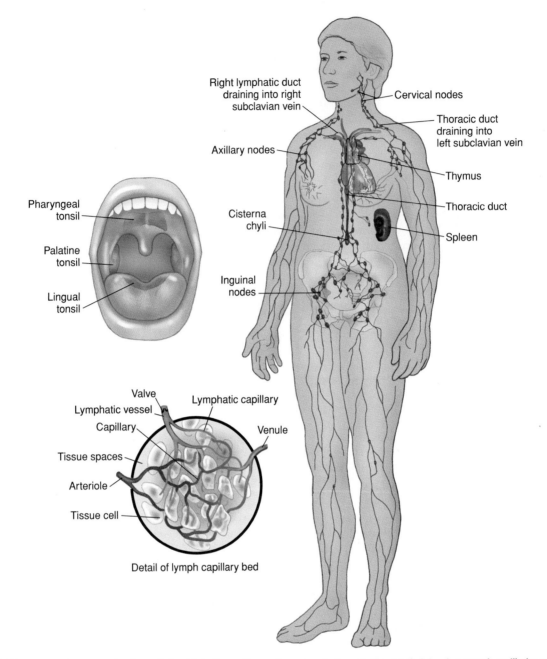

Figure 8-19 Lymphatic system. The close relationship to the cardiovascular system is shown in the detailed drawing. Lymph capillaries merge to form lymphatic vessels that join other vessels to become trunks that drain large regions of the body. The right lymphatic duct receives fluid from the upper right quadrant of the body and empties into the right subclavian vein. The thoracic duct, which begins with the cisterna chyli, collects fluid from the rest of the body and empties it into the left subclavian vein. The lymph nodes are small, bean-shaped structures distributed along the vessels. Also shown are the lymphatic organs: tonsils, thymus, and spleen.

8-89 Cells from malignant tumors may escape and be transported by the lymphatic circulation or the bloodstream to implant in lymph nodes and other organs far from the primary tumor. The process by which tumor cells spread to distant parts of the body is called metastasis (mə-tas′tə-sis). Cancer cells that wander into a lymph vessel may be trapped by the lymph nodes and begin growing there, or the cells may be carried to sites far from their origin. Lymph nodes are often examined to determine if cancer has spread to the lymphatics.

spleen	**8-90** The spleen (**splēn**), the tonsils (**ton′silz**), and the thymus (**thi′məs**) contain lymphatic tissue and are specialized lymphatic organs. The spleen is a large organ situated in the upper left part of the abdominal cavity. *Splen/ic* (**splen′ik**) refers to the _____.
spleen	Although one can live without the spleen, it performs important tasks such as defense, production of lymphocytes and plasma cells, blood storage, and destruction/recycling of red blood cells and platelets. *Spleno/lymphatic* (**sple″no-lim-fat′ik**) pertains to the _____ and the lymph nodes.
thymus	**8-91** The thymus is also called the thymus gland because it is a glandlike body. It is located in the anterior mediastinal cavity and is important in the maturation of T cells, which are involved in cell-mediated immunity. The thymus usually obtains its greatest absolute size at puberty and then becomes smaller. *Thym/ic* (**thi′mik**) means pertaining to the _____.
tonsil	**8-92** When we see the word *tonsil*, we think of the pair of small, almond-shaped masses located at the back of the throat. These are the palatine (**pal′ə-tīn**) tonsils (the palate is the roof of the mouth) and are usually what one is referring to when the term *tonsil* is used. But one should be aware that the tonsils are small masses of lymphatic tissue of several types, including the palatine and sub/lingual (*sub-*, beneath + *lingu(o)*, tongue + *-al*, pertaining to) tonsils, as well as the adenoids. *Tonsill/ar* (**ton′sĭ-lər**) means pertaining to a _____. The combining form *adenoid(o)* means adenoids.

Exercise 9

Write a word in each blank to complete this paragraph.

As blood circulates, interstitial fluid accumulates in the tissue spaces. This excess fluid is normally transported away from the tissues by a vascular network called the (1) _____ system. The system is composed of vessels, nodes, the spleen, thymus, tonsils, and a fluid called (2) _____. The fluid flows in one direction only, away from the tissue, and is eventually emptied into the subclavian
(3) _____, thus returning the fluid to the (4) _____ circulation.
   The spleen, the tonsils, and the thymus are specialized lymphatic organs. A term that means pertaining to the spleen is
(5) _____. Pertaining to the thymus is (6) _____.
Pertaining to the palatine tonsils is (7) _____.

DIAGNOSTIC TESTS AND PROCEDURES

lymphogram (**lim′fo-gram**)	**8-93** The lymphatic channels and lymph nodes can be x-rayed after injection of radiopaque material into a lymphatic vessel. This procedure is called <u>lympho/graphy</u> (**lim-fog′rə-fe**). Write a word that means the picture produced in lymphography: _____.
nodes	**8-94** The lymphatic vessels are the focus of study in <u>lymph/angio/graphy</u> (**lim-fan″je-og′rə-fe**), radiology of the lymphatic vessels after the injection of a contrast medium. In lymphadeno/graphy, the lymph _____ are the focus of study. Imaging of lymphoid organs can also be accomplished using computed tomography, magnetic resonance imaging, and nuclear magnetic imaging.
lymph	**8-95** <u>Biopsies of the lymph nodes</u> are important tools for diagnosis of the spread of cancer and are routine after many surgeries in which cancerous organs are removed. Examination of the lymph nodes is important because cancer cells are often carried to the lymph nodes via _____. Blood tests provide additional information about the lymphatic system, especially tests related to immunity and specialized studies of B and T lymphocytes.

Exercise 10

Write a word in each blank to complete these sentences.

1. Radiography of the lymphatic vessels and nodes after injection of radiopaque material is

_____.

2. The lymphatic vessels are the focus of study in lymphangiography, whereas the lymph nodes are the focus in

_____.

3. Removal of tissue from the lymph nodes to determine if cancer has spread from a nearby organ is called

_____ of the lymph nodes.

PATHOLOGIES

8-96 <u>Lymph/edema</u> (lim″fə-de′mə) means swelling of the subcutaneous tissue of an extremity as a result of obstruction of the lymphatics. The meaning of *lymphedema* is implied. You will need to remember that *lymphedema* means swelling of an extremity owing to obstruction of the

lymphatics

_____. <u>Primary lymphedema</u> is hypoplasia and maldevelopment of the lymphatic system resulting in swelling and sometimes grotesque distortion of the extremities (Figure 8-20).

  <u>Acquired lymphedema</u> results from trauma to the lymphatic ducts, such as surgical removal of lymph channels in mastectomy, obstruction of lymph drainage by malignant tumors, or the infestation of lymph vessels with parasites (see Figure 3-2). <u>Elephantiasis</u> (el″ə-fən-ti′ə-sis) is a disease in which swelling of the lymphatics causes monstrous enlargements of parts of the body, such as the legs. The lymphatics are clogged by the parasites that cause the disease, and lymph/edema results.

lymph

<u>Lympho/stasis</u> (lim-fos′tə-sis) is stoppage of _____ flow.

8-97 <u>Lymph/aden/itis</u> (lim-fad″ə-ni′tis) is inflammation of a lymph

node

_____. This inflammatory condition can result from a bacterial infection or other inflammatory condition, and the location of the affected note is indicative of the site of the infection. For example, inflammation of a cervical lymph node indicates infection of a tooth; of the mouth, throat, or ear; or somewhere in the head (Figure 8-21). Antibiotics are generally indicated when bacterial infection is present.

  Swelling of several lymph glands is characteristic of infectious mononucleosis, an acute viral infection that was discussed in the previous chapter.

8-98 <u>Lymph/adeno/pathy</u> (lim-fad″ə-nop′ə-the) is any disorder characterized by a localized or generalized enlargement of the lymph nodes or lymph vessels.

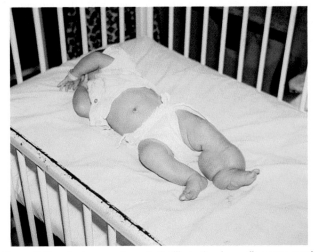

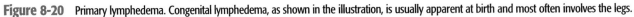

Figure 8-20   Primary lymphedema. Congenital lymphedema, as shown in the illustration, is usually apparent at birth and most often involves the legs.

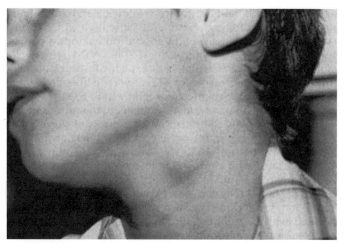

Figure 8-21   Lymphadenitis. The cervical lymph node is enlarged, firm, painless, and freely movable. The node may resolve without treatment or may eventually rupture and drain.

lymphatic

Literal interpretation of lymph/oma (**lim-fo′mə**) is a _____ tumor. A lymphoma is a type of neoplasm (tumor) of lymphoid tissue that originates in the system itself and is usually malignant. Two main types of lymphomas are Hodgkin's disease and non-Hodgkin's lymphoma (NHL).

Not all malignancies of the lymphatic system originate in the system itself. Cancer cells may be brought to the lymphatics via lymph and result in lymphatic carcinoma.

lymphatic

8-99 Lymph/ang/itis (**lim″fan-ji′tis**) is inflammation of a _____ vessel. (Note the spelling of lymphangitis, which uses the combining forms for lymph, vessel, and inflammation. Some of the vowels are omitted in the spelling of lymphangitis to facilitate pronunciation.)

Lymphangitis is often the result of an acute streptococcal infection of one of the extremities (Figure 8-22).

8-100 Thrombo/lymphang/itis (**thromb″bo-lim″fan-ji′tis**) is inflammation of a lymph_____ resulting from a blood clot.

vessel
splenopathy
(sple-nop′ə-the)
enlargement
spleen

Any disease of the spleen is called a _____.

8-101 Spleno/megaly (**sple″no-meg′ə-le**) is _____ of the spleen. Spleno/rrhagia (**sple″no-ra′jə**) is hemorrhage from the _____.

Because of its anatomic location, the spleen is often injured in abdominal trauma. Rupture of the spleen can occur from a blunt blow, such as trauma from a car accident.

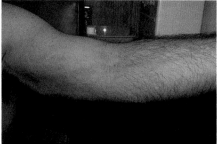

Figure 8-22   Streptococcal lymphangitis. This type of inflammatory condition of the lymph nodes is caused by streptococcal bacteria. Examination of the area distal to the affected node usually reveals the source of the infection.

splenoptosis
(sple″nop-to′sis)

thymopathy
(thi-mop′ə-the)

adenoiditis
(ad″ə-noid-i′tis)

Combine *splen(o)* and *-ptosis* to write a term that means a downward displacement (sagging) of the spleen: _____.

8-102 A <u>thym/oma</u> (thi-mo′mə) is a tumor, usually benign, of the thymus. Any disease of the thymus is a _____.

8-103 <u>Tonsill/itis</u> (ton″sǐ-li′tis) is inflammation of the palatine tonsils. Inflammation of the adenoids is _____. When the adenoids are enlarged as a result of frequent infection, they can obstruct the passageway and removal may be indicated.

Exercise 11

Match pathologies in the left column with the correct terms in the right column.

_____ 1. enlarged spleen

_____ 2. inflammation of a lymph vessel

_____ 3. inflammation of a lymph node

_____ 4. inflammation of the palatine tonsils

_____ 5. tumor originating in the lymphatics

A. lymphadenitis
B. lymphangitis
C. lymphoma
D. splenomegaly
E. tonsillitis

SURGICAL AND THERAPEUTIC INTERVENTIONS

excision

radiation

splenectomy
(sple-nek′tə-me)
thymectomy
(thi-mek′tə-me)
tonsillectomy
(ton″sǐ-lek′tə-me)

8-104 <u>Penicillin</u> and <u>hot soaks</u> are usually prescribed for lymphangitis. Infected lymph nodes often respond to <u>antibiotic therapy</u> or resolve on their own. <u>Lymphaden/ectomy</u> (lim-fad″ə-nek′tə-me) is _____ of a lymph node. This term is often accompanied by an adjective referring to the location of the node that is removed, such as cervical lymphadenectomy.

8-105 Treatment of lymphoma is determined by the type of lymphoma but can include intensive <u>radiotherapy</u>, <u>chemotherapy</u>, and <u>biological therapies</u>, including interferon. Radio/therapy is treatment of tumors using _____ to kill malignant cells and deter their proliferation.

8-106 Splenoptosis (sple″nop-to′sis), prolapse of the spleen, can be corrected by surgical fixation of the spleen. This surgery is called <u>spleno/pexy</u> (sple′no-pek″se).

A ruptured spleen often requires surgical intervention. <u>Spleno/rrhaphy</u> (sple-nor′ə-fe) is suture of the spleen. Surgical removal of the spleen is _____.

8-107 Write a word that means removal of the thymus: _____.

Excision of the tonsils is a _____. A tonsillectomy is performed to treat a chronic infection of the tonsils. An <u>adenoidectomy</u> (ad″ə-noid-ek′tə-me) is performed because the adenoids are enlarged, chronically infected, or causing obstruction. They are sometimes removed at the same time as a tonsillectomy as a prophylactic measure. A tonsillectomy and adenoidectomy performed at the same time is called a <u>tonsilloadenoidectomy</u> (ton″sǐ-lo-ad″ə-noid-ek′tə-me) and is usually written T & A.

EXERCISE 12

Match interventions in the left column with the correct terms in the right column.

_____ 1. excision of the adenoids

_____ 2. excision of the lymph nodes

_____ 3. removal of the thymus

_____ 4. suture of the spleen

A. adenoidectomy
B. adenoidopathy
C. lymphadenectomy
D. lymphangiectectomy
E. splenectomy
F. splenorrhaphy
G. thymectomy
H. thymoma

SELECTED ABBREVIATIONS

AI	aortic insufficiency
ASD	atrial septal defect
ASHD	arteriosclerotic heart disease
AST (formerly SGOT)	aspartate aminotransferase (enzyme elevated after MI)
AV, A-V	atrioventricular
BP	blood pressure
CA	carcinoma
CABG	coronary artery bypass graft
CAD	coronary artery disease
CCU	critical care unit
CHF	congestive heart failure
CK (CPK)	creatine kinase (formerly called creatine phosphokinase)
CPR	cardiopulmonary resuscitation
CT, CAT	computed tomography, computerized axial tomography
ECG, EKG	electrocardiogram

ECHO	echocardiography
LA	left atrium
LCA	left coronary artery
LDH	lactate dehydrogenase (enzyme elevated after MI)
LV	left ventricle
MI	myocardial infarction
MVP	mitral valve prolapse
PAT	paroxysmal atrial tachycardia
PTA	percutaneous transluminal angioplasty
PTCA	percutaneous transluminal coronary angioplasty
PVC	premature ventricular contraction
RA	right atrium; rheumatoid arthritis
RCA	right coronary artery
RV	right ventricle
SA	sinoatrial
T & A	tonsillectomy and adenoidectomy
VSD	ventricular septal defect

CHAPTER 8 REVIEW

■ Basic Understanding

Labeling

I. Using this illustration of a capillary bed, write combining forms for the structures that are indicated. (Line 1 is done as an example.) Write two combining forms for line 2 (artery) and three combining forms for line 4 (vein), as indicated on the drawing.

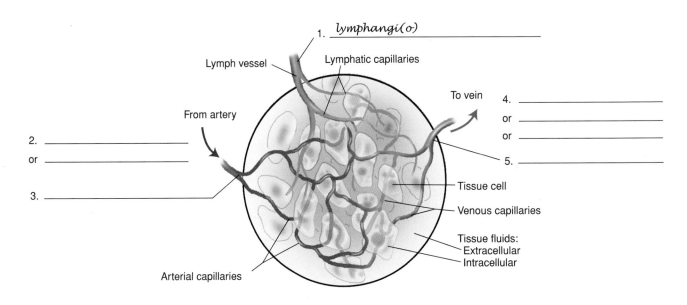

1. _lymphangi(o)_ _____

Lymph vessel   Lymphatic capillaries

From artery

To vein

4. _____
   or _____
   or _____

2. _____
   or _____

5. _____

3. _____

Tissue cell

Venous capillaries

Tissue fluids:
Extracellular
Intracellular

Arterial capillaries

II. Write combining forms for the structures of the lymphatic system structures that are indicated on the diagram.

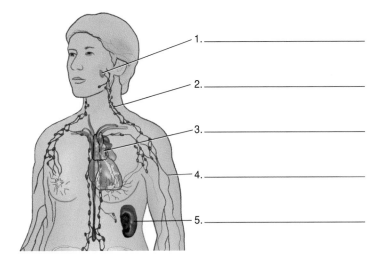

1. _____

2. _____

3. _____

4. _____

5. _____

Matching

III. Use all selections to match terms in the left column with their descriptions in the right column.

_____ 1. arterioles

_____ 2. aorta

_____ 3. atria

_____ 4. capillaries

_____ 5. pulmonary arteries

_____ 6. pulmonary veins

_____ 7. veins

_____ 8. venae cavae

_____ 9. venules

_____ 10. ventricles

A. lower chambers of the heart
B. the largest artery
C. two large veins that communicate with the right atrium
D. upper chambers of the heart
E. vessels that carry blood from the heart to the lungs
F. vessels that carry blood from the lungs to the heart
G. vessels that convey blood from the venules toward the heart
H. vessels that join arteries and capillaries
I. vessels that join arterioles and venules
J. vessels that join capillaries and veins

IV. Match terms in the left column with their descriptions in the right column.

_____ 1 cardiac septum

_____ 2. endocardium

_____ 3. mediastinum

_____ 4. myocardium

_____ 5. pericardium

A. area in the chest cavity that contains the heart
B. cardiac muscle tissue
C. inner lining of the heart
D. sac which encloses the heart
E. wall between the left and right sides of the heart

Listing

V. Name three functions of the lymphatic system.

1. _____

2. _____

3. _____

VI. Circle the correct answer for each of the following questions.

1. Charlie, a 60-year-old male, has just been diagnosed as having a coronary occlusion. He is most at risk for which of the following? (atrioventricular block, congenital heart disease, myocardial infarction, rheumatic fever)

2. Charlie is told that he has a form of arteriosclerosis in which yellowish plaque has accumulated on the walls of the arteries. What is the name of this form of arteriosclerosis? (aortostenosis, atherosclerosis, cardiomyopathy, coarctation)

3. Charlie's physician advises surgery. Which surgery is generally prescribed for coronary occlusion? (automatic implantable cardiopulmonary bypass, cardioverter, coronary artery bypass, pericardiocentesis)

4. Kristen, a 28-year-old female, is told she has inflammation of the lining of the heart. What is the medical term for this heart pathology? (coronary heart disease, endocarditis, myocarditis, pericarditis)

5. Jayne suffered ventricular fibrillation during coronary angiography. What procedure did the physician use to stop fibrillation? (atherectomy, endarterectomy, cardiopulmonary resuscitation, defibrillation)

6. Jim developed a blood clot in a coronary artery. What is Jim's condition called? (myocardial infarction, coronary artery bypass, coronary thrombosis, fibrillation)

7. Baby Seth is born with cyanosis and a heart murmur. Which congenital heart disease does the neonatologist think is more likely? (atrial septal defect, atrioventricular block, megalocardia, pericarditis).

8. Ten-year-old Zack had a sore throat for several days before he developed painful joints and a fever. Which disease does the physician suspect that can cause damage to the heart valves? (aortic valve sclerosis, aortic valve stenosis, mitral valve prolapse, rheumatic fever)

9. Uncle Ed experiences pain in his legs that is caused by blockage of arteries in the lower extremities. What is the name of his condition? (angiocarditis, lymphangioma, peripheral artery disease, varicose veins)

10. Angie has an angiogram that shows a ballooning out of the wall of a cerebrovascular artery. Which condition does Angie have? (aneurysm, angioma, arteriosclerosis, coronary thrombosis)

Writing Terms

VII. *Write one word for each of the following clues:*

1. a tumor of the thymus   _____

2. abnormal hardening of the aorta   _____

3. absence of a heartbeat   _____

4. agent that causes dilation of blood vessels   _____

5. increased blood pressure   _____

6. increased pulse   _____

7. inflammation of a lymphatic vessel _____

8. narrowing of the diameter of a vessel   _____

9. removal of the tonsils   _____

10. suture of the spleen   _____

■ Greater Comprehension

Health Care Report

VIII. Read the following consultation report and answer the questions that follow the report. Although you may be unfamiliar with some of the terms, you should be able to answer the questions by determining the meanings of word parts.

MID-WEST MEDICAL CENTER

222 Medical Center Drive   Main City, US 63017-1000   Phone: (555) 434-0000
                                                                      Fax (555) 434-0001

HISTORY AND PHYSICAL

PATIENT'S NAME: Dwight Moore   **PT #** 20031   **Date:** 10/08/xxxx

CHIEF COMPLAINT: Increased lethargy

HISTORY OF PRESENT ILLNESS: 68-year-old male with history of multiple CVAs in last year with increased lethargy and swallowing dysfunction. CT scan revealed a new cerebello-pontine ischemic CVA. Cardiac work-up did not reveal atrial fibrillation or other significant arrhythmia on telemetry. INR: 2.8-3.0. Hypercoagulable work-up was unremarkable.

MEDICAL HISTORY: Hypertension, Congestive Heart Failure, Myocardial Infarction, Coronary Artery Disease, Atherosclerotic Heart Disease, Multiple CVAs, Hypercholesterolemia

SURGICAL HISTORY: Right and left carotid endarterectomies

SOCIAL HISTORY: Married with supportive family

OCCUPATIONAL HISTORY: Retired Engineer

REVIEW OF SYSTEMS:
      HEENT: No jugular vein distention
      CARDIOPULMONARY: Lungs—bibasilar crackles; heart—regular rate and rhythm
      GASTROINTESTINAL: Abdomen soft with bowel sounds
      MUSCULOSKELETAL: Extremities—no edema
      NEUROMUSCULAR: Left hemiparesis, left facial droop

John Wilson, M.D.
John Wilson, M.D.

JW:aba
D: 10/09/xxxx
T: 10/09/xxxx

---

1. Describe the meaning of Mr. Moore's present illness, ischemic CVA:

_____

_____

2. Describe the diagnostic test that was used to diagnose the present illness:

_____

_____

3. Is the patient experiencing atrial fibrillation? _____

Define atrial fibrillation:

_____

_____

4. Is the patient experiencing arrhythmia? _____

Define arrhythmia:

_____

_____

5. Define telemetry:

_____

_____

6. Define right and left carotid endarterectomies:

_____

_____

7. Mr. Moore's medical history indicates several diseases or disorders. Describe the following:

hypertension: _____

congestive heart failure: _____

myocardial infarction: _____

coronary artery disease: _____

atherosclerotic heart disease: _____

hypercholesterolemia: _____

IX. Read the case study and define the underlined words or abbreviations.

CASE STUDY

Pt: H. I. Wilson (male, age 60)
Sx: Mid-sternal chest pain radiating to both shoulders
Patient history: Unremarkable
Family history: Both parents deceased. Father, <u>myocardial infarction</u> at age 68; mother had mid-life <u>hypertension</u> and <u>hypercholesterolemia</u>.
Physical exam: BP 160/94; apical heart rate 100 and regular; R 24. Lungs clear to <u>auscultation</u>.
ECG: Normal
Labs: Cardiac enzymes normal; cholesterol 250
Thallium stress test: Showed chest pain with increased cardiac activity; demonstrated need for <u>cardiac catheterization</u>.
Cardiac Cath: <u>Coronary angiography</u> showed blockage in three main coronary arteries.
Diagnosis: Hypercholesterolemia; <u>CAD</u>; <u>angina pectoris</u>
Plan: <u>CABG</u> in AM

---

1. myocardial infarction   _____

2. hypertension   _____

3. hypercholesterolemia   _____

4. auscultation   _____

5. ECG   _____

6. cardiac catheterization _____

7. coronary angiography   _____

8. CAD   _____

9. angina pectoris   _____

10. CABG   _____

Spelling
X. Circle all incorrectly spelled terms and write their correct spelling:

adenoidectomy   athrosclerosis   diastole   iskemia   mediastinum

Interpreting Abbreviations
XI. Write the meaning of these abbreviations:

1. ASHD _____

2. A-V   _____

3. CA   _____

4. CHF   _____

5. CK   _____

6. CPR   _____

7. LV   _____

8 MI   _____

9. RA   _____

10. VSD   _____

Pronunciation
XII. The pronunciation is shown for several medical words. Indicate the primary accented syllable with an ′.

1. cardiomyopathy (kahr de o mi op ə the)

2. lymphadenopathy (lim fad ə nop ə the)

3. lymphography (lim fog rə fe)

4. pericardial (per ĭ kahr de əl)

5. vasodilation (vas o, va zo di la shən)

Categorizing Terms

XIII. Classify the terms in the left column (1-10) by selecting A, B, C, D, or E.

_____ 1. angiography

_____ 2. angiostenosis

_____ 3. atrioseptoplasty

_____ 4. aortosclerosis

_____ 5. lymphoma

_____ 6. lymphangitis

_____ 7. lymphography

_____ 8. phlebectomy

_____ 9. vasodilators

_____ 10. venule

A. anatomy
B. diagnostic test or procedure
C. pathology
D. surgery
E. therapy

(Check your answers with the solutions in Appendix VI.)

LISTING OF MEDICAL TERMS

Use the practice CD to review the terms that have been presented. Look closely at the spelling of each term as it is pronounced, and be sure you know the meaning of each term.

adenoidectomy	aortitis	atrioventricular block	carotid endarterectomy
adenoiditis	aortogram	atrium	catheter
adenoids	aortography	axillary node	catheterization
aneurysm	aortosclerosis	B-cell lymphocyte	cerebrovascular accident
aneurysmal	arrhythmia	balloon angioplasty	cervical lymph node
angiectomy	arterial	beta blockers	cholesterol
angina pectoris	arteriogram	bicuspid valve	cisterna chyli
angiocardiography	arteriograph	bradycardia	coarctation of the aorta
angiocarditis	arteriography	bypass	computed tomography
angiogram	arteriole	calcium channel blockers	congenital heart disease
angiography	arteriopathy	cardiac angiography	congestive heart failure
angioma	arteriosclerosis	cardiac catheterization	coronary
angioplasty	arteriosclerotic heart	cardiac pacemaker	coronary arteriography
angiostenosis	disease	cardiac tamponade	coronary artery
angiostomy	arteritis	cardiomegaly	coronary artery bypass
angiotomy	artery	cardiomyopathy	coronary artery bypass
anoxia	asystole	cardioplegia	graft
antiarrhythmic	atherosclerosis	cardioplegic solutions	coronary artery disease
antihypertensive	atherosclerotic	cardiopulmonary	coronary occlusion
antilipidemic	cardiovascular disease	cardiopulmonary	coronary stent
aorta	atrial fibrillation	resuscitation	coronary thrombosis
aortic	atrial septal defect	cardiovalvulitis	creatine phosphokinase
aortic insufficiency	atriomegaly	cardiovascular	test
aortic regurgitation	atrioseptoplasty	cardioversion	cuspid valve
aortic stenosis	atrioventricular	cardioverter	cyanosis

defibrillation
defibrillator
diastole
diastolic
digital subtraction
   angiography
digoxin
diuretic
Doppler echocardiography
dysrhythmia
echocardiogram
echocardiography
edema
effusion
electrocardiogram
electrocardiograph
electrocardiography
electrophysiologic studies
elephantiasis
embolectomy
embolus
endarterectomy
endocardial
endocarditis
endocardium
endothelium
epicardium
extracorporeal
fibrillation
flutters
heart block
heart murmur
hemangioma
hematoma
hemopericardium
hemorrhoids
heparin
high-density lipoprotein
Hodgkin's disease
Holter monitor
hypertension
hypoplasia
hypotension
hypovolemia
infarct
infarction
inguinal node
interstitial fluid
ischemia

lactate dehydrogenase test
laser angioplasty
lipid
lipoprotein
low-density lipoprotein
lymph
lymph node
lymphadenectomy
lymphadenitis
lymphadenopathy
lymphangiography
lymphangioma
lymphangitis
lymphatics
lymphedema
lymphocyte
lymphogenous
lymphogram
lymphography
lymphoma
lymphostasis
macrophage
mediastinum
metastasis
microcardia
mitral valve
mitral valve prolapse
murmur
myocardial
myocardial infarction
myocarditis
myocardium
necrosis
nitroglycerin
non-Hodgkin's lymphoma
occlusion
oxygenation
pacemaker
palatine tonsils
palpitation
parietal pericardium
paroxysmal atrial
   tachycardia
patent ductus arteriosus
percutaneous transluminal
   angioplasty
pericardial
pericardial cavity
pericarditis

pericardium
peripheral vascular disease
phlebectomy
phlebitis
phleboplasty
phlebostasis
phlebotomist
phlebotomy
plaque
plasma cell
positron emission
   tomography
premature ventricular
   contraction
pulmonary
pulmonary circulation
pulse
Purkinje fibers
radiotherapy
rheumatic heart disease
sclerosis
semilunar valve
septal
septum
shock
shunt
sinoatrial node
sinus rhythm
sphygmomanometer
spleen
splenectomy
splenic
splenolymphatic
splenomegaly
splenopathy
splenopexy
splenoptosis
splenorrhagia
splenorrhaphy
stenosis
stethoscope
stricture
subclavian vein
systemic circulation
systole
systolic
T-cell lymphocyte
tachycardia
tetralogy of Fallot

thallium stress test
thoracic cavity
thoracic duct
thromboembolic
thrombolymphangitis
thrombolytic therapy
thrombophlebitis
thrombosis
thrombus
thymectomy
thymic
thymoma
thymus
tonsil
tonsillar
tonsillectomy
tonsillitis
tonsilloadenoidectomy
tourniquet
treadmill stress test
tricuspid valve
triglyceride
ultrasonography
valval
valvar
valvate
valvular
valvular stenosis
valvulitis
varicose veins
vascular
vasoconstriction
vasoconstrictor
vasodilation
vasodilator
vasomotor center
vein
vena cava
venipuncture
venous
venous thrombosis
ventricle
ventricular
ventricular fibrillation
ventricular septal defect
venular
venule
visceral pericardium

español ENHANCING SPANISH COMMUNICATION

ENGLISH	SPANISH (PRONUNCIATION)
artery	arteria (ar-TAY-re-ah)
blood pressure	presión sanguínea (pray-se-ON san-GEE-nay-ah)
capillary	capilar (cah-pe-LAR)
catheter	catéter (cah-TAY-ter)
cholesterol	colesterol (co-les-tay-ROL)
high blood pressure	hipertensión, presión alta (e-per-ten-se-ON, pray-se-ON AHL-tah)
narrow	estrecho (es-TRAY-cho)
obstruction	obstrucción (obs-trooc-se-ON)
pulse	pulso (POOL-so)
rhythm	ritmo (REET-mo)
spleen	bazo (BAH-so)
tonsil	tonsila (ton-SEE-lah), amígdala (ah-MEEG-dah-lah)
varicose veins	venas varicosas (VAH-nahs vah-re-CO-sas)
vein	vena (VAY-nah)
weakness	debilidad (day-be-le-DAHD)

CHAPTER 9

Respiratory System

LEARNING GOALS

In this chapter, you will learn to do the following:

Basic Understanding

1. Recognize names of the structures of the respiratory system and define terms associated with these structures.
2. Sequence the flow of air from the atmosphere through the respiratory structures.
3. Distinguish between structures of the upper respiratory tract and the lower respiratory tract.
4. Identify the functions of external respiration.
5. Name heart disease as the leading cause of death in the United States and cancer of the lungs and bronchi as the second leading cause of death.
6. Write the meanings of word parts associated with the respiratory system and use them to build and analyze terms.

Greater Comprehension

7. Use word parts from this chapter to define terms in a health care report.
8. Spell the terms accurately.
9. Pronounce the terms correctly.
10. Write the meanings of the abbreviations.
11. Categorize terms as anatomy, diagnostic test or procedure, pathology, surgery, or therapy.

THESE ARE THE MAJOR SECTIONS IN THIS CHAPTER:

❑ **Anatomy and Physiology**
  Upper Respiratory Passageways
  Lower Respiratory Passageways
❑ **Diagnostic Tests and Procedures**

❑ **Pathologies**
  Disordered Breathing
  Upper Respiratory Abnormalities
  Lower Respiratory Abnormalities
  Death and Cancer Statistics
❑ **Surgical and Therapeutic Interventions**

FUNCTION FIRST

The primary function of the respiratory system is to provide oxygen for the body and to remove carbon dioxide. Secondary functions are maintaining the acid-base balance, producing speech, facilitating smell, and maintaining the body's heat and water balances.

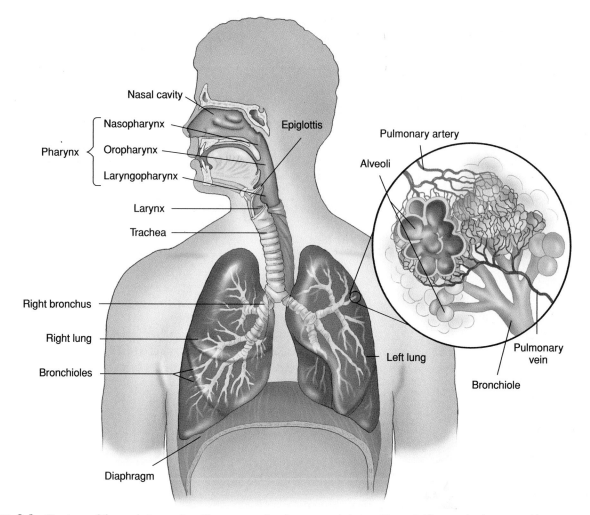

Figure 9-1   Structures of the respiratory system. The nose, nasal cavity, paranasal sinuses (shown in Figure 9-2), pharynx, and larynx comprise the upper respiratory tract. The trachea, bronchi, bronchioles, alveoli, and lungs comprise the lower respiratory tract.

ANATOMY AND PHYSIOLOGY

oxygen

9-1 The respiratory (**res′pĭ-rə-tor″e**) system cooperates with the circulatory system to provide _____ for body cells and to expel waste carbon dioxide by breathing. The exchange of these gases is involved in both internal and external respiration.

    This chapter focuses on external respiration, the processes involved in breathing, the ventilation of the lungs, and the exchange of oxygen (O_2) and carbon dioxide (CO_2) between the air in the lungs and the blood. The delivery of oxygen by the blood to body cells with the removal of carbon dioxide is internal respiration.

inspiration

9-2 Breathing is alternate inspiration (**in″spĭ-ra′shən**) and expiration (**ek″spĭ-ra′shən**) of air into and out of the lungs. Inspiration (*in, into* + *spir[o]*, to breathe + *-ation*, process) is the process of breathing in. The drawing of air into the lungs is _____. It is also called in/halation.

    Expelling air from the lungs, the act of breathing out or letting out one's breath, is expiration. This is the same as exhalation.

lungs	**9-3** In studying the respiratory system, you will often see breathing referred to as pulmonary **(pool′mo-nar″e)** ventilation,* or simply, ventilation. You learned earlier that *pulmon/ary* pertains to the _____.

The respiratory tract is the complex of organs and structures that perform pulmonary ventilation and the exchange of oxygen and carbon dioxide between the air and the blood as it circulates through the lungs. See the names and locations of the structures in Figure 9-1.

9-4 The conducting passages of this system are known as the upper respiratory tract and the lower respiratory tract. The nose, nasal cavity, paranasal **(par″ə-na′zel)** sinuses, pharynx **(far′inks)**, and larynx **(lar′inks)** comprise the upper respiratory tract (URT). The trachea **(tra′ke-ə)**, bronchi **(brong′ki)**, bronchioles **(brong′ke-ōlz)**, alveoli **(al-ve′o-li)**, and lungs belong to the

lower	_____ respiratory tract (LRT).

Study the following word parts and be sure you know their meanings.

Word Parts for Respiratory Anatomy and Physiology

Upper Respiratory Tract

COMBINING FORM	MEANING	COMBINING FORM	MEANING
epiglott(o)	epiglottis	pneumon(o), pulm(o), pulmon(o)	lungs
nas(o), rhin(o)	nose	phren(o)	diaphragm or mind
laryng(o)	larynx	thorac(o)	chest
palat(o)	palate	trache(o)	trachea
pharyng(o)	pharynx		

Lower Respiratory Tract

Word Parts Used to Describe Function

COMBINING FORM	MEANING	COMBINING FORM	MEANING
alveol (o)	alveoli	acid(o)	acid
bronch(o), bronchi(o)	bronchi	alkal(o)	alkaline; basic
bronchiol(o)	bronchioles	-capnia	carbon dioxide
lob(o)	lobe	ox(i)	oxygen
pleur(o)	pleura	phas(o)	speech
pneum(o)	lungs or air	phon(o)	voice
		spir(o)	to breathe

■ *Upper Respiratory Passageways*

nose	**9-5** Looking back at Figure 9-1, trace the passage of air through the respiratory system by writing the names of respiratory structures in the blanks: Air first enters the body through the _____, where it is warmed, moistened, and filtered. Regardless of whether air is taken in by the nose or the mouth, it passes to the pharynx, a muscular tube about 13 cm (5 inches) long in an adult. The pharynx also functions as part of the digestive system in the swallowing of food. Air then passes over the vocal cords in the larynx before reaching the trachea, also known as the windpipe. The trachea divides into two primary bronchi, which divide further
bronchioles	into many _____. Oxygen and carbon dioxide are exchanged within the alveoli.

9-6 The respiratory tract is lined with mucous membranes. Organs of the upper respiratory tract filter, moisten, and warm the air as it is inhaled. The combining forms *nas(o)* and *rhin(o)* mean

nose	_____. Already knowing that *laryng(o)* means larynx should help
pharynx	you remember that *pharyng(o)* means _____. Common names for the larynx and pharynx are voice box and throat, respectively.

The external part of the nose contains two openings, the nostrils, also called the nares **(na′rēz)**. The hollow interior of the nose is separated into right and left cavities by the nasal septum. Literal

near	interpretation of *para/nasal sinuses* means the air cavities _____

---

*Ventilation (Latin: *ventilare*, to fan).

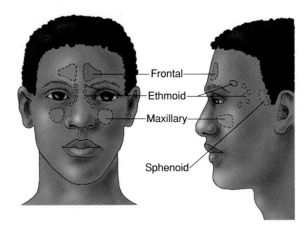

Frontal
Ethmoid
Maxillary
Sphenoid

Figure 9-2   Paranasal sinuses. These air-filled, paired cavities in various bones around the nose are lined with mucous membranes. Their openings into the nasal cavity are easily obstructed.

the nose. The paranasal sinuses are pairs of air-filled cavities in various bones that surround the nasal cavity and open into it. The types of paranasal sinuses are shown in Figure 9-2.

9-7 Both cartilage and bone give structure to the nose. The nasal septum is composed of cartilage. Build a word using *endo-* that means inside (within) the nose: _____. *Retro/nasal* (**ret″ro-na′zəl**) and *supra/nasal* (**soo″prə-na′səl**) mean behind the nose and above the nose, respectively.

The anterior portion of the palate (**pal′ət**), or roof of the mouth, separates the nasal cavity and the oral cavity. *Or/al* means pertaining to the mouth, and *nas/al* (**na′zəl**) means pertaining to the _____. The palate consists of bone and the membrane that covers it. Because the anterior portion contains bone, it is called the hard palate. The soft palate is the fleshy posterior portion of the palate. The pendant, fleshy tissue that hangs from the soft palate, is the palatine uvula (**u′vu-lə**). The combining form *palat(o)* means palate. *Palatine* (**pal′ə-tīn**) refers to the _____.

9-8 The naso/lacrimal (**na″zo-lak′rĭ-məl**) duct also opens into the nasal cavity. The nasolacrimal duct is a tubular passage that carries fluid (tears) from the eye to the _____ cavity. Now you can understand why the nose fills with fluid when a person cries. *Lacrimal* pertains to tears.

The nose has nerve endings that detect many odors. *Olfactory** (**ol-fak′tə-re**) pertains to the sense of smell. Olfaction (**ol-fak′shən**), the sense of smell, is a function of the nose.

9-9 The pharynx serves as a passageway for both the respiratory and digestive tracts. In referring to parts of the pharynx, three divisions are recognized (see Figure 9-1): the nasopharynx (**na″zo-far′inks**), the oropharynx (**or″o-far′inks**), and the laryngopharynx (**lə-ring″go-far′ənks**). The naso/pharynx is that part of the pharynx that lies behind the nose. The oro/pharynx lies behind the _____. The laryngopharynx is that part of the pharynx that lies near the larynx.

9-10 The nasopharynx is the upper part of the pharynx and is continuous with the nasal passages. The auditory tube, formerly called the eustachian (**u-sta′ke-ən**) tube, is a narrow channel connecting the middle ear and the nasopharynx. The opening to the auditory tube is in the nasopharynx. The adenoids are also located in the nasopharynx.

Naso/pharyng/eal (**na″zo-fə-rin′je-əl**) pertains to the _____.

Left margin answers:

endonasal
(en″do-na′zəl)

nose

palate

nasal

mouth

nasopharynx

---

*Olfactory (Latin: *olfacere*, to smell).

pharynx	*Pharyng/eal* (fə-rin′je-əl) means pertaining to the pharynx. *Oro/pharyngeal* (or″o-fə-rin′je-əl) means pertaining to the mouth and _____. This term also pertains to the oropharynx. The oropharynx contains the palatine tonsils, which are visible when the mouth is open wide. The lowest part of the pharynx is called the laryngopharynx. It is here that the pharynx divides into the larynx and the esophagus. Air passes through the larynx, and food passes through the esophagus.
larynx; pharynx	**9-11** *Laryngeal* means pertaining to the larynx. *Laryngo/pharyng/eal* (lə-ring″go-fə-rin′je-əl) refers to the _____ and the _____.
glottis	The glottis (glot′is) is the vocal apparatus of the larynx. It consists of the vocal cords and the opening between them. The vocal cords, also called vocal folds, are a pair of strong bands of elastic tissue with a mouthlike opening through which air passes, creating sound. These vocal folds are part of the vocal apparatus of the larynx called the _____.
	Muscles open and close the glottis during inspiration and expiration, and they regulate the vocal cords during the production of sound. Muscles also close off a lidlike structure that covers the glottis during swallowing. The lidlike structure, the epiglottis (ep″ĭ-glot′is), is composed of cartilage and covers the larynx during the swallowing of food.
aspiration	**9-12** Aspiration is the drawing in or out as by suction. Foreign bodies may be aspirated into the nose, throat, or lungs on inspiration. *Aspiration* also refers to the withdrawing of fluid from a cavity by means of suction. Drawing in or out by suction is called _____.
	If a person inspires while attempting to swallow, food may be accidentally aspirated into the larynx. Spontaneous coughing is the body's effort to clear the obstructed airway. Respiration stops if complete obstruction of the airway occurs.
epiglottis	In usual situations, food does not enter the larynx but passes on to the esophagus. Food does not enter the larynx because a lidlike structure, the _____, is closed. Epiglottides (ep″ĭ-glot′ĭ-dēs) is the plural of epiglottis, hence the term epiglottiditis (ep″ĭ-glot″ĭ-di′tis).

■ *Lower Respiratory Passageways*

	9-13 Infections of the upper respiratory tract are common and often spread to the lower respiratory tract. The lower respiratory tract, a continuation of the upper respiratory tract, begins with the trachea. *Trache/al* (tra′ke-əl) means pertaining to the trachea. *Endo/tracheal* (en″do-tra′ke-əl), abbreviated ET, means within the trachea.
	In addition to the trachea, the lower respiratory tract includes two primary bronchi and several secondary bronchi, bronchioles, alveolar ducts, and alveoli. The two lungs are composed of millions of alveoli and their related ducts, bronchioles, and bronchi.
bronchi	The trachea branches into the right and left primary _____. Bronchi are lined with cilia, hairlike projections that propel mucus up and away from the lower airway. Bronchi branch to become bronchioles, structures that lead to alveolar ducts. At the ends of the ducts are the alveoli, small pockets where carbon dioxide and oxygen are exchanged between the inspired air and capillary blood.
	9-14 Most of the lower respiratory passageways are located in the chest cavity. The mediastinum is the middle portion of the thoracic cavity between the two lungs. In the mediastinum, the trachea (windpipe) divides into the right and left primary bronchi; *bronch(o)* and *bronchi(o)* mean bronchi. *Bronchial tubes* is another term for bronchi (singular is bronchus). *Bronchi/al* means pertaining to
bronchi	the_____.
	Bronchioles are small airways that extend from the bronchi into the lungs. Translated literally, *bronchi/ole* means little bronchus.
interalveolar (in″tər-al-ve′o-lər)	*Alveolar* means pertaining to the alveoli. *Broncho/alveolar* (brong″ko-al-ve′ə-lər) means pertaining to a bronchus and alveoli. Write a word that means between alveoli: _____.

apex

9-15 The two lungs are composed of millions of alveoli and their related ducts, bronchioles, and bronchi. Normal lungs are highly elastic and fill the chest cavity during inspiration, pressing down on the diaphragm. The muscular diaphragm (di′ə-fram) contracts and increases the size of the thoracic cavity during inspiration.

Each lung is conical and has an apex (uppermost portion) and a base (lower portion). Observe in Figure 9-1 that the left lung has two lobes and the right lung has three lobes. *Apical* (ap′ĭ-kəl) refers to the _____, or the uppermost portion of the lung. The depression where blood vessels enter and leave the lung is called the hilum.

lungs

9-16 Each lung is surrounded by a membrane called the pleura (ploor′ə) (plural is pleurae). One layer of the membrane, the visceral pleura, covers the lung's surface. The other layer, the parietal (pə-ri′ə-təl) pleura, lines the walls of the thoracic cavity. *Visceral** means pertaining to the viscera, the large internal organs enclosed within a body cavity, especially the abdominal cavity. *Parietal†* pertains to the outer wall of a cavity or organ.

Two types of pleura are the visceral pleura and the parietal pleura. The visceral pleura surrounds the _____; the parietal pleura lines the walls of the thoracic cavity. Between the two pleurae is a space called the pleural cavity, which contains a thin film of pleural fluid that acts as a lubricant as the lungs expand and contract during respiration.

pleura
outside

9-17 The combining form *pleur(o)* means pleura. *Pleur/al* (ploor′əl) pertains to the _____.

Extrapleural (eks″trə-ploor′əl) means _____ the pleural cavity.

lungs

9-18 Both *pulmonary* and *pulmonic* mean pertaining to the _____ or the respiratory system, but *pulmonary* is more commonly used.

below

Extrapulmonary (eks″trə-pool′mo-nar″e) means outside, or not connected with, the lungs. *Sub/pulmonary* (səb-pool′mo-nar″e) means _____ the lung.

diaphragm

9-19 The diaphragm is the muscular partition that separates the thoracic and abdominal cavities. The formal anatomic name for the diaphragm is diaphragma (di″ə-frag′mə). *Diaphragma/tic* (di″ə-frag-mat′ik) means pertaining to the _____. Long ago, people believed that the midriff was the seat of emotions; the Greek word *phren* was applied to this area as a structure, as well as the center of emotions. For this reason diaphragm and mind have the same combining form, *phren(o)*. The diaphragm is pierced by several openings through which pass the aorta, the vena cava, and the esophagus. It aids respiration by moving up and down as we exhale and inhale (Figure 9-3).

Phren/ic (fren″ik) has two meanings, either pertaining to the diaphragm or pertaining to the mind. *Sub/phrenic* (səb-fren′ik) means located beneath the diaphragm. When studying respiration, *phren(o)* probably refers to the muscular partition that separates the chest and abdominal cavities,

diaphragm

the _____.

Exercise 1

Write the names of respiratory structures to complete these sentences.

1. The structure that is commonly called the throat is the _____.

2. The structure that is commonly called the windpipe is the _____.

3. The hollow interior of the nose is separated into two cavities by the nasal _____.

4. The glottis is the vocal apparatus of the _____.

5. The upper respiratory tract consists of the nose, nasal cavity, paranasal _____, pharynx, and larynx.

*Visceral (Latin: *viscus*, internal organ).
†Parietal (Latin: *paries*, wall).

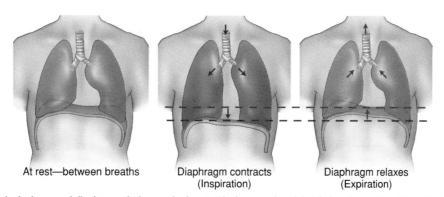

At rest—between breaths   Diaphragm contracts (Inspiration)   Diaphragm relaxes (Expiration)

Figure 9-3   Changes in the lungs and diaphragm during respiration. **A,** Diaphragm relaxed, just before inspiration. **B,** Inspiration. The diaphragm contracts, moving downward and increasing the size of the thoracic cavity. Inspiration is also aided by contraction of the intercostal muscles, which are between the ribs. Air moves into the lungs until pressure inside the lungs equals atmospheric pressure. **C,** Expiration. Respiratory muscles relax, and the chest cavity decreases in size as air moves from the lungs out into the atmosphere.

6. The lower respiratory tract begins with a structure called the _____.

7. Bronchi branch to become _____.

8. Tiny structures of the respiratory system where carbon dioxide and oxygen are exchanged between the inspired air and

   capillary blood are _____.

9. The uppermost part of the lung is called the _____.

10. Each lung is surrounded by a membrane called the _____.

DIAGNOSTIC TESTS AND PROCEDURES

nasal

9-20 Physical assessment of the respiratory structures often begins with examination of the nose and throat, often using a nasal speculum for examination of the interior of the nose. A naso/scope (na′zo-skōp) is a speculum that is used for inspecting the _____ cavity.

The color of the mucous membranes and the presence of swelling, bleeding, or discharge are noted. One finding is septal deviation, a structural defect of the nasal septum in which it is shifted toward one side of the nose or the other (Figure 9-4).

polyp

pharynx

9-21 It may also be possible to see a nasal polyp with the help of a nasoscope. A polyp (pol′ip) is a growth or mass protruding from a mucous membrane. Polyps are usually (but not always) benign. They can grow on almost any mucous membrane. If such a growth occurs in the nasal cavity or in the sinuses, it is called a nasal _____.

A pharyngo/scope (fə-ring′go-skōp) is an instrument for examining the lining of the structure that is commonly called the throat, the _____.

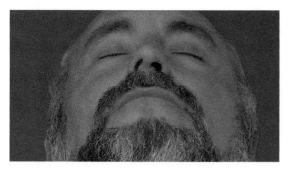

Figure 9-4   Deviated septum. This shifted partition of the nasal cavity may obstruct the nasal passages. Severe septal deviation may be corrected by rhinoplasty or septoplasty.

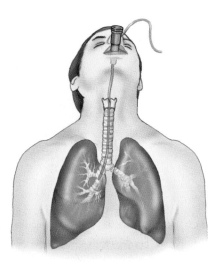

Figure 9-5 Bronchoscopy. Visual examination of the tracheobronchial tree using a bronchoscope. Other uses for this procedure include suctioning, obtaining a biopsy specimen or fluid, and removing foreign bodies.

---

instrument

9-22 Laryngo/scopy (lar″ing-gos′kə-pe), examination of the larynx with an endoscope, is generally performed by a specialist. A laryngoscope (lə-ring′gə-skōp) is the _____ used in laryngoscopy.

If further study is needed, a physician may order a radiographic examination of the larynx, laryngography (lar″ing-gog′rə-fe). This procedure usually includes the pharynx, as well as the larynx.

tracheoscopic

bronchoscope
(brong′ko-skōp)

9-23 Viewing the interior of the trachea is a tracheoscopy (tra″ke-os′kə-pe). This is also called a _____ examination.

Add a suffix to *bronch(o)* to form a word that means an instrument for viewing the bronchi: _____.

Broncho/scopy (brong-kos′kə-pe) or broncho/scopic (brong″ko-skop′ik) examination is direct viewing of the bronchi (Figure 9-5). Broncho/graphy (brong-kog′rə-fe) involves the use of x-rays after instillation of an opaque solution. The film obtained by broncho/graphy is a _____. This procedure is seldom used, having been replaced by computed tomography.

bronchogram
(brong′ko-gram)

mediastinoscope
(me″de-ə-sti′no-skōp)

9-24 Mediastino/scopy (me″de-as″tĭ-nos′kə-pe) is examination of the mediastinum by means of an endoscope inserted through an incision of the chest. This procedure allows direct inspection of the mediastinum and biopsy of tissue, using an instrument called a _____.

9-25 Radiography of the chest, commonly called a chest x-ray, is a valuable tool in studying the lungs as well as nearby structures. Examine the chest x-ray in Figure 9-6 and study the relationship of the lungs with other structures in the chest cavity. The air in the lungs appears black. Notice also the white appearance of bone (collarbone, breastbone, and ribs). The breasts and other soft tissue appear gray. In looking at the respiratory structures, it is understandable why the trachea and bronchial branches are referred to as the tracheobronchial tree.

The muscular structure that contracts and relaxes during inspiration and expiration is the

diaphragm

_____.

vessels

9-26 Pulmonary angio/graphy (an″je-og′rə-fe) is radiology of the _____ of the lungs after injection of a contrast medium. Pulmonary angiography is primarily performed on patients with suspected thrombo/embolic (throm″bo-em-bol′ik) disease. A thrombus is an internal blood clot. If part of it breaks off, the clot fragment can travel in the bloodstream to another site. Any foreign object that circulates in the bloodstream and becomes lodged in a vessel is called an embolus. *Thrombo/embol/ic* pertains to obstruction of a blood vessel with material from a blood clot that is carried by the bloodstream from its site of origin.

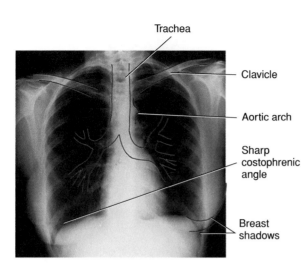

Trachea

Clavicle

Aortic arch

Sharp
costophrenic
angle

Breast
shadows

Figure 9-6   A normal radiograph of the chest. The diaphragm and several important parts of the lower respiratory tract are labeled.

Other diagnostic radiologic studies of respiratory organs include <u>computed tomography</u>, <u>magnetic resonance imaging</u>, and <u>lung scans</u>. A lung scan uses radioactive material to test blood flow or air distribution in the lungs. Information about the flow of blood in the lungs is helpful in diagnosing pulmonary embo/lism, the presence of an embolus in the lungs.

9-27 The lung volume in normal quiet breathing is approximately 500 ml; however, forced maximum inspiration raises this level considerably. <u>Spiro/metry</u> (**spi-rom′ə-tre**) is a measurement of the amount of air taken into and expelled from the lungs (Figure 9-7). The combining form *spir(o)* as used here means breath or breathing. The instrument used is a

_____.

**spirometer
(spi-rom′ə-tər)**

The largest volume of air that can be exhaled after maximal inspiration is the <u>vital capacity</u> (VC). A reduction in vital capacity often indicates a loss of functioning lung tissue.

Spirometry measures ventilation (the ability of the lungs to move air) and is one type of <u>pulmonary function test</u> (PFT) that helps determine the capacity of the lungs to exchange oxygen and carbon dioxide effectively.

9-28 A <u>pulse oxi/meter</u> (**ok-sim′ə-tər**) is a photo/electric device for determining the oxygen saturation of the blood in a pulsating capillary bed (Figure 9-8). The <u>finger probe</u> is most commonly used for monitoring the patient's oxygenation status in a hospital, during pulmonary rehabilitation programs, or during stress testing; however, an <u>ear oximeter</u> is sometimes used. The name of the procedure that determines the oxygen saturation of the blood in a pulsating capillary bed is pulse

_____.

oximetry

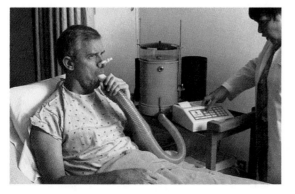

Figure 9-7   Spirometry. Evaluation of the air capacity of the lungs uses a spirometer, such as the one shown. The spirometer is used to assess pulmonary function by measuring and recording the volume of inhaled and exhaled air.

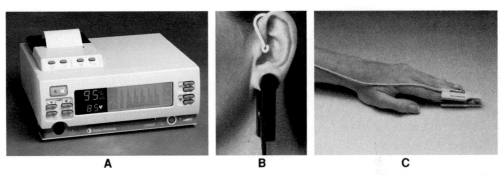

A   **B**   **C**

Figure 9-8   Oximetry, noninvasive monitoring of oxygen saturation. **A,** The oximeter shows a reading of SaO₂% = 95. **B,** The earlobe is a common site for measurement during exercise. **C,** The finger probe is most commonly used for stationary measurements.

9-29 The use of percussion, described in Chapter 6, is helpful in assessing the lungs (see Figure 6-13, C). Chest auscultation (see Figure 6-13, B), listening to breath sounds, provides information about the flow of air through the tracheo/bronchial tree. Abnormal sounds that are heard during inspiration include rhonchi (**rong'ki**), wheezes, crackles (formerly called rales [**rahlz**]), and friction rub (Figure 9-9).

Abnormal sounds can be heard when a stethoscope is used to evaluate the sound of air moving in and out of the lungs. This procedure is called _____.

auscultation	

9-30 A rhonchus (**rong'kəs**)* is an abnormal sound consisting of a continuous rumbling sound that clears on coughing. A wheeze is a musical noise that sounds like a squeak. Crackles are discontinuous bubbling noises during inspiration that are not cleared by coughing. A friction rub is a dry, grating sound. If the friction rub is heard over the pleural area, it may be a sign of lung disease, although it may be normal if heard over another area such as the liver.

Practice enables the ability to distinguish these abnormal sounds. Another sound, _stridor_,† means an abnormal high-pitched musical sound caused by an obstruction in the trachea or larynx, most

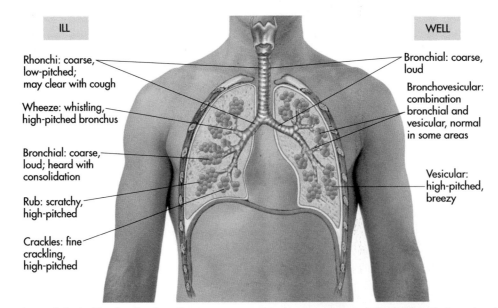

ILL

WELL

Rhonchi: coarse, low-pitched; may clear with cough

Wheeze: whistling, high-pitched bronchus

Bronchial: coarse, loud; heard with consolidation

Rub: scratchy, high-pitched

Crackles: fine crackling, high-pitched

Bronchial: coarse, loud

Bronchovesicular: combination bronchial and vesicular, normal in some areas

Vesicular: high-pitched, breezy

Figure 9-9   Breath sounds in the ill and well patient. Common terms used to describe sounds heard in the ill patient are rhonchi, wheeze, friction rub, and crackles, as well as coarse, loud bronchial sounds heard with consolidation. _Consolidation_ means the process of becoming solid, as when the lungs become firm and inelastic in pneumonia.

*Rhonchus (Greek: _rhonchos_, snore).
†Stridor (Latin: _stridor_, harsh sound).

stridor

often heard during inspiration. Write the term that is an abnormal high-pitched sound associated with an obstruction in the trachea or larynx: _____.

arterial

9-31 Arterial blood gas (ABG) analysis is a blood test that measures the amount of oxygen, carbon dioxide, and pH in a blood sample collected from an artery. ABG is an abbreviation for _____ blood gas.

Other laboratory tests include cultures for bacteria or fungi in sputum or material collected from throat swabs. Phlegm (**flem**) is abnormally thick mucus secreted by the membranes of the respiratory passages. Sputum is phlegm or other material that is coughed up from the lungs.

Exercise 2

Match these structures with the instrument or procedure that is used to study them.

_____ 1. blood vessels of the lungs

_____ 2. nose

_____ 3. throat

_____ 4. voice box

_____ 5. windpipe

A. laryngoscope
B. nasoscope
C. pharyngoscope
D. pulmonary angiography
E. tracheoscope

☤ PATHOLOGIES

■ *Disordered Breathing*

apnea (ap'ne-ə)

9-32 Disorders of the respiratory system are a major cause of illness and death. Acute or chronic respiratory problems can progress rapidly and become life-threatening emergencies. Chronic lung disease often causes heart disease because of the lungs' functional role in circulation.

You learned earlier that *-pnea* is a suffix that means breathing. Choose either *a-* or *an-* to write a word that means absence of spontaneous breathing: _____.

9-33 Sleep apnea is a sleep disorder characterized by transient periods of cessation of breathing. The two primary types are central sleep apnea (resulting from failure of stimulation by the nervous system) and obstructive sleep apnea (resulting from collapse or obstruction of the airway).

Cheyne-Stokes (**chān stōks**) respiration (CSR) is an abnormal pattern of respiration that is characterized by alternating periods of apnea and deep, rapid breathing, occurring more frequently during sleep.

breathing

9-34 Remembering that *dys-* means bad or difficult, dys/pnea (**disp'ne-ə**) is labored or difficult _____. *Dys/pne/ic* (**disp-ne'ik**) is an adjective that means pertaining to or caused by dyspnea.

An/ox/ia (**ə-nok'se-ə**) means an absence or deficiency of oxygen in body tissues below the level needed for proper functioning. Anoxia is more severe than hypoxia, but both mean oxygen deficiency. Asphyxia* (**as-fik'se-ə**) or asphyxiation (**as-fik"se-a'shən**) is a condition caused by insufficient intake of oxygen. Extrinsic† causes, those originating outside the body, include drowning, crushing injuries of the chest, and inhalation of carbon monoxide. Intrinsic‡ causes include hemorrhage into the lungs or pleural cavity, foreign bodies in the throat, and diseases of the air passages.

oxygen

Asphyxia is caused by lack of _____.

---

*Asphyxia (*a-*, no + Greek: *phyxis*, pulse).
†Extrinsic (Latin: *extrinsecus*, situated on the outside).
‡Intrinsic (Latin: *intrinsecus*, situated on the inside).

9-35 Cyanosis, dyspnea, and tachycardia accompanied by mental disturbances are seen in asphyxia. In extreme cases, convulsions, unconsciousness, and death may occur. *Tachy/cardia* (*tachy-*, fast + *-cardi(o)*, heart + *-ia*, condition) means an increased heart rate.

Write the term that means a condition caused by insufficient intake of oxygen (be careful with the spelling): _____.

asphyxia or asphyxiation

9-36 Hyper/pnea (hi″pər-, hi″pərp-ne′ə) is an exaggerated deep or rapid respiration. It occurs normally with exercise and abnormally in several conditions, including pain, fever, hysteria, or inadequate oxygen. The latter can occur in cardiac or respiratory disease. A literal translation of hyper/pnea is excessive_____.

breathing

Hyper/pnea may lead to hyper/ventilation (hi″pər-ven″tĭ-la′shən)—excessive aeration of the lungs—which commonly reduces carbon dioxide levels in the body. Carbon dioxide contributes to the acidity of body fluids, and if too much carbon dioxide is lost, alkalosis results. Alkal/osis (al″kə-lo′sis) is a pathologic condition resulting from the accumulation of basic substances or from the loss of acid by the body. Transient alkalosis can be caused by hyperventilation. *Transient** means not lasting or of brief duration.

9-37 The abbreviation *pH* means potential hydrogen, a calculated scale that represents the relative acidity or alkalinity of a solution, in which a value of 7.0 is neutral, below 7.0 is acidic, and above 7.0 is alkaline. The normal pH of body fluids (plasma, intracellular, and interstitial fluids) is 7.35 to 7.45. Is normal plasma slightly acid or alkaline? _____

alkaline

Cellular metabolism produces substances such as excess carbon dioxide that would upset the pH were it not for buffer systems of the blood, along with respiratory and urinary functions that help keep the pH constant. The state of equilibrium of the blood pH is called the acid-base balance. The expelling of carbon dioxide during exhalation is part of the regulatory mechanism that maintains the constancy of the pH—that is, the acid-base balance.

9-38 The combining form *alkal(o)* means alkaline or basic. Alkal/osis is an alkaline condition. Alkal/emia (al″kə-le′me-ə) is increased alkalinity of the blood. Alkal/emia is an aspect of alkalosis, the general term for accumulation of basic substances in the body fluids. The opposite of alkalosis is acid/osis. The combining form *acid(o)* means acid. A pathologic condition that results from accumulation of acid or depletion of alkaline substances is called

_____.

acidosis (as″ĭ-do′sis)

9-39 The suffix *-capnia* refers to carbon dioxide. Hyper/capnia (hi″pər-kap′ne-ə) means greater than normal amounts of carbon dioxide in the blood. Carbon dioxide contributes to the acidity of blood. Does hypercapnia result in lowering or increasing the blood pH?

_____

lowering

Within minutes, the lungs begin to compensate for any acid-base imbalance by increasing the excretion of carbon dioxide through faster or deeper breathing.

9-40 Hypo/capnia (hi″po-kap′ne-ə) is the opposite of *hypercapnia* and means an abnormally low level of carbon dioxide in the blood. A/capnia (ă-kap′ne-ə) is a synonym for *hypocapnia*, although in its strictest sense *a/capnia* means _____ of carbon dioxide.

Would hyperventilation lead to hypercapnia or hypocapnia? _____

absence
hypocapnia

9-41 Acid/emia (as″ĭ-de′me-ə) is an arterial blood pH below 7.35, whereas alkal/emia is recognized as a blood pH above 7.45. Either of these conditions can be considered an acid-base imbalance. Look at some conditions listed in Table 9-1 that can lead to an acid-base imbalance.

Asphyxia leads to which condition, alkalemia or acidemia? _____

acidemia

---

*Transient (Latin: *trans*, to go by).

TABLE 9-1 Potential Causes of Acid-Base Imbalances

Acidemia	Alkalemia
Ingestion of highly acidic drugs	Ingestion of alkaline drugs
Severe diarrhea	Intense hyperventilation
Severe diabetes	Vomiting of gastric acid
Asphyxia	Metabolic problems
Vomiting of lower intestinal contents	
Disease, particularly respiratory or kidney failure	

9-42 <u>Acute respiratory failure</u> is a sudden inability of the lungs to maintain normal respiratory function. It may be caused by an obstruction in the airways or failure of the lungs. Respiratory failure leads to <u>hyp/ox/ia</u>. Hypoxia (**hi-pok′se-ə**) is a reduction of oxygen in body tissues to levels below those required for normal metabolic functioning. Note the spelling of hyp/ox/ia (the *o* of *hypo-* has been dropped). <u>Acute (or adult) respiratory distress syndrome</u> (ARDS) is severe pulmonary congestion characterized by respiratory insufficiency and hypoxemia and can result in acute respiratory failure.

blood

    <u>Hyp/ox/emia</u> (**hi″pok-se′me-ə**) is decreased oxygen in the _____. Once again, notice the spelling. You learned earlier that asphyxia is caused by insufficient intake of oxygen. This leads to hypoxemia, hypercapnia, loss of consciousness, and death if not corrected.

9-43 In <u>ortho/pnea</u> (**or″thop-ne′ə**), breathing is difficult except in an upright position. Analyze *ortho/pnea* (*orth[o]*, straight + *-pnea*, breathing). In orthopnea, the person must sit or stand to breathe deeply or comfortably. Write this term that means a condition in which breathing is difficult except in an upright position: _____. Two comfortable positions that help orthopneic patients breathe more comfortably are shown in Figure 9-10.

orthopnea

9-44 Individuals normally have a respiration rate of about 12 to 15 breaths per minute. <u>Eu/pnea</u> (**ūp-ne′ə**) means normal breathing. If a person were breathing at a rate of 25 breaths per minute at rest, this would be <u>tachypnea</u>. The word *tachy/pnea* (**tak″ip-ne′ə; tak″e-ne′ə**) means _____ breathing.

fast

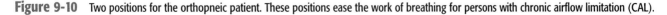

Figure 9-10   Two positions for the orthopneic patient. These positions ease the work of breathing for persons with chronic airflow limitation (CAL).

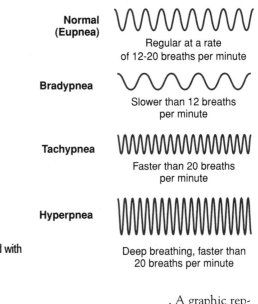

Normal (Eupnea)
Regular at a rate of 12-20 breaths per minute

Bradypnea
Slower than 12 breaths per minute

Tachypnea
Faster than 20 breaths per minute

Hyperpnea
Deep breathing, faster than 20 breaths per minute

Figure 9-11 Selected patterns of respiration. An example of normal respiration is compared with those seen in bradypnea, tachypnea, and hyperpnea.

bradypnea (**brad″e-ne′ə, brad-ip′ne-ə**)

The opposite of this is slow breathing, or _____. A graphic representation of various patterns of breathing are shown in Figure 9-11.

In another condition, hypo/pnea (**hi-pop′ne-ə**), the breathing is shallow, in addition to being slow. This may be appropriate in a well-conditioned athlete but can occur if it is painful to breathe or if there is damage to the brain stem.

9-45 Abnormalities in the diaphragm will affect breathing, because the diaphragm normally moves downward as the lungs expand during inspiration. Phreno/dynia (**fren″o-din′e-ə**) is pain in the diaphragm. Paralysis of the diaphragm is phreno/plegia (**fren″o-ple′jə**). Phreno/ptosis (**fren″op-to′sis**) is a prolapsed or downward displacement of the diaphragm. Use *phren(o)* to write a word that means inflammation of the diaphragm: _____.

phrenitis (**frə-ni′tis**)

Exercise 3

Write a word in each blank to complete these sentences.

1. Absence of spontaneous breathing is _____.

2. Labored or difficult breathing is _____.

3. Asphyxia is a condition caused by insufficient intake of _____.

4. Exaggerated deep or rapid breathing is _____.

5. Increased aeration of the lungs is _____.

6. A pathologic condition that results from the accumulation of basic substances or from the loss of acid by the body is

   _____.

7. Greater than normal amounts of carbon dioxide is _____.

8. A term for an arterial blood pH below 7.35 is _____.

9. The condition in which an individual must sit upright or stand to breathe deeply or comfortably is

   _____.

10. Paralysis of the diaphragm is _____.

■ *Upper Respiratory Abnormalities*

respiration (or breathing)

9-46 An upper airway obstruction is any significant interruption in the airflow through the nose, mouth, pharynx, or larynx. Laryngoscopy may be helpful in locating and removing the cause of the obstruction. If the cause is not removed, <u>respiratory arrest</u> occurs. Respiratory arrest is cessation of

_____.

9-47 During infections and allergies, swelling may block the passages and cause fluid to accumulate in the sinuses. A sinus headache can result from the pressure within the sinuses. Sinus/itis (si″nə-si′tis) is _____ of one or more paranasal sinuses. A structural defect of the nose can also result in sinusitis.

inflammation	

9-48 Build a word using *rhin(o)* that means inflammation of the mucous membranes of the nose: _____. Acute rhinitis is also called coryza* (ko-ri′zə), meaning a profuse discharge of the mucous membranes of the nose. This is usually what is meant when speaking of an upper respiratory infection (URI).

rhinitis (ri-ni′tis)

Rhino/rrhea (ri″no-re′ə) is discharge from the _____. This is commonly called a runny nose.

nose

9-49 Nosebleed has many causes, including irritation of the nasal membranes, fragility of these membranes, violent sneezing, trauma, high blood pressure, vitamin K deficiency, or particularly in children, picking the nose. *Rhinorrhagia* (ri″no-ra′je-ə) means profuse bleeding from the nose. Literal translation of *rhino/rrhagia* is _____ from the nose. Another medical term for nosebleed is *epistaxis* (ep″ĭ-stak′sis).

hemorrhage

9-50 A rhino/lith (ri′no-lith) is a calculus or stone in the _____. A calculus consists of inorganic substances, such as calcium and phosphate, that crystallize to form a hard mass resembling a pebble. A rhino/lith is a _____ calculus. The presence of nasal stones is rhino/lith/iasis (ri″no-lĭ-thi′ə-sis).

A rhinolith can interfere with breathing through the nose, making it more comfortable to breathe through the mouth.

nose

nasal

9-51 Canker sores, also called fever blisters, in the roof of the mouth are one cause of palatitis (pal″ə-ti′tis). Palat/itis is inflammation of the hard palate, the bony portion of the roof of the mouth.

Pharyng/itis (far″in-ji′tis) is inflammation or infection of the pharynx, usually causing symptoms of a sore throat. Sore throat (pharyngeal pain) is pharyngo/dynia (fə-ring″go-din′e-ə) or pharyng/algia (far″in-gal′jə).

Tonsill/itis (ton″sĭ-li′tis) is one reason for a sore throat. The tonsils are located in the oropharynx. Enlarged tonsils can fill the space behind the nares and may completely block the passage of air from the nose into the throat.

9-52 Other causes of a sore throat include strepto/coccal infections, herpes simplex virus (HSV), and infectious mono/nucleosis. It is important to receive an antibiotic for strep infections, because untreated infections sometimes lead to rheumatic fever (see Chapter 8). Herpes simplex, caused by a herpes simplex virus, usually produces small, transient, irritating, and sometimes fluid-filled blisters on the skin and mucous membranes. Infections tend to occur particularly around the nose and mouth.

Inflammation of the nasopharynx is _____. Various infectious organisms cause pharyngitis or nasopharyngitis.

nasopharyngitis (na″zo-far″in-ji′tis)

9-53 Pharyngo/myc/osis (fə-ring″go-mi-ko′sis) is a fungal condition of the _____.

Write a word that means any disease of the pharynx: _____.

pharynx

pharyngopathy (far″ing-gop′ə-the)

9-54 Build a word that means inflammation of the larynx: _____. This condition would probably result in temporary loss of voice. Inflammation of the larynx may be caused not only by infectious microorganisms but also by overuse of the voice, allergies, or irritants.

laryngitis (lar″in-ji′tis)

A person with laryngitis often suffers only minor discomfort. If the larynx becomes painful, the person has laryng/algia (lar″in-gal′jə), which is pain of the _____. You may be wondering if you could combine *laryng(o)* with *-dynia*, which also means pain. Although some people would know what you mean, this term is not generally found in the dictionary.

larynx

---

*Coryza (Greek: *koryza,* catarrh).

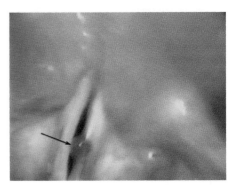

Figure 9-12   A laryngeal polyp. This hemorrhagic polyp *(arrow)* on the vocal cord occurs most commonly in adults who smoke, have many allergies, live in dry climates, or abuse the voice.

9-55 A/phonia **(a-fo′ne-ə)** is a condition characterized by the inability to produce normal speech sounds that results from overuse of the vocal cords, organic disease, or emotional problems, such as anxiety. The combining form *phon(o)* means voice. Laryngitis may result in absence of voice, which

aphonia
difficult (weak)

is called _____.
    Dys/phonia **(dis-fo′ne-ə)** means _____ voice. Dysphonia is not related to the ability to pronounce words. It is the same as hoarseness and may precede aphonia.

speech

9-56 The combining form *phas(o)* means speech. Literal translation of *dys/phas/ia* is difficult _____. Dysphasia **(dis-fa′zhə)** is impairment of speech, characterized by a lack of coordination and an inability to arrange words in their proper order, a problem resulting from a brain lesion. Difficulty in speech caused by a brain lesion is called

dysphasia

_____.

absence

9-57 A/phasia **(ə-fa′zhə)** is the _____ of speech. Aphasia is an inability to communicate through speech, writing, or signs as a result of dysfunction of the brain. A person who has aphasia is said to be aphasic **(ə-fa′zik)**.

9-58 You learned earlier that a polyp is a tumorlike growth, usually benign, that projects from a mucous membrane. A growth of this type on the vocal cords is called a laryngeal

polyp

_____ (Figure 9-12).
    Although painless, laryngeal polyps cause hoarseness. They are generally caused by smoking, allergies, or abuse of the voice, and eliminating the cause often relieves the hoarseness. If an individual smokes, smoking cessation adjuncts may help remove the desire to smoke. Surgery can be performed using direct laryngoscopy if rest does not correct the problem.

9-59 Laryngo/plegia **(lə-ring″go-ple′je-ə)** is paralysis of the muscles of the

larynx

_____. Spasmodic closure of the larynx (spasm of the larynx) is laryngospasm **(lə-ring′go-spaz″əm)**. Any disease of the larynx is a laryngopathy **(lar-ing-gop′ə-the)**.
    The epiglottis prevents food from entering the larynx and the trachea while swallowing.

inflammation

Epiglott/itis **(ep″ĭ-glŏ-ti′tis)** or epiglottid/itis is _____ of the epiglottis.

9-60 The common cold is a contagious viral infection of the upper respiratory tract. Some of its major characteristics are rhinitis **(ri-ni′tis)**, rhinorrhea **(ri″no-re′ə)**, tearing and eye discomfort, and sometimes low-grade fever. Rhin/itis is inflammation of the nasal membranes. Rhino/rrhea is

discharge

_____ from the nasal membranes. Rest, fluids, analgesics, and decongestants are recommended.
    The barking cough of croup **(kro͞op)** is often accompanied by difficulty in breathing and stridor. Croup is an acute viral infection of the upper and lower respiratory tract that occurs primarily in infants and young children.

9-61 Diphtheria (dif-thēr′e-ə) and pertussis (pər-tus′is) are two acute contagious respiratory diseases. They are both caused by specific pathogenic bacteria and are both preventable by vaccination. Immunization for diphtheria and pertussis are usually given in conjunction with tetanus immunization early in infancy. The exotoxin of the tetanus bacillus affects the nervous system, resulting in paralysis. For this reason, the common name of tetanus is lockjaw. It is easy to misspell the term *diphtheria*. Write the term here: _____.

Pertussis is commonly called whooping cough, named for the coughing that ends in a loud whooping inspiration. It occurs primarily in infants and young children who have not been immunized.

9-62 A new corona/virus (kə-ro′nə-vi″rəs), named for its appearance using an electron microscope, has been identified as the organism responsible for severe acute respiratory syndrome (SARS). It is spread by close contact with an infected person. Illness generally begins with a fever and body aches, and some people experience mild respiratory symptoms. After 3 to 7 days, a lower respiratory phase begins and patients may develop a dry cough and have trouble breathing.

Severity of the disease ranges from mild illness to death. The Centers for Disease Control and Prevention report a fatality rate of approximately 3%. SARS is the abbreviation for _____ acute respiratory syndrome.

9-63 Influenza is a highly contagious respiratory infection that is caused by various strains of influenza virus. Three main types (type A, type B, and type C) have been identified, but new strains emerge at regular intervals (for example, Asian flu virus). Influenza is characterized by fever, sore throat, cough, muscle ache, and weakness. Yearly vaccination is recommended for health care personnel, the elderly, and debilitated persons.

This highly contagious disease that is characterized by fever, respiratory systems, muscle aches, and weakness is _____.

(margin terms: diphtheria, severe, influenza)

Exercise 4

Match terms in the left column with the clues in the right column.

_____ 1. coryza

_____ 2. laryngitis

_____ 3. pertussis

_____ 4. pharyngitis

_____ 5. rhinolithiasis

A. sore throat usually accompanies this condition
B. acute rhinitis
C. formerly called whooping cough
D. sometimes results in temporary loss of voice
E. the presence of nasal calculi

■ Lower Respiratory Abnormalities

9-64 The lower respiratory tract is a common site of infections, obstructive conditions, and malignancies. Fatigue is common in chronic respiratory conditions. Malaise (mah-lāz′) is a vague feeling of bodily discomfort and fatigue. Lethargy (leth′ər-je), more severe than fatigue, is a state of dullness, sluggishness, or prolonged sleepiness or drowsiness. A person suffering lethargy is said to be lethargic (lə-thar′jik). Clubbing, most easily seen in the fingers, is an abnormal enlargement of the distal fingers and toes, often associated with advanced chronic pulmonary disease (Figure 9-13).

Several unnatural surface features of the chest can be observed during a physical examination. Both pigeon chest and funnel chest are skeletal abnormalities of the chest. The breastbone has a prominent anterior projection in pigeon chest, and it is depressed in funnel chest (Figure 9-14). Breathing is generally not affected in either of these structural defects. A prominent anterior projection of the breastbone is characteristic of which skeletal abnormality, pigeon chest or funnel chest? _____ chest

(margin term: pigeon)

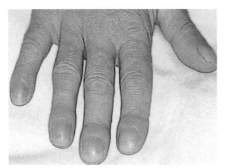

Figure 9-13   Clubbing. Abnormal enlargement of the distal phalanges is seen in advanced chronic pulmonary disease but may be associated with other disorders, such as cyanotic heart disease.

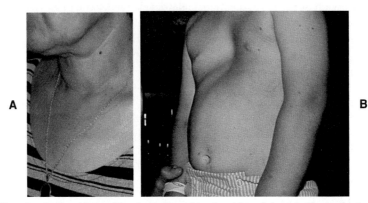

A   B

Figure 9-14   Comparison of two structural problems of the chest, pigeon breast and funnel chest. **A,** Pigeon chest, a congenital structural defect characterized by prominent sternal protrusion. **B,** Funnel chest, indentation of the lower sternum.

9-65 Flail chest occurs when multiple rib fractures cause instability of the chest wall. The lung underlying the injury contracts and bulges with each inspiration and expiration. This condition must be surgically corrected to prevent hypoxia.

barrel

Barrel chest—a large, rounded thorax—may be normal in some individuals but may also be a sign of pulmonary emphysema. The common name for a large, rounded thorax is _____ chest.

9-66 The suffix *-plasia* means formation or development. <u>A*plasia*</u> (ə-pla′zhə) means absence of formation or development. Incomplete formation or development of the lung is the same as

aplasia

_____ of the lung.

9-67 <u>Respiratory distress syndrome</u> (RDS) is an acute lung disease of the newborn that occurs most often in premature babies. In most cases, the infant dies only a few days after birth or recovers with no after affects. <u>Sudden infant death syndrome</u> (SIDS) is the unexpected and sudden death of an apparently normal and healthy infant that occurs during sleep and may be linked with respiration.

infant

SIDS means sudden _____ death syndrome.

Learn the meanings of the word parts in the following list.

Word Parts to Describe Respiratory Pathologies

COMBINING FORM	MEANING		PREFIX	MEANING
atel(o)	imperfect or incomplete		meta-	change; next, as in a series
anthrac(o)	coal			
coni(o)	dust		SUFFIX	MEANING
embol(o)	embolus		-ation	process
fibr(o)	fiber or fibrous		-pnea	breathing
thromb(o)	thrombus		-ptosis	prolapse
			-ptysis	spitting
			-stenosis	narrowing

<table>
<tbody>
<tr><td>inflammation</td><td></td></tr>
</tbody>
</table>

inflammation	

9-68 *Laryngo/trache/al* (lə-ring″go-tra′ke-əl) means pertaining to the larynx and the trachea. *Laryngotracheitis* (lə-ring″go-tra″ke-i′tis) means _____ of the larynx and trachea. If the larynx, trachea, and bronchi are inflamed, it is called laryngo/tracheo/bronch/itis (lə-ring″go-tra″ke-o-brong-ki′tis).

Tracheo/malacia (tra″ke-o-mə-la′shə) is softening of the trachea, and tracheo/stenosis (tra″ke-o-stə-no′sis; *trache(o)* + *-stenosis*, narrowing) is narrowing of the lumen of the trachea. *Trache/algia* (tra″ke-al′jə) means a _____ trachea.

painful

9-69 *Broncho/pulmonary* (brong″ko-pul′mə-nar″e) pertains to the bronchi and lungs. Build a word that means inflammation of the bronchi by combining *bronch(o)* and *-itis*:

_____.

bronchitis (brong-ki′tis)
bronchopathy (brong-kop′ə-the)
bronchi

Bronchogenic (brong-ko-jen′ik) means originating in a bronchus. Use *bronch(o)* to write a word that means any disease of the bronchi: _____.

Broncho/lith/iasis (brong″ko-lĭ-thi′ə-sis) is a condition in which stones are present in the

_____.

dilation

9-70 Literal translation of bronchi/ectasis (brong″ke-ek′tə-sis) is _____ of the bronchi; however, bronchiectasis is an abnormal condition of the bronchial tree that is characterized by irreversible dilation and destruction of the bronchial walls. Symptoms include chronic sinusitis, a constant cough producing a great deal of sputum, hemoptysis (*hem[o]*, blood + *-ptysis*, spitting), and persistent crackles.

9-71 *Broncho/spasm* (brong′ko-spaz″əm) means bronchial spasm. Bronchospasm brings about broncho/constriction (bron″ko-kən-strik′shən), resulting in an acute narrowing and obstruction of the respiratory airway. There is usually a cough with generalized wheezing, a chief characteristic of asthma and bronchitis.

Asthma is characterized by recurring episodes of paroxysmal wheezing and dyspnea, constriction of the bronchi, coughing, and viscous bronchial secretions. It is also called bronchial asthma.

bronchioles

9-72 Bronchiol/ectasis (brong″ke-o-lek′tə-sis) is dilation of the

_____.

Bronchiolitis (brong″ke-o-li′tis) means inflammation of the bronchioles.

lungs

9-73 The two highly elastic lungs are the main components of the respiratory system. *Pneumon/ia* (noo-mo′ne-ə), or *pneumonitis* (noo″mo-ni′tis), means inflammation of the

_____. Several types of bacteria, viruses, rickettsiae (rĭ-ket′se-e), and fungi have been identified as causes of pneumonia, but the disease is often caused by pneumo/cocci, a type of pathogenic coccal bacteria. This type of pneumonia is called pneumo/coccal pneumonia. A vaccine is available for pneumococcal pneumonia and is recommended for persons over 65 years of age and those with immunodeficiencies.

Lobar pneumonia involves one or more of the five major lobes of the lungs. Broncho/pneumon/ia (brong″ko-noŏ-mo′ne-ə) involves both the bronchi and the lungs and usually is a result of the spread of infection from the upper to the lower respiratory tract.

9-74 A pulmonary abscess (lung abscess) is a complication of an infection of the lung. A localized cavity containing pus and surrounded by inflamed lung tissue is a lung

_____.

abscess

9-75 Pleural effusion (ə-fu′zhən) is a collection of nonpurulent fluid in the

_____ cavity (Figure 9-15). *Non/purulent* means not containing pus. If pleural effusion contains pus, it is called pyothorax or empyema (em″pi-e′mə). This condition is an extension of infection from nearby structures. Empyema is when the

_____ effusion contains pus.

pleural

pleural

Untreated empyema can lead to pulmonary fibrosis, also called fibrosis of the lungs. The combining form *fibr(o)* means fiber or fibrous (tough, threadlike). Pulmonary fibrosis is a

_____ condition of the connective tissue of the lungs, resulting from the formation of scar tissue.

fibrous

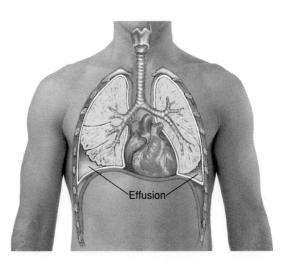

Figure 9-15 Pleural effusion. Abnormal accumulation of fluid in the pleural space is characterized by fever, chest pain, dyspnea, and nonproductive cough.

chest	**9-76** <u>Hydrothorax</u> (hi″dro-thor′aks) is a noninflammatory accumulation of fluid in one or both pleural cavities. Literal interpretation of *hydro/thorax* is watery _____.
hemothorax	An accumulation of blood and fluid in the pleural cavity is called <u>hemo/thorax</u> (he″mo-thor′aks). Trauma, such as a knife wound, is the most common cause of hemothorax, but it can occur as a result of inflammation or tumors. Write this new term that means blood and fluid in the pleural cavity: _____.
blood	**9-77** <u>Pneumo/thorax</u> (noo″mo-thor′aks) is air or gas in the pleural cavity; it leads to collapse of the lung. This may be the result of an open chest wound that permits the entrance of air, rupture of a vesicle on the surface of the lung, or a severe bout of coughing; it may even occur spontaneously without apparent cause. (Both pneumothorax and hemothorax are illustrated in Figure 9-16.) <u>Pneumo/hemo/thorax</u> (noo″mo-he″mo-thor′aks) is an accumulation of air and _____ in the pleural cavity.
pleura	**9-78** <u>Pleur/itis</u> (ploo-ri′tis) is inflammation of the _____. <u>Pleurisy</u> (ploor′ĭ-se) is another name for pleuritis. Pleurisy may be caused by an infection, injury, or tumor, or it may be a complication of certain lung diseases. A sharp pain on inspiration is characteristic of pleurisy. A pleural friction rub may be heard on auscultation.
pleuritis	*Pleurisy* is another name for _____.
lungs	**9-79** <u>Pleuro/pneumon/ia</u> (ploor″o-noo-mo′ne-ə) is a combination of pleurisy and pneumonia. You will need to remember that pleuropneumonia is inflammation of both the pleura and the _____.
pleura	**9-80** <u>Pleuro/dynia</u> (ploor″o-din′e-ə) is pain of the pleura. This can be caused by inflammation of the pleura or by <u>pleural adhesions</u>, in which the pleural membranes stick together or to the wall of the chest and produce pain on movement or breathing. *Adhesion* means a sticking together of two surfaces that are normally separated. Pleural adhesion may be associated with pleur/itis, which is inflammation of the _____.
lung	**9-81** <u>Pulmonary edema</u> is an accumulation of extravascular fluid in _____ tissue. Pulmonary edema also involves the alveoli and progresses to fluid entering the bronchioles and bronchi. Dyspnea on exertion is one of the earliest symptoms of pulmonary edema. As the condition becomes more advanced, the patient may become orthopneic. Acute pulmonary edema is an emergency situation. Congestive heart failure is the most common cause of pulmonary edema.

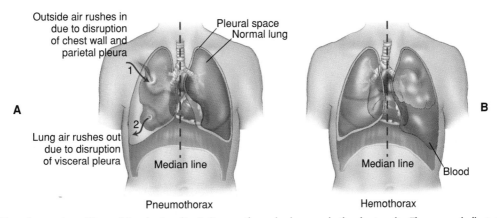

Figure 9-16 Two abnormal conditions of the chest cavity. **A,** Pneumothorax is air or gas in the chest cavity. The *arrows* indicate the two situations that result in pneumothorax. *Arrow 1* represents an open chest wound that permits the entrance of air into the pleural space. *Arrow 2* represents a tear within the lung, which allows air to enter the pleural space. **B,** Hemothorax, blood in the pleural cavity, below the left lung. The massive hemothorax shown has caused much of the left lung to collapse.

	In congestive heart failure, the work demanded of the heart is greater than its ability to perform. Decreased output of blood by the left ventricle produces congestion and engorgement of the pulmonary vessels with escape of fluid into pulmonary tissues. Congestive heart failure can result in a
pulmonary	lung disorder, _____ edema.
	9-82 A <u>pulmon/ary embolus</u> (**em′bo-ləs**) is an obstruction of the
pulmonary	_____ artery or one of its branches. Obstruction of a large pulmonary vessel can cause sudden death. The pulmonary arteries carry blood to the lungs. An embolus (plural is emboli) is a plug, usually part of a thrombus, obstructing a vessel. <u>Embolism</u> (**em′bə-liz-əm**) is the sudden blocking of an artery by a clot or foreign material that has been brought to its site of lodgment by the circulating blood. *Embol/ism (embol[o], embolus + -ism, condition)* is a general term and does not designate what constitutes the embolus or where the embolus has lodged.
	9-83 The lungs of a baby are pink. The adult lung darkens as a result of inhalation of dust and soot. <u>Pneumo/coni/osis</u> (**noo″mo-ko″ne-o′sis**) is any disease of the lung caused by chronic inhalation of dust, usually mineral dust of either occupational or environmental origin. The combining form *coni(o)* means dust. Pneumo/coni/osis is a condition (disease) of the lungs
dust	caused by inhalation of _____.
	9-84 <u>Anthrac/osis</u> (**an-thrə-ko′sis**), <u>asbest/osis</u> (**as″bes-to′sis**), and <u>silic/osis</u> (**sil″ĭ-ko′sis**) are three kinds of pneumoconiosis. The combining form *anthrac(o)* means coal. <u>Anthrac/osis</u> is a chronic lung
coal	disease characterized by the deposit of _____ dust in the lungs. It occurs in coal miners and is aggravated by cigarette smoking. <u>Asbest/osis</u> is a chronic lung disease that results from prolonged exposure to
asbestos	_____. It may occur in asbestos miners and workers or those exposed to asbestos building materials. <u>Mesothelioma</u> (**mez″o-the″le-o′mə**), a rare malignant tumor, sometimes develops and is almost always fatal. The mesothelium is a layer of epithelial cells that covers the pleura and the peritoneum. <u>Silic/osis</u> is a lung disorder caused by long-term inhalation of silica dust, which is found in sands, quartzes, and many other stones. This lung disorder is a type of
pneumoconiosis	_____.
	9-85 <u>Chronic obstructive pulmonary disease</u> (COPD), also called <u>chronic obstructive lung disease</u> (COLD), is a nonspecific designation that includes a group of progressive and irreversible respiratory problems in which dyspnea and often chronic coughs are prominent features. The mechanism of

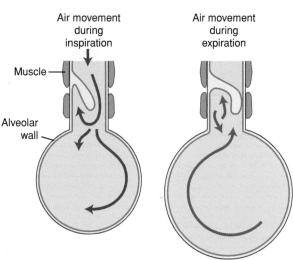

Figure 9-17   Mechanisms of air trapping in chronic obstructive pulmonary disease. Air trapping is the result of an inefficient expiratory effort. As the rate of respiration increases, breathing becomes more shallow and the amount of trapped air increases.

air trapping is explained in Figure 9-17. Airflow obstruction ultimately occurs. Emphysema, chronic bronchitis, asthmatic bronchitis, bronchiectasis, and cystic fibrosis are often included in this group. COPD is aggravated by cigarette smoking and air pollution.

Emphysema (em″fə-se′mə),* characterized by overinflation and destructive changes in alveolar walls, is probably the most severe COPD. Permanent hyperinflation of the lungs occurs as alveoli are destroyed, and alveolar air is trapped, thus interfering with exchange of carbon dioxide and oxygen.

Overinflation and destruction of the alveolar walls are major characteristics of

emphysema

_____.

9-86 <u>Cystic fibrosis</u> is an inherited disorder of the exocrine glands that involves the lungs, pancreas, and sweat glands. Heavy secretion of thick mucus clogs the bronchi and leads to a chronic cough and persistent upper respiratory infections. Excessive salt loss (three to six times the normal concentrations) in the perspiration of persons who have cystic fibrosis forms the basis of the sweat test, a laboratory test to determine the amount of sodium and chloride excretion from the sweat glands.

The disease is usually diagnosed in infancy or early childhood. The sweat test is performed to

fibrosis

diagnose cystic _____.

9-87 <u>Atel/ectasis</u> (*atel[o]*, imperfect + *-ectasis*, stretching) (at″ə-lek′tə-sis) is an abnormal condition characterized by the collapse of all or part of a lung. Failure of the lungs to expand fully at birth is called primary atelectasis. Other causes of atelectasis include obstructions of the airways, compression of the lung as a result of fluid or air, and pressure from a tumor.

Write the name of this abnormal condition in which there is incomplete expansion of a lung at

atelectasis

birth or airlessness of a lung that once functioned: _____.

9-88 <u>Tuberculosis</u> (too-ber″ku-lo′sis) (TB) is an infectious disease that often is chronic and commonly affects the lungs, although it may occur in other parts of the body. <u>Pulmonary tuberculosis</u>

lungs

affects the _____.

Resistance to tuberculosis depends a great deal on a person's general health. Early symptoms of tuberculosis (loss of energy, appetite, and weight) may go unnoticed. Fever, night sweats, and spitting up of bloody or purulent sputum may not occur until a year or more after the initial exposure to the disease. The disease is named after <u>tubercles</u> (too′bər-kəlz), which are small, round nodules produced in the lungs by the infective bacteria.

*Emphysema (Greek: *en*, inside; *physema*, a blowing).

9-89 Liquefaction of the tubercles not only results in tubercular cavities in the lungs but can also cause the production of a large quantity of highly infectious sputum that is raised when the infected person coughs.

out

To ex/pectorate (**ek-spek′tə-rāt**) is to cough up and spit _____
material from the lungs and air passages. (The material coughed up from the lungs is sputum.) Blood-stained sputum is often produced in tuberculosis. Hemo/ptysis (**he-mop′tĭ-sis**) is the spitting of blood or blood-stained sputum.

Exercise 5

Match the following unnatural chest features with their outstanding characteristics.

_____ 1. barrel chest

_____ 2. flail chest

_____ 3. funnel chest

_____ 4. pigeon chest

A. contracting and bulging of the lung during inspiration and expiration
B. depression of the breastbone
C. prominent anterior projection of the breastbone
D. rounded chest

Exercise 6

Circle the correct answer to complete each sentence.

1. Narrowing of the lumen of the trachea is (tracheitis, tracheomalacia, tracheostenosis, tracheotomy).
2. The presence of bronchial stones is (bronchiectasis, bronchoconstriction, bronchogenic, broncholithiasis).
3. Pneumonia that involves only one lobe of the lungs is called (bronchial, lobar, pleural, pneumococcal) pneumonia.
4. A collection of nonpurulent fluid in the pleural cavity is (pleural effusion, pneumothorax, pulmonary abscess, pyothorax).
5. *Pleurisy* means the same as (pleuritis, pleurodynia, pleuropneumonia, plumonary edema).
6. Sudden blocking of an artery by material that has been brought to its site of lodgment by the circulating blood is called (embolism, thrombosis, hemothorax, hydrothorax).
7. Any disease of the lung caused by chronic inhalation of dust is called (anthracosis, asbestosis, pneumoconiosis, silicosis).
8. Overinflation and destructive changes in alveolar walls are characteristics of (congenital atelactasis, emphysema, mesothelioma, pleuropneumonia).

■ *Death and Cancer Statistics*

9-90 The National Center for Health Statistics lists <u>heart disease</u> as the number 1 cause of adult deaths in the United States, and <u>cancer</u> is listed as number 2. Cancer deaths accounted for 23.90% of all deaths in 2000. In spite of the growing optimism with improvements in prevention, early detection, and treatment of many forms of cancer, the total number of recorded cancer deaths in the United States continues to increase slightly due to the aging and expanding population.

heart

The main cause of adult deaths in the United States is _____
disease, and the second leading cause of death is cancer.

Although cancer is sometimes regarded as a disease of older individuals, it is also the second leading cause of death among children ages 1 to 14 years in the United States, with accidents being the most common cause of death.

9-91 Each year the American Cancer Society (ACS) estimates the number of new cancer cases and deaths expected in the United States. Most <u>skin cancers</u> and most <u>in situ cancers</u> are not included in cancer predictions and statistics about cancer deaths. *In situ* is Latin and means localized and not invad-

localized

ing the surrounding tissue. A word that means in situ is _____.The incidence of cancer and cancer death varies by type in adult males and females. Look at estimated incidences and deaths for males and females in Table 9-2. Look first at the estimated new cases in

prostate

American males. The _____ is the site of the greatest number of estimated new cancer cases in males.

TABLE 9-2 Estimated New Cases and Cancer Deaths for Adults by Gender, U.S., 2004

Adult males	Adult females
Estimated New Cases for the Three Major Causes	
Prostate (33%)	Breast (32%)
Lung and bronchus (13%)	Lung and Bronchus (12%)
Colon and rectum (11%)	Colon and rectum (11%)
Estimated Deaths for the Three Major Causes	
Lung and bronchus (32%)	Lung and bronchus (25%)
Prostate (10%)	Breast (15%)
Colon and rectum (10%)	Colon and rectum (10%)

Excludes basal and squamous cell skin cancers and in situ carcinomas. Data from Cancer Statistics, 2004, CA, *A Cancer Journal for Clinicians* 54:1, 2004.

breast
lung

In females, what is the site of the greatest number of estimated new cancer cases?

_____

   Notice that cancer of the _____ and bronchus rank number 1 in estimated deaths from cancer for all adults.

9-92 <u>Lung cancer</u> remains a highly lethal disease, although significant improvements in treatment have occurred in the last decade. The most important cause of lung cancer is tobacco smoking. Besides cigarettes, exposure to airborne asbestos, uranium, radon, and high doses of ionizing radiation have been linked to increased incidence of lung cancer, according to the American Cancer Society. However, the greatest cause of lung cancer is _____.

cigarettes
 (or smoking)

   Cigarette smoking increases the risk of lung cancer more than the risk of cancer at any other site, but cigarette smoking—as well as pipe smoking—also multiplies the risk of cancer of the lip, mouth, tongue, and pharynx.

9-93 Elimination of tobacco use is the surest route to reducing the risk of premature mortality from lung cancer. At the time of this writing, the ACS does not recommend testing for early lung cancer detection in asymptomatic individuals. However, they maintain that patients at high risk for lung cancer (due to significant exposure to tobacco smoke or occupational exposures) and their physicians may decide to have screening tests done on an individual basis.

tobacco

   The surest way to reduce the risk of lung cancer is elimination of the use of

_____.

9-94 The ACS recommends screening tests for breast, cervical, endometrial, prostate, and colorectal cancers at various ages, depending on the type. There is growing optimism with improvements in prevention, early detection, and treatment of many forms of cancer, but the number of people living with cancer is expected to double between the years 2000 and 2050.

lung

   It is important to remember that the most common cause of cancer death is cancer of the _____ and bronchus, accounting for approximately one fourth of all cancer deaths.

SURGICAL AND THERAPEUTIC INTERVENTIONS

9-95 Asphyxiation, the inability to breathe, requires immediate corrective measures to prevent damage or death. Removal of a foreign body in the airway may be needed before oxygen and artificial respiration are administered. One method of dislodging food or other obstruction from the windpipe is the <u>Heimlich</u> (**hīm′lik**) <u>maneuver</u> (Figure 9-18).

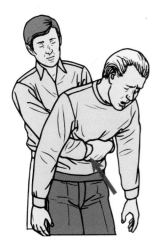

Figure 9-18   Heimlich maneuver. The rescuer grasps the choking person from behind, placing the fist below the victim's xiphoid process with the other hand placed firmly over the fist. Abruptly pulling the fist firmly upward will often force the obstruction up the windpipe.

Artificial respiration may be manual, as in the lifesaving procedure cardiopulmonary resuscitation (CPR), or provided by a mechanical ventilator, a device used to provide assisted respiration and usually temporary life support. CPR consists of artificial respiration and external cardiac massage.

An emergency tracheo/stomy (tra″ke-os′tə-me), surgical creation of an

opening

_____ in the trachea, may be necessary in upper airway obstruction. A tracheostomy requires a tracheo/tomy (tra″ke-ot′ə-me), an incision into the trachea through the neck below the larynx.

9-96 A tracheostomy is not always an emergency procedure and can be temporary or permanent. A tracheostomy is performed after a laryngectomy (lar″in-jek′tə-me) or when prolonged mechanical ventilation is needed. A tube is inserted through an incision in the neck into the trachea. There are many types of tracheostomy tubes; some permit speech.

A stoma (sto′mə) is a mouthlike opening, particularly one that is kept open for drainage or other purposes. Sometimes a person has a stoma at the base of the neck. Surgical creation of this type of opening into the trachea is called a tracheostomy. A general term for a mouthlike opening is a

stoma

_____ .

9-97 In COPD or other problems in hypoxic patients, oxygen therapy may be prescribed by the physician. Oxygen is sometimes administered after general surgery.

In patients who can breathe but are hypoxic, oxygen is delivered through tubing via a simple face mask, nasal prongs, a Venturi mask, or trans/tracheal (trans-tra′ke-əl) oxygen delivery. A Venturi mask and a transtracheal oxygen system deliver a more consistent and accurate oxygen concentration. Compare the four types of airway management shown in Figure 9-19. The term nasal cannula (kan′u-lə) refers to either of the two small tubes that are inserted into the nares. Other types of cannulas (cannulae) may be inserted into a duct or cavity to deliver medication or drain fluid. The nasal cannula shown in Figure 9-19, B, delivers oxygen. Transtracheal oxygen (TTO) delivers oxygen to the lungs through a flexible catheter that is inserted directly into the trachea.

9-98 Oxygen is administered in hypoxic patients to increase the amount of oxygen in circulating blood. It is also administered during anesthesia, because oxygen functions as a carrier gas for the delivery of anesthetic agents to the tissues of the body. An overdose of oxygen can have toxic effects, which include respiratory depression and damage to the lungs. Using hyp/ox/emia as a model, write a word that means increased oxygen content of the blood:

**hyperoxemia
(hi″pər-ok-se′me-ə)**

_____ .

9-99 Endo/tracheal intubation is the management of the patient with an airway catheter inserted through the mouth or nose into the trachea. An endotracheal tube may be used to maintain a patent (open and unblocked) airway or to maintain a closed system with a ventilator.

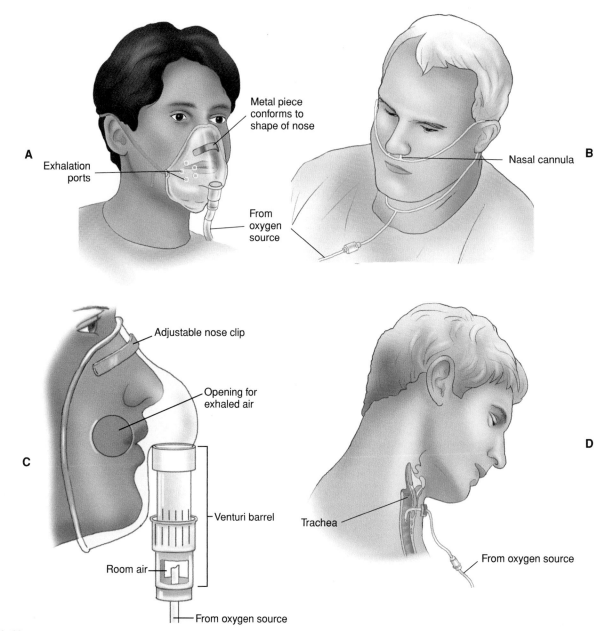

Figure 9-19   Four means of administering oxygen. **A,** A simple oxygen mask delivers high concentrations of oxygen and is used for short-term oxygen therapy or in an emergency. **B,** The nasal cannula, a device that delivers oxygen by way of two small tubes that are inserted into the nostrils. **C,** The Venturi mask, a face mask designed to allow inspired air to mix with oxygen. **D,** Transtracheal oxygen is a long-term method of delivering oxygen directly into the lungs.

Naso/tracheal **(na″zo-tra′ke-əl)** intubation is insertion of a tube through the nose into the trachea. Orotracheal **(or″o-tra′ke-əl)** intubation is insertion of a tube through the mouth into the trachea. Compare these two types of intubation with a tracheostomy tube that is used for prolonged airway management (Figure 9-20).

9-100 *Oxygenation* means the act, process, or result of oxygenating. *Extra/corpor/eal* means outside the body. Extracorporeal membrane oxygenation (ECMO) is a technique used in a hospital for providing respiratory support by circulating the blood through an artificial lung. It is used in newborns and occasionally in adults with acute respiratory distress syndrome.

lung

Pneumo/centesis **(noo″mo-sən-te′sis)** is surgical puncture of a _____ to drain fluid contents.

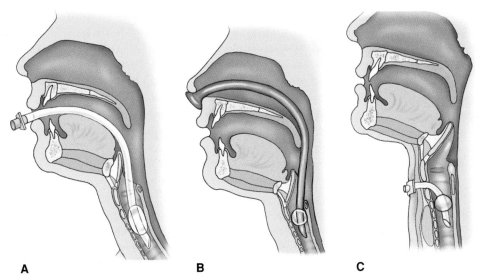

A   **B**   **C**

Figure 9-20 Comparison of endotracheal intubation and a tracheostomy tube. **A,** Orotracheal intubation for short-term airway management. **B,** Nasotracheal intubation for short-term airway management. **C,** Tracheostomy tube for longer maintenance of the airway.

9-101 The term _thoracentesis_ (**thor″ə-sen-te′sis**) is a shortened form of the term _thoracocentesis_ (**thor″ə-ko-sən-te′sis**). Thora/centesis is surgical puncture of the chest wall and pleural space with a needle to aspirate fluid or to obtain a specimen for biopsy. It has both therapeutic and diagnostic uses.

puncture

Thora/centesis is surgical _____ of the chest wall and can be used in the treatment of pleural effusion (Figure 9-21).

Thoracentesis is sometimes called _pleurocentesis_ (**ploor″o-sen-te′sis**).

9-102 A _pneumonectomy_ (**noo″mo-nek′tə-me**), either partial or complete, is usually required for treating lung cancer. Removal of a lung requires an open surgery that will provide full access to structures in the chest cavity. _Pneum/ectomy_ (**noo-mek′tə-me**) has the same meaning as pneumonectomy. Write a term that means a surgical incision into the chest:

thoracotomy

_____.

Radiation and chemo/therapy are used to destroy remaining tumor cells or for certain types of localized malignancies.

9-103 A total pneumon/ectomy is removal of an entire lung. If only part of the lung is removed, the surgery is called a partial pneumonectomy.

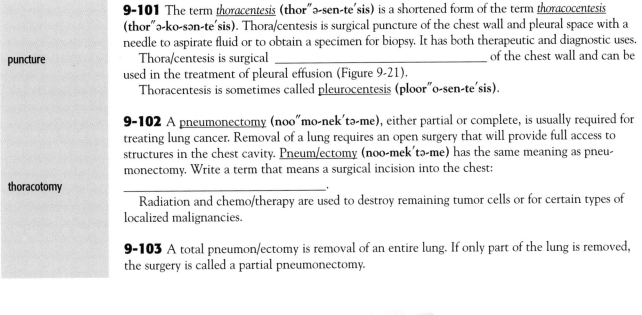

Visceral pleura
Lung tissue
Parietal pleura
Rib
Thoracentesis needle
Pleural effusion

Figure 9-21 Insertion of the needle in thoracentesis. The actual site for insertion depends on the location of the effusion and the material that has escaped into the pleural space. _Thoracocentesis_ means the same as thoracentesis, but the latter term is used more often.

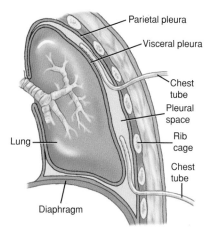

Parietal pleura

Visceral pleura

Chest tube

Pleural space

Rib cage

Chest tube

Lung

Diaphragm

Figure 9-22   Placement of chest tubes. A chest tube is a catheter that is inserted through the thorax into the pleural space and is attached to a water-seal chest drainage device. The chest tube is used to remove fluid or air after chest surgery and lung collapse.

lung

A lob/ectomy is an excision of a single lobe. Because other organs, such as the liver and brain, also have lobes, one has to specify pulmonary lobectomy, unless it is clear that the lobectomy refers to the _____.

A thoraco/stomy is an incision made into the chest wall to provide an opening for a chest tube. A chest tube is inserted into the pleural space to remove air and/or fluid and is commonly used after chest surgery (Figure 9-22).

9-104 Trauma often requires plastic surgery of various respiratory organs. However, rhino/plasty (ri′no-plas″te) is usually done for cosmetic reasons. Rhino/plasty is plastic surgery in which the

nose

structure of the _____ is changed.

Palato/plasty (pal′ə-to-plas″te) is surgical repair (reconstruction) of the palate. Palatoplasty, along with additional plastic surgery, is used to correct cleft palate, a congenital defect characterized by a fissure in the midline of the palate. Write this term that means plastic surgery of the palate:

palatoplasty

_____.

septorhinoplasty (sep″to-ri′no-plas″te)

9-105 Tracheoplasty (tra′ke-o-plas″te) is plastic surgery to repair the trachea. Write a term using sept(o), rhin(o), and -plasty: _____. This new term means plastic surgery of the nasal septum and the external nose. Surgical reconstruction of the nasal septum is septoplasty (sep′to-plas″te).

Thoraco/plasty (thor′ə-ko-plas″te) is a surgical procedure that involves removing ribs and allowing the chest wall to collapse a lung. The procedure was formerly done as a therapeutic measure and is sometimes still done to gain access during thoracic surgery. The procedure done to collapse a lung

thoracoplasty

is called a _____.

9-106 For mild sleep apnea, weight loss or a change in sleeping position may reduce or correct the problem. A common nonsurgical method to prevent airway collapse is the use of continuous positive airway pressure (CPAP ventilation, commonly called C Pap). A small electric compressor delivers positive pressure through a face mask during sleep.

Surgical intervention for sleep apnea may involve an adenoid/ectomy (ad″ə-noid-ek′tə-me),

adenoids

excision of the _____, uvul/ectomy (u″vu-lek′tə-me) (excision of the uvula, the pendant tissue in the back of the pharynx), or surgical repair of the posterior oropharynx. Both conventional and laser surgeries are used for this purpose.

9-107 Many malignant lesions are curable if detected in the early stage. Treatment selection depends on the site, stage of the cancer, and unique characteristics of the individual. Some anti/cancer treatments include surgery, irradiation, and chemotherapy with antineoplastic agents.

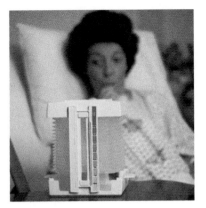

Figure 9-23 Incentive spirometry. A therapeutic means of encouraging deep breathing using a specially designed spirometer that provides visual feedback.

neoplasms

An <u>anti/neoplas/tic</u> is a treatment that acts against _____. These treatments are designed to kill or prevent the spread of cancer cells. Irradiation uses radiant energy such as x-ray and radioactive substances to treat cancer.

9-108 A method of encouraging voluntary deep breathing after surgery or with patients who have chronic air obstruction involves use of an <u>incentive spirometer</u>, a small apparatus that provides visual feedback about the inspired volume of air (Figure 9-23).

Nebulizers and inhalers are used to administer medications that are inhaled. <u>Broncho/dilators</u> (**brong″ko-di′la-torz**) are medications used in asthma and other respiratory conditions that constrict air passages. A bronchodilator expands the bronchi and other air passages. An agent that

bronchodilator

dilates the bronchi is a _____.

9-109 Respiratory infections are generally treated with <u>antibiotics</u>, along with other medications that individual patients need. For example, <u>decongestants</u>* cause vasoconstriction of the nasal membranes, thereby eliminating or reducing swelling or congestion.

<u>Anti/histamines</u> (**an″te-, an″tĭ-his′tə-mēnz**) are also used to treat colds and allergies.

against

Antihistamines act _____ histamine to reduce its effects. Histamine brings about many of the symptoms that occur with the common cold.

against

9-110 <u>Anti/tussive</u> (**an″te-, an″ti-tus′iv**) means _____ coughing. In other words, <u>antitussive</u>† means preventing or relieving coughing, or an agent that does so.

Use *muc(o)* plus a suffix to write a word that means destroying or dissolving mucus:

mucolytic (mu″ko-lit′ik)

_____. <u>Mucolytic</u> is a term that also means an agent that destroys or dissolves mucus. An abundance of mucus is produced in certain respiratory disorders, such as emphysema. Mucolytics and bronchodilators are often used in treating these patients to open their breathing passages.

Exercise 7

Write words in the blanks to complete these sentences. The first letters of the answers are given as clues.

1. The inability to breathe is a _____.

2. Artificial respiration and external cardiac massage are administered in cardiopulmonary r_____.

3. In a hospital setting, artificial respiration is supplied by a mechanical v_____.

---

*Decongestant (*de-*, away or remove; Latin: *congerere*, to pile up).
†Antitussive (*anti-*, against; Latin: *tussis*, cough).

4. Surgical creation of an opening into the trachea is called a t_____.

5. COPD means chronic o_____ pulmonary disease.

6. TTO is the abbreviation for t_____ oxygen, which is a means of delivering oxygen to the lungs.

7. Insertion of a tube through the mouth into the trachea is called o_____ intubation.

8. Pneumocentesis is surgical puncture of a l_____ to drain fluid contents.

9. A t_____ is an incision made into the chest wall to provide an opening for a chest tube.

10. An agent that prevents coughing is called an a_____.

11. The number 1 cause of death in the United States is h_____ disease.

12. The second leading cause of death in the United States is c_____.

13. The site of the greatest number of estimated new cancers in adult American males is the p_____.

14. The site of the greatest number of estimated new cancers in adult American females is the b_____.

15. The greatest number of estimated cancer deaths in adults is cancer of the l_____ and bronchus.

SELECTED ABBREVIATIONS

ABG	arterial blood gas		**LUL**	left upper lobe
ACS	American Cancer Society		**O₂**	oxygen
AFB	acid-fast bacillus (some types cause tuberculosis)		**PFT**	pulmonary function test
ARDS	acute or adult respiratory distress syndrome		**pH**	potential hydrogen
C Pap, CPAP	continuous positive airway pressure (for sleep apnea)		**PO₂**	oxygen partial pressure
			R	respiration
CAL	chronic airflow limitation		**RDS**	respiratory distress syndrome
CO₂	carbon dioxide		**RLL**	right lower lobe
COLD	chronic obstructive lung disease		**RUL**	right upper lobe
COPD	chronic obstructive pulmonary disease		**SARS**	severe acute respiratory syndrome
CPR	cardiopulmonary resuscitation		**SIDS**	sudden infant death syndrome
CSR	Cheyne-Stokes respiration		**SOB**	shortness of breath
ECMO	extracorporeal membrane oxygenation		**TB**	tuberculosis
ET	endotracheal		**TTO**	transtracheal oxygen
HSV	herpes simplex virus		**URI**	upper respiratory infection
LLL	left lower lobe		**URT**	upper respiratory tract
LRT	lower respiratory tract		**VC**	vital capacity

CHAPTER 9 REVIEW

■ Basic Understanding

Matching

I. Match structures in the left column (1-7) with their characteristics or functions in the right column (A-G).

_____ 1. alveolus

_____ 2. bronchus

_____ 3. diaphragm

_____ 4. larynx

_____ 5. nose

_____ 6. pharynx

_____ 7. trachea

A. a branch of the trachea
B. a muscular partition that facilitates breathing
C. commonly called the windpipe
D. connected with the paranasal sinuses
E. contains the palatine tonsils
F. contains the vocal cords
G. where oxygen and carbon dioxide exchange occurs

II. Match diseases or disorders in the left column (1-7) with their characteristics in the right column (A-H):

_____ 1. anthracosis

_____ 2. asthma

_____ 3. atelectasis

_____ 4. COPD

_____ 5. cystic fibrosis

_____ 6. emphysema

_____ 7. pertussis

A. accumulation of coal dust in the lungs
B. can result from disorders such as chronic bronchitis and chronic asthma
C. chronic respiratory infection and disorders of the pancreas and sweat glands
D. congenital, incomplete expansion of a lung or a portion of a lung
E. destruction of the alveolar walls that leads to hindered gas exchange
F. paroxysmal cough, ending in a whooping inspiration
G. paroxysmal dyspnea accompanied by wheezing

Labeling

III. Label structures in the diagram with the corresponding combining form. The first one is done as an example. Note that number 2 and number 6 have two answers.

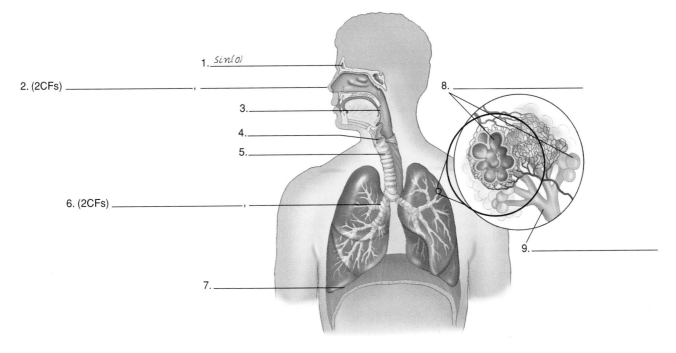

1. _Sin(o)_

2. (2CFs) _____ , _____

3. _____

4. _____

5. _____

6. (2CFs) _____ , _____

7. _____

8. _____

9. _____

Sequencing

IV. *Number the following structures to show the sequence of passage of air from the nose to the lungs. The first one is done as an example.*

nasal cavity___1___   bronchi_____   larynx_____   pharynx_____

trachea_____   alveoli_____   bronchioles_____

Listing

V. *List five functions of the respiratory system.*

1. _____

2. _____

3. _____

4. _____

5. _____

Matching

VI. *Write URT (for upper respiratory tract) or LRT (lower respiratory tract) to identify the locations of these structures.*

1. alveolus   _____

2. bronchiole _____

3. bronchus   _____

4. larynx   _____

5. nose   _____

6. pharynx   _____

7. trachea   _____

Multiple Choice

VII. *Circle one answer for each of the following multiple choice questions.*

1. Mrs. Smith's doctor tells her that she has pneumonia. What is another name for her diagnosis? (congestive heart disease, pneumonitis, pulmonary edema, pulmonary insufficiency)

2. Which term means coughing up and spitting out sputum? (expectoration, expiration, exhalation, extrapleural)

3. John R. is told that he suffers periodic absence of breathing. What is the name of his condition? (apnea, dyspnea, hyperpnea, hypopnea)

4. Which of the following activities is the respiratory system's greatest contribution to the acid-base balance? (exchange of CO_2 for O_2, maintaining body temperature, regulating water loss, taking in water)

5. What is the serous membrane that lines the walls of the thoracic cavity? (parietal pleura, rhinorrhea, silicosis, visceral pleura)

6. What is the correct sequence for the first and second leading causes of adult deaths in the United States? (cancer and heart, heart and cancer, heart and colon cancer, lung cancer and colon cancer)

7. Mrs. Sema has difficulty breathing except when sitting in an upright position. What is the term for her condition? (anoxia, hypocapnia, inspiration, orthopnea)

8. What is the term for reduced acidity of the body fluids, such as may occur in hyperventilation? (acid-base balance, acid-base compensation, acidosis, alkalosis)

9. The pulmonary specialist orders a test to measure the amount of air taken into and expelled from the lungs? What is the name of the test? (laryngoscopy, mediastinoscopy, spirometry, thoracometry)

10. What is effusion of fluid into the air spaces and tissue spaces of the lungs called? (pleuropneumonia, pneumonitis, pulmonary edema, pulmonary insufficiency)

Writing Terms
VIII. *Write a term for each of the following:*

1. an internal blood clot _____

2. difficult or weak voice _____

3. direct visualization of the bronchi _____

4. drawing in or out as by suction _____

5. inflammation of the throat _____

6. presence of nasal calculi _____

7. pertaining to the air sacs of the lung _____

8. radiographic examination of the larynx _____

9. profuse nosebleed _____

10. within the nose _____

■ Greater Comprehension

Health Care Report
IX. *Define the underlined terms or abbreviations in the following respiratory care note.*

DATE: 3/06/2004
TIME: 0600
THERAPY ORDERED: Nebulizer treatment with 1.0 ml albuterol and 0.5 mg Atrovent every 4 hours
GOAL OF THERAPY: Treat hypoventilation/hypoxemia; relieve bronchospasm; bronchodilation; mucus clearance
and patient education.
ASSESSMENT: Bilateral lobes—decreased breath sounds prior to treatment. Pt had coughing spell during treatment
with some dyspnea noted. Treatment stopped at patient request. Oxygen saturation level 95% on 1.5 L O_2 per nasal
cannula after treatment.

MID-CITY MEDICAL CENTER   **RESPIRATORY CARE NOTES**
PT. NAME: Faye Schmidt   **DIAGNOSIS:** COPD

---

1. nebulizer _____

2. hypoventilation _____

3. hypoxemia _____

4. bronchospasm _____

5. bronchodilation _____

6. dyspnea_____

7. COPD _____

X. Read the following case study and answer the questions that follow it.

PHYSICAL EXAMINATION
COUNTY MEDICAL CENTER

666 Medical Center Drive   Anytown, US 391-333-3333

PATIENT: M. A. Gordon (female, age 63)

DATE: 05/04/2004

SYMPTOMS: Fever; dyspnea; mild, productive cough; malaise; loss of appetite.

HISTORY: Bronchitis, myocardial infarction (status post-CABG 1 year ago), and deep venous thrombosis with pulmonary embolism.

FAMILY HISTORY: Mother, age 85 with congestive heart failure; father deceased with a history of COLD and diabetes.

PHYSICAL EXAM: T 100.8; P 98, R 28; BP 160/94; fine crackles bilateral lung bases with some wheezes; increased dyspnea on exertion; O_2 saturation level 92% on 2 L O_2.

LABORATORY DATA: WBC 24.6

CHEST X-RAY: Increased right lung density; no pneumothorax or pleural effusion. Increasing rt. lung infiltrate with masslike density rt. hilum.

DIAGNOSIS: Community-acquired pneumonia.

TREATMENT PLAN: IV antibiotic pending sputum culture, bronchodilator such as Alupent, and expectorant such as guaifenesin.

Write the answer from the report that corresponds to each of these descriptions.

1. a vague feeling of discomfort and fatigue   _____

2. abnormal accumulation of fluid in the pleural space   _____

3. abnormal musical respiratory sounds   _____

4. abnormal respiratory sounds that consist of discontinuous bubbling noises   _____

5. the presence of air or gas in the pleural space   _____

6. inflammation of the bronchi   _____

7. labored or difficult breathing   _____

8. the blockage of a pulmonary artery by a substance brought by the circulating blood _____

9. therapeutic agent that relaxes the bronchioles   _____

10. therapeutic agent that assists in the coughing up of sputum   _____

Spelling

XI. Circle all incorrectly spelled terms and write their correct spelling:

acapnia   auscultation   bronchiectasis   laryngografy   pnumonitis

Pronunciation

XII. *The pronunciation is shown for several medical words. Indicate which syllable has the primary accent by marking it with an ´.*

1. laryngopathy (lar ing gop ə the)

2. parietal (pə ri ə təl)

3. pharyngeal (fə rin je əl)

4. spirometer (spi rom ə tər)

5. tracheostomy (tra ke os tə me)

Interpreting Abbreviations

XIII. *Write the meaning of these abbreviations:*

1. ABG _____

2. ECMO _____

3. HSV _____

4. SARS _____

5. URT _____

Categorizing Terms

XIV. *Classify the terms in the left column (1-10) by selecting category A, B, C, D, or E.*

_____ 1. anthracosis   A. anatomy

                                  B. diagnostic test or procedure

_____ 2. antitussives   C. pathology

                                  D. surgery

_____ 3. bronchography   E. therapy

_____ 4. coryza

_____ 5. epiglottis

_____ 6. nares

_____ 7. oximeter

_____ 8. palatoplasty

_____ 9. percussion

_____ 10. rhoncus

(Check your answers with the solutions in Appendix VI.)

LISTING OF MEDICAL TERMS

Use the practice CD to review the terms that have been presented. Look closely at the spelling of each term as it is pronounced, and be sure you know the meaning of each term.

acapnia	bronchoscopy	hyperventilation	neoplasm
acid-base balance	bronchospasm	hypocapnia	olfaction
acidemia	bronchus	hypopnea	olfactory
acidosis	canker	hypoxemia	oropharyngeal
acute	cannula	hypoxia	oropharynx
adenoidectomy	cardiopulmonary	incentive spirometer	orotracheal intubation
alkalemia	Cheyne-Stokes respiration	influenza	orthopnea
alkaline	chronic	inhalation	orthopneic
alkalosis	congestive heart failure	inhaler	oxygenation
alveolar	coronavirus	inspiration	palate
alveolus	coryza	interalveolar	palatine
anoxia	crackle	intrinsic	palatine tonsil
anthracosis	croup	lacrimal	palatitis
antiasthmatic	cyanosis	laryngalgia	palatoplasty
anticancer	cystic fibrosis	laryngeal	paranasal sinus
antihistamine	decongestant	laryngectomy	parietal pleura
antineoplastic	diaphragm	laryngitis	patent
antitussive	diaphragmatic	laryngography	percussion
apex	diphtheria	laryngopathy	pertussis
aphasia	dysphasia	laryngopharyngeal	pharyngalgia
aphasic	dysphonia	laryngopharynx	pharyngeal
aphonia	dyspnea	laryngoplegia	pharyngitis
apical	dyspneic	laryngoscope	pharyngodynia
aplasia	embolism	laryngoscopy	pharyngomycosis
apnea	embolus	laryngospasm	pharyngopathy
asbestosis	emphysema	laryngotracheal	pharyngoscope
asphyxia	empyema	laryngotracheitis	pharynx
asphyxiation	endonasal	laryngotracheobronchitis	phlegm
aspiration	endotracheal	larynx	phrenic
asthma	endotracheal intubation	lethargic	phrenitis
atelectasis	epiglottiditis	lethargy	phrenodynia
auditory tube	epiglottis	lobar pneumonia	phrenoplegia
auscultation	epiglottitis	lobectomy	phrenoptosis
bradypnea	epistaxis	malaise	pleura
bronchi	eupnea	mediastinoscope	pleural
bronchiectasis	eustachian tube	mediastinoscopy	pleural adhesion
bronchiole	exhalation	mediastinum	pleural cavity
bronchiolectasis	expectorate	mesothelioma	pleural effusion
bronchiolitis	expiration	mesothelium	pleurisy
bronchitis	extrapleural	mucolytic	pleuritis
bronchoalveolar	extrapulmonary	mucus	pleurocentesis
bronchoconstriction	extrinsic	nares	pleurodynia
bronchodilator	glottis	nasal cannula	pleuropneumonia
bronchogenic	Heimlich maneuver	nasal polyp	pneumectomy
bronchogram	hemoptysis	nasal septum	pneumocentesis
bronchography	hemothorax	nasolacrimal duct	pneumococci
broncholithiasis	herpes simplex virus	nasopharyngeal	pneumoconiosis
bronchopathy	hilum	nasopharyngitis	pneumohemothorax
bronchopneumonia	hydrothorax	nasopharynx	pneumonectomy
bronchopulmonary	hypercapnia	nasoscope	pneumonia
bronchoscope	hyperoxemia	nasotracheal intubation	pneumonitis
bronchoscopic	hyperpnea	nebulizer	pneumothorax

polyp
pulmonary
pulmonary angiography
pulmonary edema
pulmonary embolus
pulmonary fibrosis
pulmonary lobectomy
pulmonary ventilation
pulmonic
pulse oximeter
pulse oximetry
pyothorax
rale
respiration
respiratory
resuscitation
retronasal
rhinitis

rhinolith
rhinolithiasis
rhinoplasty
rhinorrhagia
rhinorrhea
rhonchus
septal deviation
septorhinoplasty
severe acute respiratory
    syndrome
silicosis
sinusitis
spirometer
spirometry
sputum
stoma
stridor
subphrenic

subpulmonary
supranasal
tachycardia
tachypnea
thoracentesis
thoracocentesis
thoracoplasty
thoracostomy
thoracotomy
thorax
thromboembolic
thrombus
tonsillitis
trachea
tracheal
trachealgia
tracheomalacia
tracheoplasty

tracheoscopic
tracheoscopy
tracheostenosis
tracheostomy
tracheotomy
transtracheal
tubercle
tuberculosis
uvula
uvulectomy
ventilation
Venturi mask
visceral pleura
vital capacity
wheeze

español ENHANCING SPANISH COMMUNICATION

ENGLISH	SPANISH (PRONUNCIATION)
acidity	acidez (ah-se-DES)
asphyxia	asfixia (as-FEEC-se-ah)
asthma	asma (AHS-mah)
breathe	alentar (ah-len-TAR), respirar (res-pe-RAR)
breathing	respiración (res-pe-rah-se-ON)
cancer	cáncer (CAHN-ser)
cough	tos (tos)
diaphragm	diafragma (de-ah-FRAHG-mah)
erect, straight	derecho (day-RAY-cho)
imperfect	imperfecto (im-per-FEC-to)
influenza	gripe (GREE-pay)
lobe	lóbulo (LO-boo-lo)
lung	pulmón (pool-MON)
nose	nariz (nah-REES)
nostril	orificio de la nariz (or-e-FEE-se-o day lah nah-REES)
obstruction	obstrucción (obs-trooc-se-ON)
paralysis	parálisis (pah-RAH-le-sis)
pneumonia	neumonía (nay-oo-mo-NEE-ah), pulmonía (pool-mo-NEE-ah)
respiration	respiración (res-pe-rah-se-ON)
throat	garganta (gar-GAHN-tah)
tonsil	tonsila (ton-SEE-lah), amígdala (ah-MEEG-dah-lah)
trachea	tráquea (TRAH-kay-ah)
voice	voz (vos)

CHAPTER 10

Digestive System

FUNCTION FIRST

Four major functions of the digestive system are ingestion of food, digestion of food, absorption of nutrients, and elimination of wastes. Accessory organs of digestion have additional functions, including the production or storage of secretions that aid in the chemical breakdown of food, filtration of the blood and breakdown of toxic compounds, storage of iron and certain vitamins, synthesis of plasma proteins, and regulation of blood glucose levels.

ANATOMY AND PHYSIOLOGY

intestines

10-1 The digestive system is known by many names, including the digestive tract, the alimentary (al″ə-men′tər-e) tract, and the gastrointestinal (gas″tro-in-tes′tĭ-nəl) or GI system. *Gastro/intestin/al* refers to the stomach and the _____.

The digestive tract is a long, muscular tube, lined with mucous membrane, that extends from the mouth to the anus. The upper GI (UGI) tract consists of the mouth, pharynx (far′inks) (called the throat in non-medical language), esophagus, and stomach. The lower GI tract is made up of the small and large intestines. The accessory organs (salivary glands, liver, gallbladder, and pancreas) secrete fluids that aid in digestion and absorption of nutrients.

■ *Digestion and Nutrition*

10-2 Nutrition is the sum of the processes involved in the taking in, digestion, absorption, and use of food substances by the body. The digestive system provides the body with water, nutrients, and minerals, and eliminates undigested food particles.

The first function of digestion is ingestion, the way in which the body takes in nutrients. In humans, ingestion (in-jes′chən) is orally taking substances into the body. *Ingestion* means swallowing the substances; in other words, the substance is taken into the body through the

mouth

_____.

10-3 Digestion, the second function, is the conversion of food into substances that can be absorbed in the GI tract. The two types of digestion are mechanical and chemical digestion. Mechanical digestion begins in the mouth with chewing and continues with churning actions in the stomach. Carbohydrates, proteins, and fats are transformed into smaller molecules through chemical digestion. The accessory organs contribute digestive fluids to aid this process.

digestion

The second activity of nutrition, called _____, consists of both mechanical and chemical processes that break down the food.

10-4 After swallowing, the digestive system moves the food particles along the digestive tract and mixes them with enzymes and other fluids. These movements are brought about by the contractions of smooth muscles of the digestive system. Be aware that some texts list movement of the food particles along the digestive tract as an additional function.

around

The movement of food particles through the digestive tract is called peristalsis (per″ĭ-stawl′sis). You learned earlier that *peri-* means _____. The suffix *-stalsis* means contraction. The presence of food in the digestive tube stimulates a coordinated, rhythmic muscular contraction called peristalsis.

10-5 Absorption, the third function, is the process in which the digested food molecules pass through the lining of the small intestine into the blood or lymph capillaries. This passage of the simple molecules from the lining of the small intestine into the blood or lymph is called

absorption

_____. Assimilation is the process of incorporating nutritive material into living tissue and occurs after or simultaneously with absorption.

10-6 The fourth function, elimination, is removal of undigested food particles (waste). Wastes are excreted (eliminated) through the anus in the form of feces. The anus is the opening of the large intestine to the outside. This last function of the digestive system is called

elimination

_____.

The elimination of undigested food particles is only one type of elimination of body wastes. Other body wastes include carbon dioxide excreted by the lungs, and excess water and other substances excreted in the urine and through perspiration.

nutrition

10-7 Alimentation (al″ə-men-ta′shən) is the process of providing nourishment, or nutrition,* for the body. Good nutrition is essential for metabolism (mə-tab′ə-liz″əm), the sum of all the physical and chemical processes that take place in living organisms and result in growth, generation of energy, elimination of wastes, and other body functions as they relate to the distribution of nutrients in the blood after digestion.

Alimentation means providing _____ for the body.

dietary

10-8 A balanced diet is one that is adequate in energy-providing substances (carbohydrates and fats), tissue-building compounds (proteins), inorganic chemicals (water and mineral salts), vitamins, and certain other substances, such as bulk for promoting movement of the contents of the digestive tract. The recommended dietary allowances (RDAs) are the levels of daily intake of essential nutrients that are considered adequate to meet nutritional needs. RDA means recommended _____ allowance.

Homeo/stasis is the state of dynamic equilibrium of the internal environment of the body. Homeostasis is maintained even though the amounts of various food substances and water that we take in vary. Learn the meanings of the following word parts that are used in discussing digestion and nutrition.

Word Parts for Digestion and Nutrition

Substances COMBINING FORMS	MEANING	Functions SUFFIXES	MEANING
amyl(o)	starch	-dipsia	thirst
bil(i), chol(e)	bile or gall	-orexia	appetite
glyc(o)	sugar	-pepsia	digestion
lact(o)	milk	-stalsis	contraction
lip(o)	fats		
prote(o)	protein		

sugar

10-9 Carbohydrates, fats, and proteins are the three major classes of nutrients. Carbohydrates, the basic source of energy for human cells, include starches and sugars.

The combining form glyc(o) means sugar. Glyco/lysis (gli-kol′ə-sis) is the breaking down of _____.

glucose

10-10 Glucose (gloo′kōs), a simple sugar, is the major source of energy for the body's cells. It is found in certain foods, especially fruits, and is also formed when more complex sugars and starches are broken down by the digestive system. The concentration of glucose in the blood in healthy individuals is maintained at a fairly constant level.

The type of sugar that is the main source of energy for the body is _____.

destruction

10-11 Starches, a second type of carbohydrate, break down easily and are eventually reduced to glucose before being absorbed into the blood. The combining form amyl(o) means starch. The digestive process whereby starch is converted into sugars is called amylolysis (am″ə-lol′ə-sis). The literal translation of amylo/lysis is _____ of starch.

protein

10-12 Proteins are nitrogenous compounds that provide amino acids and building material for development, growth, and maintenance of the body. The combining form prote(o) means protein. Proteo/lysis (pro″te-ol′ĭ-sis) is breaking down (destruction, digestion) of _____. Proteolysis is necessary for digestion, because proteins must be chemically broken down before they can be absorbed.

*Nutrition (Latin: nutriens, food that nourishes).

10-13 Fats, also called lipids, serve as an energy reserve. When stored in fat cells, they form lipoid tissue that helps to cushion and insulate vital organs. The combining form *lip(o)* means fats. Although lipids also include steroids, waxes, and fatty acids, *lip(o)* usually refers to fats. *Lip/oid* (**lip′oid**) means resembling _____.

fats

Calories are units that are used to denote the energy value of food or the heat expenditure of an organism. Proteins, carbohydrates, and fats contain calories. Having about twice as many calories per gram as carbohydrates and proteins, fats are well suited for storage of unused calories.

10-14 Bile is a digestive chemical that breaks fats into smaller particles, preparing them for further digestion and absorption. Two combining forms mean bile, *chol(e)* and _____.

bil(i)

10-15 Digestive enzymes act upon food substances, causing them to break down into simpler compounds. Enzymes are usually named by adding *-ase* (meaning enzyme) to the combining form of the substance on which they act. For example, lip/ase (**lip′ās, li′pās**) breaks down lipids.

The combining form *lact(o)* means milk. Remembering that *-ose* means sugar, write a new word that means the main sugar in milk (milk sugar): _____. The enzyme, lact/ase, breaks down lactose. Lactose intolerance is a disorder caused by inadequate production of, or defect in, the enzyme lactase.

lactose

Amylase (**am′ə-lās**) is an enzyme that breaks down starch. Proteinase (**pro′tēn-ās**) or protease (**pro′te-ās**) is an enzyme that breaks down protein.

10-16 Thirst is the desire for fluid, especially for water. Not only does water serve to transport food in the digestive tract, but it is also the principal medium in which chemical reactions occur. The suffix that means thirst is _____.

-dipsia

10-17 The normal desire for food is called the appetite. The suffix that you will use to write words about the appetite is _____.

-orexia
-pepsia

The suffix that means digestion is _____. Normal digestion is eu/pepsia (**u-pep′se-ə**).

Exercise 1

Write the meanings of these word parts:

1. amyl(o) _____

2. chol(e) _____

3. glyc(o) _____

4. lact(o) _____

5. lip(o) _____

6. prote(o) _____

7. -dipsia _____

8. -orexia _____

9. -pepsia _____

10. -stalsis _____

■ *Major Structures of the Digestive System*

10-18 Label the structures in Figure 10-1 as you read the following information.

Digestion begins in the mouth (1). The teeth grind and chew the food before it is swallowed. The mass of chewed food is called a bolus.

The pharynx (2) passes the bolus to the esophagus (3), which leads to the stomach (4), where food is churned and broken down chemically and mechanically.

The liquid mass, called chyme, is passed to the small intestine, where digestion continues and absorption of nutrients occurs. The three parts of the small intestine are shown: duodenum (5), jejunum (6), and ileum (7).

Undigested food passes to the large intestine (8), where much of the water is absorbed. It is stored in the rectum until it is eliminated through the anus (9).

10-19 The structures that you labeled make up the muscular tube portion of the digestion tract, which consists of the upper GI tract and the _____ GI tract.

The salivary glands, liver, gallbladder, and pancreas (the accessory organs) are already labeled. Note their locations in relation to the other structures. Learn the meanings of the following word parts.

lower

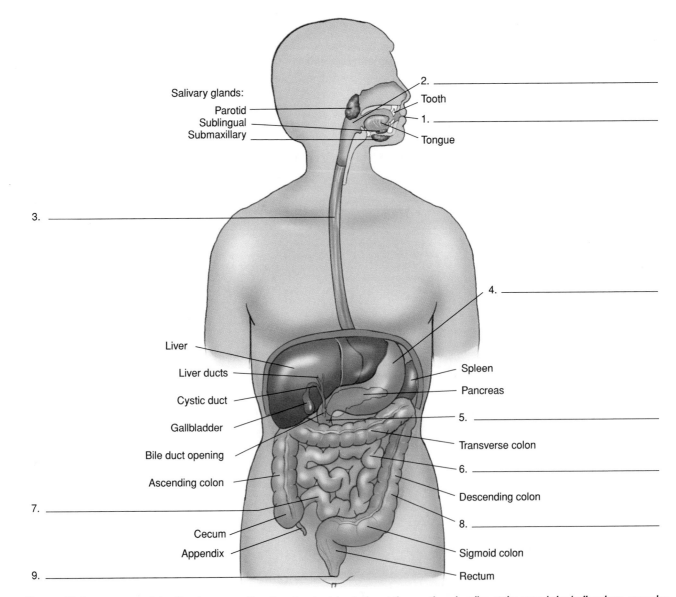

Figure 10-1   Structures of the digestive system. The alimentary tract, beginning at the mouth and ending at the anus, is basically a long, muscular tube. Several accessory organs (salivary glands, liver, gallbladder, and pancreas) are also shown.

Word Parts for Major Structures of the Digestive System

Upper GI Tract

STRUCTURES	COMBINING FORMS
mouth	or(o), stomat(o)
esophagus	esophag(o)
stomach	gastr(o)

Lower GI Tract

STRUCTURES	COMBINING FORMS
small intestine	enter(o)*
duodenum	duoden(o)
jejunum	jejun(o)
ileum	ile(o)
large intestine	col(o), colon(o)†
rectum	rect(o)
anus	an(o)

Accessory Organs of Digestion

STRUCTURES	COMBINING FORMS
gallbladder	cholecyst(o)
common bile duct	choledoch(o)
liver	hepat(o)
pancreas	pancreat(o)
salivary glands	sialaden(o)‡

*Enter(o) sometimes means the intestines in general.
†Col(o) and colon(o) sometimes refer specifically to the colon, the larger portion of the large intestine.
‡Sometimes sial(o).

---

mouth

10-20 You already know the combining forms for several structures that you labeled. *Or/al* means pertaining to the _____.

A second combining form that means mouth is *stomat(o)*. In general, *or(o)* is used in terms that describe the mouth as a structure and *stomat(o)* is used to write other terms, such as diagnostic and surgical terms. *Pharyngeal* (**fə-rin′je-əl**) means pertaining to the _____.

pharynx

Oropharyngeal (**or″o-fə-rin′je-əl**) means pertaining to the mouth and pharynx or pertaining to the oropharynx, the part of the pharynx posterior to the mouth.

10-21 The esophagus is a long, muscular canal that extends from the pharynx to the stomach. *Gastric* (**gas′trik**) means pertaining to the stomach. *Gastro/intestinal* (**gas″tro-in-tes′tĭ-nəl**) means pertaining to the _____ and intestines.

stomach

10-22 Both *intestin/al* and *enter/ic* (**en-ter′ik**) mean pertaining to the _____. Most medical words concerning the intestines are formed using *enter(o)*, but a few terms use *enter(o)* to specifically mean the small intestine (for example, enter/itis).

intestine

10-23 *Enter/al* (**en′tər-əl**) means within, by way of, or pertaining to the small intestine. Although *enter(o)* is used to write terms about the small intestine, you need to remember that *enter(o)* means either the small intestine or the _____ in general. Enter/al tube feeding introduces food directly into the gastrointestinal tract.

intestines

10-24 The combining form *col(o)* means the large intestine. This combining form can also mean the colon, the structure that comprises most of the large intestine and where much of the water is absorbed as the wastes are moved along to the rectum. An adjective that means pertaining to the colon uses *colon(o)*. Join *colon(o)* and -ic to write this term: _____.

colonic (ko-lon′ik)

Colic (**kol′ik**) means pertaining to the large intestine, but it also means spasm in any hollow or tubular soft organ accompanied by pain. You may be most familiar with infantile colic, which is colic occurring in infants, principally during the first few months.

10-25 The rectum (**rek′təm**) is the lower part of the large intestine. The anus (**a′nəs**) is the outlet of the rectum, and it lies in the fold between the buttocks. The anal canal is about 4 cm long. Solid wastes are eliminated via the anus. *Rectal* and *anal* mean pertaining to the rectum and anus, respectively.

The digestive tract is lined with a mucous membrane, which secretes mucus for lubrication. Mucus is the slippery material produced by mucous membranes. The adjective used to describe a

resembling	membrane that secretes mucus is *mucous* (mu′kəs). Mucosa (mu-ko′sə) is the same as a mucous membrane. *Muc/oid* means _____ mucus.

Exercise 2

Write the meaning of these combining forms.

1. an(o)   _____

2. cholecyst(o)   _____

3. choledoch(o)   _____

4. col(o)   _____

5. duoden(o)   _____

6. enter(o)   _____

7. gastr(o)   _____

8. hepat(o)   _____

9. ile(o)   _____

10. jejun(o)   _____

11. or(o)   _____

12. pancreat(o)   _____

13. rect(o)   _____

14. sialaden(o)   _____

15. stomat(o)   _____

■ *Upper Digestive Tract*

stomach	**10-26** The oral cavity is the beginning of the digestive tract and, along with the esophagus and _____, comprises the upper digestive tract. The mouth contains many structures that hold the food in place and facilitate chewing (Figure 10-2). Learn the following word parts that pertain to structures of the upper digestive tract.

Word Parts for Structures of the Upper Digestive Tract

COMBINING FORMS	MEANING	COMBINING FORMS	MEANING
or(o), stomat(o)	mouth	maxill(o)	maxilla
		pharyng(o)	pharynx
Structures of the Mouth		sial(o)	saliva, salivary glands
COMBINING FORMS	MEANING	sialaden(o)	salivary gland
bucc(o)	cheek		
cheil(o)	lip	**Other Structures**	
dent(i), dent(o), odont(o)	teeth	COMBINING FORMS	MEANING
gingiv(o)	gums	esophag(o)	esophagus
gloss(o), lingu(o)	tongue	gastr(o)	stomach
palat(o)	palate	pylor(o)	pylorus
mandibul(o)	mandible	vag(o)	vagus nerve

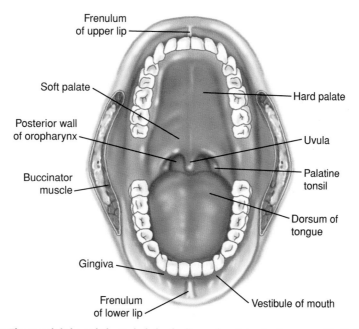

Frenulum
of upper lip

Soft palate

Posterior wall
of oropharynx

Buccinator
muscle

Hard palate

Uvula

Palatine
tonsil

Dorsum of
tongue

Gingiva

Frenulum
of lower lip

Vestibule of mouth

Figure 10-2   Mouth structures. The mouth is bounded anteriorly by the lips and contains the tongue and teeth. The roof of the mouth is the hard palate. Other aspects of the mouth include the gums, the uvula (the fleshy appendage in the back of the throat), the oropharynx, and the buccinator muscle, the main muscle of the cheek that is involved in chewing.

lower upper	**10-27** The mandible (**man′dĭ-bəl**) is the lower jaw, and the maxilla (**mak-sil′ə**) is the upper jaw. *Mandibul/ar* (**man-dib′u-lər**) means pertaining to the mandible, the _____ jaw. *Maxill/ary* (**mak′sĭ-lar″e**) means pertaining to the maxilla, or _____ jaw.
palate	**10-28** The roof of the mouth is formed by the bony arch of the hard palate and the fibrous soft palate. *Palat/ine* (**pal′ə-tīn**) pertains to the _____. The combining form *bucc(o)* means cheek, and the *bucc/al* (**buk′əl**) *cavity* pertains to the area between the teeth and the cheeks.
lip	The combining form *cheil(o)* means the _____.
gums	**10-29** The mucous membrane that provides support for the teeth is the gum. Another name for the gum is gingiva. *Gingiv/al* (**jin′jĭ-vəl**) pertains to the _____.
under	**10-30** Both *gloss(o)* and *lingu(o)* mean the tongue; therefore, *gloss/al* (**glos′əl**) and *lingual* (**ling′gwəl**) mean pertaining to the tongue. Most words involving the tongue use the combining form *gloss(o)*. However, both *hypo/glossal* (**hi″po-glos′əl**) and *sub/lingual* (**səb-ling′gwəl**) mean _____ the tongue. Some medications are designed to be placed under the tongue, where they dissolve.
tongue	**10-31** *Glosso/pharyng/eal* (**glos″o-fə-rin′je-əl**) refers to the _____ and the throat (or pharynx).
teeth	**10-32** Three combining forms mean the teeth: *dent(i)*, *dent(o)*, and *odont(o)*. *Dent/al* pertains to the teeth. *Inter/dental* (**in″tər-den′təl**) means between the _____. The *dent-* in denture refers to teeth. A *dent/ure* (**den′chər**) refers to a set of teeth, either natural or artificial, but is ordinarily used to designate artificial ones.
teeth	*Denti/lingual* (**den″tĭ-ling′wəl**) pertains to the _____ and the tongue.

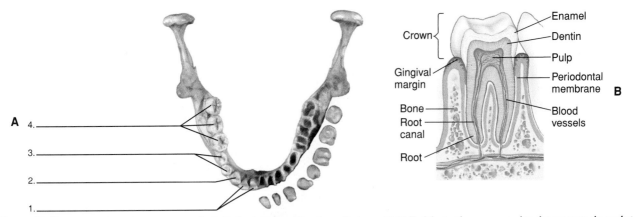

Figure 10-3   Designations of permanent teeth. **A,** Teeth of the lower jaw (mandibular arch). Half of the teeth are removed to demonstrate the sockets. **B,** Section of a molar tooth. All teeth follow a basic plan, consisting of two basic parts: the crown and the root or roots (embedded in the bony socket). The central cavity contains the root canal and tooth pulp, which are richly supplied with blood and lymph vessels, as well as nerves. The chief substance of the tooth, dentin, is similar to bone but harder and more compact. Dentin is covered by enamel on the crown. Enamel is the hardest substance in the body and is composed mainly of calcium phosphate. The cementum is a bonelike connective tissue that provides support to the tooth.

10-33 The primary or deciduous teeth, often called "baby teeth," begin to fall out and to be replaced with permanent teeth when the child is about 6 years of age. The wisdom teeth are the last teeth to erupt, generally between 17 and 25 years of age.

There are 32 permanent teeth in a full set. The mouth has an upper and a lower dental arch, the curving shape formed by the arrangement of a normal set of teeth in the jaw. A complete set has 16 teeth in each dental arch. Observe the dental arch in Figure 10-3, A. Note that the illustration shows the teeth of the lower jaw, or _____ arch. The eight teeth on each side of the dental arch make up a quadrant. Label the teeth in a quadrant as you read the information that follows.

There are two incisors **(in-si′zorz)** (1), one cuspid **(kus′pid)** (2), two bicuspids (3), and three molars (4). Anterior teeth generally fall out and are replaced sooner than posterior ones. The last molar, which is posterior to all other teeth, is known as the wisdom tooth.

10-34 The structure of a molar is shown in Figure 10-3, B. All teeth consist of two basic parts: the crown and the root or roots (embedded in the bony socket). A socket is a hollow or depression into which another part fits—in this case, the tooth. The part that projects above the gum is the

_____.

The exposed part of the crown is covered by enamel, the hardest substance in the body. The soft tissue inside the tooth is the dental pulp, also called the endodontium **(en″do-don′she-əm)**. When the word _endodontium_ is broken down into its component parts, its parts mean a membrane _____ the tooth, but you need to remember that it means dental pulp.

10-35 The tissue investing and supporting the teeth is peri/odont/ium **(per″e-o-don′she-əm)**. You learned that _peri-_ means around, so peri/odont/ium is the tissue _____ the teeth. _Peri/odont/al_ **(per″e-o-don′təl)** means around a tooth, or pertaining to the periodontium.

10-36 Dentistry is the art and science of diagnosing, preventing, and treating diseases and disorders of the teeth and surrounding structures of the oral cavity. There are several dental specialties, each requiring additional training after graduating from dental school.

Orth/odont/ics is concerned with irregularities of alignment of _____ and associated facial problems. One who specializes in orthodontics, often using braces to straighten the teeth, is an orthodontist. One o is dropped when _orth(o)_ is combined with _odont(o)_ to facilitate pronunciation. You will see that one o is generally dropped when _odont(o)_ is joined with prefixes or other combining forms that also end in o.

10-37 A peri/odont/ist **(per″e-o-don′tist)** specializes in the study and treatment of the periodontium. This specialty concerns the gingival tissue, as well as the other tissue that supports the teeth. What is the specialty of a periodontist? _____

Margin notes (left column):

mandibular

crown

inside

around

teeth

periodontics
(per″e-o-don′tiks)

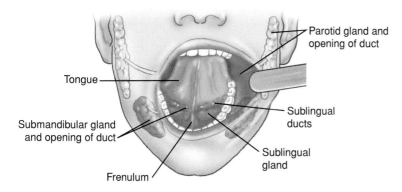

Tongue

Parotid gland and opening of duct

Submandibular gland and opening of duct

Sublingual ducts

Sublingual gland

Frenulum

Figure 10-4   Salivary glands. Three pairs of salivary glands (parotid, sublingual, and submandibular glands) consist of numerous lobes connected by vessels and ducts.

An endodontist is a dentist who specializes in the prevention and treatment of conditions that affect the dental pulp, tooth root, and surrounding tissue and the associated practice of root canal therapy. The specialty is endodontics (**en″do-don′tiks**).

10-38 A dentist who specializes in ped/odontics (**pe-do-don′tiks**) treats

children

_____. Pedodontics is a branch of dentistry that deals with tooth and mouth conditions of children. A specialist in pedodontics is a pedodontist.

10-39 Ger/odont/ics (**jer″o-don′tiks**) is a branch of dentistry that deals with the dental problems of older persons. Note that the vowel is dropped from _ger(o)_ when it is combined with _odont(o)_. A

dental

ger/odont/ist is a dentist specializing in the _____ problems of older persons.

10-40 Salivary glands, which are accessory organs of digestion, secrete saliva into the oral cavity. The mouth tastes what we consume and performs other functions of digestion by mixing the food with saliva, chewing, and voluntarily swallowing it. In addition, saliva contains amylase, which

starch

begins digestion of _____ in the mouth.

The salivary glands are three paired glands (Figure 10-4). Their names indicate their locations. The par/ot/id glands, the largest salivary glands, are near the _____. The

ears

suffix _-id_ means either having the shape of or a structure. The sub/lingual glands are located under the tongue. The sub/maxillary glands are located beneath the mandible, rather than beneath the maxilla, as the name implies.

10-41 Food that is swallowed passes from the mouth to the pharynx and the esophagus. Both the pharynx and the esophagus are muscular structures that move food along on its way to the stomach.

The esophagus is a muscular canal, about 24 cm (about 9.5 inches) long, extending from the pharynx to the stomach. The esophagus secretes mucus to facilitate the movement of food into the stomach, which also is lined with mucous membrane. Upper and lower esophag/eal sphincters control the movement of food into and out of the esophagus. A sphincter* (**sfingk′tər**) consists of circular muscle that constricts a passage or closes a natural opening in the body.

esophagus

Esophag/eal means pertaining to the _____.

10-42 The circular esophageal muscle that controls movement of food from the pharynx into the esophagus is called the upper esophageal sphincter. The lower esophageal

sphincter

_____ controls the movement of food into the stomach. This sphincter is also called the cardiac sphincter because the name of the portion of the stomach near the upper opening is the cardiac region. The region was so named because of its proximity to the heart.

behind

Post/esophag/eal (**pōst-ə-sof″ə-je′əl**) means situated _____ the esophagus.

*Sphincter (Greek: _sphincter_, that which binds tight).

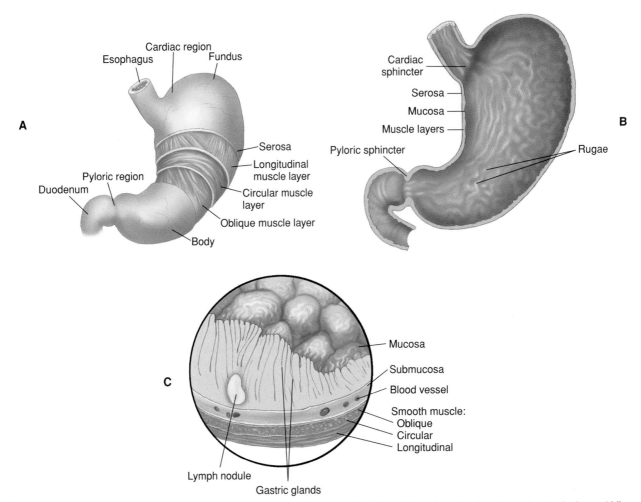

Figure 10-5   Features of the stomach. **A,** External view: The stomach is composed of the cardiac region, a fundus or round part, a body or middle portion, and a pyloric portion, which is the small distal end. The stomach has a serous coat (serosa) and three muscular layers. **B,** Internal view: The cardiac sphincter guards the opening of the esophagus into the stomach and prevents backflow of material into the esophagus. The stomach ends with the pyloric sphincter, which regulates outflow. The lining of the stomach, the mucosa, is arranged in temporary folds called rugae (visible in the empty stomach), which allow expansion as the stomach fills. **C,** Structure of the stomach wall: Longitudinal, circular, and oblique smooth muscle lie just beneath the serosa. All stomach layers are richly supplied with blood vessels and nerves. Gastric glands secrete gastric juice through gastric pits, tiny holes in the mucosa.

10-43 Examine Figure 10-5, A, to learn more about the structure of the stomach. Regions of the stomach are the cardiac region, the fundus (**fun′dəs**), the body, and the pyloric (**pi-lor′ik**) region.

The cardiac region lies near the upper opening from the esophagus. The round and most superior region of the stomach is the fundus. The main portion of the stomach is called the body. As the body of the stomach approaches the lower opening, it narrows and is called the

_____ region.

The stomach ends with the pyloric sphincter, which regulates the outflow of stomach contents into the duodenum, the first part of the small intestine.

pyloric

10-44 Look again at Figure 10-5, B. The mucosa that lines the stomach is arranged in temporary folds called rugae (**roo′je**). _Ruga_ (singular of _rugae_) means ridge, wrinkle, or fold. The rugae, most apparent when the stomach is empty, allow the stomach to expand as it fills.

The outer layer of the stomach is the _____. This type of visceral peritoneum holds the stomach in position by folding back on and over the structure.

Three muscle layers are present in the stomach, rather than two, which are found in other structures of the digestive tract.

serosa
(sēr-o′sə, sēr-o′zə)

endogastric
(en″do-gas′trik)

10-45 *Gastr/ic* (**gas′trik**) means pertaining to the stomach. Place a prefix before *gastric* to write a word that means pertaining to the inside (interior) of the stomach: _____.

The stomach is a temporary reservoir for food and is the first major site of digestion. After digestion, the stomach gradually feeds liquefied food (chyme) into the small intestine.

Exercise 3

Write a word in each blank to complete the following sentences. The first letter of each answer is given as a clue.

1. Another name for the mouth is the o_____ cavity.

2. The lower jaw is the m_____.

3. The upper jaw is the m_____.

4. The roof of the mouth is the p_____.

5. The buccal cavity pertains to the area between the teeth and the c_____.

6. Another name for the gum is g_____.

7. Glossal means pertaining to the t_____.

8. Sublingual means beneath the t_____.

9. Another name for the throat is the p_____.

10. Dental pulp is called e_____.

11. The tissue that invests and supports the teeth is p_____.

12. The dental specialty that is concerned with irregularities of the alignment of teeth and associated facial problems is o_____.

13. The branch of dentistry that deals with the tooth and mouth conditions of children is p_____.

14. The branch of dentistry that specializes in dental problems of older persons is g_____.

15. The three paired glands that secrete saliva into the oral cavity are the s_____ glands.

16. The muscular canal that extends from the mouth to the stomach is the e_____.

17. A circular muscle that constricts a passage or closes a natural opening in the body is called a s_____.

18. The lower region of the stomach is called the p_____ region.

■ *Lower Digestive Tract*

small

10-46 The intestines make up the lower digestive tract. The intestines are sometimes called the bowels.

Extending from the pyloric opening to the anus, the intestinal tract is about 7.5 to 8.5 meters (24.5 to 28 feet) long. The intestines are divided into the small intestine and large intestine. The adult small intestine, comprising more than three fourths of the length of the intestines, is 6 to 7 meters (about 20 to 23 feet) long. The large intestine is so named because it is larger in diameter than the small intestine, but it is less than one fourth as long. Which is longer, the small intestine or the large intestine? _____ intestine

absorption

10-47 The small intestine finishes the process of digestion, absorbs the nutrients, and passes the residue on to the large intestine. In other words, the small intestine is responsible for two successive processes, digestion and _____, before passing the residue to the large intestine.

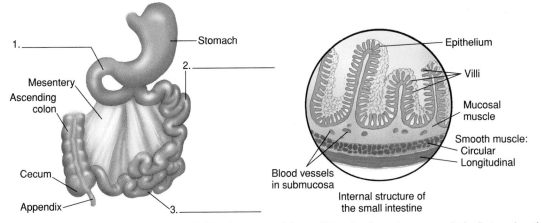

Figure 10-6   Characteristics of the small intestine. Label the three parts of the small intestine (1 to 3) as you read. The first portion, the duodenum *(1)*, begins at the pyloric sphincter and is the shorter section. The second portion is the jejunum *(2)*, which is continuous with the third portion, the ileum *(3)*. The ileum is the longest of the three parts of the small intestine. Note that the small intestine decreases in diameter from beginning at the duodenum to its ending, at the ileum. The internal structure is similar throughout its length. The wall *(inset)* has an inner lining of mucosa, two layers of muscle, and an outer layer of serosa.

villi (vil′i)*

serosa

duodenum

jejunum
ileum

large

10-48 The small intestine consists of three parts: the duodenum (**doo″o-de′nəm, doo-od′ə-nəm**), the jejunum (**jə-joo′nəm**), and the ileum (**il′e-əm**). The structure of the small intestine is shown in Figure 10-6. Read the information that accompanies the drawing and label the three parts of the small intestine.

Study the layers of the wall of the small intestine to write answers in these blanks. The innermost membrane is called the mucosa. Both the mucosa and submucosa have many folds and fingerlike projections called _____. Both these features increase the surface area of the mucosa. In addition, the villi function to absorb nutrients.

There are two layers of muscle and an outer membrane called the _____.

10-49 The duodenum is short, less than a foot long. *Duoden/al* (**doo″o-de′nəl**) means pertaining to the _____.

10-50 The part of the small intestine below the duodenum is the jejunum. It is about 2.4 meters (8 feet) long and joins the ileum, which is the twisted end of the small intestine. *Jejun/al* means pertaining to the _____.

Both *ile/ac* and *ile/al* mean pertaining to the _____.

10-51 The large intestine is only about 1.5 meters (5 feet) long. The combining forms *col(o)* and *colon(o)* mean the colon (**ko′lən**) or the _____ intestine. The colon is only that portion of the large intestine extending from the cecum to the rectum, but *colon* is sometimes used to mean the large intestine in general.

The large intestine is anatomically divided into the cecum, colon, rectum, and anal canal. Learn the combining forms for the following structures.

Word Parts for the Large Intestine

Structures COMBINING FORMS	MEANING	Pathology COMBINING FORMS	MEANING
col(o), colon(o)	large intestine or colon	diverticul(o)	diverticula
cec(o)	cecum		
append(o), appendic(o)	appendix		
proct(o)	anus, rectum		
sigmoid(o)	sigmoid colon		

*Villus, pl. villi (Latin: tuft of hair).

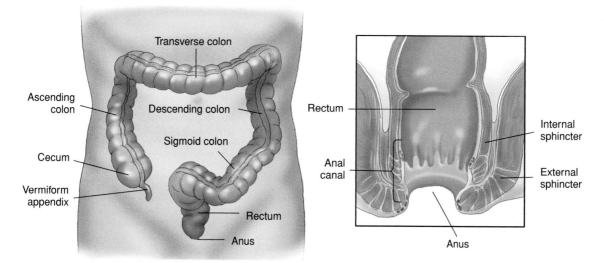

Figure 10-7 Features of the large intestine: the cecum, appendix, colon, and rectum. The colon is anatomically divided into four parts. The first part rises upward and is called the ascending colon. The transverse colon is the part that crosses the abdomen. The colon then descends on the left side of the abdomen and thus is called the descending colon. The last part is S-shaped and is called the sigmoid colon. The internal structure of a portion of the rectum and the anus are shown.

cecum

10-52 Study the location of the parts of the large intestine in Figure 10-7.

The cecum (**se′kəm**) forms the first portion of the large intestine and is located just distal to the ileum. The combining form *cec(o)* means cecum. The ileo/cecal (**il″e-o-se′kəl**) valve is located between the ileum and the _____. *Retro/cecal* (**ret″ro-se′kəl**) means behind the cecum.

appendix

10-53 The vermiform appendix is a wormlike structure that opens into the cecum. An *appendix* simply means an appendage, but its most common usage is in referring to the vermiform appendix just described. *Appendicular* means either pertaining to an appendage or pertaining to the vermiform _____.

sigmoid

around

10-54 The colon makes up most of the 5 feet of large intestine. Different parts of the colon are designated as the ascending, transverse, descending, and sigmoid (**sig′moid**) colon. The last part of the colon is the _____ colon.

Retro/colic (**ret″ro-kol′ik**) means behind the colon. Remembering that *peri-* means around, the literal translation of peri/col/ic (**per″ĭ-ko′lik**) is _____ the colon. *Pericolic* means pertaining to the tissue around the colon. In this term, "the tissue around the structure" is implied.

rectum

10-55 The lower part of the large intestine is the rectum, which terminates in a narrow anal canal. This canal in turn opens to the exterior at the anus. Feces is body waste that is discharged from the bowels by way of the anus. Feces is also called stool, or fecal material. Defecation (**def″ə-ka′shən**) is the elimination of feces from the rectum.

Colo/rectal (**ko″lo-rek′təl**) means pertaining to or affecting the colon and the _____.

rect(o)

10-56 The combining form *proct(o)* refers to the anus (**a′nəs**) or rectum. You have now learned two combining forms for rectum: *proct(o)* and _____. A procto/logist (**prok-tol′ə-jist**) specializes in treating disorders of the colon, rectum, and anus.

anus

Most medical terms that refer to the anus use *proct(o)*, but you need to remember that *an(o)* also means anus. *An/al* (**a′nəl**) refers to the _____, as in the phrases "anal opening" and "anal canal."

intestines

10-57 The combining form *enter(o)* means intestines, sometimes referring to the small intestine only, but the term *gastro/entero/logy* is the study of the stomach and _____ and associated diseases.

10-58 Structural features of both the small intestine and large intestine are well suited for their roles in the digestive system. As you studied earlier, the small intestine is responsible for further digestion of the chyme and absorption of nutrients. The large intestine also has several important functions:

- While moving wastes along its length, the large intestine absorbs water, sodium, and chloride. The large intestine is capable of absorbing 90% of the water and sodium it receives.
- The large intestine secretes mucus, which binds fecal particles into a formed mass and lubricates the mucosa.
- Bacteria in the large intestine are responsible for the production of several vitamins.
- Feces is formed and expelled from the body.

Exercise 4

Match the structures in the left column with either A, small intestine, or B, large intestine.

_____ 1. anal canal

_____ 2. cecum

_____ 3. colon

_____ 4. duodenum

_____ 5. ileum

_____ 6. jejunum

_____ 7. rectum

A. small intestine
B. large intestine

■ Accessory Organs of Digestion

accessory

10-59 The liver, gallbladder, pancreas, and salivary glands produce substances that are needed for proper digestion and absorption of nutrients and are considered to be

_____ organs to the digestive system.

  These organs lie outside the digestive tract, yet they produce or store secretions that aid in the chemical breakdown of food.

10-60 The accessory organs have secretions that are conveyed to the digestive tract by ducts. The liver, gallbladder, and pancreas are located near the other digestive structures within the abdominal cavity. See these structures in Figure 10-8.

liver

  The liver is the largest organ in the body and is essential for the maintenance of life. *Hepat/ic* (hə-pat′ik) means pertaining to the _____.

10-61 Production of bile is a major function of the liver. The bile is then transported to the gall-bladder for storage. The liver has several other important functions:

- breakdown of toxic compounds
- involvement in the regulation of blood glucose
- lipid metabolism
- synthesis of plasma proteins
- storage of iron and certain vitamins
- filtering of the blood
- excretion of bile pigments from the breakdown of hemoglobin
- excretion of hormones and cholesterol

bile

  A major function of the liver is the production of _____, which is transported to the gallbladder for storage. Bile aids in the digestion of fats.

liver

10-62 *Hepato/lytic* (hep″ə-to-lit′ik) means destructive to the _____. (The term *hepatolytic* is less common than *hepatotoxic* (hep′ə-to-tok″sik), which means essentially the same thing.)

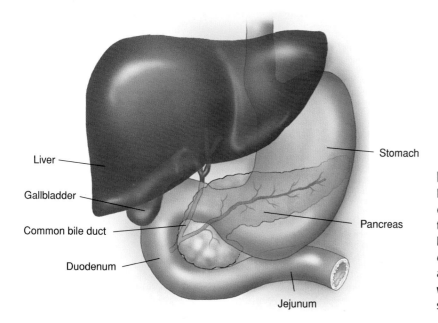

Liver

Gallbladder

Common bile duct

Duodenum

Stomach

Pancreas

Jejunum

Figure 10-8 Accessory organs of digestion. The liver, gallbladder, and pancreas are accessory digestive organs. The liver and pancreas have additional functions as well. More than 500 functions of the liver have been identified. The formation and excretion of bile for digestion of fats is one of its most commonly known activities. Bile is stored in the gallbladder and released when fats are ingested. The pancreas secretes many substances, including digestive enzymes and insulin.

liver

Extrahepatic (**eks″trə-hə-pat′ik**) means situated or occurring outside the _____. *Supra/hepatic* (**soo″prə-hə-pat′ik**) means above the liver.

bile

10-63 The combining forms *chol(e)* and *bil(i)* refer to bile or gall. *Biliary* (**bil′e-ar-e**) means pertaining to _____, but *chol(e)* is used more often to write terms. The organs and ducts that participate in the secretion, storage, and delivery of bile make up the biliary tract.

10-64 Bile leaves the liver by the hepatic duct and is taken to the gallbladder for storage until it is needed. The combining form *cholecyst(o)* often forms part of a term that refers to the gallbladder (GB). *Cholecyst/ic* (**ko″lə-sis′tik**) means pertaining to the gallbladder.

gallbladder

Cholecysto/gastric (**ko″lə-sis″to-gas′trik**) pertains to the _____ and the stomach.

duct

10-65 A few words contain the combining form *choledoch(o)*, which means the common bile duct. *Choledoch/al* (**ko-led′ə-kəl**) means pertaining to the common bile_____.

pancreas

10-66 The pancreas has both digestive and hormonal functions. *Pancreat/ic* (**pan″kre-at′ik**) means pertaining to the _____.
Pancreatic juice plays an important role in the digestion of all classes of food. Pancreatic juice contains lipase, amylase, and several other enzymes that are essential to normal digestion. The pancreas also produces hormones (including insulin) that play a primary role in regulation of carbohydrate metabolism.

blood

10-67 Clusters of cells in the pancreas, the islets of Langerhans, produce glucagon (**gloo′kə-gon**) and insulin (**in′sə-lin**). Glucagon increases blood glucose levels, and insulin lowers blood glucose levels. The two hormones, glucagon and insulin, work together to regulate blood glucose. Secretion of glucagon is stimulated by hypo/glycemia. Hypo/glycemia (**hi″po-gli-se′me-ə**) is a decreased level of glucose in the _____. Small amounts of insulin are secreted continuously in the fasting state, but secretion rises in response to an increase in blood glucose levels.
Hyper/glyc/emia (**hi″pər-gli-se′me-ə**) is a greater than normal amount of sugar in the blood. This condition is most often associated with diabetes mellitus (**di″ə-be′tēz mel′lĕ-təs, mə-li′tis**) (DM). This disorder is primarily a result of insufficient production or improper use of insulin.

Exercise 5

Write adjectives that mean pertaining to the following structures.

1. common bile duct _____

2. bile _____

3. gallbladder _____

4. liver _____

5. pancreas _____

DIAGNOSTIC TESTS AND PROCEDURES

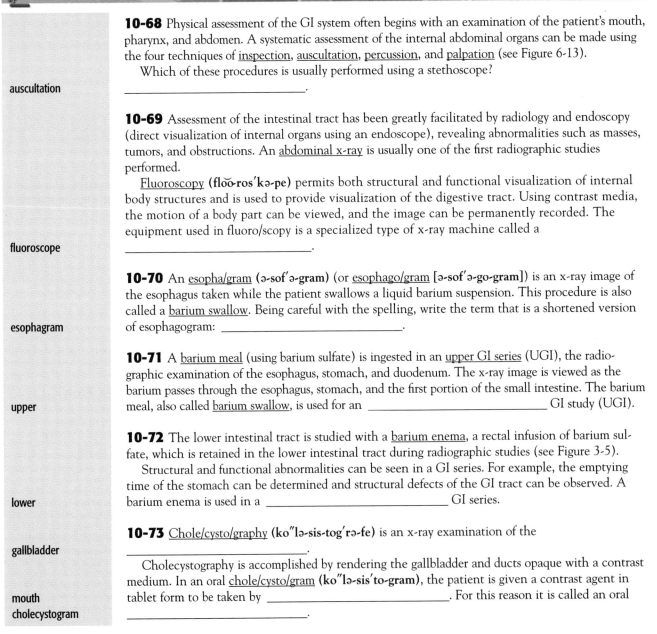

auscultation

10-68 Physical assessment of the GI system often begins with an examination of the patient's mouth, pharynx, and abdomen. A systematic assessment of the internal abdominal organs can be made using the four techniques of <u>inspection</u>, <u>auscultation</u>, <u>percussion</u>, and <u>palpation</u> (see Figure 6-13).

Which of these procedures is usually performed using a stethoscope?

_____.

10-69 Assessment of the intestinal tract has been greatly facilitated by radiology and endoscopy (direct visualization of internal organs using an endoscope), revealing abnormalities such as masses, tumors, and obstructions. An <u>abdominal x-ray</u> is usually one of the first radiographic studies performed.

<u>Fluoroscopy</u> (floo-ros′kə-pe) permits both structural and functional visualization of internal body structures and is used to provide visualization of the digestive tract. Using contrast media, the motion of a body part can be viewed, and the image can be permanently recorded. The equipment used in fluoro/scopy is a specialized type of x-ray machine called a

fluoroscope

_____.

10-70 An <u>esopha/gram</u> (ə-sof′ə-gram) (or <u>esophago/gram</u> [ə-sof′ə-go-gram]) is an x-ray image of the esophagus taken while the patient swallows a liquid barium suspension. This procedure is also called a <u>barium swallow</u>. Being careful with the spelling, write the term that is a shortened version of esophagogram: _____.

esophagram

10-71 A <u>barium meal</u> (using barium sulfate) is ingested in an <u>upper GI series</u> (UGI), the radiographic examination of the esophagus, stomach, and duodenum. The x-ray image is viewed as the barium passes through the esophagus, stomach, and the first portion of the small intestine. The barium meal, also called <u>barium swallow</u>, is used for an _____ GI study (UGI).

upper

10-72 The lower intestinal tract is studied with a <u>barium enema</u>, a rectal infusion of barium sulfate, which is retained in the lower intestinal tract during radiographic studies (see Figure 3-5).

Structural and functional abnormalities can be seen in a GI series. For example, the emptying time of the stomach can be determined and structural defects of the GI tract can be observed. A barium enema is used in a _____ GI series.

lower

10-73 <u>Chole/cysto/graphy</u> (ko″lə-sis-tog′rə-fe) is an x-ray examination of the

gallbladder

_____.

Cholecystography is accomplished by rendering the gallbladder and ducts opaque with a contrast medium. In an oral <u>chole/cysto/gram</u> (ko″lə-sis′to-gram), the patient is given a contrast agent in tablet form to be taken by _____. For this reason it is called an oral

mouth
cholecystogram

_____.

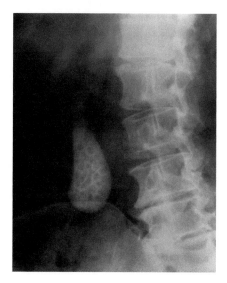

Figure 10-9 Oral cholecystogram. Numerous gallstones are evident on this cholecystogram. In oral cholecystography, radiography of the gallbladder is obtained 12 to 15 hours after ingestion of contrast medium. Because nausea, vomiting, and diarrhea are fairly common with this means of diagnosing biliary disease, it has been largely replaced by ultrasound.

Examine the appearance of several gallstones in Figure 10-9. Oral cholecystograms were the principal method for investigating the presence of gallstones until the advent of ultrasound.

10-74 Computed tomography (CT) and endoscopic procedures are also used to detect gallstones. Endo/scopy (**en-dos′kə-pe**) is direct visualization of the interior of organs and cavities using a flexible fiberoptic endo/scope. Fiberoptic materials are flexible glass or plastic fibers that transmit light and permit visual images around corners. Each of the instruments used in endoscopy is specially designed for the examination of particular organs. The instruments used in endoscopy are called

endoscopes   _____.

Other instruments can be inserted through the endoscope to remove small pieces of tissue, collect samples of tissue for study, to inject agents, or to perform laser surgery.

10-75 Cholangio/graphy (**ko-lan″je-og′rə-fe**) is radiography of the major bile ducts and is useful in demonstrating gallstones and tumors. One type of cholangiography is performed during surgery to detect residual calculi in the biliary tract, after the gallbladder has been removed. This radiographic

cholangiography   procedure is called operative _____, and the contrast material is injected into the common bile duct.

10-76 Operative cholangiography is performed by injecting a contrast medium into the common bile duct through a catheter called a T-tube. This allows residual stones in the bile ducts to be seen.

operative   This type of angiography is called _____ cholangiography. It is not unusual for the incision to be closed with the T-tube left temporarily in the common bile duct and extending through the skin. The T-tube allows for drainage and postoperative study.

10-77 Pancreato/graphy (**pan″kre-ə-tog′rə-fe**) means visualization of the pancreas. This can be accomplished by various means, including CT and sonography. Various methods of imaging of the

pancreatography   pancreas are called _____.

10-78 The salivary ducts can also be studied by injecting radiopaque substances into the ducts in a procedure called a sialography (**si″ə-log′rə-fe**). This procedure sometimes demonstrates the presence of calculi in the salivary ducts. Write a word that means salivary calculus:

sialolith (**si″al′o-lith**)   _____.

10-79 Esophago/gastro/scopy (**ə-sof″ə-go-gas-tros′kə-pe**) refers to examination of the esophagus and

stomach   the _____.

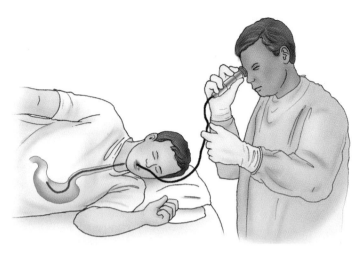

Figure 10-10 Esophagogastroduodenoscopy. If the focus of the examination is the esophagus, the procedure is called esophagoscopy. If the stomach is the focus, the procedure is called gastroscopy.

gastroscope
(gas′tro-skōp)

Write the name of the instrument used to examine (inside) the stomach:

_____.

10-80 In an <u>esophago/gastro/duodeno/scopy</u> (ə-sof″ə-go-gas″tro-doo″od-ə-nos′kə-pe) (EGD), the esophagus, stomach, and duodenum are examined (Figure 10-10). If the esophagus is the focus of the examination, the procedure is called <u>esophagoscopy</u> (ə-sof″ə-gos′ko-pe). If the stomach is the focus, the procedure is called _____.

gastroscopy
(gas-tros′kə-pe)

pylorus

10-81 <u>Pyloroscopy</u> (pi″lor-os′kə-pe) is visual inspection of the_____, the pyloric region of the stomach.

<u>Duodenoscopy</u> (doo″o-də-nos′kə-pe) is endoscopic examination of the _____. The fiberoptic instrument used to inspect the duodenum is called a <u>duodenoscope</u> (doo″o-de′no-skōp).

duodenum

colon

10-82 <u>Colonoscopy</u> (ko″lən-os′kə-pe) is visual examination of the mucosal lining of the _____. <u>Coloscopy</u> (ko-los′ko-pe) means the same as colonoscopy, but the former is more commonly used in naming this procedure (Figure 10-11). The instrument used is a <u>colonoscope</u> (ko-lon′o-skōp). The physician may also obtain tissue biopsy specimens or remove polyps through the colonoscope.

<u>Procto/sigmoido/scopy</u> (prok″to-sig″moi-dos′kə-pe) is endoscopic examination of the rectum and sigmoid colon. This procedure uses a <u>sigmoido/scope</u> (sig-moi′do-skōp) and is also called <u>sigmoidoscopy</u> (sig″moi-dos′kə-pe).

10-83 <u>Sonography</u> is less invasive than endoscopy and can be used to image soft tissues, such as the liver, the spleen, and the pancreas.

<u>Nuclear imaging</u> can be used to evaluate the size of organs and vessels, as well as to detect the presence of tumors or abscesses. One of the more common tests of this type is a liver scan, which involves intravenous injection of a radioactive compound that is readily absorbed by certain cells of the liver. The radiation emitted by the compound provides information about the size, shape, and consistency of the _____.

liver

10-84 Several blood tests provide information about functions of the liver, and these are aptly named <u>liver function tests</u> (LFTs). Examples include <u>serum bilirubin</u>, <u>alkaline phosphatase</u>, <u>SGO transaminase</u> (SGOT), and <u>alanine aminotransferase</u> (ALT or SGPT). Increased values of these laboratory tests often indicate liver disease. LFT is an abbreviation for _____ function test.

liver

10-85 Additional blood tests are helpful in the diagnosis of disorders of the liver, as well as other organs of the digestive system. Urine tests and stool examinations are also used, as in testing for <u>occult blood</u>. Occult blood is blood that is not obvious on examination but can be detected by chemical tests, <u>guaiac tests</u> (for example, the <u>Hemoccult test</u>). Blood that cannot be seen but can be detected by a chemical test is called _____ blood.

occult

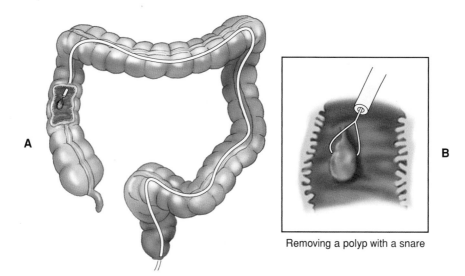

A   B

Removing a polyp with a snare

Figure 10-11   Colonoscopy. **A,** Endoscopic examination of the colon using a flexible colonoscope. **B,** Colonic polyps can often be removed with the use of a snare (wire noose) that fits through the colonoscope.

An occult blood test of the stool in healthy individuals is usually negative. The presence of occult blood in the stool indicates gastrointestinal bleeding, a finding associated with ulcers, ulcerative colitis, or cancer.

10-86 <u>Stool samples</u> are tested for fats as an indication of pancreatic disease or mal/absorption, impaired absorption. Fat is normally absorbed in the small intestine, giving a negative test for fecal fats. The presence of fat in stool samples is an abnormal finding. Literal translation of malabsorption is poor or _____ absorption.

bad

Stool samples are also tested for ova and parasites to aid in the diagnosis of parasitic infection.

Exercise 6

Match the diagnostic test, procedure, or instrument in the left column with the digestive structure in the right column that is the focus of study. (Use all terms once.)

_____ 1. cholangiography

_____ 2. cholecystography

_____ 3. duodenoscopy

_____ 4. esophagram

_____ 5. gastroscope

_____ 6. pancreatography

_____ 7. pyloroscopy

_____ 8. sialography

A. bile ducts
B. duodenum
C. esophagus
D. gallbladder
E. lower region of the stomach
F. pancreas
G. salivary ducts
H. stomach

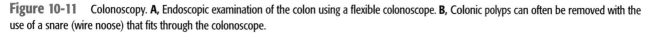

PATHOLOGIES

10-87 <u>Malaise</u> (**mah-lāz´**) is a feeling of body weakness, distress, or discomfort. Many disturbances of the digestive system can give a feeling of malaise. Basic functions, such as eating, can be severely impaired by problems of the digestive system, but not all eating or nutritional disorders are caused by malfunction of the digestive system. For example, anorexia nervosa is a sometimes life-

without

threatening illness that is self-induced starvation. Literal translation of <u>an/orexia</u> is
_____ appetite.

This clinical syndrome occurs primarily in females, with onset most often during adolescence. There is often an intense fear of losing control of eating and becoming fat. Unless there is intervention, <u>anorexia nervosa</u> results in <u>emaciation</u> (**e-ma″she-a′shən**), excessive leanness caused by disease or lack of nutrition.

bulimia

10-88 <u>Bulimia</u> (**boo̅-le′me-ə**) is another eating disorder that occurs predominantly in females, with onset usually in adolescence or early adulthood. The derivation of the term *bulimia* from Greek is *bous*, ox, and *limos*, hunger. This disorder is characterized by episodes of binge eating that often end in purging and depression. Purging is accomplished by self-induced vomiting or the use of laxatives. The name of this disorder that is characterized by binge eating and purging is _____.

poor

10-89 If something interferes with eating or the digestion of food, body cells will lack needed nutrients and mal/nutrition will result. <u>Malnutrition</u> (**mal″noo-trish′ən**) means improper or _____ nutrition.

<u>Mal/absorption</u> (**mal″əb-sorp′shən**) is improper absorption of nutrients into the bloodstream from the intestines. This will eventually result in malnutrition. Malabsorption syndrome is subnormal absorption of dietary constituents and can be caused by a number of disorders, including several inborn errors of metabolism, such as celiac disease. Malabsorption is characterized by anorexia, weight loss, abdominal bloating, muscle cramps, and the presence of fat in stool samples.

vomiting

10-90 Excessive vomiting, unless treated with an anti/emetic (**an″te-ə-met′ik**), can also lead to malnutrition. <u>Emesis</u> (**em′ə-sis**) means vomiting. <u>Hyper/emesis</u> (**hi″pər-em′ə-sis**) is excessive _____. <u>Nausea</u> usually accompanies vomiting.

<u>Hemat/emesis</u> (**he″mə-tem′ə-sis**) is vomiting of blood and indicates upper GI bleeding as that caused by an ulcer of the esophagus or stomach.

obesity

10-91 <u>Obesity</u> (**o-bēs′ĭ-te**) is an abnormal increase in the proportion of fat cells of the body, and a person is regarded as medically obese if he or she is 20% above desirable body weight for the person's age, sex, height, and body build. The calculated body mass index (BMI) using weight-to-height ratios is an index of obesity or altered body fat distribution. An abnormal increase in the proportion of fat cells of the body is called _____.

<u>Exo/gen/ous</u> (**ek-soj′ə-nəs**) <u>obesity</u> is caused by a greater caloric intake than that needed to meet the metabolic needs of the body. <u>Endo/gen/ous</u> (**en-doj′ə-nəs**) <u>obesity</u> originates from within the body, as seen in hormonal disorders such as uncontrolled diabetes. Breaking exo/gen/ous into its component parts, *exo-* means outside, *gen(o)* means origin, and *-ous* means pertaining to.

excessive

10-92 <u>Poly/phag/ia</u> (**pol″e-fa′jə**) means _____ eating. Excessive eating over a long period generally leads to weight gain as a result of taking in more calories than the number needed for normal body metabolism. The amount of fuel or energy in food is measured in calories.

difficult

10-93 <u>Dys/phagia</u> (**dis-fa′je-ə**) means _____ eating. Canker sores on the mouth could cause dysphagia.

thirst

10-94 <u>Poly/dips/ia</u> (**pol″e-dip′se-ə**) is excessive _____. It is characteristic of several different conditions, including those in which there is increased excretion of fluid because of increased urination, which leads to thirst. Polydipsia is a common occurrence in untreated <u>diabetes mellitus</u>. See Chapter 17, The Endocrine System, to learn more about this disorder and tests used to diagnose diabetes mellitus.

absence

<u>A/dips/ia</u> (**ə-dip′se-ə**) is _____ of thirst.

difficult

10-95 Literal translation of <u>dys/pepsia</u> (**dis-pep′se-ə**) is bad or _____ digestion. Dyspepsia, imperfect or painful digestion, is not a disease in itself but symptomatic of other diseases or disorders. It means the same as indigestion. <u>Eructation</u> (**ə-rək-ta′shən**),* or belch-

*Eructation (Latin: *eructare*, to belch).

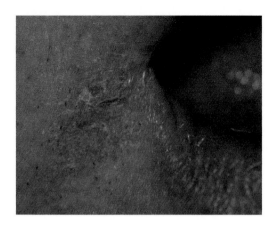

Figure 10-12   Cheilosis. This disorder of the lips and mouth is characterized by splitting of the lips and skin around the mouth.

ing, results from the act of drawing up air from the stomach and expelling it through the mouth. Eructation and hiccups sometime accompany dyspepsia. A <u>hiccup</u> is produced by the involuntary contraction of the diaphragm, followed by rapid closure of the glottis (opening between the vocal cords). Other causes of hiccups include rapid eating and certain types of surgery.

■ *Upper Digestive Tract*

10-96 Diseases of the upper digestive tract include those diseases or disorders that affect the mouth, the esophagus, and the stomach.

eating

Literal translation of <u>a/phag/ia</u> (ə-fa′jə) is absence of _____, but you will need to remember that *aphagia* means an inability to swallow as a result of an organic or psychological cause. This differs from anorexia nervosa, a disorder characterized by self-imposed starvation.

10-97 *Dysphagia* means difficult eating. Stomat/itis makes eating difficult because the mouth is painful. <u>Stomatitis</u> (sto″mə-ti′tis) is _____ of the mouth.

inflammation

<u>Stomato/dynia</u> (sto″mə-to-din′e-ə) means painful mouth. A familiar cause of stomatodynia is <u>canker</u> (kang′kər) <u>sores</u>. The term *canker* has several definitions, but when associated with humans, it means an <u>ulcer</u> (ul′sər), particularly in the mouth. Ulcers are defined, craterlike lesions. Ulcerations on the lips are often called cold sores or fever blisters (usually caused by the <u>herpes simplex virus</u> [HSV] type 1).

10-98 Any oral disease caused by a fungus is <u>stomatomycosis</u>. Stomato/myc/osis (sto″mə-to-mi-ko′sis) is a fungal condition of the _____.

mouth

Candida albicans is a yeast type of fungus that is part of the normal flora of the oral cavity (see Figure 7-11, *B*). Because antibiotic therapy destroys the normal bacteria that usually prevent fungal infections, candidiasis (an infection caused by *Candida*, usually *C. albicans*) can result. Also, patients receiving chemo/therapy often develop candidiasis, because chemotherapy diminishes the ability of the immune system to prevent infection.

lips

10-99 <u>Cheil/osis</u> (ki-lo′sis) is a condition of the _____. In cheilosis there is splitting of the lips and angles of the mouth (Figure 10-12). Cheilosis is a characteristic of riboflavin deficiency in the diet.

cheilitis (ki-li′tis)

10-100 Inflammation of the lip is _____.

<u>Cheilitis</u> often produces pain when one attempts to eat. Cheilitis and other abnormal conditions of mouth structures can result in poor nutrition.

10-101 <u>Gingivo/stomat/itis</u> (jin″ji-vo-sto″mə-ti′tis) is inflammation of the gums and

mouth

_____. Inflammation of the gum is <u>gingivitis</u> (jin″ji-vi′tis).

painful

10-102 <u>Gingiv/algia</u> (jin″ji-val′jə) is _____ gums. <u>Gingivo/gloss/itis</u> (jin″ji-vo-glos-i′tis) is inflammation of the tongue and gums.

glossopathy (glos-op′ə-the)	**10-103** Any disease of the tongue is a _____. <u>Gloss/itis</u> (**glos-i′tis**) is inflammation of the tongue. <u>Glossoplegia</u> (**glos″o-ple′je-ə**) means paralysis of the tongue.
tongue	**10-104** <u>Glosso/pyr/osis</u> (**glos″o-pi-ro′sis**) is an abnormal sensation of pain, burning, and stinging of the tongue without apparent lesions or cause. The combining form *pyr(o)*, which means fire, in glosso/pyr/osis refers to the stinging sensation of the _____.
pulp	**10-105** <u>Dent/algia</u> (**den-tal′jə**) means a toothache. Dentalgia is often caused by caries that have extended into the tooth pulp. <u>Caries</u>* (**kar′ēz, kar′e-ēz**) means decay. Neglected dental caries, over time, invades and inflames pulpal tissues. <u>End/odont/itis</u> means inflammation of the endodontium, or the tooth _____. <u>Halitosis</u>† is an offensive breath resulting from poor oral hygiene, dental or oral infections, use of tobacco, ingestion of certain foods such as garlic, or some systemic diseases such as the odor of acetone in diabetes or ammonia in liver disease.
periodontium **pus**	**10-106** <u>Peri/odont/itis</u> (**per″e-o-don-ti′tis**) is inflammation of the _____, the structure that supports the tooth. <u>Pyorrhea</u> (**pi″o-re′ə**) is one type of periodontal disease. Pyorrhea is an inflammation of the gingiva and the periodontal ligament, the fibrous connective tissue that anchors the tooth to the base. Literal interpretation of pyo/rrhea is discharge of _____.
straighten	**10-107** An impacted tooth is one that is unable to erupt because of crowding by adjacent teeth or mal/position of the tooth. <u>Mal/occlusion</u> (**mal″o-kloo′zhən**), or improper bite, is abnormal contact of the teeth of the upper jaw, the maxilla, with the teeth of the lower jaw, the mandible. Ortho/dontic braces are used to move the teeth into alignment—in other words, to _____ the teeth.
temporomandibular	**10-108** <u>TMJ pain dysfunction syndrome</u> is an abnormal condition that interferes with eating and is believed to be caused by a defective or dislocated temporo/mandibular (**tem″pə-ro-mən-dib′u-lər**) joint (TMJ), one of a pair of joints connecting the mandible to the skull. Often called TMJ syndrome, this condition is characterized by facial pain and clicking sounds while chewing. Malocclusion, ill-fitting dentures, and a variety of conditions can cause TMJ syndrome. TMJ refers to the _____ joint.
cheek	**10-109** The mouth is examined for <u>oral cancer</u> during a routine dental examination. Tumors of the oral cavity can cause pain and change aspects of talking, swallowing, or chewing. Oral tumors can be classified as pre/malignant (precancerous), malignant, or benign. <u>Leuko/plakia</u> (**loo″ko-pla′ke-ə**) is a precancerous, slowly developing change in a mucous membrane characterized by white patches with sharply defined edges that are slightly raised. Leukoplakia may occur on the genitals or the lips and buccal mucosa (Figure 10-13). The buccal mucosa is the mucous membrane that lines the inside of the _____.
inflammation	**10-110** Tumors of the salivary glands are rare. More common disorders affecting the salivary glands are <u>sial/adenitis</u> (**si″əl-ad″ə-ni′tis**) or <u>sialo/lithiasis</u> (**si″ə-lo-lĭ-thi′ə-sis**). Sialo/lithiasis is the presence of one or more calculi in a salivary gland. Sial/adenitis is _____ of a salivary gland, often following conditions associated with a decrease in production of saliva. The microorganisms that are generally present in saliva usually compete with pathogens and prevent infection of the salivary glands.

*Caries (Latin: *decay*).
†Halitosis (Latin: *halitus*, breath).

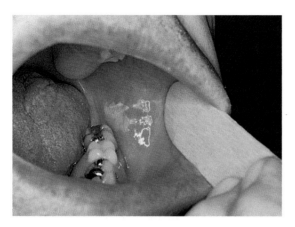

Figure 10-13   Leukoplakia. This slowly developing change in a mucous membrane characterized by white, sharply circumscribed patches is a precancerous lesion.

10-111 <u>Parot/itis</u> (**par″o-ti′tis**) is inflammation of the parotid gland. Epidemic or infectious parotitis is another name for mumps, a contagious viral disease that can generally be prevented by immunization.

<u>Mumps</u> is an acute viral infection that is characterized by swelling of the parotid glands and may affect one or both glands. The parotid gland is a salivary gland located

near   _____ the ear.

10-112 <u>Cleft palate</u>, often associated with cleft lip, is a congenital defect in which there is a division of the palate, resulting from the failure of the two sides of the palate to fuse during development. <u>Cleft lip</u> is one or more clefts in the upper lip. Surgical repair in infancy is generally recommended for both of these congenital defects.

Failure of the two sides of the palate to fuse during development results in

cleft   _____ palate.

10-113 The esophagus is susceptible to a variety of inflammatory, structural, and neoplastic (*ne[o]*, new + *-plastic*, repair) disorders. A <u>neo/plasm</u> is an abnormal growth of new tissue and can be benign or malignant.

<u>Esophag/itis</u> (**ə-sof″ə-ji′tis**) is inflammation of the mucosal lining of the esophagus, caused by infection, backflow of gastric juice from the stomach, or irritation from a naso/gastric tube. A naso-

stomach   gastric tube is a tube passed through the nose into the _____ and is used to both remove and introduce substances.

<u>Esophago/malacia</u> (**ə-sof″ə-go-mə-la′shə**) is a morbid softening of the esophagus. <u>Esophago/dynia</u>

pain   (**ə-sof″ə-go-din′e-ə**) is _____ of the esophagus.

10-114 <u>Gastroesophageal reflux disease</u> (GERD) is a dysfunction that involves a backflow of the

esophagus   contents of the stomach into the _____. The cause is often a weak cardiac sphincter. Repeated episodes of reflux can result in esophagitis, stricture (narrowing) of the esophagus, or an esophageal ulcer (craterlike lesion). Treatment of the disorder in its early stages is elevation of the head of the bed, avoidance of acid-stimulating foods, and use of ant/acids or anti/ulcer medications.

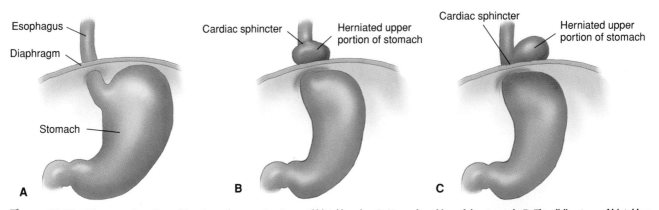

Figure 10-14   The normal position of the stomach versus two types of hiatal hernias. **A,** Normal position of the stomach. **B,** The sliding type of hiatal hernia accounts for 85% to 90% of hiatal hernias. The upper portion of the stomach slides up and down through the opening in the diaphragm. **C,** The rolling type of hiatal hernia accounts for 10% to 15% of hiatal hernias. The upper portion of the stomach is found alongside the esophagus, above the diaphragm.

10-115 GERD is one of the major symptoms of a hiatal (**hi-a′təl**) hernia, protrusion of a portion of the stomach upward through a defect in the diaphragm. Figure 10-14 shows two types of hiatal hernias.

As much as 40% of the population may have hiatal hernia, but most are asymptomatic. Diagnosis is generally confirmed by radiology, and surgery is seldom necessary. This type of herniation is called a _____ hernia.

hiatal

10-116 Esophageal achalasia (**ak″ə-la′zhə**) is an abnormal condition in which the lower esophageal sphincter fails to relax properly. It is characterized by dysphagia. Regurgitation, the return of swallowed food into the mouth, may also occur. Changes in diet and certain drugs may be helpful, but dilation of the esophagus with progressively larger sizes of dilators is also used. Write the name of the condition in which the lower esophageal sphincter fails to relax appropriately in response to swallowing: esophageal _____.

achalasia

10-117 Esophageal atresia (**ə-tre′zhə**), usually a congenital abnormality, is an esophagus that ends in a blind pouch or narrows so much that it obstructs continuous passage of food to the stomach. Write this term that is a congenital abnormality that results in a blind pouch or narrowing of the esophagus: esophageal _____. Narrowing may be improved by progressively larger dilators, or corrective surgery may be necessary.

atresia

10-118 Esophageal varices (singular, varix) are enlarged and swollen veins at the lower end of the esophagus, which are especially susceptible to hemorrhage. These large and swollen veins are called _____.

varices

Upper gastrointestinal bleeding is usually caused by esophageal varices, gastritis, ulcerations, or cancer of either the esophagus or stomach (Figure 10-15).

10-119 Gastr/itis (**gas-tri′tis**), one of the most common stomach disorders, is inflammation of the lining of the stomach. Causes of gastritis include medicines, food allergies, and toxins of microorganisms. Chronic gastritis can be a sign of another disease, such as cancer of the stomach or peptic ulcer.

Peptic ulcers occur in the stomach, duodenum, and occasionally the esophagus. The ulcerations are breaks in the continuity of the mucous membrane that comes in contact with the acids of the stomach. They usually occur near the pyloric opening (Figure 10-16). These types of ulcers cause stomachache, also called gastr/algia (**gas-tral′jə**). The literal interpretation of gastralgia is _____ of the stomach.

pain

10-120 Most peptic ulcers eventually heal, and the pain is controlled with drugs that either neutralize or block secretion of acid. However, some peptic ulcers are caused by a bacterium and can be treated with an antibiotic.

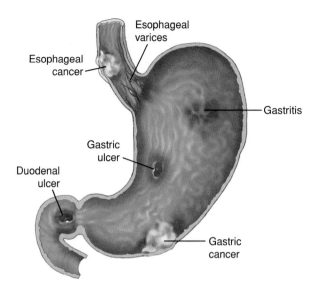

Esophageal varices

Esophageal cancer

Gastritis

Gastric ulcer

Duodenal ulcer

Gastric cancer

Figure 10-15   Common causes of upper gastrointestinal bleeding.

A small percentage of patients with ulcers need surgery to remove the affected part of the stomach or to sever a branch of the vagus nerve to reduce the amount of gastric acid produced.

10-121 Any disease of the stomach is a <u>gastropathy</u> (gas-trop′ə-the). *Gastromalacia* (gas″tro-mə-la′shə) means a morbid _____ of the stomach.

softening

Gastromegaly (gas″tro-meg′ə-le) means abnormal enlargement of the stomach or abdomen.

<u>Gastric carcinoma</u> is _____ of the stomach.

cancer

10-122 <u>Pyloric stenosis</u> is narrowing of the pyloric sphincter. The condition is a congenital defect, and it interferes with the flow of food into the small intestine.

This condition in which there is narrowing of the pyloric sphincter is pyloric _____.

stenosis

10-123 <u>Gastr/ectasis</u> (gas-trek′tə-sis) is abnormal _____ of the stomach. This may be caused by overeating, a hernia, or obstruction of the pyloric opening.

stretching

10-124 Some prominent signs and symptoms of gastric dysfunction are pain, excessive belching, flatulence, nausea, vomiting, blood in the stool, and diarrhea. <u>Flatulence</u> is excessive gas in the stomach or intestines. <u>Diarrhea</u> is frequent passage of watery bowel movements, often accompanied by cramping.

Write the term that means excessive gas in the stomach or intestines: _____.

flatulence

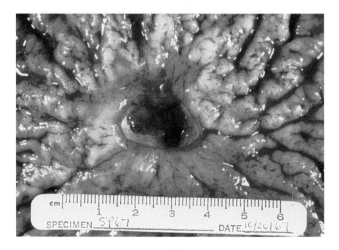

Figure 10-16   Photograph of a peptic ulcer. This peptic ulcer is located in the lesser curvature of the stomach.

Exercise 7

Match the pathologies of the upper digestive tract in the left column with their meanings or characteristics in the right column.

_____ 1. cheilosis

_____ 2. dyspepsia

_____ 3. esophageal achalasia

_____ 4. esophageal atresia

_____ 5. esophageal varices

_____ 6. gastritis

_____ 7. gingivitis

_____ 8. glossitis

_____ 9. hematemesis

_____ 10. leukoplakia

_____ 11. polydipsia

_____ 12. polyphagia

_____ 13. pyorrhea

_____ 14. sialadenitis

_____ 15. stomatodynia

_____ 16. stomatomycosis

A. a purulent inflammation of tissue around the teeth
B. enlarged and swollen veins of the esophagus
C. esophageal sphincter fails to relax properly
D. esophagus ends in a blind pouch or narrows
E. excessive hunger
F. excessive thirst
G. fungal condition of the mouth
H. indigestion
I. inflammation of the stomach
J. inflammation of a salivary gland
K. inflammation of the gums
L. inflammation of the tongue
M. painful mouth
N. precancerous change in a mucous membrane
O. splitting of the lips and angles of the mouth
P. vomiting of blood

■ Lower Digestive Tract

peritonitis

10-125 Intestinal disorders can be classified as inflammatory or noninflammatory. Similar symptoms may make it difficult to differentiate inflammatory and infectious disorders.

Periton/itis is an acute inflammation of the peritoneum (the lining of the abdominal cavity). Causes of peritonitis include rupture of abdominal organs such as the appendix, peptic ulcers, or perforations of an organ in the GI tract. Without treatment, it becomes a life-threatening illness.

A rupture or perforation of an organ in the GI tract may lead to

_____.

appendix

10-126 Three examples of acute inflammatory bowel problems are appendicitis, gastroenteritis, and dysentery. Appendic/itis (ə-pen″dĭ-si′tis) is acute inflammation of the vermiform

_____.

intestines

water

10-127 Gastro/enteritis (gas″tro-en″tər-i′tis) means inflammation of the stomach and

_____. It primarily affects the small intestine and can be either viral or bacterial. Intestinal flu (or influenza) is a viral gastroenteritis.

Symptoms of gastroenteritis are anorexia, nausea, vomiting, abdominal discomfort, diarrhea, and possibly fever. The feces may contain blood, mucus, pus, or excessive amounts of fat. Untreated severe diarrhea may lead to rapid dehydration. Dehydration is excessive loss of

_____ from body tissues.

Dysentery (dis′ən-ter″e) is an inflammation of the intestine, especially of the colon, that may be caused by bacteria, protozoa, parasites, or chemical irritants. It is characterized by abdominal pain and frequent and bloody stools.

10-128 Literal translation of col/itis is inflammation of the large intestine. Ulcerative col/itis and Crohn's disease are two of the more common chronic inflammatory bowel diseases (IBD).

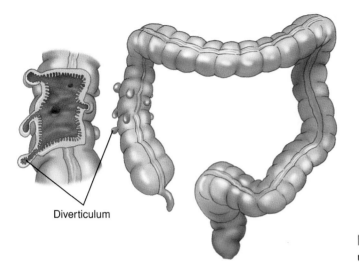

Diverticulum

Figure 10-17   Diverticulosis. Several abnormal outpouchings (diverticula) in the wall of the intestine.

Ulcerative colitis is a chronic inflammatory disorder of the colon or rectum, characterized by profuse, watery diarrhea containing mucus, blood, and pus. The chronic inflammation results in a loss of the mucosal lining and ulceration or abscess formation.

This type of chronic inflammatory bowel disease is called ulcerative

colitis   _____.

10-129 Crohn's disease (**krōnz dǐ-zēz′**) is another inflammatory bowel disease that can affect any part of the GI tract, from the mouth to the anus. Like ulcerative colitis, the cause is unknown. The lesions of Crohn's disease are patchy and often extend through all bowel layers.

Abnormal passages between internal organs or abnormal communications leading from internal organs to the body surface are called fistulas.* Fistulas can occur between the bowel and almost any adjacent structures. An <u>anal fistula</u> (**fis′tu-lə**) is an abnormal opening near the

anus   _____.

10-130 Diverticular disease includes <u>diverticul/itis</u> and <u>diverticu/losis</u>. A diverticulum (**di″vər-tik′u-ləm**) is a pouchlike herniation through the muscular wall of a tubular organ. A diverticulum (plural is diverticula) is most commonly present in the colon but also can occur in the esophagus, stomach, or small intestine (Figure 10-17). The combining form *diverticul(o)* refers to diverticula.

If diverticula are present in the colon without inflammation or symptoms, the condition is called diverticulosis (**di″vər-tik″u-lo′sis**). Diverticula generally do not cause a problem. Diverticul/itis

inflammation   (**di″vər-tik″u-li′tis**) is _____ of one or more diverticula.

10-131 A <u>fissure</u> (**fish′ər**) is a cleft or a groove or a cracklike lesion of the skin. A painful linear ulceration or tear at the anal opening is called an anal _____. Fissures

fissure   are sometimes associated with constipation, diarrhea, or Crohn's disease (Figure 10-18, A).

10-132 Parasites and pathogenic bacteria or viruses can invade the GI tract. <u>Food poisoning</u> results when a person ingests toxic substances or infectious organisms in food, but unlike gastroenteritis, food poisoning cannot be passed directly to another person. Mushroom poisoning is a type of

food   _____ poisoning.

Some common types of food poisoning include <u>staphylococcal infection</u>, *Escherichia coli* (commonly called *E. coli*) infection, and <u>botulism</u>. All these types of food poisoning are caused by pathogenic bacteria. Another bacterium, *Salmonella*, causes <u>salmonell/osis</u> (**sal″mo-nəl-o′sis**), and some forms of salmonella infection cause acute gastroenteritis.

*Fistula (Latin: *fistula*, pipe).

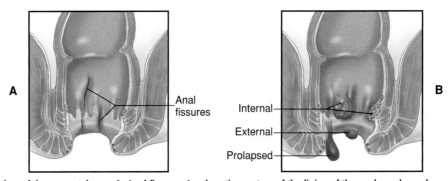

Figure 10-18   Two disorders of the anorectal area. **A,** Anal fissures. An ulceration or tear of the lining of the anal canal may be caused by excessive tissue stretching. These tears are very tender and tend to reopen when stool is passed. **B,** Hemorrhoids. Three types of hemorrhoids are shown: internal, external, and prolapsed. Internal hemorrhoids lie above the anal sphincter and cannot be seen on inspection of the anal area. External hemorrhoids lie below the anal sphincter and can be seen on inspection of the anal region. Hemorrhoids that enlarge, fall down, and protrude through the anus are called prolapsed hemorrhoids.

duodenum

stomach

10-133 A duodenal ulcer, the most common type of peptic ulcer, is one that occurs in the _____. Inflammation of the duodenum is <u>duodenitis</u> (**doo-od″ə-ni′tis**). Inflammation of the ileum is ileitis (**il″e-i′tis**).

    <u>Gastro/duoden/itis</u> (**gas″tro-doo″o-də-ni′tis**) is inflammation of the _____ and duodenum.

10-134 Noninflammatory intestinal disorders include malignant diverticulosis, tumors, obstructions, malabsorption, and trauma. <u>Irritable bowel syndrome</u> (IBS), also called spastic colon, spastic bowel, and mucous colitis, is a common chronic noninflammatory intestinal disorder. The cause is unknown, and it primarily involves increased motility of the intestines, diarrhea, and pain in the lower abdomen. Most of those affected are young adults. The pain is usually relieved by passing flatus (gas passed through the rectum) or stool.

irritable

    This noninflammatory intestinal disorder is called _____ bowel syndrome.

hemorrhoids

10-135 Rectal bleeding may be indicative of an intestinal disorder. <u>Hemorrhoids</u> (**hem′ə-roidz**), a common cause of rectal bleeding, are masses of dilated veins of the anal canal that lie just inside or outside the rectum. Several types are shown in Figure 10-18, *B*. They are often accompanied by pain, itching, and bleeding.

    Hemorrhoids are commonly called piles. This condition is aggravated by constipation, difficulty in passing stool or infrequent passage of hard stools. Constipation, straining to defecate (**def′ə-kāt**), and prolonged sitting contribute to the development of _____.

impaction

10-136 An accumulation of hardened feces in the rectum or sigmoid colon that the individual cannot expel is <u>impaction</u> (**im-pak′shən**).

    Write this term that means the presence of a large or hard fecal mass in the rectum or colon: _____.

enterostasis

10-137 Impaction leads to colonic stasis, also called <u>entero/stasis</u> (**en″tər-o-sta′sis**). When enterostasis occurs, there is a delay or a stopping of the movement of food in the intestinal tract.

    Colonic stasis, also called _____, is a stagnation of the normal flow of contents of the colon.

polyps

10-138 Common causes of rectal bleeding are shown in Figure 10-19. <u>Colonic polyps</u>, small, tumorlike growths, can arise from the mucosal surface of the colon. They may be seen during a colonoscopy. Some types of colonic polyps are closely linked to colorectal cancer, and for this reason are removed. Polyp/ectomy (**pol″ĭ-pek′tə-me**), removal of a polyp, can be performed during a colonoscopy if the polyp is small.

    Small, tumorlike growths on the mucosal surface of the colon are called colonic _____.

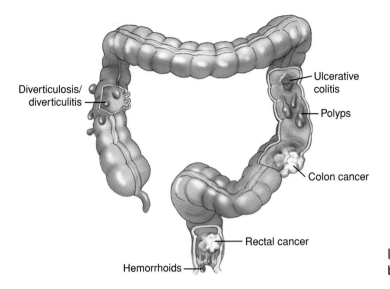

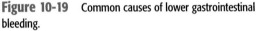

Figure 10-19   Common causes of lower gastrointestinal bleeding.

10-139 Intestinal obstruction occurs when intestinal contents cannot pass through the GI tract. The obstruction may be partial or complete and can occur anywhere in the intestinal tract. Figure 10-20 shows several causes of intestinal obstruction. Look closely at the illustration as you read about the different types of bowel obstructions.

Adhesions are bands of scar tissue that bind surfaces that normally are separated. They most commonly form in the abdomen after abdominal surgery, inflammation, or injury. Write this term that means scar tissue that binds surfaces together that are normally separate:

_____.

adhesion

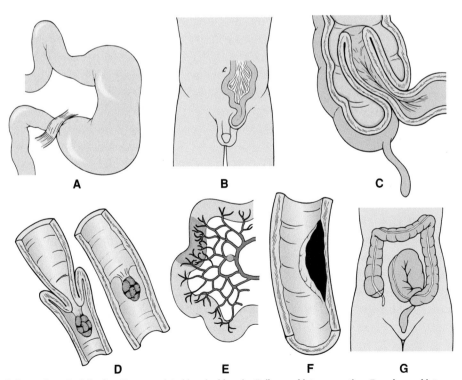

Figure 10-20   Bowel obstructions. **A,** Adhesion; **B,** strangulated inguinal hernia; **C,** ileocecal intussusception; **D,** polyp and intussusception; **E,** mesenteric occlusion; **F,** neoplasm; **G,** volvulus of the sigmoid colon.

10-140 <u>Inguinal hernias</u> develop because of a weakness in the abdominal muscle wall or a widened space at the inguinal ligament (see Figure 6-12, B). In a <u>strangulated hernia</u>, the blood vessels become so constricted by the neck of the hernial sac that circulation is stopped in the constricted area. Surgical intervention is necessary. A hernia in which the blood vessels are constricted by the neck of the hernial sac is called a _____ hernia.

strangulated

10-141 <u>Intussusception</u> (in″tə-sə-sep′shən) is a telescopic folding back of the bowel into itself. Mesenteric occlusion is a binding or closing off of a segment of the intestine by the mesentery, the peritoneum that suspends the intestine from the abdominal wall. A twisting of the bowel is called volvulus, and a folding back of the bowel onto itself is called _____. (Be careful with the spelling of this term.)

intussusception

　　Neoplasms or tumors are the most common cause of obstruction of the large intestine. Surgery is usually necessary to correct obstructions of the bowel.

10-142 <u>Mal/absorption syndrome</u> is a disorder in which one or multiple nutrients are not digested or absorbed. Literal translation of mal/absorption is _____ absorption.

poor

　　The nutrient that is not absorbed well depends on which abnormality exists. Various deficiencies can lead to malabsorption of fats, various vitamins, lactose, or iron. <u>Lipo/penia</u> (lip″o-pe′ne-ə) is a deficiency of _____.

fats

Exercise 8

Write a word in each blank to complete these sentences. The first letter of the word is given as a clue.

1. Inflammation of the stomach and intestines is g_____.

2. Inflammation of the colon that is characterized by abdominal pain and frequent and bloody stools is d_____.

3. An abnormal passage between two internal organs is a f_____.

4. The presence of diverticula in the colon without inflammation is called d_____.

5. A painful linear ulceration or tear at the anal opening is an anal f_____.

6. A common noninflammatory intestinal disorder has many names, including spastic bowel, mucous colitis, spastic colon, and i_____ bowel syndrome.

7. Masses of dilated veins that are varicose and lie just inside or outside the rectum are h_____.

8. An accumulation of feces that the individual cannot expel is called an i_____.

9. A telescopic folding back of one part of the intestine into itself is i_____.

10. A twisting of the bowel is called v_____.

■ *Accessory Organs of Digestion*

10-143 The liver is one of the most vital internal organs. Degeneration of the liver may lead to severe consequences, including <u>ascites</u> (accumulation of abdominal fluid), defects in coagulation of the blood, jaundice, neurologic symptoms, and hepatic and renal failure.

　　<u>Hepato/renal syndrome</u> is a type of kidney failure that is associated with hepatic failure. In hepat/ic failure, the _____ cannot perform its vital functions for the body. Hepatorenal syndrome has a poor prognosis, because both the kidneys and liver fail.

liver

10-144 <u>Hepat/itis</u> (hep″ə-ti′tis) is _____ of the liver. It is characterized by jaundice, <u>hepatomegaly</u> (hep″ə-to-meg′ə-le), anorexia, abnormal liver function, clay-colored stools, and tea-colored urine.

inflammation

　　<u>Jaundice</u> (jawn′dis) is a yellow discoloration of the skin, the mucous membranes, and the whites of the eyes, caused by greater than normal amounts of bilirubin in the blood. Bilirubin is the yellow-orange pigment of bile. *Hepato/megaly* means an _____ liver.

enlarged

10-145 Hepatitis may result from bacterial or viral infections or other causes, such as medications, toxins, or alcohol. <u>Viral hepatitis</u> is generally one of five major types. Other types of hepatitis are less common or generally have mild symptoms. The major types of viral hepatitis and their associated viruses are:

- hepatitis A (hepatitis A virus [HAV])
- hepatitis B (hepatitis B virus [HBV])
- hepatitis C (hepatitis C virus [HCV])
- hepatitis D (hepatitis D virus [HDV])
- hepatitis E (hepatitis E virus [HEV])

virus

Hepatitis A is caused by HAV, the abbreviation for hepatitis A _____. Hepatitis A and hepatitis E can be acquired by ingestion of contaminated food, but the other types are acquired only by contact with an infected person or infected materials. Most types of viral hepatitis can be acquired by contaminated blood, sexual contact, or the use of contaminated needles and instruments. Immunization is available for some types of hepatitis. Read more about viral hepatitis in the Sexually Transmitted Diseases section of Chapter 13.

liver

10-146 <u>Cirrhosis</u> (sĭ-ro′sis) is a chronic, progressive liver disease that is characterized by degeneration of liver cells with eventual increased resistance to flow of blood through the liver. Cirrhosis is a disease of what organ? _____.
   <u>Alcoholic cirrhosis</u> occurs in approximately 20% of chronic alcoholics. Unless alcohol is avoided, coma, gastrointestinal hemorrhage, and kidney failure may occur. In addition to alcohol, nutritional deficiencies, poisons, toxic drugs, some types of heart disease, or prior viral hepatitis can lead to cirrhosis.

enlargement

10-147 Any disease of the liver is a <u>hepato/pathy</u> (hep″ə-top′ə-the). <u>Hepato/spleno/megaly</u> (hep″ə-to-sple″no-meg′ə-le) is _____ of the liver and spleen.

hepatoma
(hep″ə-to′mə)

10-148 A tumor of the liver is a _____. This term is usually reserved for a specific type of primary liver carcinoma.
   Tumors of the liver may be benign or malignant. Cancer of the liver is called hepatic

carcinoma

_____. Malignancy in the liver that is spread from another source is many times more common than primary tumor of the liver.

bile

10-149 Bile is produced by the liver, stored in the gallbladder, and released into the duodenum via the common bile duct when needed for digestion. Anything that interferes with the flow of bile interferes with digestion. <u>Chole/stasis</u> (ko″le-sta′sis) is stoppage or suppression of bile flow. Obstruction of bile flow can cause inflammation of the gallbladder, the liver, or the pancreas.
   <u>Chol/angitis</u> (ko″lan-ji′tis) is inflammation of a _____ vessel, or duct. (Note that the *e* is dropped from *chol[e]* when it is combined with *angi[o]*.) This can be caused by bacterial infection or by obstruction of the ducts by calculi or a tumor.

calculus

10-150 <u>Choledoch/itis</u> (kol″ə-do-ki′tis) is inflammation of the common bile duct. <u>Choledocho/lith/iasis</u> (ko-led″ə-ko-lĭ-thi′ə-sis) is the presence of a _____ in the common bile duct.

gallstones (or calculi)

10-151 <u>Chole/lith/iasis</u> (ko″lə-lĭ-thi′ə-sis) is the presence of _____ in the gallbladder. Acute <u>cholecyst/itis</u>, inflammation of the gallbladder, is usually caused by a gallstone. If surgery is not performed to remove the gallbladder, a perforation (opening or hole) in its wall may occur. An abscess may form if the perforation is small, or peritonitis may result if the perforation is large.
   Acute cholecystitis may occur in the absence of gallstones, possibly due to bacterial invasion. A chronic form of cholecystitis, with pain following a fatty meal, may occur when there is insufficient emptying of bile by the gallbladder.

10-152 Both cholangitis and pancreatitis can occur as complications of cholecystitis, resulting from the backup of bile through the biliary tract. <u>Pancreat/itis</u> (pan″kre-ə-ti′tis) is inflammation of

pancreas

the _____. Acute pancreatitis can be life threatening, resulting in destruction of the organ by its own enzymes. Destruction of pancreatic tissue is pancreatolysis (pan″kre-ə-tol′ĭ-sis).

Several factors that contribute to acute pancreatitis include alcoholism, gallstones, trauma, tumors, peritonitis, viral infections, and drug toxicity. Chronic pancreatitis may develop after repeated episodes of acute pancreatitis (particularly that induced by alcohol abuse) or chronic obstruction of the common bile duct. A pancreatic abscess, a collection of _____ in or around the pancreas, is a serious complication of pancreatitis.

pus

10-153 Stones, tumors, or cysts can cause pancreatic obstructions. Pancreato/lithiasis (pan″kre-ə-to-lĭ-thi′ə-sis) is the presence of calculi in the pancreas or pancreatic duct. Pancreato/lith (pan″kre-at′o-lith) means a pancreatic _____.

calculus (stone)

Pancreatic carcinoma is one of the most deadly malignancies. The cancer is usually discovered in the late stages, and survival after diagnosis is usually only a few months. Pancreatic cancer is not common in North America, but it ranks fourth as a cause of cancer death because of its extremely low survival rate.

Like pancreatic carcinoma, the prognosis for cancer of the gallbladder is poor. However, cancer of the gallbladder is rare.

10-154 Three of the more likely disorders of the salivary glands are sialadenitis, sialolithiasis, and tumors. Sialadenitis (si″əl-ad″ə-ni′tis), _____ of the salivary glands, can be caused by an infectious microorganism, an allergic reaction, or irradiation. The latter may result from radiation therapy, which causes a very dry mouth and is treated with substances that stimulate saliva or substitute for saliva.

inflammation

Sialo/lithiasis (si″ə-lo-lĭ-thi′ə-sis), the presence of salivary stones, either within the gland itself or in the salivary ducts, may cause few symptoms unless the duct becomes obstructed.

Exercise 9

Match terms in the left column with their meaning or characteristics in the right column. (Use all choices once.)

_____ 1. ascites

_____ 2. cholangitis

_____ 3. cholecystitis

_____ 4. choledochitis

_____ 5. choledocholithiasis

_____ 6. cholestasis

_____ 7. cirrhosis

_____ 8. hepatoma

_____ 9. jaundice

A. accumulation of abdominal fluid
B. calculus in the common bile duct
C. chronic degeneration of liver cells
D. inflammation of a bile duct
E. inflammation of the common bile duct
F. inflammation of the gallbladder
G. stoppage or suppression of bile flow
H. tumor of the liver
I. yellow discoloration of the skin and increased bilirubin

SURGICAL AND THERAPEUTIC INTERVENTIONS

■ Upper and Lower Digestive Tracts

10-155 Patients who can digest and absorb nutrients but need nutritional support may receive enteral (en′tər-əl) nutrition. Enteral nutrition is the provision of nutrients through the GI tract when the patient cannot ingest, chew, or swallow food but can digest and absorb nutrients. This is

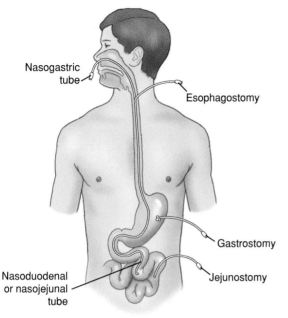

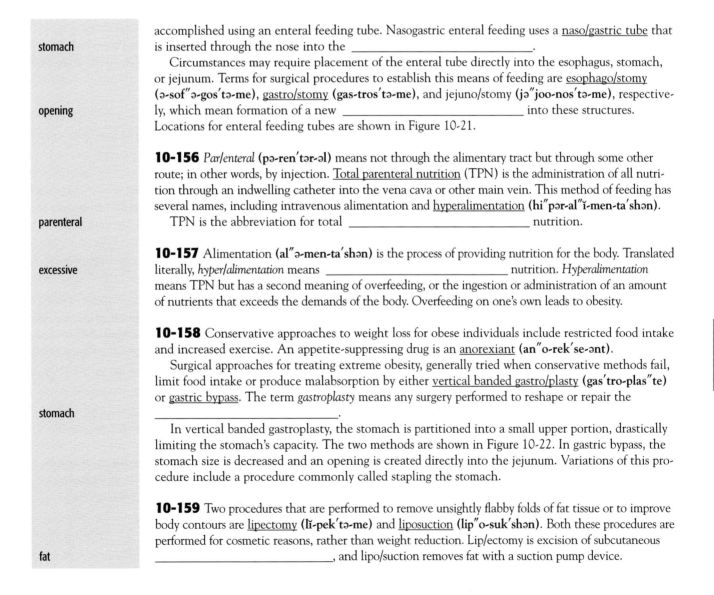

Figure 10-21 Common placement locations for enteral feeding tubes.

stomach

accomplished using an enteral feeding tube. Nasogastric enteral feeding uses a <u>naso/gastric tube</u> that is inserted through the nose into the _____.

Circumstances may require placement of the enteral tube directly into the esophagus, stomach, or jejunum. Terms for surgical procedures to establish this means of feeding are <u>esophago/stomy</u> **(ə-sof″ə-gos′tə-me)**, <u>gastro/stomy</u> **(gas-tros′tə-me)**, and jejuno/stomy **(jə″joo-nos′tə-me)**, respective-

opening

ly, which mean formation of a new _____ into these structures. Locations for enteral feeding tubes are shown in Figure 10-21.

10-156 *Par/enteral* **(pə-ren′tər-əl)** means not through the alimentary tract but through some other route; in other words, by injection. <u>Total parenteral nutrition</u> (TPN) is the administration of all nutrition through an indwelling catheter into the vena cava or other main vein. This method of feeding has several names, including intravenous alimentation and <u>hyperalimentation</u> **(hi″pər-al″ĭ-men-ta′shən)**.

parenteral

TPN is the abbreviation for total _____ nutrition.

10-157 Alimentation **(al″ə-men-ta′shən)** is the process of providing nutrition for the body. Translated literally, *hyper/alimentation* means _____ nutrition. *Hyperalimentation*

excessive

means TPN but has a second meaning of overfeeding, or the ingestion or administration of an amount of nutrients that exceeds the demands of the body. Overfeeding on one's own leads to obesity.

10-158 Conservative approaches to weight loss for obese individuals include restricted food intake and increased exercise. An appetite-suppressing drug is an <u>anorexiant</u> **(an″o-rek′se-ənt)**.

Surgical approaches for treating extreme obesity, generally tried when conservative methods fail, limit food intake or produce malabsorption by either <u>vertical banded gastro/plasty</u> **(gas′tro-plas″te)** or <u>gastric bypass</u>. The term *gastroplasty* means any surgery performed to reshape or repair the

stomach

_____.

In vertical banded gastroplasty, the stomach is partitioned into a small upper portion, drastically limiting the stomach's capacity. The two methods are shown in Figure 10-22. In gastric bypass, the stomach size is decreased and an opening is created directly into the jejunum. Variations of this procedure include a procedure commonly called stapling the stomach.

10-159 Two procedures that are performed to remove unsightly flabby folds of fat tissue or to improve body contours are <u>lipectomy</u> **(lĭ-pek′tə-me)** and <u>liposuction</u> **(lip″o-suk′shən)**. Both these procedures are performed for cosmetic reasons, rather than weight reduction. Lip/ectomy is excision of subcutaneous

fat

_____, and lipo/suction removes fat with a suction pump device.

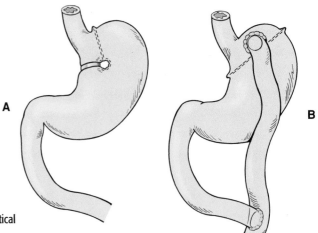

Figure 10-22 Two surgical procedures for limiting nutrient intake. **A,** Vertical banded gastroplasty; **B,** gastric bypass.

esophagus

stomach

fixation

stomach

lip

approximate

gastric

lip

10-160 Trauma or a tumor in the cardiac region of the stomach sometimes makes it necessary to create a new opening between the esophagus and stomach. <u>Esophagogastrostomy</u> (ə-sof″ə-go-gas-tros′tə-me) means creating a new opening between the _____ and the stomach.

If either the stomach or the esophagus becomes diseased near the cardiac sphincter, an <u>esopha-gogastroplasty</u> (ə-sof″ə-go-gas′tro-plas″te) may be performed. This new term means surgical repair of the esophagus and the _____.

10-161 <u>Gastro/pexy</u> (gas′tro-pek″se) is surgical _____ of the stomach. Gastropexy involves suturing (sewing) the stomach to the abdominal wall to prevent displacement.

An important feature of suture material is whether it is absorbable or nonabsorbable. Absorbable suture is gradually removed by the body's phagocytes. Catgut is one of the best examples of absorbable suture material. <u>Gastro/rrhaphy</u> (gas-tror′ə-fe), suture of the _____, would probably use absorbable suture material.

Nonabsorbable suture is either left in the body, where it becomes embedded in scar tissue, or removed when healing is complete. Silk, cotton, wire, and certain synthetic materials are not absorbed by the body and are examples of nonabsorbable sutures.

<u>Cheilo/rrhaphy</u> (ki-lor′ə-fe), suture of the _____, and <u>glosso/rrhaphy</u> (glos-or′ə-fe), suture of the tongue, would probably use nonabsorbable material because of the easy access for removal of the suture.

10-162 <u>Approximate</u> (ə-prok′sĭ-māt″) means to bring close together by suture or other means. The act of bringing closer together is approximation. Tissue approximation can be accomplished with materials other than suture, such as tape, clips, and staples. In some instances, special adhesives that bond almost instantly can be sprayed on a wound to _____ the skin, thus eliminating the need for stitches.

10-163 <u>Lavage</u> (lah-vahzh′) is irrigation or washing out of an organ, such as the stomach or bowel. Washing out of the stomach is _____ lavage, performed to remove irritants or toxic substances and before or after surgery on the stomach.

Flushing of the inside of the colon is called colonic irrigation; this is not the same as an enema. <u>Colonic irrigation</u> may be used to remove any material high in the colon, whereas an <u>enema</u> is introduction of a solution into the rectum for cleansing the rectum or is used as a treatment for constipation.

10-164 Cancer or trauma can affect any structure of the digestive system and may require plastic surgery if there is extensive damage. <u>Cheilo/plasty</u> (ki′lo-plas″te) is surgical repair of the _____.

Stomato/plasty (sto'mə-to-plas"te) is surgical repair of the mouth. Cheilo/stomato/plasty (ki"lo-sto-mat'o-plas"te) is surgical repair of the lips and mouth.

10-165 A gloss/ectomy (glos-ek'tə-me) is removal of all or part of the tongue, necessary in carcinoma of the tongue.
Surgical repair of the tongue is called_____.

glossoplasty
(glos'o-plas"te)

10-166 Write a term that means surgical excision of all or part of the esophagus: _____. This surgical procedure may be required to treat severe bleeding of the esophagus or esophageal cancer.

esophagectomy
(ə-sof"ə-jek'tə-me)

Esophago/myo/tomy (ə-sof"ə-go-mi-ot'ə-me) is an incision into the muscle of the lower part of the esophagus, performed to expedite the passage of food in esophageal achalasia. You remember from studying this term earlier that achalasia is an abnormal condition characterized by the inability of the muscle to _____.

relax

10-167 Gingiv/ectomy (jin"gĭ-vek'tə-me) is excision of the _____. Gingivectomy is surgical removal of all loose and diseased gum tissue, performed to arrest the progress of periodontal disease. This procedure is performed by a dentist or periodontist.

gums

10-168 Some types of ulcers of the stomach, esophagus, and duodenum are caused by a particular bacterium called *Helicobacter pylori* and can be treated with antibiotics. Medications can also cause ulcers. Treatment of peptic ulcer can include any of the following: antibiotic, change of a suspected medication, dietary management, and antacids to counteract the acidic gastric contents. An ant/acid (ant-as'id) is an agent used to treat gastric hyper/acidity (hi"pər-ə-sid'ĭ-te), _____ acid in the stomach. Gastric hyperacidity may lead to ulcers. (Note the omission of the *i* in *antacid*.)

excessive

10-169 Gastric secretions are controlled by the vagus (va'gəs) nerve, the tenth cranial nerve. Vago/tomy (va-got'ə-me) is _____ of certain branches of the vagus nerve to reduce the amount of gastric acid secreted. Vagotomy may be done in such a way that the branches supplying the acid-secreting glands of the stomach are severed without disturbing those branches that supply other abdominal structures.

incision

10-170 Pyloro/plasty (pi-lor'o-plas"te) is surgical repair of the pyloric sphincter. It may be done when other methods of treating peptic ulcers have not been effective. Pyloroplasty consists of surgical enlargement of the pyloric sphincter to facilitate the easy passage of the stomach contents to the duodenum. (Pyloroplasty may be necessary when there is pyloric stenosis, a narrowing of the pyloric sphincter at the outlet of the stomach.)

Pyloro/tomy (pi"lor-ot'o-me) is incision of the pylorus. Pylorotomy is often called *pyloromyotomy* (pi-lor"o-mi-ot'ə-me), which means_____ of the muscles of the pylorus, and is also done to expedite the passage of food from the stomach.

incision

10-171 Persons with ulcers who do not respond to medical treatment or who develop complications (perforation or hemorrhage) may require partial gastr/ectomy (gas-trek'tə-me), which is _____ of part of the stomach. A gastrectomy, removal of part or all of the stomach, is done also to remove a malignancy.

removal

10-172 Anastomosis* (ə-nas"tə-mo'sis) means a connection between two vessels. It may be created by surgical, traumatic, or pathologic means between two normally distinct organs or spaces. The communication (union) itself is also called an anastomosis. The verb that means to join the structures is *anastomose* (ə-nas'tə-mōs).

Study the three types of surgical anastomoses of the gastrointestinal tract in Figure 10-23 and write answers in these blanks. A gastro/entero/stomy (gas"tro-en"tər-os'tə-me) is the simplest of these three anastomoses. In a gastro/entero/stomy, the body of the stomach is joined with some part

---

*Anastomose (Greek: *anastomoien*, to provide a mouth).

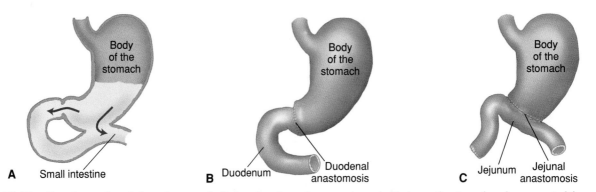

Figure 10-23   Three types of surgical anastomoses. **A,** Gastroenterostomy. A passage is created between the stomach and some part of the small intestine, often the jejunum. **B,** Gastroduodenostomy. The lower portion of the stomach is removed, and the remainder is anastomosed to the duodenum. **C,** Gastrojejunostomy. The lower portion of the stomach is removed, and the remainder is anastomosed to the jejunum. The remaining duodenal stump is closed.

small	of the _____ intestine. This term, like the other two terms, begins with the proximal organ (the organ nearest the place where nutrition begins).
	In the two other types of anastomoses, the lower portion of the stomach is removed before the gastric stump is anastomosed to either the duodenum or the jejunum.
	The terms *gastro/duodeno/stomy* (**gas″tro-doo″o-də-nos′tə-me**) and *gastro/jejuno/stomy* (**gas″tro-jə-joo-nos′tə-me**) are anastomosis of the gastric stump with the duodenum and
jejunum	_____, respectively. They may also be called gastro/duodenal (**gas″tro-doo″o-de′nəl**) anastomosis and gastro/jejunal anastomosis.
	10-173 In extensive gastric cancer, a total gastrectomy with anastomosis of the esophagus to the jejunum is the principal medical intervention. This means that all of the
stomach	_____ is removed and an esophago/jejuno/stomy (**ə-sof-ə-go-je″joo-nos′tə-me**) is performed.
	Esophago/jejuno/stomy (**ə-sof-ə-go-je″joo-nos′tə-me**) means surgical anastomosis of the
esophagus	_____ to the jejunum.
	10-174 In an *esophago/duodeno/stomy* (**ə-sof″ə-go-doo″o-de-nos′tə-me**), the anastomosis is between the esophagus and the _____.
duodenum	*Jejuno/ileo/stomy* (**jə-joo″no-il″e-os′tə-me**) is formation of an opening between the jejunum and
ileum	the _____.
	10-175 If the large intestine must be removed, a new opening is made into the ileum through the abdominal wall. Fecal material drains into a bag worn on the abdomen. Formation of an opening
ileostomy (il″e-os′tə-me)	into the ileum is _____.
	If all of the colon is removed, an *ileostomy* is necessary. An ileo/stomy is forming an ileal stoma onto the surface of the abdomen.
	10-176 *Col/ectomy* (**ko-lek′tə-me**) is excision of all, or a part, of the
colon	_____.
	A *colo/stomy* (**kə-los′tə-me**) is generally performed after partial colectomy. A colostomy is surgical creation of an artificial anus on the abdominal wall by drawing the colon out to the surface or,
colon	in other words, creating an artificial opening from the _____ on the abdominal surface. Colostomies may be permanent or temporary, perhaps to divert feces after surgery. Several locations for colostomy and an ileostomy are shown in Figure 10-24.
	The artificially created opening in a colostomy is called a stoma (**sto′mə**). The term *stoma* means any small orifice or opening, and it can refer to the opening established in the abdominal wall by a colostomy or similar surgery or the opening between two portions of the intestine in an anastomosis.

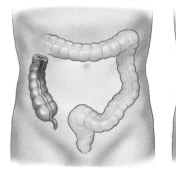
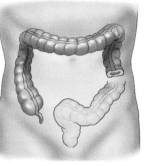
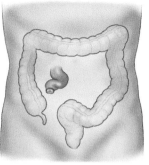

Ascending colostomy   Descending colostomy   Ileostomy

Sigmoid colostomy
single-barreled

Transverse colostomy
double-barreled

Figure 10-24   A comparison of an ileostomy and several types of colostomy. The lighter section indicates the portion of the large intestine that is removed.

intestine	**10-177** Remembering that *lapar(o)* means abdominal wall, <u>laparo/entero/stomy</u> is formation of an opening through the abdominal wall into the small _____. This procedure is done to install a tube to drain the bowel, or it may be used to supply nutrients to a patient with an upper digestive tract obstruction.
duodenostomy (doo″o-də-nos′ tə-me)	**10-178** <u>Jejuno/tomy</u> (jə″joo-not′ə-me) is surgical incision of the jejunum. An incision of the duodenum is a duodeno/tomy (doo″o-də-not′ə-me). Formation of a new opening into the duodenum is a _____.
proctoplasty (prok′to-plas″te)	**10-179** <u>Ceco/ileo/stomy</u> (se″ko-il″e-os′tə-me) is formation of a new opening between the cecum and the ileum. Using *proct(o)*, write a word that means surgical repair of the rectum and anus: _____.
diverticulum removal (excision)	**10-180** You studied the difference in diverticulosis and diverticulitis earlier in this chapter. <u>Diverticul/ectomy</u> (di″vər-tik″u-lek′tə-me), surgical excision of a _____, may be performed if repeated bouts of diverticulitis result in obstruction of the colon. In cases of acute appendic/itis, an append/ectomy is usually performed. An <u>append/ectomy</u> is _____ of the appendix.
pain	**10-181** Nonsurgical management of hemorrhoids is aimed at reducing symptoms without surgery and decreasing the likelihood that the symptoms recur. <u>Topical anesthetics</u>, application of cold packs, and soaks are used to alleviate hemorrhoid/al pain. *Topi/cal* (*top[o]*, place + *ical*, pertaining to) means pertaining to a particular place on the surface area. You have learned that an anesthetic is used to produce a loss of sensation or feeling. The purpose of a topical an/esthetic is to alleviate _____ on a particular area of the skin.

hemorrhoids

Several surgical methods are available if symptoms persist, and treatment is determined by the type of hemorrhoid. Treatments include <u>elastic band ligation</u> (lǐ-gaʹshən) and a <u>hemorrhoidectomy</u> (hem″ə-roid-ekʹtə-me). In elastic band ligation,* the hemorrhoids are bound with rubber bands, become necrotic, and eventually disappear. A hemorrhoid/ectomy is excision of

_____.

10-182 In addition to those already mentioned, several pharmaceuticals are helpful in the treatment of gastrointestinal problems. Various antibiotics are used, depending on the type of infectious microorganisms that are present.

diarrhea

<u>Anti/diarrheals</u> are used to treat _____, and <u>anti/emetics</u> are used to relieve or prevent vomiting.

<u>Stool softeners</u> are used to prevent constipation. <u>Laxatives</u> cause evacuation of the bowel by a mild action and may be prescribed to correct constipation. Purgatives or cathartics are strong medications used to promote full evacuation of the bowel, as in preparation for diagnostic studies or surgery of the digestive tract.

■ Accessory Organs of Digestion

liver

10-183 Carcinoma that has spread from another site to the liver is more common than primary liver cancer. If the tumor is localized to one portion of the liver, <u>hepatic lob/ectomy</u>, excision of a lobe of the _____, may be performed. Other surgeries and chemotherapy are also used, depending on the type of liver cancer.

hepatectomy (hep″ə-tekʹtə-me)

10-184 Surgical incision of the liver is <u>hepatotomy</u> (hep″ə-totʹə-me). Excision of part of the liver is _____. <u>Liver transplantation</u> may be performed in some cases, usually for liver disease related to chronic viral hepatitis.

pancreatectomy (pan″kre-ə-tekʹ tə-me)

10-185 <u>Pancreato/tomy</u> (pan″kre-ə-totʹə-me) is incision of the pancreas. Removal of the pancreas is _____. <u>Pancreato/lith/ectomy</u> (pan″kre-ə-to-lǐ-thekʹtə-me) is removal of pancreatic stones.

insulin

10-186 <u>Diabetes mellitus</u> results primarily from a deficiency or lack of insulin secretion by the pancreas or resistance to insulin. Some forms of diabetes are treated with diet, exercise, and weight control, and other forms require glucose-lowering agents (oral agents or insulin by injection). Diabetes mellitus results primarily from a lack of _____ secretion by the pancreas or resistance to insulin.

lithotripsy

10-187 Gallstones are a common disorder of the gallbladder and bile ducts and are usually associated with cholecystitis. Several nonsurgical approaches are available, including oral drugs that dissolve stones, <u>laser litho/tripsy</u> (lithʹo-trip″se), and <u>extracorporeal shock wave lithotripsy</u> (ESWL).

In ESWL, extracorporeal (outside the body) shock wave _____, a lithotriptor uses high-energy shock waves to disintegrate the stone. The patient is positioned over a shock wave generator (lithotriptor) by means of a table that moves upward and downward, forward and backward, and side to side. Particles slough off the gallstone as the lithotriptor is fired, and the particles pass through the biliary ducts and are eliminated. The name of the shock wave generator

lithotriptor

in biliary lithotripsy is a _____ (Figure 10-25).

*Ligation (Latin: *ligare*, to bind).

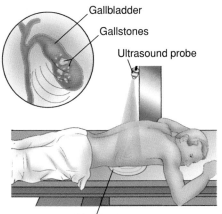

Gallbladder
Gallstones
Ultrasound probe

Lithotriptor

Figure 10-25   Biliary lithotripsy. The gallbladder is positioned over the lithotriptor; then the lithotriptor is fired and particles slough off the gallstones until they are fragmented and can pass through the biliary ducts.

10-188 <u>Lithotripsy</u> is nonsurgical management of gallstones and can sometimes be an alternative to cholecystectomy (ko″lə-sis-tek′tə-me), surgical removal of the gallbladder. The gallbladder stores bile but is not essential for life, because bile is produced continuously.

Endoscopic removal of biliary stones is called <u>endoscopic sphinctero/tomy</u>, because the endoscope is passed to the duodenum, and then the sphincter muscle is incised to reach and retrieve the stone.

<u>Laparo/scopic cholecystectomy</u>, removal of the gallbladder through a small incision in the

abdominal

_____ wall, is performed more often than the traditional, open cholecystectomy. Laparoscopic cholecystectomy is commonly done as an outpatient surgery. The gallbladder is excised with laser and removed through the small opening.

10-189 Write a term that means surgical incision of the gallbladder:

**cholecystotomy
(ko″lə-sis-tot′ə-me)**

_____.

This new term means incision of the gallbladder for the purpose of exploration, drainage, or removal of stones.

Laparo/cholecysto/tomy (lap″ə-ro-ko″lə-sis-tot′ə-me) means incision into the gallbladder through the abdominal wall.

10-190 <u>Choledocho/litho/tripsy</u> (ko-led″o-ko-lith′o-trip″se) means the crushing of gallstones in the common bile duct. <u>Choledocho/stomy</u> (ko-led″ə-kos′tə-me) is surgical formation of an

opening

_____ into the common bile duct through the abdominal wall. This is commonly done for temporary drainage of the duct after cholecystectomy.

<u>Choledocho/jejuno/stomy</u> (ko-led″ə-ko-jə-joo-nos′tə-me) is surgical formation of a new opening

jejunum

between the common bile duct and the _____.

10-191 Treatment of infected salivary glands includes antibiotics and warm compresses. If the flow of saliva is obstructed by a stone, the duct's opening may be dilated and massaged. If these measures fail, surgery may be necessary to remove the stone.

Tumors of the salivary glands, either benign or malignant, are excised. However, radiation therapy may be used for highly malignant or very large tumors or for recurrence of a tumor after surgery.

Exercise 10

Match the procedures listed on this surgery schedule with their descriptions. (Use all terms once only.)

_____ 1 cheilorrhaphy

_____ 2. cholecystectomy

_____ 3. colostomy

_____ 4. esophagogastroplasty

_____ 5. esophagogastrostomy

_____ 6. gastrectomy

_____ 7. gastric bypass

_____ 8. gastroenterostomy

_____ 9. gastropexy

_____ 10. lipectomy

A. a type of gastroplasty
B. creation of a new opening between the esophagus and stomach
C. excision of subcutaneous fat
D. excision of the gallbladder
E. formation of an artificial anus on the abdominal wall
F. joining of the stomach with some part of the small intestine
G. removal of part or all of the stomach
H. surgical repair of the esophagus and stomach
I. suture of the lip
J. suture of the stomach to the abdominal wall

SELECTED ABBREVIATIONS

ALT	alanine transferase		**HSV**	herpes simplex virus
ALP	alkaline phosphatase (liver function test)		**IBD**	inflammatory bowel disease
BM	bowel movement		**IBS**	irritable bowel syndrome
BMI	body mass index		**IC**	irritable colon
DM	diabetes mellitus		**lap**	laparotomy
EGD	esophagogastroduodenoscopy		**LFT**	liver function test
ESWL	extracorporeal shock wave lithotripsy		**NG tube**	nasogastric tube
GB	gallbladder		**RDA**	recommended dietary allowance
GERD	gastroesophageal reflux disease		**SGOT**	serum glutamic-oxaloacetic transaminase (enzyme test of heart and liver function)
GI	gastrointestinal			
HAV	hepatitis A virus		**SGPT**	serum glutamic-pyruvic transaminase (enzyme test of liver function, now called ALT)
HBV	hepatitis B virus			
HCV	hepatitis C virus		**TPN**	total parenteral nutrition
HDV	hepatitis D virus		**UGI**	upper gastrointestinal (or upper GI) series
HEV	hepatitis E virus			

CHAPTER 10 REVIEW

■ Basic Understanding

Labeling

I. Label the structures (1 through 13) in the diagram with the corresponding combining form. (Write two combining forms for numbers 2 and 6.)

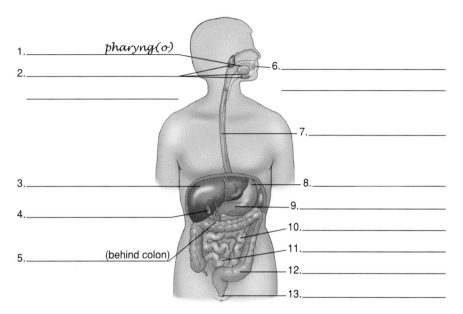

1._____ *pharyng(o)*

2._____

_____

6._____

_____

7._____

3._____

8._____

4._____

9._____

10._____

11._____

5._____ (behind colon)

12._____

13._____

Matching

II. Match the major functions of the digestive tract in the left column with their descriptions in the right column.

_____ 1. absorption

_____ 2. digestion

_____ 3. elimination

_____ 4. ingestion

A. eating food
B. mechanically and chemically breaking down food
C. passing nutrient molecules into blood or lymph
D. removing wastes

III. Match structures of the digestive system with their descriptions in the right column.

_____ 1. duodenum

_____ 2. esophagus

_____ 3. gallbladder

_____ 4. ileum

_____ 5. jejunum

_____ 6. liver

_____ 7. mouth

_____ 8. pancreas

_____ 9. stomach

_____ 10. transverse colon

A. connects with the cecum
B. first major site of digestion
C. its lower end connects with the stomach
D. its upper end connects with the stomach
E. midsection of the three parts of the small intestine
F. part of the large intestine
G. produces bile
H. produces insulin
I. stores bile
J. where the buccal cavity is located

IV. *pathologies on the left with meanings on the right.*

_____ 1. caries

_____ 2. fissure

_____ 3. esophageal atresia

_____ 4. esophageal achalasia

_____ 5. esophageal varices

_____ 6. fistula

_____ 7. hernia

_____ 8. malocclusion

_____ 9. sialadenitis

_____ 10. ulcer

A. abnormal passage
B. cleft or cracklike lesion
C. decay
D. improper bite
E. inflammation of a salivary gland
F. enlarged and swollen veins at the lower end of the esophagus
G. lower esophageal sphincter fails to relax properly
H. esophagus ends in a blind pouch or is too narrow
I. open sore or lesion
J. protrusion of an organ through the wall of a cavity

Listing

V. *List the three classes of nutrients and explain their functions.*

1. _____

2. _____

3. _____

VI. *List the four accessory organs of digestion and write their combining form(s).*

1. _____ = _____

2. _____ = _____

3. _____ = _____

4. _____ = _____

Multiple Choice

VII. *Circle the correct answer for each of the following multiple choice questions:*

1. Mrs. Vogel's physician tells her that she needs to see a specialist for the problem that she's been having with her colon. What is the name of the specialty practiced by the physician Mrs. Vogel should see? (cardiology, gastroenterology, gynecology, urology)

2. Cal Stone has radiography of the gallbladder. What is the name of this diagnostic test? (barium enema, barium meal, cholecystography, esophagogastroscopy)

3. Tests show that Cal Stone has a gallstone in the common bile duct. Which of the following is a noninvasive conservative procedure to alleviate Cal's problem? (cholecystostomy, choledochostomy, choledochojejunostomy, extracorporeal shock wave lithotripsy)

4. Linda M., a 16-year-old female, is diagnosed as having self-induced starvation. Which of the following is the name of the disorder associated with Linda's problem? (anorexia nervosa, aphagia, malaise, polyphagia)

5. Unless there is intervention for Linda's self-induced starvation, which condition will result? (adipsia, atresia, emaciation, volvulus)

6. A 70-year-old male is diagnosed with cancer of the colon. Which term indicates a surgical intervention for this condition? (colectomy, colonoscopy, colonic irrigation, colonic stasis)

7. Baby Jake is born with a narrowing of the muscular ring that controls the outflow of food from the stomach. What is the name of this disorder? (pyloric sphincter, pyloric stenosis, pyloroplasty, pyloromyotomy)

8. What is the name of the valve that regulates movement of intestinal contents from the small intestine into the large intestine? (cecorectal valve, ileocecal valve, jejunocecal valve, pyloric valve)

9. Mary suffers from GERD. The physician explains to her that radiography indicates that a portion of the stomach is protruding upward through the diaphragm. What is the name of this disorder? (anorexia nervosa, caries, cholelith, hiatal hernia)

10. Jane is scheduled for a cheilostomatoplasty. What structures are involved in her surgery? (gums and mouth, lips and mouth, mouth and stomach, tongue and mouth)

11. A 70-year-old woman has an obstruction that has led to stagnation of the normal movement of food in the intestinal tract. What is the name of this condition? (duodenitis, enterostasis, peptic ulcer, peristalsis)

12. Which of the following is an instrument designed for passage into the stomach to permit examination of its interior? (gastric lavage, gastroscope, gastrotome, gastrorrhaphy)

13. Which of the following is the main source of energy for body cells? (fats, glucose, lactose, starches)

14. Which of the following is a disorder characterized by episodes of binge eating that are terminated by abdominal pain, sleep, self-induced vomiting, or purging with laxatives? (anorexia nervosa, bulimia, Crohn's disease, malabsorption syndrome)

15. Which of the following is the name of the procedure in which the stomach is anastomosed with the small intestine? (gastrectasis, gastrectomy, gastroenterostomy, gastropexy)

Writing Terms

VIII. *Write a term for each of the following.*

1. absence of thirst _____

2. any disease of the stomach _____

3. enzyme that breaks down starch _____

4. excessive vomiting _____

5. excision of the gallbladder _____

6. incision of the vagus nerve _____

7. inflammation of the stomach _____

8. pertaining to the throat _____

9. poor digestion _____

10. visual inspection of the duodenum _____

■ Greater Comprehension

Health Care Report

IX. Read this operative report and answer the questions that follow it. Although you may be unfamiliar with some of the terms, you should be able to decide their meaning by determining the word parts.

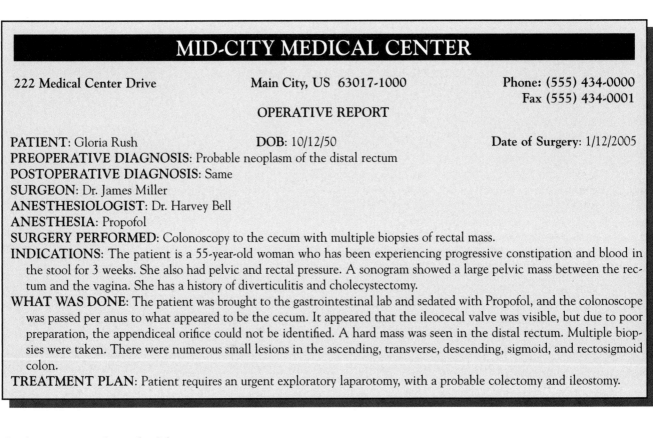

MID-CITY MEDICAL CENTER

222 Medical Center Drive   Main City, US 63017-1000   Phone: (555) 434-0000
                                                                      Fax (555) 434-0001

OPERATIVE REPORT

PATIENT: Gloria Rush   **DOB**: 10/12/50   **Date of Surgery**: 1/12/2005

PREOPERATIVE DIAGNOSIS: Probable neoplasm of the distal rectum

POSTOPERATIVE DIAGNOSIS: Same

SURGEON: Dr. James Miller

ANESTHESIOLOGIST: Dr. Harvey Bell

ANESTHESIA: Propofol

SURGERY PERFORMED: Colonoscopy to the cecum with multiple biopsies of rectal mass.

INDICATIONS: The patient is a 55-year-old woman who has been experiencing progressive constipation and blood in the stool for 3 weeks. She also had pelvic and rectal pressure. A sonogram showed a large pelvic mass between the rectum and the vagina. She has a history of diverticulitis and cholecystectomy.

WHAT WAS DONE: The patient was brought to the gastrointestinal lab and sedated with Propofol, and the colonoscope was passed per anus to what appeared to be the cecum. It appeared that the ileocecal valve was visible, but due to poor preparation, the appendiceal orifice could not be identified. A hard mass was seen in the distal rectum. Multiple biopsies were taken. There were numerous small lesions in the ascending, transverse, descending, sigmoid, and rectosigmoid colon.

TREATMENT PLAN: Patient requires an urgent exploratory laparotomy, with a probable colectomy and ileostomy.

Circle one answer for each of these questions.

1. To which body structure does the diagnosis pertain? (gallbladder, large intestine, small intestine, stomach)

2. Which of the following describes the rectum in the preoperative diagnosis? (abnormal new growth, enlarged, inflamed, impacted with feces).

3. The patient has a history of cholecystectomy. Which organ is removed in a cholecystectomy? (colon, gallbladder, liver, small intestine)

4. What structure is incised in a laparotomy? (abdominal wall, cecum, ileum, umbilicus)

5. All or part of which structure is excised in a colectomy? (large intestine, small intestine, stomach, umbilicus)

6. Where is the stoma created in an ileostomy? (abdomen, anus, colon, umbilicus)

Write T for True or F for False for each of these statements.

7. The procedure involved a visible inspection of the large intestine. ___

8. The procedure involved excising tissue from a hard mass that was seen. ___

9. The history indicates that the patient had experienced upper gastrointestinal bleeding. ___

10. The patient has a history of diverticula with accompanying inflammation. ___

11. The surgeon identified the opening to the appendix. ___

12. The surgeon examined most of the small intestine. ___

X. Read this consultation report and answer the questions that follow it. Although you may be unfamiliar with some of the terms, you should be able to decide their meanings by determining the word parts.

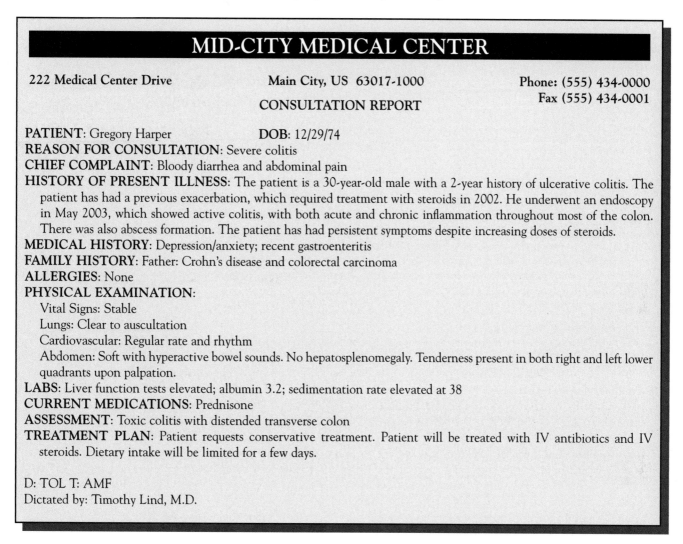

MID-CITY MEDICAL CENTER

222 Medical Center Drive   Main City, US 63017-1000   Phone: (555) 434-0000
                                   CONSULTATION REPORT   Fax (555) 434-0001

PATIENT: Gregory Harper   **DOB:** 12/29/74
REASON FOR CONSULTATION: Severe colitis
CHIEF COMPLAINT: Bloody diarrhea and abdominal pain
HISTORY OF PRESENT ILLNESS: The patient is a 30-year-old male with a 2-year history of ulcerative colitis. The patient has had a previous exacerbation, which required treatment with steroids in 2002. He underwent an endoscopy in May 2003, which showed active colitis, with both acute and chronic inflammation throughout most of the colon. There was also abscess formation. The patient has had persistent symptoms despite increasing doses of steroids.
MEDICAL HISTORY: Depression/anxiety; recent gastroenteritis
FAMILY HISTORY: Father: Crohn's disease and colorectal carcinoma
ALLERGIES: None
PHYSICAL EXAMINATION:
    Vital Signs: Stable
    Lungs: Clear to auscultation
    Cardiovascular: Regular rate and rhythm
    Abdomen: Soft with hyperactive bowel sounds. No hepatosplenomegaly. Tenderness present in both right and left lower quadrants upon palpation.
LABS: Liver function tests elevated; albumin 3.2; sedimentation rate elevated at 38
CURRENT MEDICATIONS: Prednisone
ASSESSMENT: Toxic colitis with distended transverse colon
TREATMENT PLAN: Patient requests conservative treatment. Patient will be treated with IV antibiotics and IV steroids. Dietary intake will be limited for a few days.

D: TOL T: AMF
Dictated by: Timothy Lind, M.D.

Circle the correct answer in the following questions.

1. Which structure is the focus of the consultation? (gallbladder, large intestine, liver, small intestine)

2. Which adjective describes the patient's ulcerative colitis? (acute, cancerous, chronic, noninflammatory)

3. To which category does the term *endoscopy* belong? (anatomy, diagnostic procedure, radiology, therapy)

4. Which of the following terms is associated with the presence of an abscess? (anorexia, emesis, malaise, pus)

5. Which of the following is not included in the family history? (cancer of the lower GI tract, colonic obstruction, Crohn's disease, inflammatory bowel disease)

Define the following terms.

6. colorectal carcinoma: _____

7. diarrhea: _____

8. gastroenteritis: _____

9. hepatosplenomegaly: _____

10. transverse colon: _____

Spelling
XI. *Circle all incorrectly spelled terms and write their correct spelling.*

emaciation   enteral   glossorhaphy   nasogastrik   varices

Interpreting Abbreviations
XII. *Write the meaning of these abbreviations.*

1. BMI _____

2. GI _____

3. HBV _____

4. HSV _____

5. TPN _____

Pronunciation
XIII. *The pronunciation is shown for several medical words. Indicate which syllable has the primary accent by marking it with an ʹ.*

1. cholecystogastric (ko lə sis to gas trik)

2. choledochal (ko led ə kəl)

3. dysentery (dis ən ter e)

4. fistula (fis tu lə)

5. hemorrhoidectomy (hem ə roid ek tə me)

Categorizing Terms
XIV. *Classify the terms in the left column (1-10) by selecting A, B, C, D, or E.*

_____ 1. achalasia

_____ 2. antiemetics

_____ 3. cholecystogram

_____ 4. choledochal

_____ 5. diverticulosis

_____ 6. esophagogram

_____ 7. esophagoduodenostomy

_____ 8. gingivoglossitis

_____ 9. jaundice

_____ 10. sialolithiasis

A. anatomy
B. diagnostic test or procedure
C. pathology
D. surgery
E. therapy

LISTING OF MEDICAL TERMS

Use the practice CD to review the terms that have been presented. Look closely at the spelling of each term as it is pronounced and be sure you know the meaning of each term.

absorbable suture	cheiloplasty	diverticulectomy	exogenous
absorption	cheilorrhaphy	diverticulitis	extracorporeal shock wave
achalasia	cheilosis	diverticulosis	lithotripsy
adhesion	cheilostomatoplasty	diverticulum	extrahepatic
adipsia	cholangitis	duodenal	feces
alimentary tract	cholecystectomy	duodenitis	fissure
alimentation	cholecystic	duodenoscope	fistula
amylase	cholecystitis	duodenoscopy	flatulence
amylolysis	cholecystogastric	duodenostomy	flatus
anal	cholecystography	duodenotomy	fluoroscope
anastomose	cholecystotomy	duodenum	fluoroscopy
anastomosis	choledochal	dysentery	fundus
anorexia nervosa	choledochitis	dyspepsia	gastralgia
anorexiant	choledochojejunostomy	dysphagia	gastrectasis
antacid	choledocholithiasis	E. coli infection	gastrectomy
antidiarrheal	choledocholithotripsy	elimination	gastric
antiemetic	choledochostomy	emaciation	gastric bypass
anus	cholelithiasis	emesis	gastric carcinoma
aphagia	cholestasis	enamel	gastric lavage
appendectomy	chyme	endodontics	gastritis
appendicitis	cirrhosis	endodontist	gastroduodenal
appendicular	cleft lip	endodontitis	anastomosis
approximate	cleft palate	endodontium	gastroduodenitis
approximation	colectomy	endogastric	gastroduodenostomy
ascending colon	colic	endogenous	gastroenteritis
ascites	colitis	endoscope	gastroenterology
atresia	colon	endoscopic	gastroenterostomy
auscultation	colonic	sphincterotomy	gastroesophageal reflux
barium enema	colonic irrigation	endoscopy	disease
barium meal	colonic polyps	enema	gastrointestinal
barium swallow	colonic stasis	enteral	gastrojejunal anastomosis
bile	colonoscope	enteral feeding	gastrojejunostomy
biliary	colonoscopy	enteric	gastromalacia
bilirubin	colorectal	enteritis	gastromegaly
bolus	coloscopy	enterostasis	gastropathy
buccal cavity	colostomy	eructation	gastropexy
buccal mucosa	constipation	esophageal	gastrorrhaphy
bulimia	Crohn's disease	esophagoduodenostomy	gastroscope
calorie	cuspid	esophagodynia	gastroscopy
Candida albicans	defecation	esophagogastroduodeno-	gerodontics
candidiasis	dehydration	scopy	gerodontist
canker sores	dental	esophagogastroplasty	gingiva
carbohydrates	dental caries	esophagogastroscopy	gingival
cardiac region	dentalgia	esophagogastrostomy	gingivalgia
cardiac sphincter	dentilingual	esophagogram	gingivectomy
caries	denture	esophagojejunostomy	gingivitis
cathartic	descending colon	esophagomalacia	gingivoglossitis
cecoileostomy	diabetes mellitus	esophagoscopy	gingivostomatitis
cecum	diarrhea	esophagram	glossal
celiac disease	digestion	esophagus	glossectomy
cheilitis	disease	eupepsia	glossitis

glossopathy
glossoplasty
glossoplegia
glossopyrosis
glossorrhaphy
glucagon
glucose
glucose-lowering agent
guaiac test
halitosis
hematemesis
hemorrhoid
hemorrhoidectomy
hepatectomy
hepatic
hepatic lobectomy
hepatitis
hepatolytic
hepatoma
hepatomegaly
hepatopathy
hepatorenal syndrome
hepatosplenomegaly
hepatotomy
hepatotoxic
hernia
herpes simplex virus
hiatal hernia
homeostasis
hyperacidity
hyperalimentation
hyperemesis
hyperglycemia
hypoglossal
hypoglycemia
ileac
ileal
ileal stoma
ileitis
ileocecal valve
ileostomy
ileum
impaction
incisor
inflammatory bowel
   disease
influenza
ingestion
inguinal hernia
insulin
interdental
intestinal

intussusception
irritable bowel syndrome
islets of Langerhans
jaundice
jejunal
jejunoileostomy
jejunotomy
jejunum
lactase
lactose
lactose intolerance
laparocholecystotomy
laparoenterostomy
laparoscopic
   cholecystectomy
lavage
laxative
leukoplakia
ligation
lingual
lipase
lipectomy
lipid
lipoid
lipopenia
liposuction
lithiasis
lithotripsy
lithotriptor
malabsorption syndrome
malaise
malnutrition
malocclusion
mandible
mandibular
maxilla
maxillary
mesenteric occlusion
metabolism
molar
mucoid
mucosa
mucous
mucous colitis
mucus
nasogastric
nasogastric tube
neoplasm
neoplastic
nonabsorbable suture
nutrition
obesity

occult blood
oropharyngeal
orthodontics
orthodontist
palatine
palpation
pancreatectomy
pancreatic
pancreatitis
pancreatography
pancreatolith
pancreatolithectomy
pancreatolysis
pancreatotomy
parenteral
parietal peritoneum
parotid
parotid gland
parotitis
pedodontics
pedodontist
peptic ulcer
percussion
pericolic
periodontal
periodontics
periodontist
periodontitis
periodontium
peristalsis
peritoneum
peritonitis
pharyngeal
pharynx
polydipsia
polypectomy
polyphagia
postesophageal
precancerous
premalignant
proctologist
proctoplasty
proctosigmoidoscopy
protease
proteinase
proteolysis
purgative
purging
pyloric region
pyloric sphincter
pyloric stenosis
pyloromyotomy

pyloroplasty
pyloroscopy
pylorotomy
pylorus
pyorrhea
rectal
rectum
regurgitation
retrocecal
retrocolic
rugae
saliva
salivary gland
salmonellosis
serosa
sialadenitis
sialography
sialolith
sialolithiasis
sigmoid colon
sigmoidoscope
sigmoidoscopy
spastic colon
sphincter
stoma
stomatitis
stomatodynia
stomatomycosis
strangulated hernia
stricture
sublingual
sublingual gland
submaxillary gland
suprahepatic
temporomandibular joint
topical anesthetic
total parenteral nutrition
transverse colon
ulcer
ulceration
ulcerative colitis
vagotomy
vagus nerve
varices
vermiform appendix
vertical banded
   gastroplasty
villi
viral hepatitis
visceral peritoneum
volvulus

español ENHANCING SPANISH COMMUNICATION

ENGLISH	SPANISH (PRONUNCIATION)
appetite	apetito (ah-pay-TEE-to)
belch	eructo (ay-ROOK-to)
chew, to	masticar (mas-te-CAR)
constipation	estreñimiento (es-tray-nye-me-EN-to)
defecate	evacuar (ay-vah-coo-AR)
diabetes	diabetes (de-ah-BAY-tes)
digestion	digestión (de-hes-te-ON)
enzyme	enzima (en-SEE-mah)
esophagus	esófago (ay-SO-fah-go)
excretion	excreción (ex-cray-se-ON)
feces	excremento (ex-cray-MEN-to)
gallbladder	vesícula biliar (vay-SEE-coo-la be-le-AR)
gallstone	cálculo biliar (CAHL-coo-lo be-le-AR)
glucose	glucosa (gloo-CO-sah)
gum, gingiva	encía (en-SEE-ah)
hunger	hambre (AHM-bray)
insulin	insulina (in-soo-LEE-nah)
laxative	purgante (poor-GAHN-tay)
lips	labios (LAH-be-os)
milk	leche (LAY-chay)
pancreas	páncreas (PAHN-cray-as)
rectum	recto (REK-to)
saliva	saliva (sah-LEE-vah)
starch	almidón (al-me-DON)
swallow	tragar (trah-GAR)
teeth	dientes (de-AYN-tays)
thirst	sed (sayd)

CHAPTER 11

Urinary System

FUNCTION FIRST

The urinary system plays an important role in maintaining homeostasis by constantly filtering the blood to remove urea and other waste products, maintaining the proper balance of water, salts, and other substances by removing or reabsorbing them as needed, and excreting the waste products via the urine. Other, less known roles are production of renin, erythropoietin, and prostaglandins, as well as degrading insulin and metabolizing vitamin D to its active form.

ANATOMY AND PHYSIOLOGY

11-1 There are several excretory routes through which the body eliminates wastes. The lungs eliminate carbon dioxide. The digestive system provides a means of expelling solid wastes. The skin serves as an excretory (eks′krə-tor-e) organ by eliminating wastes in the form of perspiration. Another important mode of excretion is performed by the kidneys, which are part of the urinary system.

The combining form *urin(o)* means urine. *Urin/ary* (u′rĭ-nar″e) means pertaining to _____. The organs and ducts that are involved in the secretion and elimination of urine from the body are referred to as the urinary tract.

urine

■ Anatomy of Major Urinary Structures

11-2 You learned in an earlier chapter that *ur(o)* means urinary system or urine. In terms that use the combining form *ur(o)*, you will need to decide which meaning is intended.

The urinary system consists of paired kidneys, one on each side of the spinal column, a ureter **(u-re′tər)** for each kidney, a bladder, and a urethra **(u-re′thrə)**. Although the terms *ureter* and *urethra* sound similar, notice the difference in their spellings. The body has two kidneys, two ureters, one bladder, and only one _____.

urethra

11-3 Figure 11-1 shows the location of these structures in the body. Read all the information that accompanies Figure 11-1. Complete the blank lines 1 through 4 by reading the following information.

Urine is formed in the kidneys. Label the left kidney (1). The ureters carry the urine to the urinary bladder. Label the left ureter (2). The bladder (3) is a temporary reservoir for the urine until it is excreted via the urethra (4).

The information that accompanies Figure 11-1 explains that blood is transported to the kidneys by vessels of the cardio/vascular (*cardi[o]*, heart + *vascul[o]*, vessel + *-ar*, pertaining to) system. These vessels that carry blood to the kidneys are renal _____.

arteries

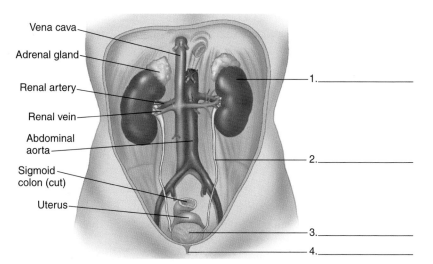

Figure 11-1 The urinary system. Adjacent vessels of the cardiovascular system are also shown. The right and left renal arteries branch off the abdominal aorta to transport blood to the kidneys. Urine, formed in the kidneys, leaves by way of the ureters and passes to the bladder, where it is stored. When voluntary control is removed, urine is expelled through the urethra. When blood is filtered, wastes are removed, but much of the water and other substances are reabsorbed. They enter the renal vein and are returned to the bloodstream via the inferior vena cava.

Learn the following word parts for major structures of the urinary system.

Word Parts Pertaining to Urinary Structures

WORD PART	MEANING
ur(o)	urine, urinary tract
-uria	urine or urination

Major Urinary Structures

WORD PART	MEANING
cyst(o)	bladder (also cyst or fluid-filled sac)
ureter(o)	ureter
urethr(o)	urethra
vesic(o)	bladder or blister

Internal Structures of the Kidneys

WORD PART	MEANING
glomerul(o)	glomerulus
pyel(o)	renal pelvis

Other

WORD PART	MEANING
gon(o)	genitals or reproduction
thromb(o)	thrombus (internal blood clot)

11-4 Most of the work of the urinary system takes place in the kidneys. The average adult kidney is about 11 cm long by 6 cm wide (about 4 1/2 by 2 1/3 inches) and weighs about 145 grams (less than half a pound). Although the kidneys are best known for their life-maintaining function of filtering the blood and regulating the volume and composition of blood plasma, they also produce renin (assists regulation of blood pressure), erythro/poietin (ə-rith″ro-poi′ə-tin) (erythrocyte production), and prostaglandins (pros″tə-glan′dinz) (fatty acid derivatives that have effects on many organs). They are also involved in degrading insulin and metabolizing vitamin D.

red

Erythr(o) means _____, and *-poietin* means that which causes production. Erythropoietin is a substance that causes the production of red blood cells.

11-5 *Ren/al* (re′nəl) means pertaining to the kidney. Use *supra-* to write a term that means above a kidney: _____.

suprarenal

(soo″prə-re′nəl)

Inter/renal (in″tər-re′nəl) means between the kidneys.

11-6 Urine leaves the kidney by way of the right and left ureters, which take it to the bladder. *Ureter/al* (u-re′tər-əl) means pertaining to a ureter. A ureteral dysfunction is a disturbance of the

ureters

normal flow of urine through one or both _____.

11-7 The combining form *cyst(o)* means cyst, bladder, or fluid-filled sac. The term *cystic* (sis′tik)

bladder

pertains to a *cyst*, the gallbladder, or the urinary _____. *Extra/cystic* (eks″trə-sis′tik) means outside a cyst or outside the bladder.

Vesic/al (ves′ĭ-kəl) means pertaining to a fluid-filled sac, usually the urinary bladder. *Vesico/ureter/al* (ves″ĭ-ko-u-re′ter-əl) means pertaining to the urinary bladder and a

ureter

_____. *Vesico/vaginal* (ves″ĭ-ko-vag′ĭ-nəl) means pertaining to the urinary bladder and the vagina.

11-8 Urine leaves the bladder by way of the urethra and is expelled from the body. *Urethr/al*

urethra

(u-re′thrəl) means pertaining to the _____.

The urethra is about 3 cm long in women and lies anterior to the vagina. In men the urethra is about 20 cm long and serves as a passageway for semen and as a canal for urine.

11-9 Anatomic features of the kidney are shown in Figure 11-2. The kidney is encased in a fibrous (*fibr[o]*, fiber + *-ous*, characterized by) (fi′brəs) capsule. *Fibrous* means consisting mainly of fibers. The fibrous capsule provides protection for the delicate internal parts of the kidney. The ribs and muscle also provide protection from direct trauma.

The notch or depression on the inner border of the kidney where the renal artery, renal vein, lymphatics, and nerves enter or leave the kidney is called the hilum (hi′ləm).

The renal pelvis is a funnel-shaped structure located in the center of each kidney. The combin-

pyel(o)

ing form for renal pelvis is _____.

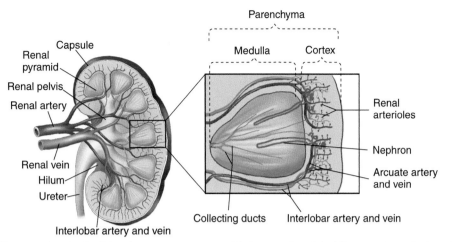

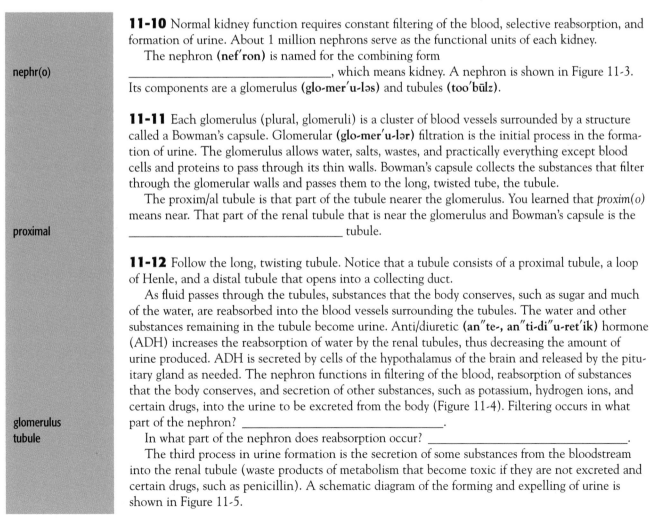

Figure 11-2   The kidney (sectioned). The kidney has a convex contour with the exception of the hilus, a notch on the inner border. A longitudinal section shows two distinct regions: the outer cortex and the inner medulla. The medulla has 10 to 15 triangular wedges called renal pyramids, made up of collecting ducts, lymphatics, and blood vessels. Cortical and medullary regions of each kidney contain approximately 1 million nephrons, the functioning units. A normal person can survive, although with difficulty, with less than 20,000 functioning nephrons.

■ *Formation and Excretion of Urine*

11-10 Normal kidney function requires constant filtering of the blood, selective reabsorption, and formation of urine. About 1 million nephrons serve as the functional units of each kidney.

nephr(o)

The nephron (**nef′ron**) is named for the combining form _____, which means kidney. A nephron is shown in Figure 11-3. Its components are a glomerulus (**glo-mer′u-ləs**) and tubules (**too′bŭlz**).

11-11 Each glomerulus (plural, glomeruli) is a cluster of blood vessels surrounded by a structure called a Bowman's capsule. Glomerular (**glo-mer′u-lər**) filtration is the initial process in the formation of urine. The glomerulus allows water, salts, wastes, and practically everything except blood cells and proteins to pass through its thin walls. Bowman's capsule collects the substances that filter through the glomerular walls and passes them to the long, twisted tube, the tubule.

proximal

The proxim/al tubule is that part of the tubule nearer the glomerulus. You learned that *proxim(o)* means near. That part of the renal tubule that is near the glomerulus and Bowman's capsule is the _____ tubule.

11-12 Follow the long, twisting tubule. Notice that a tubule consists of a proximal tubule, a loop of Henle, and a distal tubule that opens into a collecting duct.

As fluid passes through the tubules, substances that the body conserves, such as sugar and much of the water, are reabsorbed into the blood vessels surrounding the tubules. The water and other substances remaining in the tubule become urine. Anti/diuretic (**an″te-, an″ti-di″u-ret′ik**) hormone (ADH) increases the reabsorption of water by the renal tubules, thus decreasing the amount of urine produced. ADH is secreted by cells of the hypothalamus of the brain and released by the pituitary gland as needed. The nephron functions in filtering of the blood, reabsorption of substances that the body conserves, and secretion of other substances, such as potassium, hydrogen ions, and certain drugs, into the urine to be excreted from the body (Figure 11-4). Filtering occurs in what

glomerulus
tubule

part of the nephron? _____.

In what part of the nephron does reabsorption occur? _____.

The third process in urine formation is the secretion of some substances from the bloodstream into the renal tubule (waste products of metabolism that become toxic if they are not excreted and certain drugs, such as penicillin). A schematic diagram of the forming and expelling of urine is shown in Figure 11-5.

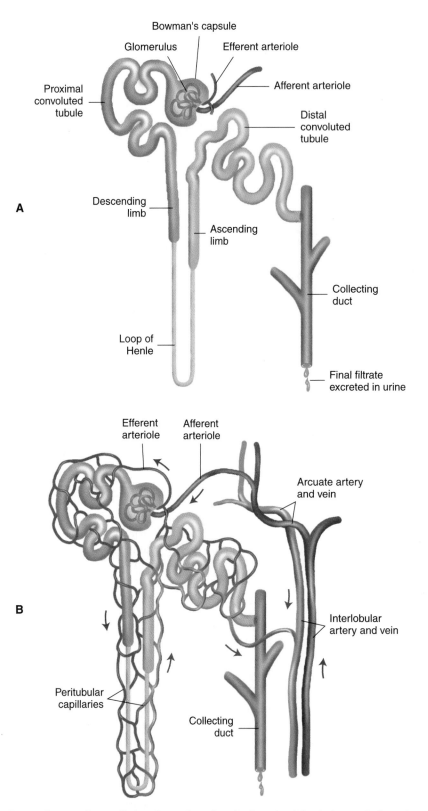

Figure 11-3 **A,** A nephron and surrounding capillaries. The renal arteries arise from the abdominal aorta. Each renal artery branches as it enters the hilum and after branching several times gives rise to the afferent arteriole. This terminates in capillary tufts called a glomerulus. Blood leaves the glomerulus through the efferent arteriole, which subdivides into peritubular capillaries. As the glomerular filtrate flows through the tubules, most of its water and varying amounts of solutes are reabsorbed into the peritubular capillaries. These capillaries join others and become the arcuate vein and eventually the renal vein, whereby blood leaves the kidney. **B,** As the filtrate passes through the tubular portion of the nephron, variable quantities of water, electrolytes, and other substances are reabsorbed into the body. Reabsorption occurs across the tubule walls into blood capillaries nearby (peritubular capillaries are shown).

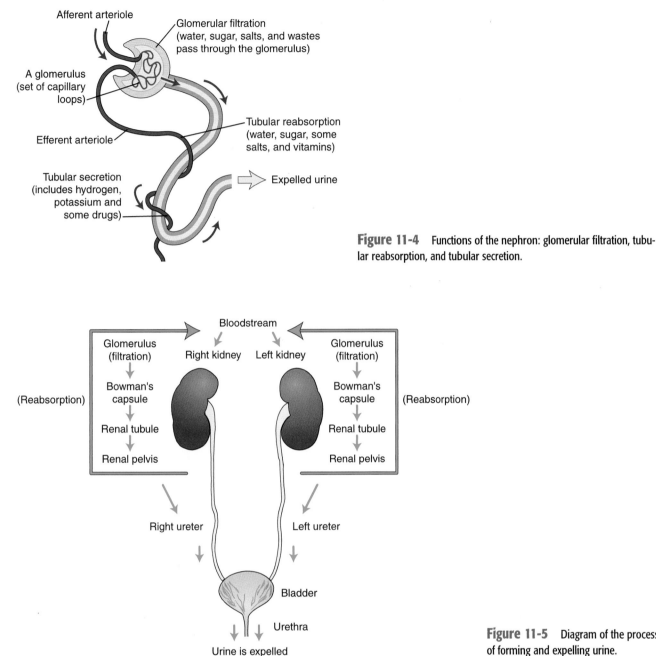

Figure 11-4   Functions of the nephron: glomerular filtration, tubular reabsorption, and tubular secretion.

Figure 11-5   Diagram of the process of forming and expelling urine.

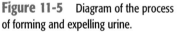

ureter

11-13 Waste products and some of the water remaining in the tubules after reabsorption combine to become urine, which passes to the collecting duct. Thousands of collecting ducts deposit urine in the renal pelvis, the large central reservoir of the kidney.

After urine collects in the renal pelvis, it drains to the bladder by passing through a tube called the _____.

The urinary bladder is a collapsible muscular bag that serves as a reservoir for urine until it is expelled. It has a storage capacity in health of about 500 ml (1 pint) or more. *Micturition* (**mik″tu-rĭ-′shən**), or *voiding*, means urination, expelling urine from the bladder.

11-14 The glomerular filtration rate (GFR) is a calculated volume of fluid filtered by the glomeruli. GFR decreases with advancing age, and the decline in the filtration rate is more rapid in persons with diabetes or hypertension (elevated blood pressure). GFR forms the basis of a test for how well the kidneys are functioning.

glomerular

This calculated volume of fluid filtered by the glomeruli is called _____ filtration rate.

bladder

11-15 Decide which meaning of cystic is implied in the term *abdomino/cystic* (**ab-dom″ĭ-no-sis′tik**), which means pertaining to the abdomen and the urinary _____. This term means the same as abdomino/vesical (**ab′dom″i-no-ves′ĭ-kəl**).

Filling of the bladder with urine stimulates receptors, producing the desire to urinate. Voluntary control prevents urine from being released. When the control is removed, urine is expelled through the urethra. The opening to the outside from the urethra is called the urinary meatus (**me-a′təs**).

urethra

11-16 *Recto/urethr/al* (**rek″to-u-re′thrəl**) pertains to the rectum and the _____. *Urethro/rect/al* (**u-re″thro-rek′təl**) also means pertaining to the urethra and rectum; however, not all words can be reversed like this!

Urethro/vaginal (**u-re″thro-vaj′ĭ-nəl**) means pertaining to the urethra and the vagina. *Genito/urinary* (**jen″ĭ-to-u′rĭ-nar-e**) (GU) or *uro/genital* (**u″ro-jen′ĭ-təl**) pertains to the genitals, as well as to the urinary organs.

Exercise 1

Write the names of the structures to complete these sentences.

1. The cavity in the kidney that collects urine from many collecting ducts is the renal _____.

2. A tube that carries urine to the bladder is a _____.

3. The tube that carries urine from the bladder is the _____.

4. The _____ is the functional unit of the kidney.

5. The _____ is the reservoir for urine until it is expelled.

6. The filtering structure of the kidney is the _____.

7. Reabsorption occurs in structures called the _____.

8. The external opening of the urethra is the urinary _____.

DIAGNOSTIC TESTS AND PROCEDURES

palpation

11-17 Physical assessment of the kidneys, ureters, and bladder (KUB) includes abdominal inspection, auscultation, palpation, and percussion (see Figure 6-13). Which of these procedures makes use of the examiner's hands to assess the texture, size, consistency, and location of the kidneys and bladder? _____. Laboratory tests, biopsies, radiography, and endoscopy (**en-dos′kə-pe**) are helpful in diagnostic assessment of the urinary system.

■ Laboratory Tests

urinalysis

11-18 Several urine tests are used to evaluate the status of the urinary system. A urinalysis (**u″rĭ-nal′ĭ-sis**) is usually part of a physical examination but is particularly useful for patients with suspected urologic disorders. The urin/alysis is an examination of urine. Urin/alysis was originally called urine analysis. It is often abbreviated UA or U/A. Examination of the urine is called

_____.

The complete urinalysis generally includes a physical, chemical, and microscopic examination performed in the clinical laboratory.

11-19 The urine specimen is physically examined for color, turbidity, and specific gravity. Ideally, the urine is collected at the first morning's voiding. Freshly voided urine is normally clear and straw-colored. Changes in the color of urine may indicate dilute or concentrated urine. Dark red or brown urine may indicate blood in the urine, and other color changes may result from diet or medications. In a urinalysis, the specific gravity is the density of urine compared with the density of water. The specific gravity of water is 1.0, and urine is normally 1.010 to 1.025. Dilute urine has a low specific gravity, and concentrated urine has a high specific gravity.

Specific gravity can be measured by various means, including the use of a chemical dipstick or with a urino/meter (u″rĭ-nom′ə-tər), an instrument that measures the specific gravity of

urine

_____.

11-20 Chemical analysis of urine may be performed to measure the pH and to identify and measure the levels of ketones (ke′tōnz), sugar, protein, blood components, and many other substances. Urea (u-re′ə), ammonia, creatinine (kre-at′ĭ-nin), and salts are important waste products in urine. Urea is a nitrogen compound that is the final product of protein metabolism.

Several substances are not present in normal urine, and their presence indicates various pathologic states. Some abnormal components of urine are sugar, albumin, ketones, and blood. The presence of these substances can be detected in which part of the urinalysis, the physical, chemical, or

chemical

microscopic part? The _____ part. Learn the meaning of the following word parts.

Word Parts Pertaining to Urine

WORD PART	MEANING		Other	
urin(o)	urine		WORD PART	MEANING
			noct(i), nyct(o)	night
Abnormal Substances in Urine			olig(o)	few, scanty
WORD PART	MEANING			
albumin(o)	albumin			
glyc(o), glycos(o)	sugar			
ket(o), keton(o)	ketone bodies			
prote(o), protein(o)	protein			

11-21 Sugar in the urine is glycos/uria (gli″ko-su′re-ə). The combining forms *glyc(o)* and *glycos(o)* mean sweet or sugar, and you'll need to remember that *glycos(o)* is combined with *-uria*. Sugar should not be detected in the chemical testing of urine, because glucose is generally reabsorbed in the renal tubules. When the blood glucose rises above a certain level, the renal threshold for reabsorption is exceeded and glucose is excreted in the urine. Glycosuria may indicate diabetes and

sugar

requires further testing. *Glycosuria* means _____ in the urine.

blood

11-22 *Hemat/uria* (he″mə-, hem″ə-tu′re-ə) means _____ in the urine. Blood should not be present in the urine, so hematuria is considered an abnormal condition. (Of course, urine can be contaminated by menstrual blood in voided urine of women.)

protein

11-23 *Protein/uria* (pro″te-nu′re-ə) is _____ in the urine, usually albumin. *Albumin/uria* (al″bu-mĭ-nu′re-ə) is albumin in the urine.

Ketone bodies are end products of lipid (fat) metabolism in the body. Excessive production of ketone bodies, however, leads to urinary excretion of ketones. Under normal conditions, ketones are not present in urine. *Keton/uria* (ke″to-nu′re-ə) is the presence of ketones in the

urine

_____.

Ketone bodies are acids, and ketones are found in the urine when the body's fat stores are metabolized for energy, thus providing an excess of metabolic end products. This can occur in uncontrolled diabetes mellitus because of a deficiency of insulin. *Keto/acid/osis* (ke″to-as″ĭ-do′sis) means acidosis accompanied by an accumulation of ketones in the body and results from faulty carbohydrate metabolism. It occurs primarily as a complication of diabetes mellitus. Write this term that means acidosis

ketoacidosis

accompanied by an accumulation of ketones: _____.

11-24 A microscopic study is generally part of a complete urinalysis. Body cells, crystals, and bacteria are some of the particles present in a microscopic study (Figure 11-6). These are generally

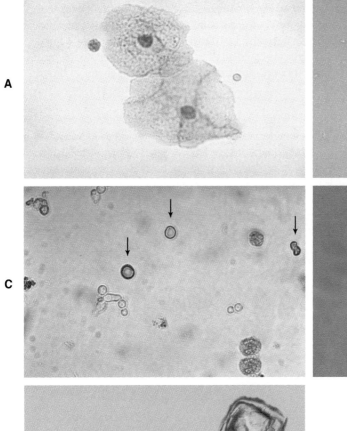

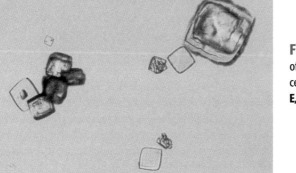

Figure 11-6 Structures seen in a microscopic examination of urine. **A**, Squamous epithelial cells; **B**, waxy cast; **C**, red blood cells (arrows); **D**, white blood cells (the nucleated cells shown); **E**, uric acid crystals.

high

urine

reported as number/high power field (HPF). *HPF* means a microscopic _____ power field.

    Very few white cells are normally present in urine. The presence of a large number of white blood cells may be indicative of an infectious or inflammatory process somewhere in the urinary tract. For example, there is usually a large number of white blood cells/HPF in most urinary tract infections.

    Pus cells, necrotic white blood cells, are a major component of pus. For this reason, *py/uria* (pi-u′re-ə) means the presence of an excessive number of white blood cells in the _____.

11-25 Only a few red blood cells are normally present in urine. If several red blood cells/HPF are present, it may indicate a variety of abnormalities, including a tumor, urinary stones, infection, or a bleeding disorder.

    Urinary casts are gelatinous structures that take the shape of the renal tubules. Casts are described by the type of element in the structure (for example, WBC cast, RBC cast, granular cast, waxy cast).

kidney

There are usually few casts to none, so the presence of several casts in urine generally indicates renal disease or urinary calculi. *Renal disease* means disease of a _____.

11-26 There are normally very few bacteria in freshly collected urine. The presence of many bacteria may indicate a urinary tract infection. If the patient has symptoms of a urinary tract infection, a <u>urine culture</u> is used to determine the types of pathogenic bacteria present. When bacteria are present in significant numbers, another test (an <u>antibiotic sensitivity test</u>) is used to determine which antibiotics are effective against that particular pathogen.

culture

The two tests are often ordered together as culture and sensitivity testing. The cultivation of microorganisms in the laboratory on special culture medium is called a bacterial _____, and testing to determine which drugs are effective in killing or stopping the growth of the bacteria is a sensitivity test.

voids (or urinates)

11-27 Urine specimens are collected according to the laboratory or physician's instructions. A <u>voided specimen</u> is one in which the patient _____ into a container supplied by the laboratory or physician's office. Because improperly collected urine may yield incorrect test results, voided urine should always be collected using the <u>clean-catch midstream</u> technique. This technique is based on the concept that the tissues adjacent to the urethral meatus must be cleansed prior to collection to avoid contamination of the specimen, and only the middle portion of the urine stream is collected.

A <u>catheterized urine specimen</u> is obtained by placing a catheter* (**kath′ə-tər**) into the bladder and withdrawing urine. This may be necessary to obtain an uncontaminated urine specimen.

creatinine

11-28 Creatinine is a substance formed in normal metabolism and is commonly found in blood, urine, and muscle tissue. Creatinine is measured in blood and urine as an indicator of kidney function. A <u>serum creatinine test</u> is a measurement of the creatinine level in the blood. A creatinine clearance test is a diagnostic test that measures the rate at which creatinine is cleared from the blood by the kidney. This kidney function test is called a _____ clearance test, one example of a renal clearance test. <u>Renal clearance tests</u> determine the efficiency with which the kidneys excrete particular substances.

A <u>24-hour urine collection</u> is collection of all of the urine voided in a 24-hour period. This type of collection may be ordered to measure levels of various substances in the urine, such as calcium or creatinine.

11-29 In addition to blood creatinine levels, <u>blood urea nitrogen</u> (BUN) is directly related to the metabolic function of the liver and the excretory function of the kidney. BUN is a measure of the amount of urea in the blood. Urea forms in the liver as the end product of protein metabolism and is excreted by the kidneys in urine. A critically elevated BUN level indicates serious impairment of renal function.

urea

BUN, a blood test that measures the excretory function of the kidney, means blood _____ nitrogen.

■ *Urinary Catheterization*

catheter

11-30 In <u>urinary catheterization</u> (**kath″ə-tər-ĭ-za′shən**), a catheter is inserted through the urethra and into the bladder for temporary or permanent drainage of urine. Urinary catheterization may be done to collect a urine specimen, and for other reasons, including urinary testing, instillation of medications into the bladder, and drainage of the bladder during many types of surgeries or in cases of urinary obstruction or paralysis.

<u>Catheters</u> are hollow, flexible tubes that can be inserted into a vessel or cavity of the body. They vary in type and size, and the type that is used varies with the size of the individual and the purpose of catheterization (Figure 11-7). The hollow tube that is used in catheterization is a _____.

*Catheter (Greek: *katheter*, something lowered).

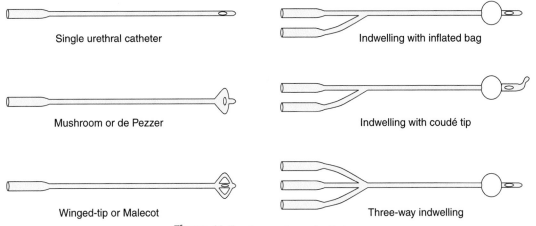

Single urethral catheter

Mushroom or de Pezzer

Winged-tip or Malecot

Indwelling with inflated bag

Indwelling with coudé tip

Three-way indwelling

Figure 11-7   Commonly used catheters.

11-31 Four methods are used for urinary tract catheterizations. They are urethral, ureteral, and suprapubic **(soo″prə-pu′bik)** and use of a nephrostomy **(nə-fros′tə-me)** tube. The four types of urinary catheterization are shown in Figure 11-8.

urethral

The most common means is insertion of the catheter through the external meatus into the urethra and then to the bladder. Insertion of the catheter through the urethra and into the bladder is _____ catheterization.

11-32 An indwelling catheter is designed to be left in place for a prolonged period. A Foley catheter is held securely in place by a balloon tip that is filled with a sterile liquid after the catheter has been placed in the bladder. This type of catheter is used when continuous drainage of the bladder is desired, such as in surgery, or when repeated urinary catheterization would be necessary if an indwelling catheter were not used.

Foley

An indwelling catheter that has a balloon tip and is left in place in the bladder is a _____ catheter.

Ureteral catheters are usually passed into the distal ends of the ureters from the bladder via a cystoscope and threaded up the ureters into the renal pelves (plural for pelvis). A ureteral catheter may also be surgically inserted through the abdominal wall into a ureter. Placement of catheters through the ureters into the renal pelves is _____ catheterization.

ureteral

Ureteral catheters may be placed temporarily as part of a diagnostic procedure called a retrograde urogram or pyelogram, which permits visualization of the renal collecting system in patients whose renal function is too limited for adequate visualization with intravenous urography.

11-33 If disease or obstruction does not allow urethral catheterization, a supra/pubic catheter can be placed into the bladder through a small incision or puncture of the abdominal wall about 1 inch above the symphysis pubis, the bony eminence that lies beneath the pubic hair. *Supra/pubic* means pertaining to a location _____ the symphysis pubis.

above

The fourth means of urinary catheterization is using a nephrostomy tube (catheter), which is inserted on a temporary basis into the renal pelvis when a complete obstruction of the ureter is present. This procedure is a per/cutaneous nephro/stomy, which means formation of a new opening into the renal pelvis through the overlying skin.

11-34 Urodynamic studies measure various aspects of the process of voiding and are used along with other procedures to evaluate problems with urine flow. Types of urodynamic studies include cystometrography, electromyography, and urethral pressure profile.

Cysto/metro/graphy (*cyst[o]*, bladder + *metr[o]*, to measure + *-graphy*, process of recording) **(sis″to-mə-trog′rə-fe)** provides information about the effectiveness of the bladder wall muscle. This procedure may incorporate the use of a urinary catheter with an attached cysto/meter (*-meter*, instrument for measuring) that measures bladder capacity in relation to changing urine pressure.

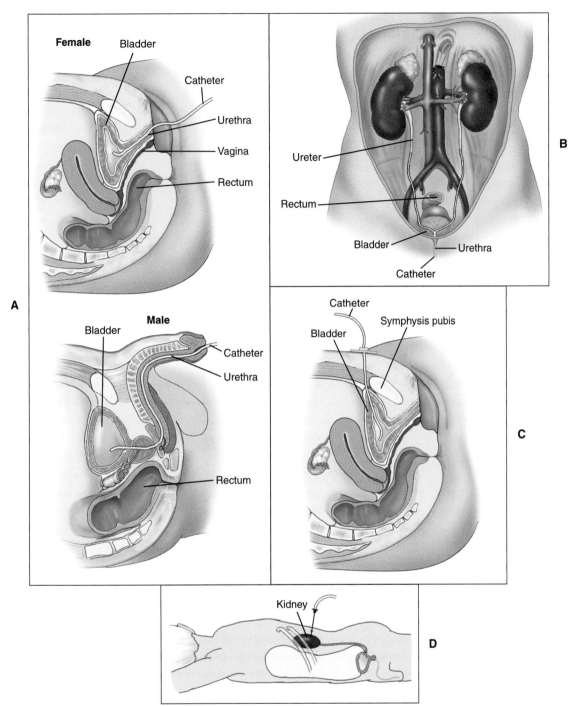

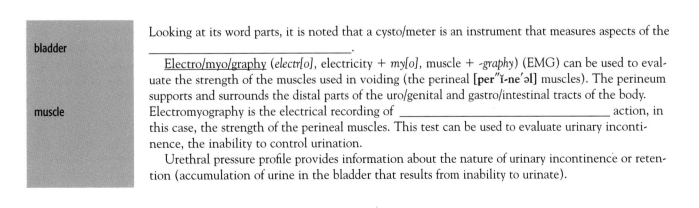

Figure 11-8 Urinary diversion. **A,** Urethral catheterization; **B,** ureteral catheterization; **C,** suprapubic catheterization; **D,** percutaneous nephrostomy.

bladder

Looking at its word parts, it is noted that a cysto/meter is an instrument that measures aspects of the

_____ .

Electro/myo/graphy (*electr[o]*, electricity + *my[o]*, muscle + *-graphy*) (EMG) can be used to evaluate the strength of the muscles used in voiding (the perineal [per″ĭ-ne′əl] muscles). The perineum supports and surrounds the distal parts of the uro/genital and gastro/intestinal tracts of the body.

muscle

Electromyography is the electrical recording of _____ action, in this case, the strength of the perineal muscles. This test can be used to evaluate urinary incontinence, the inability to control urination.

Urethral pressure profile provides information about the nature of urinary incontinence or retention (accumulation of urine in the bladder that results from inability to urinate).

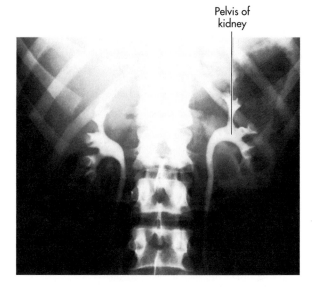

Pelvis of kidney

Figure 11-9   Intravenous pyelogram. Normal IVP. The x-ray film was taken as the contrast medium is cleared from the blood by the kidneys. The renal pelvis and ureters are clearly visible.

■ *Urinary Radiography*

11-35 A number of special radiologic procedures are used to diagnose abnormalities of the urinary system, and plain abdominal x-ray images are used to show obvious aspects of the kidneys, ureters, and bladder (KUB).

Intra/venous (**in″trə-ve′nəs**) uro/graphy (**u-rog′rə-fe**) is the making of x-ray images of the entire urinary system or part of it after the urine has been rendered opaque by a contrast medium that is injected intravenously. Various structural features can be seen on the resulting radiographs, as well as tumors or stones. Various functional abnormalities may also be diagnosed with this technique. The renal pelves and ureters are clearly visible in the normal pyelogram (**pi′ə-lo-gram**) shown in Figure 11-9.

Intravenous (IV) urography is also called intravenous pyelography (**pi″ə-log′rə-fe**), IVP, and the

pyelogram

resulting radiograph is called a _____.

11-36 Cysto/graphy (**sis-tog′rə-fe**) is radiography of the bladder, and urethrography (**u″rə-throg′rə-fe**) is radiography of the urethra after introduction of a radiopaque contrast medium. In cysto/urethro/graphy (**sis″to-u″rə-throg′rə-fe**), both the bladder and

urethra

_____ are studied. A urinary catheter is used to instill the contrast medium.

In a voiding cysto/urethro/gram (**sis″to-u-re′thro-gram**) (VCUG), radiographs are made before, during, and after voiding (urination). It allows observation of the bladder as it empties and checks for reflux of urine into the ureters.

11-37 Adequate blood circulation is essential for normal renal function. Anything that interferes with the normal circulation significantly reduces renal capabilities. Renal angio/graphy (renal arteriography) is a radiographic study to assess the arterial blood supply to the

kidneys

_____.

This procedure requires injection of a radiopaque contrast agent into the renal arteries via a catheter that is inserted into a major artery, usually a femoral artery, and threaded up the aorta under fluoroscopic control to the point where the renal arteries branch off from the aorta. A renal

arteriogram

_____ is the record of the arterial blood supply to the kidneys (Figure 11-10).

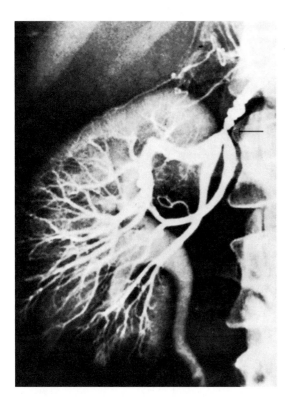

Figure 11-10 Renal arteriogram showing stenosis of the right renal artery.

kidney

11-38 A kidney scan also provides information about renal blood flow. In this procedure, radioactive material is intravenously injected and is absorbed by kidney tissue. Special equipment measures, records, and produces an image of the low-level radioactivity that is emitted.

Reno/graphy (re-nog′rə-fe) means the same as a kidney scan, because the literal translation of reno/graphy is the process of recording the _____.

11-39 _Nephro/sono/graphy_ (nef″ro-so-nog′rə-fe) is ultrasonic scanning of the kidney. Very large or very small kidneys, cysts, and kidney stones can be diagnosed using nephrosonography. _Nephro/tomo/graphy_ (nef″ro-to-mog′rə-fe) means tomography of the kidney. The film produced by nephrotomography is a _____.

nephrotomogram
(nef″ro-to′mo-gram)

■ _Endoscopy_

cystoscopy
(sis-tos′kə-pe)

11-40 Write a term for direct visual examination of the bladder: _____.
In this type of examination, a hollow metal tube is passed through the urethra and into the bladder. By means of a light, special lenses, and mirrors, the bladder mucosa is examined (Figure 11-11).

The instrument used in cystoscopy is a _cystoscope_ (sis′to-skōp). In addition to examining the interior of the bladder, cystoscopy is used to obtain biopsy specimens of tumors or other growths, to remove polyps (growths protruding from the lining of the bladder) or stones, and to pass catheters into the ureters.

11-41 Cystoscopy also generally involves _urethro/scopy_ (u″rə-thros′kə-pe), which is visualization of the urethra. This is referred to as _cysto/urethro/scopy_ (sis″to-u″re-thros′kə-pe).

Cysto/uretero/scopy (sis″to-u-re-tər-os′kə-pe) is slightly more involved than a cystoscopy, because cystoureteroscopy involves examination of the _____
and the bladder.

ureters

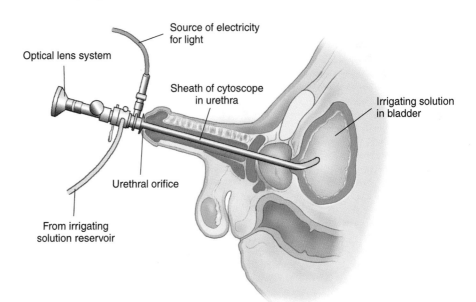

Source of electricity
for light

Optical lens system

Sheath of cytoscope
in urethra

Irrigating solution
in bladder

Urethral orifice

From irrigating
solution reservoir

Figure 11-11   A cystoscope in place
inside the male bladder.

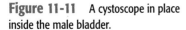
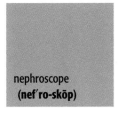

nephroscope
(nef′ro-skōp)

11-42 <u>Nephro/scopy</u> (**nə-fros′kə-pe**) allows visualization of the kidney using a fiberoptic instrument. A major use of this procedure is to remove or crush renal calculi. Nephroscopy requires the use of an instrument that is inserted through the skin into a small incision in the renal pelvis, allowing the urologist to view inside the kidney (Figure 11-12).

The instrument for nephroscopy is called a _____.

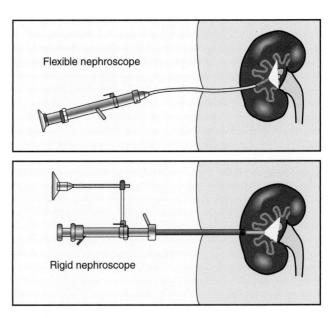

Flexible nephroscope

Rigid nephroscope

Figure 11-12   Two types of nephroscopes. The nephroscope, a fiberoptic instrument, is inserted percutaneously into the kidney. An ultrasonic probe emits high-frequency sound waves that break up calculi after they are located.

Exercise 2

Circle the correct answer for each of the following questions.

1. Which of the following is an examination of urine that is usually part of a routine physical examination? (BUN, creatinine clearance test, renal clearance test, urinalysis)
2. Which of the following is a normal component of urine? (ketone, protein, sugar, urea)
3. Which term means an excessive number of white blood cells in the urine? (albuminuria, ketoacidosis, pyuria, uremia)
4. Which term means sugar in the urine? (albuminuria, glycosuria, hematuria, ketonuria)
5. Which of the following is not a means of urinary tract catheterization? (cystometrography, ureteral, urethral, suprapubic)
6. Which of the following tests evaluates the strength of muscles used in voiding? (cystography, electromyography, intravenous urography, nephroscopy)
7. Which term means a kidney scan? (cystourethrogram, renography, nephroscopy, nephrostomy)
8. Which term means a radiographic procedure that produces layered images as if the kidney had been sliced in a plane? (intravenous urography, nephrosonography, nephrostomy, nephrotomography)

PATHOLOGIES

urinary

vessels

difficult

many

urination

oliguria

retention

11-43 A <u>uro/pathy</u> (**u-rop′ə-the**) is any disease or abnormal condition of the _____ tract. Uropathies include inflammatory, hereditary, obstructive, and renovascular disorders. In addition, some uropathies are the result of metabolic disease processes that affect renal function. <u>Reno/vascular disorders</u> are those affecting the blood _____ of the kidneys.

11-44 Discomfort during urination and unexplained change in the volume of urine are sometimes the earliest indications of a urinary problem. <u>Dys/uria</u> (**dis-u′re-ə**) is _____ or painful urination, and can be caused by a bacterial infection or an obstruction of the urinary tract.

   <u>Poly/uria</u> (**pol″e-u′re-ə**) is excretion of an abnormally large quantity of urine. Literal translation of polyuria is _____ urines or urinations. You will need to remember that *polyuria* means excretion of an abnormally large quantity of urine. This can be brought about by excessive intake of fluids or the use of medications. Two pathologies in which polyuria is common are diabetes insipidus and diabetes mellitus. Both are described later in this section.

11-45 Literal translation of <u>an/uria</u> (**an-u′re-ə**) is absence of _____. The full meaning of *anuria* is a urinary output of less than 100 ml per day. The patient who has less than 100 ml of urine output per day is described as anur/ic (**an-u′rik**).

   Compare *anuria* and <u>olig/uria</u> (**ol″ĭ-gu′re-ə**), which means diminished capacity to form urine, excreting less than 500 ml of urine per day. The combining form *olig(o)* means few or scanty. Write this term that means diminished urine production of less than 500 ml per day: _____ .

11-46 <u>Urgency</u>, <u>frequency</u>, and <u>hesitancy</u> are terms that are often used to describe urination patterns. Urgency is a sudden onset of the need to urinate immediately. Increased frequency is a greater number of urinations than expected in a given time. Hesitancy is difficulty in beginning the flow, often with a decrease in the force of the urine stream and with difficulty in starting the flow.

   <u>Retention</u> (**re-ten′shən**) means holding in place, or persistent keeping within the body of matter that is normally excreted. Incomplete emptying of the bladder is called urinary _____ . <u>Urinary reflux</u> is an abnormal backward or return flow of urine from the bladder into the ureters.

11-47 Continence* (kon′tĭ-nəns) is the ability to control bladder or bowel function. Urinary <u>incontinence</u> (in-kon′tĭ-nəns) is inability to control urination. This is loss of control of the passage of urine from the bladder. There are many causes of incontinence, such as loss of muscle tone, obesity, or unconsciousness. For the latter reason, indwelling catheters are used when patients are anesthetized.

    Enuresis (en″u-re′sis) also means the inability to control urination, and the term is applied especially to nocturnal bed-wetting. *Nocturnal* means pertaining to or occurring at night.

11-48 <u>Noct/uria</u> (nok-tu′re-ə), also called <u>nyct/uria</u> (nik-tu′re-ə), is excessive urination at night. Both *noct(i)* and *nyct(o)* mean night. Although nocturia may be a symptom of disease, it also can occur in people who drink excessive amounts of fluids before bedtime or when nearby structures put pressure on the bladder. An example of the latter is pressure on the bladder by a prolapsed uterus.

night

    Both nocturia and nycturia mean excessive urination at _____, sometimes interfering with sleep because of the need to urinate several times during the night.

11-49 When one kidney is removed, the other kidney becomes enlarged. Enlargement of the kidney is <u>nephro/megaly</u> (nef″ro-meg′ə-le).

one

    Kidney enlargement may involve one or both kidneys. Uni/lateral nephromegaly is enlargement of _____ kidney; bi/lateral nephromegaly involves both kidneys.

11-50 Because the urinary system is responsible for removing harmful waste products from the blood, anything that interferes with excretion of wastes can be dangerous. <u>Uremia</u> (u-re′me-ə) is an accumulation of toxic products in the blood. This occurs when the kidneys fail to function properly. The meaning of ur/emia (*ur[o]*, urine + *-emia*, blood) is implied.

uremia

    Write this term that means an accumulation of waste products in the blood owing to inadequate functioning of the urinary system: _____.

11-51 Inability of the kidneys to excrete wastes, concentrate urine, and function properly is <u>renal failure</u>. It may be acute or chronic. <u>Acute renal failure</u> (ARF) has symptoms that are more severe than _____ renal failure (CRF).

chronic

    Acute renal failure is characterized by oliguria and by the rapid accumulation of nitrogenous wastes in the blood, indicated by a higher than normal amount of blood urea nitrogen. Acute renal failure may be caused by nephr/itis (inflammation of the kidney), interference in blood flow to the kidney, or conditions that disrupt urinary output.

    Acute renal failure can often be reversed after the cause has been identified (for example, removal of an obstruction in the urinary tract). However, <u>chronic renal failure</u> may lead to the need for dialysis (di-al′ə-sis) if all other medical measures have not alleviated the problem.

11-52 A substance that is <u>nephro/toxic</u> (nef′ro-tok″sik) is toxic or destructive to kidney cells. Build a word that means destruction of the kidney by combining *nephr(o)* with the suffix for destruction: _____.

nephrolysis
(nə-frol′ə-sis)

    <u>Nephrolysis</u> also means freeing of a kidney from adhesions, bands of scar tissue that bind surfaces together that are normally separate.

    <u>Nephro/malacia</u> (nef″ro-mə-la′shə) is abnormal softening of the kidney.

11-53 A <u>polyp</u> (pol′ip) is any growth or mass protruding from a mucous membrane. A bladder polyp is a growth protruding from the lining of the bladder. This abnormality is one of the conditions that may be detected during cytoscopy. Polyps may occur anywhere there is mucous membrane, such as the urethra.

11-54 <u>Urethrorrhagia</u> (u-re″thro-ra′je-ə) means urethral hemorrhage. <u>Urethro/rrhea</u> (u-re″thro-re′ə)

discharge

means _____ from the urethra.

---

*Continence (Latin: *continere*, to contain).

Exercise 3

Match terms in the left column with their descriptions in the right column.

_____ 1. anuria

_____ 2. dysuria

_____ 3. hesitancy

_____ 4. nycturia

_____ 5. oliguria

_____ 6. polyp

_____ 7. polyuria

_____ 8. urgency

_____ 9. urinary incontinence

_____ 10. urinary retention

A. a decrease in the force of the urine stream
B. a mass protruding from a mucous membrane
C. difficult or painful urination
D. excessive urination at night
E. excretion of an abnormally large volume of urine
F. excretion of less than 100 ml of urine a day
G. excretion of less than 500 ml of urine a day
H. incomplete emptying of the bladder
I. loss of control of the passage of urine from the bladder
J. the sense of the need to urinate immediately

infection

urethritis

cystitis

ureteritis (u-re″tər-i′tis)

pyelitis (pi″ə-li′tis)

11-55 Bacterial infection is the most common cause of inflammation of the urinary tract, but inflammation may be attributed to other disorders, such as the presence of a stone.

A <u>urinary tract infection</u> (UTI), an infection of one or more structures in the urinary system, is one of the more common disorders of the urinary tract. A UTI may be asymptomatic but is usually characterized by urinary frequency and possibly discomfort during urination. Other signs and symptoms, particularly in severe infections, include backache, fever, and blood and/or pus in the urine. It is important to diagnose and treat urinary tract infections to prevent their spreading to another part of the body, such as the blood. <u>Septic/emia</u> (*sept[o]*, infection + *-emia*, blood) is a systemic infection in which pathogens are present in the circulating blood, having spread from an infection in another part of the body, such as the urinary tract.

UTI means urinary tract _____.

11-56 Kinds of urinary tract infections include <u>cyst/itis</u> (**sis-ti′tis**), <u>urethritis</u> (**u″rə-thri′tis**), and <u>pyelonephritis</u> (**pi″ə-lo-nə-fri′tis**). Most urinary infections are caused by bacteria (especially *Escherichia coli*), but certain fungi (*Candida*) can also cause infection. When UTIs are caused by bacteria, they are treated with an antibiotic.

The urinary tract above the urethra is normally free of microorganisms. Most of the time, UTIs are caused by ascending infection, with the area near the anus serving as a reservoir for bacteria. Organisms spread directly from the anal area (occasionally, the vagina) to the urethral meatus, where they multiply and can ascend throughout the urethra to the bladder and eventually the kidney in some cases. Infection is more likely in females than males because of the short distance separating the anus and the urethra, as well as a shorter urethra. Both catheterization and sexual intercourse promote the ascent of bacteria. Urinary tract infections are also more common in persons with structural abnormalities or lowered immunity and are a major type of hospital-acquired infections.

Write the term that means inflammation of the urethra: _____. This condition is characterized by dysuria. It may result from minor trauma or from infection. <u>Urethro/cyst/itis</u> (**u-re″thro-sis-ti′tis**) is inflammation of the urethra and bladder. This means the same as <u>cysto/urethr/itis</u> (**sis″to-u″re-thri′tis**).

Write the term that means inflammation of the bladder: _____.

11-57 Cystitis often involves inflammation of the ureters. Write a term that means inflammation of a ureter: _____. Ureteritis may also be caused by the mechanical irritation of a stone. <u>Ureteropathy</u> (**u-re″tər-op′ə-the**) means any disease of a ureter.

<u>Uretero/pyelo/nephritis</u> (**u-re″tər-o-pi″ə-lo-nə-fri′tis**) means inflammation of a ureter, renal pelvis, and the kidney. Write a word that means inflammation of the renal pelvis: _____.

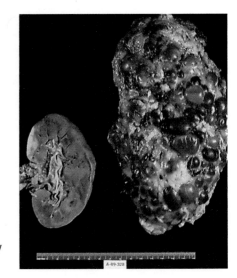

Figure 11-13 Comparison of polycystic kidney with a normal kidney. Notice the kidney enlargement and the replacement of normal tissue by numerous fluid-filled cysts.

Pyelonephritis means inflammation of the kidney and its renal pelvis. Acute pyelonephritis is usually the result of spreading of an infection from the lower urinary tract and has a rapid onset. Chronic pyelonephritis can develop after bacterial infection of the kidney that is either untreated or resistant to treatment.

11-58 Some renal disorders are hereditary. <u>Poly/cyst/ic</u> **(pol″e-sis′tik)** <u>kidney disease</u>, one of the more common hereditary renal disorders, is characterized by enlarged kidneys containing many cysts. *Poly/cystic* means containing many cysts. See Figure 11-13 for comparison of a polycystic kidney and a normal kidney.

11-59 <u>Nephr/itis</u> **(nə-fri′tis)** is one of a large group of kidney diseases that is characterized by _____ and abnormal function. The most usual form is <u>glomerulo/nephritis</u> **(glo-mer″u-lo-nə-fri′tis)**, in which glomeruli within the kidney are inflamed. Glomeruli **(glo-mer′u-li)** are clusters of capillaries that act as filters. In glomerulonephritis, there is impairment of the filtering process. Inflammation of the kidney may be caused by microorganisms or their toxins or even by toxic drugs or alcohol.

Glomerul(o) is a combining form that means glomerulus. Write a word that means any disease of the glomeruli: _____.

11-60 <u>Nephrotic</u> **(nə-frot′ik)** <u>syndrome</u> is an abnormal condition of the kidney characterized by marked proteinuria and edema. It occurs as a complication of many systemic diseases, such as diabetes mellitus.

<u>Diabetes mellitus</u> **(di″ə-be′tēz mel′lĕ-təs, mə-li′təs)** is a complex disorder of carbohydrate, fat, and protein metabolism that is primarily a result of a deficiency or lack of insulin secretion by the pancreas or a resistance to insulin. <u>Diabetic nephro/pathy</u> **(nə-frop′ĕ-the)** is a disease of the _____ resulting from diabetes mellitus. Chronic hyperglycemia and increased blood pressure accelerate the progression of the disorder. *Hyper/glycemia* means excessive glucose in the _____.

Diabetes mellitus is a major cause of end-stage renal disease in the United States and can result from either type 1 or type 2 diabetes mellitus. See Chapter 17 for additional information about this disorder.

11-61 Obstructive nephropathies are conditions that block or interfere with the flow of urine. Several causes are illustrated in Figure 11-14 and include prolapsed adjacent structures, tumors (benign or malignant), stones, narrowing of the ureters or urethra, and dysfunctions of the bladder that result from spinal cord injury or a lesion of the nervous system (neurogenic bladder).

Margin answers:

inflammation

glomerulopathy
(glo-mer″u-lop′ə-the)

kidneys

blood

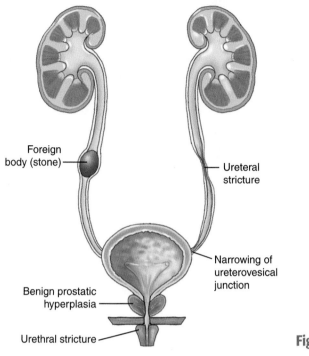

Foreign body (stone)

Ureteral stricture

Narrowing of ureterovesical junction

Benign prostatic hyperplasia

Urethral stricture

Figure 11-14 Common causes of urinary tract obstruction.

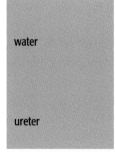

water

ureter

Hydro/nephrosis (**hi″dro-nə-fro′sis**) is distension (or distention) of the renal pelvis and kidney by urine that cannot flow past an obstruction in a ureter. The literal translation of hydronephrosis is a condition of _____ in the kidney. You will need to remember that *hydronephrosis* means distension of the renal pelvis with urine as a result of an obstruction in the upper part of a ureter.

If a stone or another obstruction occurs in the lower part of the ureter, the condition that results is called hydroureter (**hi″dro-u-re′tər**), abnormal distension of a _____ with urine or watery fluid. See Figure 11-15 for comparison of hydronephrosis and hydroureter.

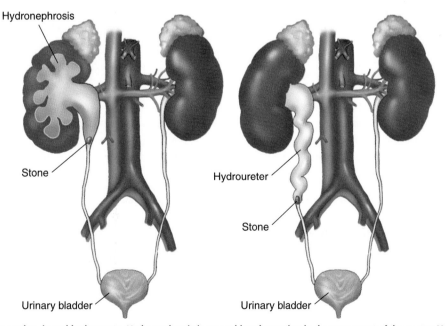

Hydronephrosis

Stone

Urinary bladder

Hydroureter

Stone

Urinary bladder

Figure 11-15 Hydronephrosis and hydroureter. Hydronephrosis is caused by obstruction in the upper part of the ureter. Hydroureter is caused by obstruction in the lower part of the ureter.

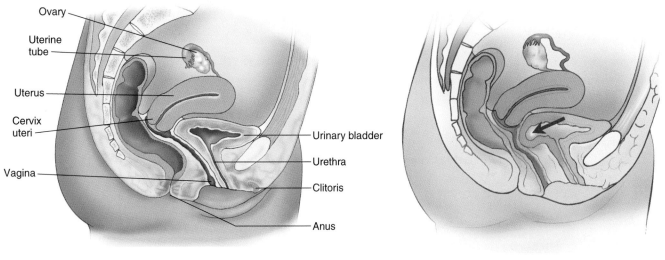

Figure 11-16   Comparison of a cystocele with the normal position of the urinary bladder. With a cystocele, the bladder is displaced downward, causing bulging of the anterior vaginal wall.

ureter

urethrocele
(u-re′thro-sēl)

cystocele
(sis′to-sēl)

11-62 <u>Uterine prolapse</u>, the loss of support that anchors the uterus, can result in pressure on the bladder and lead to urinary frequency.

Prolapse can also occur in the urinary structures themselves. <u>Uretero/cele</u> (**u-re′tər-o-sēl″**) is a prolapse or herniation of a _____. This condition may lead to obstruction of the flow of urine and hydronephrosis.

Herniation of the urethra is a _____. This is characterized by a protrusion of the female urethra through the urethral opening or encroachment of a segment of the urethral wall upon the vaginal canal.

Using -cele, write a word that means herniation of the bladder: _____. In a cystocele, the bladder hernia protrudes into the vagina (Figure 11-16).

benign

11-63 Enlargement of a nearby structure (for example, the prostate) also puts pressure on urinary structures. The prostate is a gland in men that surrounds the neck of the bladder. <u>Benign prostatic hyperplasia</u> (BPH) is a nonmalignant, noninflammatory enlargement of the prostate and is common among men over 50 years of age. It may lead to urethral obstruction and interference with urine flow, causing frequency, dysuria, nocturia, and urinary tract infections.

Prostatic hyperplasia results in enlargement of the prostate. This is not a malignant disease, as noted by its name, _____ prostatic hyperplasia.

urolithiasis
(u″ro-lĭ-thi′ə-sis)

kidney

ureterolith
(u-re′tər-o-lith)

11-64 Knowing that *lith(o)* means stone, build the word that means formation of urinary calculi by using *ur(o)*, *lith(o)*, and *-iasis*: _____.

Urinary stones are often named according to their location: kidney, ureter, or bladder. They vary greatly in size, from small enough to pass through the ureter, to large stones that occupy the entire renal pelvis, and have roughly the shape of a deer antler (<u>staghorn calculi</u>). <u>Nephro/lith/iasis</u> (**nef″ro-lĭ-thi′ə-sis**) is a condition marked by the presence of _____ stones. A kidney stone is also called a renal calculus or a <u>nephro/lith</u> (**nef′ro-lith**).

<u>Uretero/lith/iasis</u> (**u-re″tər-o-lĭ-thi′ə-sis**) is the presence of a stone in a ureter. If a nephro/lith is a kidney stone, build a word that means stone in a ureter: _____.
A <u>cystolith</u> (**sis′to-lith**) means a calculus in the urinary bladder.

11-65 A <u>ureteral or urethral stricture</u> is a narrowing of the lumen (inner space) of the ureter or urethra. A narrowing can also occur at the place where the ureter joins the bladder. This is called

bladder	narrowing of the uretero/vesical junction. Uretero/vesical pertains to the ureter and the _____.
stricture (narrowing)	Urethro/stenosis (u-re″thro-stə-no′sis) is a stricture of the urethra, and a uretero/stenosis (u-re″tər-o-stə-no′sis) is _____ of a ureter. Stenosis is narrowing of an opening or passageway of a vessel.
	These strictures may lead to urinary stasis or reflux, oliguria, and eventually anuria. In some cases, the stricture is relieved or corrected by balloon or catheter dilation.
	11-66 <u>Reno/vascular disease</u>, problems of the blood vessels of the kidney, include nephrosclerosis (**nef″ro-sklə-ro′sis**), stenosis of the renal artery, and thrombosis of the renal vein.
	<u>Nephro/sclerosis</u> is hardening of the small arteries of the kidney and results in decreased blood flow and eventually necrosis of kidney cells. This condition occurs in a small number of persons with hypertension (elevated blood pressure). Treatment of nephrosclerosis is the use of medications to lower the blood pressure. Write this term that means hardening of the arteries of the kidney:
nephrosclerosis	_____.
	Renal artery stenosis is partial or complete blocking of one or both renal arteries. The pathologic changes to the renal arteries result in drastically reduced blood flow through the kidneys and lead to hypertension and damage to the kidneys. Hypertension resulting from renal artery stenosis or other kidney disorders is called renal hypertension.
	A blood clot in the renal vein is called <u>renal vein thrombosis</u>. The cause of the blood clot (the thrombus) includes compression by a nearby tumor, renal carcinoma, or renal trauma. The presence of a thrombus in the renal vein is called renal vein _____.
thrombosis	
	11-67 The characteristics of diabetes mellitus were described earlier. Another disorder that shares the name *diabetes* is <u>diabetes insipidus</u> (**di-ə-be′tēz in-sip′ĭ-dəs**). The disorder is not related to diabetes mellitus but was so named because of the large quantity of urine excreted.
	Unlike diabetes mellitus, diabetes insipidus is not related to the body's use of insulin. Its cause may be hormonal or renal, and the disorder refers to several types of polyuria in which the urinary output exceeds 3000 ml a day. Write the name of this disorder: diabetes
insipidus	_____.
	11-68 <u>Genitourinary infections</u> are those affecting both the genital and _____ structures.
urinary	A <u>sexually transmitted disease</u> (STD) is one that may be acquired as a result of sexual contact with a person who has the disease or with secretions containing the suspected organism. Sexually transmitted diseases were formerly called venereal (**və-nēr′e-əl**) diseases (VD).
	11-69 You have learned that *-rrhea* means flow or discharge, and you probably have heard of <u>gono/rrhea</u> (**gon″o-re′ə**), a sexually transmitted disease. Gonorrhea is derived from *gon(o)*, which means the genitals or reproduction. This sexually transmitted disease, caused by the bacterium *Neisseria gonorrhoeae*, is characterized by a heavy discharge from the vagina in females or from the urethra in either males or females. The discharge may be accompanied by urethritis and dysuria. See Chapter 13 for more information about gonorrhea.
gonorrhea	Write the name of the sexually transmitted disease that can cause urethritis: _____.

Exercise 4

Write a word in each blank to complete these sentences. The first letter of each answer is given as a clue.

1. Enlargement of both kidneys is called <u>b</u>_____ nephromegaly.

2. An accumulation of toxic products in the blood is <u>u</u>_____.

3. Abnormal softening of the kidney is <u>n</u>_____.

4. Discharge from the urethra is <u>u</u>_____.

5. Disorders that affect the blood vessels of the kidneys are r_____ disorders.

6. Inflammation of the bladder is c_____.

7. Inflammation of the kidney and its renal pelvis is p_____.

8. A hereditary disorder characterized by enlarged kidneys containing many cysts is called p_____ kidney disease.

9. Inflammation of the renal glomeruli is called g_____.

10. A complex disorder of carbohydrate, fat, and protein metabolism that is primarily a result of deficiency of insulin or a resistance to insulin is diabetes m_____.

11. Distension of the renal pelvis with urine, resulting from an obstruction in the upper part of a ureter, is h_____.

12. Distension of a ureter with urine or a watery fluid is h_____.

13. Hernial protrusion of the bladder into the vagina is a c_____.

14. A nonmalignant, noninflammatory enlargement of the prostate is called benign prostatic h_____.

15. A condition marked by the presence of kidney stones is n_____.

16. A hormonal or renal disorder in which the urinary output exceeds 3000 ml a day is diabetes i_____.

17. Partial or complete blocking of one or both renal arteries is renal artery s_____.

18. Blood clot in the renal vein is renal vein t_____.

🏺 SURGICAL AND THERAPEUTIC INTERVENTIONS

blood	**11-70** <u>Kidney dialysis</u> (**di-al′ə-sis**) is required when the kidneys fail to remove waste products from the blood. This is also called <u>hemo/dialysis</u> (**he″mo-di-al′ə-sis**), which means dialysis of the _____. Kidney dialysis or hemodialysis is the process of diffusing blood through a semipermeable membrane for the purpose of removing toxic materials and maintaining the acid-base balance in cases of impaired kidney function. <u>Peritoneal dialysis</u> is dialysis through the peritoneum, with the solution being introduced into and removed from the peritoneal cavity. Sometimes this type of dialysis is done as an alternative to hemodialysis.
nephrectomy **(nə-frek′tə-me)** **ureter**	**11-71** In a <u>renal transplant</u> the patient (recipient) receives a kidney from a suitable donor. The donated kidney is surgically removed from the donor. Build a word that means surgical excision of a kidney, using *nephr(o)* and the suffix for excision: _____. <u>Nephroureterectomy</u> (**nef″ro-u-re″tər-ek′tə-me**) means surgical excision of a kidney with the _____. Selected situations may allow <u>laparo/scopic</u> (**lap″ə-ro-skop′ik**) <u>nephrectomy</u>, removal of the kidney through several small incisions in the abdominal wall, rather than an open surgical excision. <u>Immuno/suppressive therapy</u>, the administration of agents that significantly interfere with the immune response of the recipient, are provided after renal transplantation to prevent rejection of the donor kidney.
kidney **bladder**	**11-72** Removal of the diseased kidney or radiation therapy is used to treat renal carcinoma. Ren/al carcinoma is cancer of a _____. Treatment for bladder cancer depends on several factors, including the size of the lesion. Tests of the urine may show atypical cells or the presence of factors associated with cancer, but cystoscopy and biopsy are generally used for confirmation. Radiation therapy, laser eradication of small lesions, chemotherapy, and cystectomy may be used. Chemotherapy can be given systemically or, in some cases, the chemical treatment is instilled directly into the bladder through a catheter. <u>Cyst/ectomy</u> (**sis-tek′tə-me**) is surgical excision of the _____. It may be a partial cystectomy, in which only a portion of the bladder is removed, or the cystectomy may be radical, in which all of the bladder is removed along with selected adjacent organs (the prostate and seminal vesicles in males; the uterus, cervix, ovaries, and urethra in females).

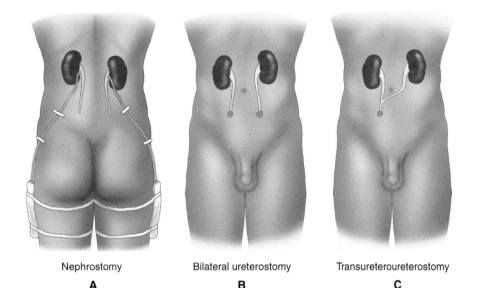

Nephrostomy   Bilateral ureterostomy   Transureteroureterostomy
A   **B**   **C**

Figure 11-17   Comparing nephrostomy and two ureterostomies. **A,** Nephrostomy. Percutaneous openings are made into the renal pelvis, and urine is diverted to bags. **B,** Bilateral ureterostomy. Both ureters are brought out onto the skin for drainage of urine into bags. **C,** Transureteroureterostomy. One ureter is surgically attached to the other ureter, which is brought out onto the skin for drainage of urine into a bag.

ureter

11-73 Various surgical procedures may be performed for urinary diversion if the bladder is removed. The ureters must be diverted into some type of collecting reservoir, opening either onto the abdomen or into the large intestine so that urine is expelled with bowel movements.

Formation of a new opening through which a ureter empties is called a <u>ureterostomy</u> (**u-re″tər-os′tə-me**) (Figure 11-17). In a bilateral or double ureterostomy, there are two pouches on the abdominal surface, one for each ureter, to receive drainage of the urine. Surgical connection of one ureter to another is called <u>trans/ureteroureterostomy</u> (**trans″u-re″tər-o-u-re″tər-os′tə-me**). In other words, one ureter is brought across and joined to the other_____.
The latter results in only one opening on the abdominal surface that serves both ureters.

skin

11-74 <u>Percutaneous nephro/stomy</u> (**nə-fros′tə-me**) is a surgical procedure in which the skin is punctured so that a catheter can be inserted into the renal pelvis for the purpose of drainage. Literal translation of nephro/stomy is formation of a new opening into the kidney. Percutaneous tells us that the _____ is punctured to gain access to the renal kidney. This procedure allows for drainage, drug instillation, and selected surgical procedures, including removal of calculi.

A nephrostomy may be performed on one or both kidneys and may be temporary or permanent. If both ureters are removed, a nephrostomy is necessary. Compare nephrostomy and the two types of ureterostomies described in the previous frame.

11-75 Cancer is one reason for urinary diversion. An obstruction lower in the urinary tract could also require formation of a new opening through which the ureter could discharge its contents.

Stones in the urinary tract are sometimes passed out through the urethra, but many are too large or do not dissolve. Stones can cause urinary obstruction, which interferes with function and can be very painful. There are several methods of dealing with stones, including <u>lithotripsy</u> and open surgery to remove the stone.

stone

Litho/tripsy (**lith′o-trip″se**) is surgical crushing of a _____.
Sometimes lithotripsy is successful with small stones and is accomplished by inserting a catheter through the urethra to the point where the stone is lodged. The stone is then crushed with an instrument called a <u>lithotrite</u> (**lith′o-trīt**).

extracorporeal

11-76 <u>Extracorporeal shock wave lithotripsy</u> (ESWL) is also used to break up stones. *Extra/corpor/eal* means outside the body. Extracorporeal shock wave lithotripsy uses ultrasonic energy from a source outside the body (Figure 11-18). This technique is used on stones that resist passage and is far less incapacitating than a full-scale surgery.

Write the name of the procedure that uses ultrasonic energy from a source outside the body to break up a stone: _____ shock wave lithotripsy.

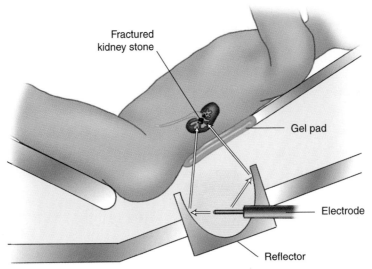

Figure 11-18   Lithotripsy, crushing of a kidney stone (calculus). Extracorporeal shock wave lithotripsy, illustrated here, is used to crush certain types of urinary stones. The reflector focuses a high-energy shock wave on the stone. The stone disintegrates into particles and is passed in the urine.

calculi (or stones)

11-77 Nephro/litho/tomy (**nef″ro-lĭ-thot′ə-me**) is removal of renal _____ by cutting through the body of the kidney. Notice that -tomy is used rather than -ectomy, because -tomy refers to incision of the kidney, and removal of the stone is only implied. Nephrolithotomy is necessary if the stone is too large to pass or break up or if it will not dissolve.

pelvis

Pyelo/lithotomy (**pi″ə-lo-lĭ-thot′ə-me**) is surgical removal of a stone from the renal _____. Literal translation of this term is incision of the renal pelvis for stones, and it is understood that the procedure is done for this purpose. Write the term:

pyelolithotomy

_____.

Ureterolithotomy (**u-re″tər-o-lĭ-thot′ə-me**) and cysto/litho/tomy (**sis″to-lĭ-thot′ə-me**) are procedures for surgical removal of a stone or stones from the ureter and the

bladder

_____, respectively. It is important that the patient have a high fluid intake after a stone is removed to prevent the formation of another stone.

11-78 Renal artery stenosis, partial blocking of one or both renal arteries, is treated by percutaneous transluminal renal angio/plasty or by using another major artery to route blood to the kidney. In percutaneous angio/plasty, the repair of the renal artery is via an incision of the

skin

_____.

Anticoagulant therapy is used in renal vein thrombosis, a blood clot in the renal vein. A thromb/ectomy may also be performed, which means surgical excision of the

thrombus

_____.

11-79 Catheter dilation is useful in treating stricture of the ureter or urethra. Severe stricture that does not respond to dilation may require ureter/ectomy (**u-re″tər-ek′tə-me**), partial or complete surgical excision of the ureter.

The section of the ureter that remains after ureterectomy is attached to a different site on the bladder. This surgical procedure is called ureterocystostomy (**u-re″tər-o-sis-tos′tə-me**). It involves surgical transplantation of the ureter to a different site on the bladder and is also called uretero/cysto/neo/stomy (**u-re″tər-o-sis″to-ne-os′tə-me**).

11-80 Ureteroplasty (**u-re′tər-o-plas″te**) means surgical repair of a ureter. Write a term that means surgical repair of the renal pelvis: _____.

pyeloplasty
(**pi′ə-lo-plas″te**)

11-81 Write another term that means surgical repair of the bladder:

cystoplasty
(**sis′to-plas″te**)

_____.

bladder	<u>Cystostomy</u> (sis-tos'tə-me) means formation of a new opening into the bladder. <u>Suprapubic</u> <u>cystotomy</u> is surgical incision of the _____ via an incision just above the symphysis pubis. <u>Cystotomy</u> (sis-tot'ə-me) means incision of the bladder.
urethrotomy (u″rə-throt'ə-me) urethra	**11-82** Surgical incision of the urethra is _____. Remembering that *trans-* means through or across, trans/urethral (**trans″u-re'thrəl**) means through the _____. Transurethral surgery is performed by inserting an instrument through or across the wall of the urethra and makes it possible to perform surgery on certain organs that lie near the urethra without having an abdominal incision. In transurethral resection (TUR), small pieces of tissue from a nearby structure are removed through the wall of the urethra.
transurethral	**11-83** One surgery of this type is a <u>transurethral resection of the prostate</u> (TURP). In a TURP, surgery is performed on the prostate gland in males by means of an instrument passed through the wall of the urethra and is sometimes done to alleviate the problems of benign prostatic hyperplasia. In a TURP, an abdominal incision is not involved, since the surgeon approaches the prostate through the urethra. Small pieces of the prostate are removed with a special instrument. Because this surgery is performed by passing the instrument through the urethra, it is called _____ resection of the prostate.

Be Careful With These!

Prostate is a frequently misspelled term.

Note the difference in spelling of *prostate* and *prostrate*, which means lying in a face-down, horizontal position.

nephropexy (nef'ro-pek″se)	**11-84** Use *nephr(o)* and *-pexy* to write a word that means surgical fixation of the kidney: _____. This type of surgery is often used to correct nephroptosis (**nef″rop-to'sis**), also called floating kidney. Nephroptosis is a gradual downward displacement of the kidney and is also called floating, hypermobile, or wandering kidney. It can occur when the kidney supports are weakened by sudden strain or a blow, or it may be present at birth.
urination	**11-85** There are several types of urinary incontinence, and treatment depends on the cause. One of the more common types, stress incontinence (leakage of urine when coughing, sneezing, or straining), is sometimes helped with the use of <u>Kegel exercises</u> to strengthen the pelvic muscles, weight loss in obese persons, drug therapy, or surgery. Incontinence resulting from spinal cord injury necessitates use of an indwelling catheter. *Urinary incontinence* means the inability to control _____. Urinary retention may require catheterization, either intermittent or indwelling. Certain medications are also helpful.
diuretic	**11-86** Treatment of urinary tract infections includes <u>antibiotics</u>, <u>analgesics</u>, and increased intake of water. Increased or excessive urination is polyuria or diuresis (**di″u-re'sis**). Sometimes diuretics (**di″u-ret'ikz**) are prescribed to increase urination. An agent that causes the body to eliminate more water in the form of urine is called a _____.
urethrospasm (u-re'thro-spaz-əm) against	**11-87** Write a term that means spasm of the urethra (actually, the muscular tissue of the urethra): _____. This may occur after certain surgical procedures such as transurethral resection of the prostate. Literal interpretation of anti/spasmodics is _____ spasms. <u>Antispasmodics</u> (**an″te-, an″ti-spaz-mod'ikz**) are drugs or other agents that prevent muscle spasms.

Exercise 5

Circle the correct answer for the following questions.

1. Which term means excision of a kidney? (nephrectomy, nephroscopy, nephrostomy, nephrotomy)
2. Which of the following terms is a type of urinary diversion? (cystometrography, glomerular filtration, hemodialysis, ureterostomy)
3. Which of the following is least likely to cause a urinary obstruction? (infection, stone, tumor, ureterolith)
4. Which of the following is not a likely treatment of a stone located in the bladder? (cystolithotomy, ESWL, lithotripsy, pyelolithotomy)
5. Which of the following may be used to treat renal vein thrombosis? (anticoagulant therapy, cystoplasty, nephropexy, shock wave lithotripsy)
6. Which term means a procedure that is performed by inserting an instrument through or across the wall of the urethra? (nephroptosis, transurethral resection, ureterocystostomy, urinary retention)

SELECTED ABBREVIATIONS

ADH	antidiuretic hormone		**IVP**	intravenous pyelogram
ARF	acute renal failure		**KUB**	kidneys, ureters, and bladder
BPH	benign prostatic hyperplasia		**pH**	potential of hydrogen
BUN	blood urea nitrogen		**PSA**	prostate-specific antigen
CRF	chronic renal failure		**TUR**	transurethral resection
EMG	electromyography		**TURP**	transurethral resection of the prostate
ESWL	extracorporeal shock wave lithotripsy		**UA, U/A**	urinalysis
GFR	glomerular filtration rate		**UTI**	urinary tract infection
GU	genitourinary		**VCUG**	voiding cystourethrogram
I & O	intake and output		**VD**	venereal disease
IV	intravenous			

CHAPTER 11 REVIEW

■ Basic Understanding

Labeling

I. Label the numbered structures with their corresponding combining form. Number 1 has two answers.

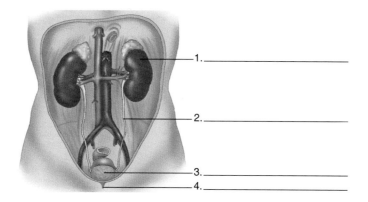

1. _____

2. _____

3. _____
4. _____

Matching

II. Match structures in the left column with their functions in the right column.

_____ 1. bladder

_____ 2. nephron

_____ 3. renal pelvis

_____ 4. ureter

_____ 5. urethra

A. cavity in the kidney that collects urine from many collecting ducts
B. carries urine from the bladder
C. carries urine to the bladder
D. functional unit of the kidney
E. reservoir for urine until it is expelled

Listing

III. List three major functions of the urinary system.

1. _____

2. _____

3. _____

True or False

IV. Several urinary substances are listed. Write T for those substances that are normally detected in urine and F for those substances that are not normally detected.

1. albumin _____

2. blood _____

3. creatinine _____

4. glucose _____

5. ketones _____

6. protein _____

7. sugar _____

8. urea _____

Multiple Choice

V. Circle the correct answer for each of the following multiple choice questions.

1. Which of the following is the filtering structure of the kidney? (glomerulus, tubule, ureter, urethra)

2. Which of the following means excision of a renal calculus from the pelvis of the kidney? (cystolithectomy, lithotripsy, pyelolithotomy, pyelostomy)

3. Which of the following means the same as nephromegaly? (floating kidney, kidney dialysis, renal enlargement, renal stone)

4. Which of the following is not a method of collecting a urine sample? (catheterization, lithotripsy, urinating, voiding)

5. Which of the following terms means making radiographic images of the urinary system after the urine has been rendered opaque by a contrast medium? (cystoscopy, cystoureteroscopy, intravenous pyelography, nephrotomography)

6. Which of the following is indicated if the blood urea nitrogen is elevated? (pyelostomy, pyuria, renal clearance, renal failure)

7. Which term means an inability to control urination? (frequency, hesitancy, incontinence, retention)

8. Which term means excretion of an abnormally large quantity of urine? (anuria, dysuria, oliguria, polyuria)

9. Which of the following is not a type of urinary tract catheterization? (endoscopy tube, nephrostomy tube, suprapubic tube, urethral tube)

10. In which of the following is an instrument passed through the urethra in order to remove small pieces of the prostate gland? (intravenous pyelogram, retrograde pyelography, transurethral resection, urethrography)

11. Which of the following is a toxic condition of the body that occurs when the kidneys fail to function properly? (nephromalacia, nephrolithiasis, uremia, urography)

12. What does pyuria indicate about a urine specimen? (excessive sugar, excessive number of white cells, increased creatinine, increased protein)

13. Which of the following terms means distension of a ureter with urine or watery fluid? (hydronephrosis, hydroureter, ureteral stricture, ureterolithiasis)

14. Which term describes partial or complete blocking of a blood vessel? (herniation, sclerosis, stenosis, thrombosis)

15. Which term means inflammation of the kidney and renal pelvis? (pyelography, pyelonephritis, pyelolithotomy, pyelostomy)

Writing Terms

VI. Write a term for each of the following:

1. any disease of the urinary tract   _____

2. between the kidneys   _____

3. blood in the urine   _____

4. herniation of the urethra   _____

5. inflammation of the renal glomeruli   _____

6. inflammation of the renal pelvis   _____

7. kidney dialysis   _____

8. outside the urinary bladder   _____

9. radiography of the bladder   _____

10. surgical crushing of a stone   _____

■ Greater Comprehension

Labeling
VII. Choose from the following list to label parts of the nephron shown (1-5):

afferent arteriole, distal convoluted tubule, glomerulus, Bowman's capsule, efferent arteriole, proximal convoluted tubule, collecting duct

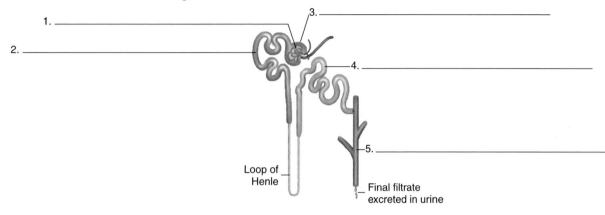

1. _____
2. _____
3. _____
4. _____
5. _____

Loop of Henle

Final filtrate excreted in urine

Health Care Record
VIII. Read the case study and answer the questions that follow.

CASE STUDY

Patient: M.A. Stewart (male, age 43)
Symptoms: Hematuria, dysuria
History: Cystitis, nephritis
Family History: Father—age 65 with history of BPH; mother—age 64 with history of renal calculi and pyelonephritis
Diagnostic Studies: KUB and IV urography show three small calculi in ureter
Labs: Urinalysis and urine culture show no evidence of UTI
Diagnosis: Ureteral urolithiasis
Plan: Ureteroscopy and possible lithotripsy

Circle one answer for each of the following.

1. Mr. Stewart's symptom of dysuria indicates what aspect of urine or urination? (blood, decreased output, difficult or painful, protein)

2. What does his history indicate? (bladder and kidney stones, inflammation of the bladder and kidney, inflammation caused by trauma, frequent urinary infections)

3. His father's history indicates problems with which of the following? (bladder, kidney, prostate, urethra)

4. Which of the following is indicated in his mother's history? (kidney stones, polycystic kidney, renal vein thrombosis, renovascular disease)

5. Which of the following is Mr. Stewart's diagnosis? (narrowing of the ureter, obstruction of the ureter, stone in the ureter, urinary infection)

What do these abbreviations mean?

6. BPH _____

7. KUB _____

8. IV _____

9. UTI _____

Health Care Record

IX. Read the case study and answer the questions that follow.

CASE STUDY

Patient: L.R. Schmitt (male, age 65)

Symptoms: Nocturia, frequency of urination, interruption of urinary stream, dribbling, urgency of urination, fatigue

History: Frequent UTIs, prostatitis

Family History: Father—deceased with history of cancer of the prostate with metastasis to the bone and nephrolithiasis; mother—age 84 with history of insulin-dependent diabetes mellitus, hypertension, and renal failure; currently on hemodialysis

Physical exam: Rectal exam demonstrated large, rubbery prostate

Lab results: UA is WNL; PSA 2.0 (normal: 0 to 4.0 nanograms/ml)

Diagnostic studies: Cystoscopy demonstrated a normal bladder and urethra
Ultrasound and biopsy of the prostate showed benign hypertrophy

Diagnosis: BPH

Plan: Conservative treatment with Proscar and Flomax. Will eventually need to have surgical intervention with TURP

Circle one answer for each of the following questions.

1. Mr. Schmitt's symptom of nocturia indicates which of the following about urination? (nighttime frequency, incontinence, painful, retention)

2. His father's history indicates which of the following? (diabetes insipidus, diabetes mellitus, frequent urinary tract infections, kidney stones)

3. His mother's health condition indicates a deficiency or improper use of which of the following? (ADH, carbohydrates, diuretics, insulin)

4. Which instrument was used for Mr. Schmitt's diagnostic study? (catheter, cystoscope, nephroscope, ultrascope)

What do these abbreviations mean?

5. UA _____

6. WNL _____

7. TURP _____

Spelling
X. *Circle all incorrectly spelled terms and write their correct spelling:*

antispasmodic   catheterization hydronefrosis ketoacidosis gonorhea

Interpreting Abbreviations
XI. *Write the meaning of these abbreviations:*

1. ARF _____

2. EMG _____

3. BUN _____

4. ESWL _____

5. VCUG _____

Pronunciation
XII. *The pronunciation is shown for several medical words. Indicate which syllable has the primary accent by marking it with an ʹ.*

1. diuresis (di u re sis)

2. lithotripsy (lith o trip se)

3. nephrolithiasis (nef ro lǐ thi ə sis)

4. pyelogram (pi ə lo gram)

5. ureteroplasty (u re tər o plast te)

Categorizing Terms
XIII. *Classify the terms in the left column (1-10) by selecting A, B, C, D, or E from the right column.*

_____ 1. cystourethrography
_____ 2. diuretics
_____ 3. genitourinary
_____ 4. glycosuria
_____ 5. hemodialysis
_____ 6. nephrectomy
_____ 7. nephrosclerosis
_____ 8. nephrosonography
_____ 9. tubule
_____ 10. ureterocele

A. anatomy
B. diagnostic test or procedure
C. pathology
D. surgery
E. therapy

LISTING OF MEDICAL TERMS

Use the practice CD to review the terms that have been presented. Look closely at the spelling of each term as it is pronounced and be sure you know the meaning of each term.

abdominal auscultation
abdominal palpation
abdominal percussion
abdominocystic
abdominovesical
albumin
albuminuria
angiogram
antihypertensive
antiinfective
antispasmodic
anuria
anuric
bacilli
bacterial culture
benign prostatic
   hyperplasia
bilateral nephromegaly
bladder
bladder polyp
blood urea nitrogen
Bowman's capsule
Bright's disease
Candida albicans
catheter
catheterized specimen
chronic
cocci
continence
creatinine
creatinine clearance
cystectomy
cystic
cystitis
cystocele
cystogram
cystography
cystolith
cystolithectomy
cystolithotomy
cystometrography
cystoplasty
cystoscope
cystoscopy
cystostomy
cystotomy
cystoureteroscopy
cystourethritis
cystourethrography
cystourethroscopy
diabetes insipidus
diabetes mellitus

diabetic nephropathy
dialysis
distal tubule
diuresis
diuretic
dysuria
electromyography
enuresis
erythropoietin
Escherichia coli
excretion
extracorporeal
extracorporeal shock wave
   lithotripsy
extracystic
fibrous
Foley catheter
frequency
genitourinary
glomerular filtration rate
glomeruli
glomerulonephritis
glomerulopathy
glomerulus
glycosuria
gonococcus
gonorrhea
hematuria
hemodialysis
hemorrhage
hesitancy
hilus
homeostasis
hydronephrosis
hydroureter
hyperglycemia
hypertension
immunosuppressive
incontinence
indwelling catheter
insulin
interrenal
intracellular
intravenous pyelogram
intravenous pyelography
intravenous urography
Kegel exercises
ketoacidosis
ketone
ketonuria
kidney dialysis
laparoscopic nephrectomy

lipid
litholysis
lithotripsy
lithotrite
loop of Henle
microbiology
microorganism
micturition
nephrectomy
nephritis
nephrolith
nephrolithiasis
nephrolithotomy
nephrolysis
nephromalacia
nephromegaly
nephron
nephropexy
nephroptosis
nephrosclerosis
nephroscope
nephroscopy
nephrosonography
nephrostomy
nephrostomy tube
nephrotic syndrome
nephrotomogram
nephrotomography
nephrotoxic
nephroureterectomy
nocturia
nycturia
obstructive nephropathy
oliguria
percutaneous
   nephrostomy
percutaneous transluminal
   angioplasty
perineal muscles
peritoneal dialysis
polycystic
polycystic kidney
polyp
polyuria
prostaglandin
prostate
proteinuria
proximal tubule
pus cells
pyelitis
pyelogram
pyelography

pyelolithotomy
pyelonephritis
pyeloplasty
pyuria
reabsorption
rectourethral
renal
renal angiography
renal artery
renal artery stenosis
renal calculus
renal carcinoma
renal clearance
renal failure
renal pelvis
renal threshold
renal transplant
renal vein
renal vein thrombosis
renin
renography
renovascular
retention
sensitivity test
sexually transmitted
   disease
specific gravity
stenosis
stress incontinence
stricture
suprapubic
suprapubic catheterization
suprapubic cystotomy
suprarenal
symphysis pubis
thrombectomy
thrombus
toxemia
transureteroureterostomy
transurethral resection
trasurethral resection of
   the prostate
tubule
urea
uremia
ureter
ureteral
ureteral catheterization
ureterectomy
ureteritis
ureterocele
ureterocystoneostomy

ureterocystostomy
ureterolith
ureterolithiasis
ureterolithotomy
ureteroneocystostomy
ureteropathy
ureteroplasty
ureteropyelitis
ureteropyelonephritis
ureterostenosis
ureterostomy
ureteroureterostomy

urethra
urethral
urethral catheterization
urethritis
urethrocele
urethrocystitis
urethrography
urethrorectal
urethrorrhagia
urethrorrhea
urethroscopy
urethrospasm

urethrostenosis
urethrotomy
urethrovaginal
urgency
urinalysis
urinary
urinary calculi
urinary cast
urinary meatus
urinary reflux
urinometer
urodynamic studies

urogenital
urography
urolithiasis
uropathy
vaginitis
venereal disease
vesical
vesicovaginal
voided specimen
voiding
voiding cystourethrogram

español ENHANCING SPANISH COMMUNICATION

ENGLISH	SPANISH (PRONUNCIATION)
acidity	acidez (ah-se-DES)
catheter	catéter (cah-TAY-ter)
dialysis	diálisis (de-AH-le-sis)
excretion	excreción (ex-cray-se-ON)
renal artery	arteria renal (ar-TAY-re-ah ray-NAHL)
renal calculus	cálculo renal (CAHL-coo-lo ray-NAHL)
urinalysis	urinálisis (oo-re-NAH-le-sis)
urinary	urinario (oo-re-NAH-re-o)
urinate	orinar (o-re-NAR)
urination	urinación (oo-re-nah-se-ON)
voiding	urinar (oo-re-NAR)

CHAPTER 12

Reproductive System

LEARNING GOALS

In this chapter, you will learn to do the following:

Basic Understanding
1. Identify and match the structures and functions of the male and female reproductive systems.
2. Name the three types of uterine tissue.
3. Write the meanings of the word parts and use them to build and analyze terms.

Greater Comprehension
4. Use word parts from this chapter to determine the meaning of terms in a health care report.
5. Spell the terms accurately.
6. Pronounce the terms correctly.
7. Write the meanings of the abbreviations.
8. Categorize terms as anatomy, diagnostic test or procedure, pathology, surgery, or therapy.

THESE ARE THE MAJOR SECTIONS IN THIS CHAPTER:

❏ **Female Reproductive System**
Anatomy and Physiology
  Ovarian and Uterine Cycles
Diagnostic Tests and Procedures
Pathologies
Surgical and Therapeutic
  Interventions

❏ **Male Reproductive System**
Anatomy and Physiology
  Spermatogenesis
Diagnostic Tests and Procedures
Pathologies
Surgical and Therapeutic
  Interventions

FUNCTION FIRST

The male and female reproductive systems include the gonads (ovaries and testes), where sex cells and hormones are produced, and other organs, ducts, and glands that transport and sustain the egg or sperm cells.

Female Reproductive System

ANATOMY AND PHYSIOLOGY

genitalia

12-1 The female reproductive system includes the ovaries, fallopian tubes, uterus, vagina, accessory glands, and external genital structures. The ovaries are the female gonads. A gonad **(go′nad)** produces the reproductive cells. Information about the breasts, often considered a part of this system, is found in Chapter 17, which covers hormones and the endocrine system.

The reproductive organs, whether male or female, are called the genitals or genitalia **(jen″ĭ-tāl′e-ə)**. The combining form *genit(o)* refers to organs of reproduction. The genitalia include both external and internal organs. Another name for genitals is _____.

Knowing that *ur(o)* means pertaining to urine or the urinary system, *uro/genit/al* or *genito/urinary* (GU) means pertaining to the urinary and the reproductive systems.

females

12-2 The combining form that means woman or female is *gynec(o)*. The medical specialty that treats diseases of the female reproductive organs is gynecology.
Gyneco/logic **(gi″nə, jin″ə-kə-loj′ik)** means pertaining to gynecology (Gyn) or study of diseases that occur only in _____.

internal

12-3 Examine Table 12-1, which lists the internal and external structures of the female genitalia. Note that the ovaries, uterus, vagina, and several glands make up the _____ structures of the female genitalia.

Label the internal structures on Figure 12-1 as you read this frame. The right ovary **(o′və-re)** and left ovary are the primary reproductive structures because they produce ova (eggs) and hormones. The singular form of ova is ovum. The drawing in Figure 12-1 is a midsagittal view of the internal genitalia, so only one ovary is shown. Label line 1 the ovary. Ovaries are about the size and shape of an almond.

One fallopian tube is associated with each ovary. Label line 2 the fallopian tube. These tubes are also called uterine tubes, because they extend laterally from the upper portion of the uterus to the region of the ovary. There is no direct connection between the ovary and the fingerlike projections of the fallopian tube, the fimbriae. When an ovum (singular form of ova) is produced, the fimbriae create currents that sweep the ovum into the tube, and it is then carried along toward the uterus over the next 5 to 7 days. The fallopian tube is the most common site of fertilization of the ovum, which disintegrates or dies within 24 to 48 hours if it is not fertilized.

The uterus **(u′tər-əs)** is a muscular organ that prepares to receive and nurture the fertilized ovum. Label line 3 the uterus. The uterus is hollow and pear shaped. The lower and narrower part that has the outlet from the uterus is the cervix uteri **(sər′viks u′tər-i)**, commonly called the uterine cervix (Cx). When used alone, the term *cervix* often means the cervix uteri. Label line 4 in the drawing the cervix uteri.

The vagina **(və-ji′nə)**, commonly called the birth canal, is muscular and capable of sufficient expansion for passage of the child during childbirth. It also serves as the repository for sperm during intercourse. The vagina is the connection between the internal genitalia and the outside through its opening called the vaginal orifice (opening). Label line 5 the vagina.

TABLE 12-1 The Female Genitalia

Internal Structures	External Structures (Vulva)
Left ovary and associated left uterine tube	Mons pubis
Right ovary and associated right uterine tube	Labia majora
Uterus	Labia minora
Vagina	Clitoris
Special glands	Prepuce
	Openings for glands

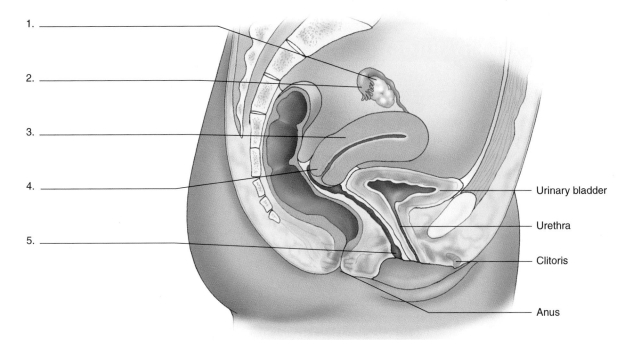

1. _____

2. _____

3. _____

4. _____

5. _____

Urinary bladder

Urethra

Clitoris

Anus

Figure 12-1   Female genitalia, midsagittal section. Identification of the genitalia is completed as you write the names of the structures in the blank lines. Structures other than the genitalia are shown with black labels and are included to show their close proximity to the reproductive structures. The urinary bladder and urethra are structures of the urinary apparatus; the anus is part of the digestive system.

Learn the following word parts that are used to write terms about the female genitalia.

Word Parts for the Female Genitalia

WORD PARTS	MEANING	OTHER WORD PARTS	MEANING
cervic(o)	neck; uterine cervix	o(o)	egg (ovum)
colp(o), vagin(o)	vagina	lapar(o)	abdominal wall
genit(o)	organs of reproduction	men(o)	month
hyster(o), uter(o)	uterus	top(o)	place or position
metr(o)	measure, uterine tissue	-tropin	that which stimulates
oophor(o), ovari(o)	ovary		
perine(o)	perineum		
salping(o)	fallopian tube		
vulv(o)	vulva		

ovary

12-4 Two words parts mean ovary: *ovari(o)* and *oophor(o)*. The combining form *ovari(o)* is generally used to write terms that describe the structure of the ovary. *Ovari/an* (**o-var′e-ən**) means pertaining to the _____.

salping(o)

12-5 Write the combining form that is used to write terms about the uterine tubes: _____.

uterus
(your answer choice)

Two combining forms that mean uterus are *uter(o)* and *hyster(o)*. You have already used the term *uterine* (**u′tər-in**), which means pertaining to the _____.

Write any word that you know that begins with *hyster(o)*: _____.

Many students will think of words such as *hysterics*, *hysterical*, or *hysterectomy*. All these words use the combining form *hyster(o)*, which means uterus. The use of *hyster(o)* as a combining form may have originated with the ancient Greeks, who believed that women were especially susceptible to emotional disorders that arose from the womb. The Greeks used the word *hysterikos* to refer to suffering in the womb and the emotional upheaval caused by this suffering.

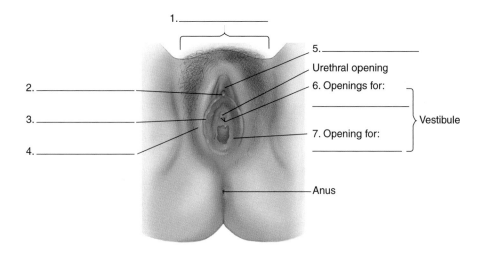

1._____

5._____
Urethral opening
6. Openings for:
_____
7. Opening for:
_____
⎫
⎬ Vestibule
⎭

2._____

3._____

4._____

Anus

Figure 12-2   Female external genitalia. These structures are external to the vagina and are also called the vulva.

vagina

vagina

12-6 The vagina is the birth canal, the receptacle for receiving sperm, and the passageway for menstrual flow. Both *vagin(o)* and *colp(o)* mean vagina. *Vaginal* (**vaj′ĭ-nəl**) is an adjective and refers to the _____.

Knowing that *cyst(o)* means bladder, colpo/cyst/itis is inflammation of the _____ and the urinary bladder.

12-7 Look again at the external structures that are listed in Table 12-1. *Vulva* refers to the external genitalia in the female, and the combining form is *vulv(o)*.

Vulv/ar (**vul′vər**) or *vulv/al* (**vul′vəl**) are terms that mean pertaining to the

vulva

_____.

12-8 Look at Figure 12-2, noting the structures that comprise the vulva. These structures are external to the vagina. Label the structures as you read the following material.

The mons* pubis (**monz pu′bis**) is a pad of fatty tissue and thick skin that overlies a bone called the symphysis pubis. The pubis is the anterior portion of the hipbones. After puberty, the mons pubis is covered with hair. Label line 1 in Figure 12-2 the mons pubis.

The clitoris (**klit′ə-ris, kli′tə-ris, klĭ-tor′is**) is a small mass of erectile tissue and nerves that has similarities to the male penis. This small mass of erectile tissue becomes erect in response to sexual stimulation. Label line 2 the clitoris.

Two pairs of skin folds, the labia (**la′be-ə**) majora and the labia minora, protect the vaginal opening.

minora

The smaller pair of skin folds is called the labia _____. Write the name of these structures on line 3 in the drawing.

majora

The larger pair of skin folds is called the labia _____. Write the name of these structures on line 4 in the drawing.

The labia minora merge and form a hood over the clitoris. This fold of skin that forms a retractable cover is called the prepuce (**pre′pūs**). Label line 5 the prepuce.

near

Label line 6 the paraurethral glands. The name of the para/urethral (**par″ə-u-re′thrəl**) glands tell us they are located _____ the urethra.

Other glands, the vestibular glands, lie adjacent to the vaginal opening. Label line 7 the vestibular glands.

12-9 Vestibule (**ves′tĭ-būl**) is any space or cavity at the entrance to a canal. The vaginal vestibule is the space between the two labia minora into which the urethra and vagina open. The greater vestibular glands (Bartholin's glands) produce a mucuslike secretion for lubrication during sexual intercourse.

*Mons (Latin: *mons,* mountain).

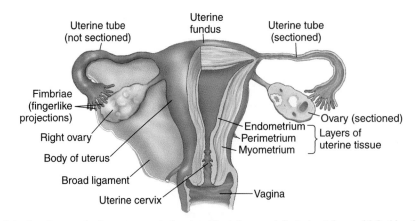

Figure 12-3   Organs of the female reproductive system, anterior view. The left ovary, left uterine tube, and left side of the uterus are sectioned to show their internal structure. Peritoneum and ligaments hold the reproductive structures in place.

perineum

Another important locational term is *perineum* (**per″ĭ-ne′əm**), the area between the vaginal opening and the anus. The combining form *perine(o)* means perineum. *Perine/al* means pertaining to the _____.

12-10 The uterus is the normal site where a fertilized ovum implants and develops. Examine the anterior view of the female genitalia in Figure 12-3.

The uterus consists of an upper portion, a large main portion, and a narrow region that connects with the vagina. The upper, bulging surface of the uterus, above the entrance of the uterine tubes, is called the uterine _____.

fundus (fun′dəs)

The large, main portion is called the body of the uterus, and the narrow region is the uterine _____.

cervix

12-11 The word *cervix* refers to the neck itself or part of an organ that resembles a neck. The cervix uteri specifically means the lower, necklike portion of the uterus, although it is common to see cervix written alone and meaning the cervix uteri. The proper name of the uterine cervix is the cervix _____.

uteri

The combining form *cervic(o)* means neck or cervix uteri. Look at other parts of a term to decide which meaning of *cervic(o)* is intended. *Colpo/cervic/al* (**kol″po-sər′vĭ-kəl**) refers to the vagina and cervix _____.

uteri

12-12 You have learned that *uter(o)* and *hyster(o)* mean uterus. A third combining form, *metr(o)*, also means the uterus, and occasionally *metr(o)* means measure.

Whenever you see *metr(o)* used in a word, you will need to decide if it means measure or _____ tissue. It is not as difficult as it might seem. For example, *metr/itis* (**mə-tri′tis**) could only refer to inflammation of _____ tissue.

uterine

uterine

12-13 The uterus consists of three layers of tissue. From the outermost layer to the innermost layer, the layers are called perimetrium (**per″ĭ-me′tre-əm**), myometrium (**mi-o-me′tre-əm**), and endometrium (**en″do-me′tre-əm**). Find these three layers of uterine tissue in Figure 12-3.

The outer layer is visceral peritoneum and is called peri/metr/ium. Analyzing its word parts, *peri* means around, *metr(o)* means _____ tissue, and *-ium* means membrane. In other words, perimetrium is a membrane that surrounds the uterus.

uterine

The myo/metr/ium (*my[o]* means muscle) is the thick muscular wall of the uterus. The inner layer, the endo/metr/ium, is a mucous membrane. Write the name of this mucous membrane that lines the uterus: _____.

endometrium

Exercise 1

Write word parts or meanings as indicated in the following blanks.

COMBINING FORM	MEANING
1. colp(o)	_____
2. genit(o)	_____
3. hyster(o)	_____
4. men(o)	_____
5. metr(o)	_____
6. o/o	_____
7. oophor(o)	_____
8. ovari(o)	_____
9. uter(o)	_____
10. vagin(o)	_____
11. _____	perineum
12. _____	cervix uteri or neck
13. _____	fallopian tube
14. _____	vulva

Exercise 2

Match terms in the left column with definitions or descriptions in the right column.

_____ 1. ovary

_____ 2. ovum

_____ 3. uterus

_____ 4. fallopian tube

_____ 5. vagina

A. a gonad
B. its endometrium sloughs off in menstruation
C. receives the sperm during intercourse
D. reproductive cell
E. usual site of fertilization

Ovarian and Uterine Cycles

12-14 During much of a female's life, the endometrium goes through a monthly cycle of growth and discharge known as the menstrual cycle. Reproductive cycles normally occur in females from shortly after the onset of menstruation to menopause.

The monthly cycle of growth and discharge of the endometrium is called the _____ cycle.

menstrual

12-15 The hypothalamus (part of the brain) and the pituitary gland, located just beneath the brain, secrete hormones that have significant roles in the control of reproductive functions. The hormones produced by these structures act on the ovaries to bring about two important functions: the production of ova and additional hormones (estrogen [es′trə-jen] and progesterone [pro-jes′tə-rōn]) and ova.

Female reproductive cycles begin at puberty (pu′bər-te) and continue for about 40 years until menopause (men′o-pawz). Puberty is that stage of development when genitalia reach maturity and secondary sex characteristics appear. The external characteristics of sexual maturity include adult distribution of hair and development of the penis or breasts and the labia. The onset of puberty normally occurs in females between 9 and 13 years of age with the development of breasts and menarche (**mə-nahr′ke**). Menarche is the first occurrence of menstruation (**men″stroo-a′shən**), the periodic bloody discharge caused by the shedding of the endometrium from the nonpregnant uterus. Write this term that means the first menstruation: _____.

Menopause, also called the climacteric (**kli-mak′tər-ik**), is the natural cessation of reproductive cycles and menstruation with the decline of reproductive hormones in later years. Menopause may occur earlier as a result of illness or surgical removal of the uterus or both ovaries. Write the term that means menopause: _____.

12-16 Paying particular attention to its spelling, write the term that means the periodic (generally monthly) bloody discharge from the shedding of the endometrium: _____.

The secretion of female reproductive hormones follows monthly cyclic patterns that affect the ovaries and uterus. Together, these cycles, called the ovarian cycle and the menstrual (uterine) cycle, make up the female reproductive cycle. The ovarian cycle reflects the changes that occur within the _____. The uterine (menstrual) cycle reflects the changes that take place in the _____. See Figure 12-4 for the correlation of events in the ovarian and uterine cycles.

12-17 The ovarian and uterine cycles begin at puberty when certain unknown stimuli cause the hypothalamus to start secreting a hormone that acts on the pituitary gland. The pituitary gland then begins to secrete two hormones, follicle-stimulating hormone (FSH) and luteinizing hormone (LH). Looking at Figure 12-4, you see that FSH and LH act on follicles in the _____.

The graafian follicle is a small ovarian recess or pit that contains fluid and surrounds an ovum (egg). Generally one ovum is released each month. The follicle produces hormones and grows in preparation for release of the ovum. These changes in the follicle are classified as the follicular phase, which is followed by the luteal phase. Find these two phases in the upper part of Figure 12-4. The follicular changes are represented by follicle development, _____, and corpus luteum.

Ovulation (**ov″u-la′shən**) is the release of the ovum from the follicle. After the ovum is released, the ruptured follicle enlarges, takes on a yellow appearance, and is called the corpus luteum, meaning yellow body. The luteal phase is named after the yellowish structure called the corpus _____.

12-18 Two important hormones that are secreted by the follicles influence the uterine cycle. During the follicular phase, increasing amounts of estrogen are secreted that stimulate repair of the endometrium. Estrogen reaches it peak near the middle of the cycle, then decreases until the next month. The corpus luteum secretes another important hormone, progesterone, which causes continued growth and thickening of the endometrium with additional preparatory activities to support a potential embryo. If fertilization (union of the ovum and sperm) does not occur, the corpus luteum begins to degenerate and the cycle starts again.

The initial hormone secreted by the ovarian follicle that causes the endometrium to thicken is _____.

This is the same hormone that brings about female secondary sex characteristics, the external physical signs of sexual maturity, such as development of the breasts and pubic hair.

A second hormone is secreted by the corpus luteum. That hormone is called _____.

12-19 The uterine cycle occurs simultaneously with the ovarian cycle and is the result of estrogen and progesterone secretion by the ovaries. Looking again at Figure 12-4, write down the phases of the uterine cycle: the menstrual phase, the proliferative phase, and the _____ phase.

The menstrual phase begins on day 1 of the cycle and continues for 3 to 5 days. The proliferative phase lasts for about 8 days. The name of this phase refers to the growth of the endometrium as it

---

Left margin terms:

menarche

climacteric

menstruation

ovaries
uterus

ovaries

ovulation

luteum

estrogen

progesterone

secretory

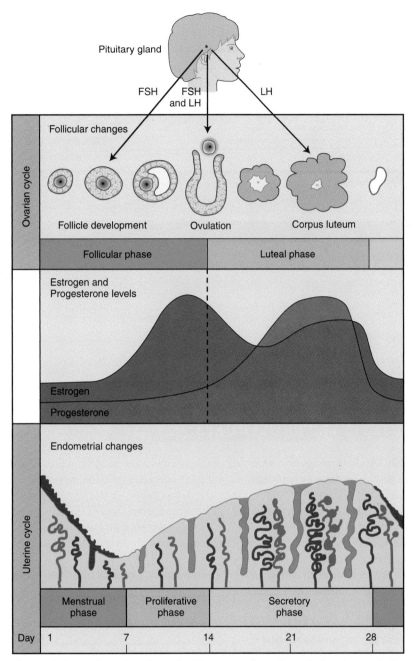

Figure 12-4   Correlation of events in the ovarian and uterine cycles. These two cycles make up the female reproductive cycle, with an average length of 28 days from the first day of bleeding of one cycle to the first day of bleeding of the next cycle.

thickens and glands and blood vessels develop in the new tissue. The endometrium continues to grow and thicken in the secretory phase, and in addition, begins to secrete glycogen, which will nourish a developing embryo if fertilization occurs.

The term *menses* means the normal flow of blood during menstruation when fertilization has not occurred. Menses and menstruation are often used interchangeably. Several of the terms pertaining to the menstrual cycle use the combining form *men(o)*, which means month. The events of the menstrual cycle are summarized in Table 12-2.

12-20 Estrogen and progesterone prepare the uterus for pregnancy. Write a word that means formation of ova, using the combining form for ovum, *o(o)*, and the suffix *-genesis*, which means origin or beginning: _____.

oogenesis
(o″o-jen′ə-sis)

TABLE 12-2 The Reproductive Cycle

Days	Ovarian Phase	Uterine (Menstrual) Phase
1-5	*Follicular phase.* Growth of the follicle. Secretion of estrogen.	Menses. Blood is shed from the vagina.
6-12	Follicular phase continues.	*Proliferative phase.* Growth of the endometrium.
13-14	*Ovulation.* Ovum is released by the follicle.	Proliferative phase continues.
15-28	*Luteal phase.* Follicle becomes corpus luteum. Secretes progesterone.	*Secretory phase.* Continued growth of endometrium, secretion of glycogen.

Exercise 3

Write a term for each description or definition.

1. another term for menses   _____

2. another term for menopause   _____

3. first occurrence of menstruation   _____

4. release of an ovum from the ovarian follicle   _____

5. initial hormone that causes thickening of the endometrium _____

DIAGNOSTIC TESTS AND PROCEDURES

12-21 Gynecologic problems and obstetric care account for one fifth of all female visits to physicians. Many diagnostic procedures and treatments are available to females with gynecologic disorders.

The physical assessment of the female reproductive system includes examination of the breasts, the external genitalia, and the pelvis. A vaginal speculum (spek′u-ləm) is an instrument that can be pushed apart after it is inserted into the vagina to allow examination of the cervix and the walls of the vagina (Figure 12-5).

A speculum is an instrument for examining body orifices (openings) or cavities. A speculum that

vaginal   is used to examine the vagina is a _____ speculum.

12-22 Specimens (scrapings) for cytology can be collected during the pelvic examination.

cells   Cyto/logy means the study of _____. Both Pap smears and endo/metrial biopsies are performed to detect cancer of the cervix.

Pap smear is an abbreviated way of saying Papanicolaou smear or test. In a Pap smear, material is collected from areas of the body that shed cells. The cells are then studied microscopically. A short-

Pap   ened way of saying Papanicolaou smear is _____ smear.

12-23 The term *Pap smear* may refer to collection of material from other surfaces that shed cells, but it usually refers to collection and examination of cells from the vagina and cervix (Figure 12-6). Early diagnosis of cancer of the cervix is possible with the Pap test. When the Pap smear is examined, malignant cells have a characteristic appearance that indicates cancer, sometimes before symptoms appear.

Cancer of the uterus may begin with a change in shape, growth, and number of cells, called dysplasia (dis-pla′zhə). The dysplasia (*dys-*, bad or difficult + *-plasia*, development) is not cancer, but cells of this type tend to become malignant. This abnormality, which can be detected before cancer

dysplasia   occurs, is called _____.

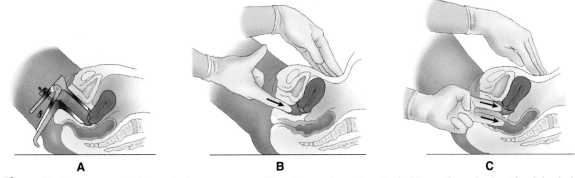

A   **B**   **C**

Figure 12-5   The gynecologic examination. **A,** Proper position of inserted speculum. **B,** The bimanual examination. The abdominal hand presses the pelvic organs toward the intravaginal hand. **C,** Rectovaginal examination. The examiner's index finger is placed in the vagina and the middle finger is inserted into the rectum. The gynecologic inspection consists of four parts: (1) Inspection of the external genitalia. (2) The speculum examination. The vaginal walls and cervix are inspected. Smears (Pap smear, for cytologic examination) are obtained. (3) Bimanual examination assesses the location, size, and mobility of the pelvic organs. (4) The rectovaginal examination is not always performed. In this examination, the posterior aspect of the genital organs and rectal tissue can be evaluated.

It is standard practice to grade Pap smears as class I, II, III, IV, or V. Class I is normal, and class V is definitely cancer. Most physicians recommend having Pap smears done on a routine basis. Regular Pap smears are an excellent method for early detection of cervical cancer, and it is possible that the lesion can be excised, thus preventing spread of cancer to other organs.

12-24 Specimens of vaginal or cervical discharge are collected and tested for the presence of micoorganisms using several techniques. Wet mounts, the direct microscopic examination of the fluid, aid in diagnosis of infections with yeast or *Trichomonas*, a vaginal and urethral parasite. Gram stain, a slide-staining technique that aids in classification and identification of bacteria, is especially useful for vaginal smears if gonorrhea is suspected. Bacterial or fungal cultures may also be helpful in identifying the cause of infections.

The Venereal Disease Research Laboratories (VDRL) test and the rapid plasma reagin (RPR) test are blood tests to detect and monitor syphilis.

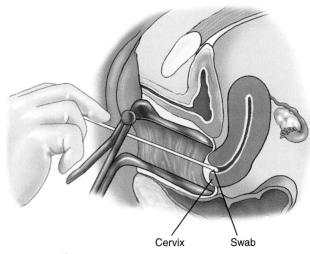

Cervix   Swab

Figure 12-6   Obtaining a cervical Pap smear.

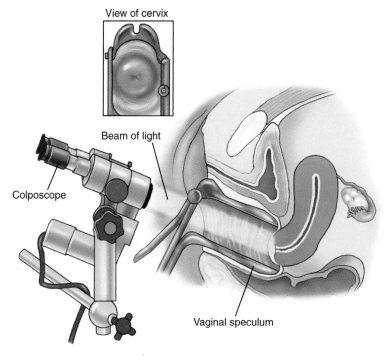

View of cervix

Beam of light

Colposcope

Vaginal speculum

Figure 12-7   Colposcopy.

Levels of hormones in the blood and urine are helpful in determining the function of the ovaries, particularly in fertility studies and pregnancy. <u>Human chorionic gonadotropin</u> (**go′nə-do-tro″pin**) (HCG) is present in body fluids of pregnant females, and blood or urine is tested to determine if pregnancy exists. *Chorion/ic* pertains to the chorion, a membrane that develops around a fertilized embryo. Gonado/tropin (*gonad(o)* + *-tropin*, that which stimulates) is a hormonal substance that stimulates the _____—in this case, the ovaries.

HCG can be detected long before other signs of pregnancy appear. This test may also be used to detect rare forms of tumors in either men or women, but more often, the test is performed to ascertain pregnancy. Write the name of the hormone that is tested for in pregnancy tests: human chorionic _____.

12-25 <u>Colposcopy</u> (**kol-pos′kə-pe**) involves the use of a low-powered microscope to magnify the mucosa of the vagina and the cervix. The instrument used is a _____ (Figure 12-7).

Suspicious cervical or vaginal lesions may be seen during colposcopy. Some findings indicate the need for a cervical or endometrial biopsy. A <u>cervical biopsy</u> is removal of tissue from the _____. An <u>endometrial biopsy</u> requires collection of tissue from the lining of the _____.

12-26 <u>Hysteroscopy</u> (**his″tər-os′kə-pe**) is direct visual inspection of the cervical canal and uterine cavity, using an <u>endoscope</u> passed through the vagina. Hysteroscopy is performed for several reasons, including the excision of cervical polyps, the collection of tissue for biopsy, and removal of an intrauterine device. Change the suffix of hysteroscopy to write the name of the endoscope: _____.

12-27 <u>Pelvic ultrasonography</u> may be helpful in detecting masses, such as ovarian cysts. <u>Computed tomography</u> (CT) may be used to detect a tumor within the pelvis.

<u>Hystero/salpingo/graphy</u> (**his″tər-o-sal″ping-gog′rə-fe**) is radiologic examination of the uterus and the _____ tubes after an injection of radiopaque material into those organs. It allows evaluation of the size, shape, and position of the organs, including tumors and certain other abnormalities, as well as obstruction of a uterine tube.

Sidebar terms:

gonads

gonadotropin

colposcope
(**kol′po-skōp**)

cervix
uterus

hysteroscope
(**his′tər-o-skōp**)

uterine or fallopian

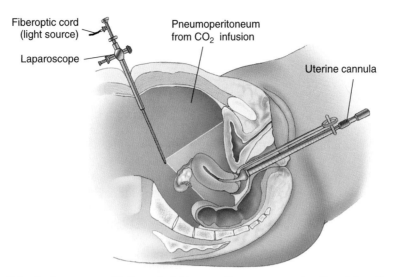

Figure 12-8 Laparoscopy. Using the laparoscope with fiberoptic light source, the surgeon can view the pelvic cavity and the reproductive organs. Further instrumentation, for example, for tubal sterilization, is possible through a second small incision. The purpose of the uterine cannula is to allow movement of the uterus during laparoscopy.

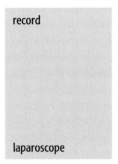

record

A <u>hysterosalpingogram</u> (**his″tər-o-sal-ping′go-gram**) is the_____ that is produced in hysterosalpingography.

12-28 <u>Laparo/scopy</u> (**lap″ə-ros′kə-pe**) is the examination of the abdominal cavity with a <u>laparoscope</u> (**lap′ə-ro-skōp**) through one or more small incisions in the abdominal wall. This surgical procedure is especially useful for inspection of the ovaries and other structures within the pelvic cavity, as well as collection of biopsy specimens or performance of tubal ligation to prevent pregnancy (Figure 12-8). Write the name of the instrument used in laparoscopy:

laparoscope

_____.

Exercise 4

Write a term in each of the blanks to complete the sentences. The first letter of each term is given as a clue.

1. An instrument that is used to examine the walls of the vagina and the cervix is a vaginal

   s_____.

2. The study of cells in a Pap test is called c_____.

3. In a Pap smear, an alteration in the shape, growth, or number of cells that is not a sign of cancer, but indicates a tendency

   of the cells to become malignant, is called d_____.

4. A hormone that is tested to ascertain pregnancy is human chorionic g_____.

5. The use of a low-powered microscope to examine the mucosa of the vagina and the cervix is called

   c_____.

6. Direct visualization of the uterus with a hysteroscope is h_____.

7. A radiographic examination of the uterus and the uterine tubes after an injection of a radiopaque contrast medium is called

   h_____.

8. Examination of the pelvic cavity after making one or more small incisions in the abdominal wall is

   l_____.

PATHOLOGIES

12-29 Menstrual disorders include painful menstruation, heavy or irregular flow, spotting, absence of or skipping periods, and premenstrual syndrome.

Build a word by combining *men(o)* and *-rrhea* (flow or discharge):

menorrhea
(men″o-re′ə)

_____. *Menorrhea* means either normal menstruation or too profuse menstruation. Because of the double meaning of menorrhea, it would be clearer to use either of the following terms to mean the normal monthly flow of blood from the genital tract:

menstruation

_____ or menses.

The second meaning of menorrhea is profuse menstruation. Build a word that is a synonym for this meaning by using the combining form for month and the suffix for hemorrhage:

menorrhagia
(men″o-ra′jə)

_____.

<u>Menorrhagia</u> is abnormally heavy or long menstrual periods.

12-30 <u>Metrorrhagia</u> **(me″tro-ra′je-ə)** is uterine bleeding other than that caused by menstruation. It may occur as spotting or outright bleeding, the period of flow sometimes being prolonged. The literal translation of metro/rrhagia is _____ of the uterus.

hemorrhage

Metrorrhagia may be caused by uterine tumors, benign or malignant, and especially cervical cancer.

12-31 <u>A/menorrhea</u> **(ə-men″o-re′ə)** is _____ of menstruation.

absence

Amenorrhea is normal before puberty, after menopause, and during pregnancy. Underdevelopment of the reproductive organs or hormonal disturbances can cause absence of the onset of menstruation

amenorrhea

at puberty. This absence of menstruation is called _____.

When menstruation has begun but then ceases, this is also called amenorrhea.

12-32 <u>Dys/menorrhea</u> **(dis-men″ə-re′ə)** is painful or difficult

menstruation

_____.

<u>Mittelschmerz</u>* **(mit′əl-shmertz)** means abdominal pain in the region of an ovary during ovulation. It is helpful in pinpointing the fertile period of the ovarian cycle.

12-33 <u>Premenstrual syndrome</u> (PMS) is nervous tension, irritability, edema, headache, and painful breasts that can occur the last few days before the onset of menstruation. Various studies indicate that many females experience some degree of PMS but fewer than half experience symptoms that

premenstrual

disrupt their lives. *PMS* means _____ syndrome.

12-34 <u>Cervic/itis</u> **(sər″vĭ-si′tis)** refers specifically to inflammation of the cervix uteri. Acute cervicitis is infection of the cervix marked by redness, bleeding on contact, and often pain, itching, or burning, and a foul-smelling discharge from the vagina. Acute cervicitis may be caused by several species of bacteria, *Chlamydia* (specialized bacteria), *Candida albicans* (yeast), or the parasite *Trichomonas vaginalis*. Some <u>sexually transmitted diseases</u> (STDs)—for example, <u>gonorrhea</u>—cause cervicitis. Diagnosis of gonorrhea can often be made by examination of a stained smear and is confirmed by culture.

cervicitis

Persistent inflammation of the cervix is called chronic _____.

12-35 <u>Vagin/itis</u> **(vaj″ĭ-ni′tis)** is inflammation of the vaginal tissues. This may be accompanied by itching, burning or discomfort during urination, and vaginal discharge, but some infections are asymptomatic. Many of these lower genital tract infections are related to sexual intercourse, which can irritate vaginal tissues and transmit microorganisms. Vaginal infections are sometimes considered a sexually transmitted disease, but an infection can also occur following childbirth or after taking antibiotics that produce changes in the vaginal tissues and allow overgrowth of normal bacterial flora such as C. *albicans*.

vaginitis

Write this term that means infection of the vagina: _____. This is the same as <u>colp/itis</u> **(kol-pi′tis)**.

---

*Mittelschmerz (German: *mittel*, mid, middle + *schmerz*, pain, suffering).

vulva

12-36 <u>Vulv/itis</u> is inflammation of the _____ and is associated with itching and burning. This can be caused by infection, contact with irritants, or systemic conditions. Irritants such as soaps and detergents or allergens can cause vulvitis, as well as dryness of the tissues and hormonal changes, particularly associated with aging. Sexually transmitted diseases should particularly be considered if lesions are present such as venereal warts or the blisters that occur with genital herpes. See information about sexually transmitted diseases in Chapter 13.

12-37 <u>Vulvo/vaginitis</u> (**vul″vo-vaj″ĭ-ni′tis**) is inflammation of the vulva and vagina. Vulvar infections can be extensions of vaginal infections. Vulvo/vagin/al candidiasis is infection of the vagina and vulva with *C. albicans*. An infection caused by *Candida* is called <u>candidiasis</u> (**kan″dĭ-di′ə-sis**). Remembering that *-iasis* means condition, write this term that means a condition caused by

candidiasis

C. albicans: _____.

disease
oophoritis
(o″of-ə-ri′tis)

12-38 Practice using *oophor(o)* to write pathologies of the ovaries.
<u>Oophoropathy</u> (**o-of″ə-rop′ə-the**) is any _____ of an ovary.
    Inflammation of an ovary is _____.

    <u>Oophor/algia</u> (**o″of-ər-al′jə**) is also called ovarian pain.

ovary

    <u>Oophoro/salping/itis</u> (**o-of″ə-ro-sal″pin-ji′tis**) is inflammation of an _____ and a fallopian tube.

12-39 <u>An/ovulation</u> (**an″ov-u-la′shən**), absence of ovulation, is failure of the ovaries to produce, mature, or release ova. Its causes include altered ovarian function or dysfunction, side effects of medications, or the result of stress or disease. Write this term that means lack of ovulation:

anovulation

_____.
    <u>Polycystic ovary syndrome</u> is a hormonal disturbance characterized by anovulation, amenorrhea, and infertility. It is caused by increased levels of testosterone (male hormone), estrogen, and luteinizing hormone and decreased secretion of FSH. Numerous cysts may develop, with the affected ovary sometimes doubling in size.

12-40 Polycystic ovary syndrome differs from what is usually meant by the term <u>*ovarian cyst*</u>, which is a globular sac filled with fluid or semisolid material that develops in or on the ovary. This type of ovarian cyst may be transient or pathologic. Benign cysts are common and may be asymptomatic, or they may cause pelvic pain and menstrual irregularities. If a female is a/symptomatic, this

without

means that she is _____ symptoms.
    <u>Ovarian cancer</u> is the leading cause of death from reproductive cancers, because the disease has usually spread to other organs by the time it is discovered (Figure 12-9). Sonography and CT may detect the ovarian mass, but diagnosis generally requires surgical exploration.

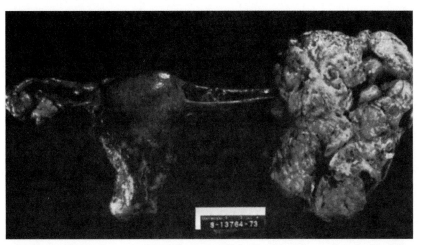

Figure 12-9   Carcinoma of the ovary. The specimen consists of the uterus with both uterine tubes and ovaries. The left ovary is enormously enlarged by a tumor; the right ovary shows a white area that also contains a tumor. Note the asymmetry of the body of the uterus (a congenital abnormality in this patient that is not related to ovarian carcinoma).

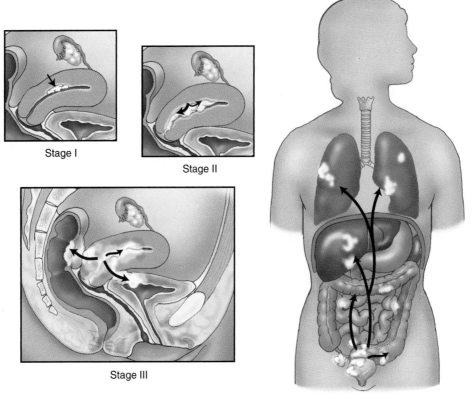

Stage I

Stage II

Stage III

Stage IV

Figure 12-10   Staging uterine cancer. Stage I: Tumor is confined to the uterine corpus. Stage II: The cancer has invaded the cervix also. Stage III: The cancer has spread beyond the uterus but remains confined to the pelvis, such as in the bladder or rectum. Stage IV: The highest level of invasiveness; the cancer has spread beyond the pelvis, causing metastatic disease and large masses, such as in the liver or lungs.

---

fallopian (or uterine)

salpingitis
(sal″pin-ji′tis)

12-41 <u>Salpingo/cele</u> (**sal-ping′go-sēl**) is hernial protrusion of a
_____ tube.
  Inflammation of a fallopian tube is _____.

An <u>ectopic</u> (**ek-top′ik**) <u>pregnancy</u> is one in which a fertilized ovum implants somewhere outside the uterine cavity. *Ectopic* (*ect[o]*, outside + *top[o]*, position + *-ic*, pertaining to) means situated in an unusual place, away from its normal location. The abnormal implantation site is usually in the fallopian tube, and this is called a <u>tubal pregnancy</u>. Treatment is generally removal of the pregnancy, often with removal of the fallopian tube.

pelvic

12-42 The fallopian tubes are usually infected in <u>pelvic inflammatory disease</u> (PID). Without treatment, the tubes can become obstructed and cause infertility. Pelvic inflammatory disease is any infection that involves the upper genital tract beyond the cervix. Untreated gonococcal or staphylococcal infections, for example, can spread along the endometrium to the fallopian tubes and cause an acute salpingitis. If untreated or treated inadequately, the tubes can become obstructed. *PID* means _____ inflammatory disease.
  <u>Septicemia</u> (*sept[o]*, infection + *-emia*, blood) and other severe complications rarely occur in PID as they do in <u>toxic shock syndrome</u> (TSS). A sudden high fever, headache, confusion, acute renal failure, and abnormal liver function are characteristic of TSS. This acute disease is caused by a type of *Staphylococcus* species and is most common in menstruating women who use tampons.

hysteropathy
(his″tə-rop′ə-the)

12-43 Cancer can occur in any of the reproductive structures and spread to other organs. The stage of <u>uterine cancer</u> is identified by the extent to which it has spread to other organs (Figure 12-10). Early removal of cancerous tissue is vital for preventing the spread of cancer. Write a word that means any disease of the uterus: _____.

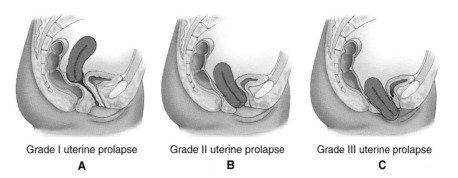

Grade I uterine prolapse
A

Grade II uterine prolapse
B

Grade III uterine prolapse
C

Figure 12-11   Three stages of uterine prolapse of increasing severity. Uterine prolapse may be congenital or may be caused by heavy physical exertion or other situations that weaken the pelvic supports. **A,** The uterus bulges into the vagina but does not protrude through the entrance. **B,** The uterus bulges farther into the vagina and the cervix protrudes through the entrance. **C,** The body of the uterus and the cervix protrude through the entrance to the vagina.

**hysteroptosis
(his″tər-op-to′sis)**

12-44 The uterus is normally held in its proper alignment with the vagina and the uterine tubes by ligaments that hold each structure in its proper place. Weakening of the ligaments causes a prolapsed uterus. Using *-ptosis*, write a word that means uterine prolapse:
_____.

A prolapsed uterus can be congenital or caused by heavy physical exertion. It is classified according to its severity (Figure 12-11).

12-45 The uterus normally lies midline in the pelvis; however, some variations, called uterine displacements, occur (Figure 12-12). Mild degrees of these four types of displacements are common, may or may not cause symptoms, and may be determined by the position of the cervix when the pelvic examination is performed. Use the information in Figure 12-12 to complete these sentences.

**anteversion
(an″te-vər′zhən)**

A forward displacement of the body of the uterus toward the pubis, the anterior portion of the hipbone, is _____.

**backward
anteflexion
(an-te-flek′shən)**

Retro/version (**ret″ro-ver′zhən**) is a common condition in which the uterus is tipped _____ and is the opposite of anteversion.
A bending forward of the uterus is called _____, and a bending backward of the uterus is retroflexion (**ret″ro-flek′shən**).

12-46 A uterine leiomyoma (*leio-*, smooth + *my[o]*, muscle + *-oma*, tumor) (**li″o-mi-o′mə**) is a benign tumor occurring in the uterus and is also called a uterine fibroid. Large tumors may cause a general enlargement of the lower abdomen. Write the name of this type of uterine tumor:
_____.

leiomyoma

Cervical polyps are benign lesions attached to the cervix, often by a stalk, and can sometimes be seen in a gynecologic examination.

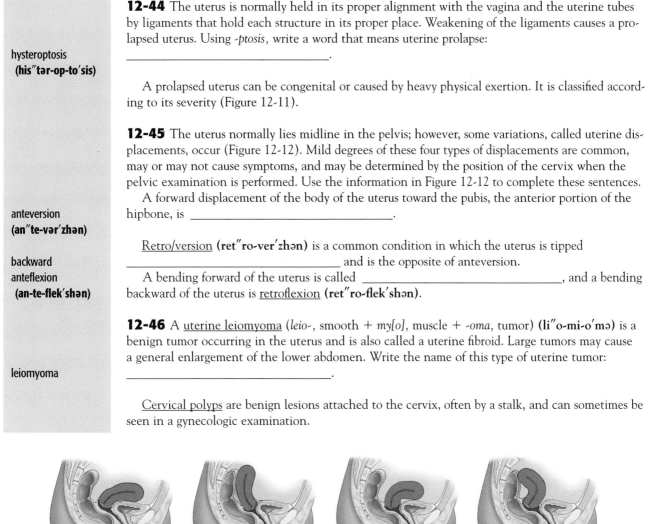

Anteversion
A

Retroversion
B

Anteflexion
C

Retroflexion
D

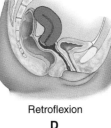

Figure 12-12   Normal versus abnormal (forward or backward) displacements of the uterus. **A,** Anteversion, forward displacement of the body of the uterus toward the pubis, with the cervix tilted up; **B,** retroversion, tipped backward, the opposite of anteversion; **C,** anteflexion, bending forward; **D,** retroflexion, bending backward.

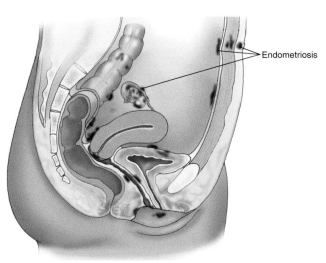
→ Endometriosis

Figure 12-13   Common sites of endometriosis. The abnormal location of endometrial tissue is often the ovaries and less commonly other pelvic structures.

myometritis
(mi″o-mə-tri′tis)

12-47 Write a term that means inflammation of the myometrium:
_____.

Endometritis (en″do-me-tri′tis) is inflammation of the endometrium and is generally produced by bacterial invasion of the endometrium.

Endometriosis (en″do-me″tre-o′sis), however, is an abnormal condition in which tissue that contains typical endometrial elements is present outside the uterus, usually within the pelvic cavity. See the common sites of endometriosis in Figure 12-13.

Endometrial tissue that is located outside the uterine lining responds to hormonal changes and goes through cyclic changes of bleeding and proliferation. Scarring and adhesions result. An adhesion is an abnormal adherence of structures that are not normally joined. A condition in which endometrium occurs in other places besides the uterus is called

endometriosis

_____.

vulvitis (vəl-vi′tis)

12-48 Write a term that means inflammation of the vulva: _____.

12-49 Leuko/rrhea (loo″ko-re′ə) normally occurs in the adult female and is somewhat increased before and after the menstrual period. It may be abnormal if there is an increase in amount or a change in color or odor.

white

Literal translation of *leuko/rrhea* is _____ discharge. This new term specifically refers to a white, viscid discharge from the vagina and the uterine cavity.

vagina

12-50 Colpo/dynia (kol″po-din′e-ə) is pain of the _____.
Use *colp(o)* to write a word that means hemorrhage from the vagina:

colporrhagia
(kol″po-ra′jə)

_____.

urethra

12-51 Vaginal fistulas are abnormal openings between the vagina and the urethra, the bladder, or the rectum. Urethro/vaginal (u-re″thro-vaj′ĭ-nəl) fistulas occur between the _____ and the vagina. A rectovaginal (rek″to-vaj′ĭ-nəl) fistula is one that occurs between the rectum and the vagina.

Knowing that *vesic(o)* means bladder, a vesicovaginal (ves″ĭ-ko-vaj′ĭ-nəl) fistula occurs between the urinary _____ and the vagina. (See the locations of these types of fistulas in Figure 12-14.)

bladder

12-52 A cysto/cele (*cyst[o]*, bladder + *-cele*, herniation) (sis′to-sēl), protrusion of the urinary bladder through the wall of the vagina, occurs when support is weakened between the two structures. A recto/cele (*rect[o]*, rectum) occurs from weakening between the vagina and rectum. Both problems are common and often asymptomatic. A large cystocele can interfere with emptying the bladder, and a large rectocele can interfere with emptying the rectum. (Compare these two types of herniations in Figure 12-15.)

Herniation of the urinary bladder through the wall of the vagina is called a

cystocele

_____.

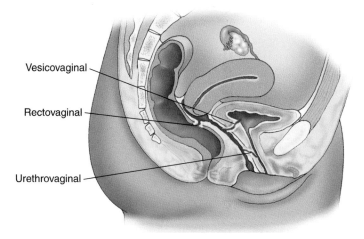

Vesicovaginal

Rectovaginal

Urethrovaginal

Figure 12-14 Sites of vaginal fistulas. Abnormal openings between the vagina and the bladder, rectum, and urethra are shown. These abnormal openings are called vesicovaginal fistula, rectovaginal fistula, and urethrovaginal fistula, respectively.

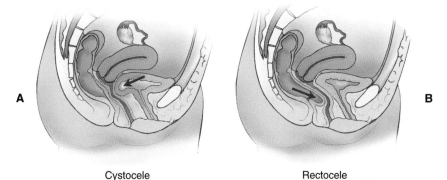

A

B

Cystocele

Rectocele

Figure 12-15 Comparison of a cystocele and a rectocele. **A,** Cystocele. The urinary bladder is displaced downward, causing bulging of the anterior vaginal wall. **B,** Rectocele. The rectum is displaced, causing bulging of the posterior vaginal wall.

Exercise 5

Match menstrual disorders in the left column with their descriptions in the right column.

_____ 1. amenorrhea

_____ 2. dysmenorrhea

_____ 3. menorrhagia

_____ 4. metrorrhagia

A. abnormally heavy or long menstrual periods
B. absence of menstruation
C. painful or difficult menstruation
D. uterine bleeding other than menstruation

Exercise 6

Write words in the blanks to complete these sentences.

1. *PMS* means _____ syndrome.

2. *Mittelschmerz* means pain in the region of the ovary during _____.

3. Failure of the ovaries to produce, mature, or release ova is _____.

4. The leading cause of death from reproductive cancer is _____ carcinoma.

5. *PID* means _____ inflammatory disease.

6. Weakening of the ligaments that hold the uterus in place is uterine _____.

7. A common uterine condition in which it is tipped backward is _____.

8. A uterine fibroid is also called a _____.

9. An abnormal opening between the rectum and the vagina is called a rectovaginal _____.

10. Herniation of the urinary bladder through the wall of the vagina is a _____.

SURGICAL AND THERAPEUTIC INTERVENTIONS

12-53 Contra/ceptives (*contra-*, against) are used to prevent conception—in other words, pregnancy. Read about the various methods of preventing pregnancy in Chapter 13.

Some of the most common gynecologic problems for which females seek treatment are vaginal discharge, bleeding, and pain. Dysmenorrhea, painful _____ flow, is caused by uterine cramping and can usually be alleviated with aspirin or antiinflammatory drugs such as ibuprofen. Advil is a common over-the-counter ibuprofen.

Other medications and changes in diet may be recommended for premenstrual syndrome.

menstrual

12-54 After the cause of amenorrhea is established, it is treated by surgical and pharmaceutical means (hormone replacement and stimulation of the ovaries, for example).

Menopause, though, is a natural termination of menstruation, and many women experience few if any unpleasant symptoms of hot flashes and night sweats. Hormone replacement therapy (HRT), a combination of estrogen and progesterone, is the primary intervention for women who suffer the symptoms of transition or those at high risk for osteoporosis, abnormal loss of bone density and deterioration of bone tissue. There is not agreement on the value versus risk of HRT: prevention of osteoporosis, heart disease, and Alzheimer's disease (progressive mental deterioration) versus the risks of breast and endometrial cancer. *HRT* means _____ replacement therapy.

hormone

12-55 Treatment of vulvitis can sometimes be as simple as avoiding contact with irritants, such as soaps or detergents. Therapeutic interventions for infections of the vulva, vagina, and cervix depend on the causative organism. Oral or topical antibiotics, vaginal creams, and suppositories (sə-poz′ĭ-tor-ēz) are prescribed according to the type of infection. Oral antibiotics are taken by _____. Topical (*top[o]*, position or place) medications, such as antibiotic ointments or gynecologic creams, are applied directly to the affected area. Vaginal suppositories are easily melted medicated materials that are inserted into the vagina.

Laser therapy may be performed for persistent vulvitis. Vulv/ectomy (vəl-vek′tə-me), _____ of the vulva, is characteristically used to treat cancer of the vulva.

mouth

excision

12-56 Vaginal and vulvar cancer are not common and occur mainly in women older than 50 years. Two terms that mean the removal of all or a part of the vagina are *vaginectomy* (vaj″ĭ-nek′tə-me) and _____. (In vaginal cancer, this surgical procedure may be part of a radical hysterectomy—removal of ovaries, fallopian tubes, lymph nodes, and lymph channels, as well as the uterus and cervix).

Remembering that *-rrhaphy* means suture, colporrhaphy (kol-por′ə-fe) is _____ of the vagina.

Surgical repair of the vagina is _____.

colpectomy
(kol-pek′tə-me)

suture
colpoplasty
(kol′po-plas″te)

12-57 The combining form *oophor(o)* is used to write most surgical terms concerning the ovaries. Using *oophor(o)*, write a word that means surgical fixation to correct an ovary that has lost its normal support: _____.

oophoropexy
(o-of′ə-ro-pek″se)

If benign ovarian cysts become large enough to cause pressure in the pelvis, they produce variable symptoms, including pain, menstrual irregularities, and urinary frequency. The cysts may be removed surgically, either using a laparoscope or open (abdominal) surgery, and in general, saving as much of the ovary as possible.

Removal of an adult female's ovaries prohibits reproduction and prevents further production of ovarian hormones. Oophor/ectomy (o″of-ə-rek′tə-me), surgical

excision

_____ of the ovaries, in a girl who has not reached puberty prevents development of secondary sex characteristics.

12-58 Treatment of ovarian cancer includes a combination of surgical removal of the uterus, ovaries, and uterine tubes, either preceding or following chemotherapy. A hyster/ectomy (his″tər-ek′tə-me) is removal of the _____. A hysterectomy and bilateral oophorosalpingectomy (o-of″ə-ro-sal″pin-jek′tə-me) is removal of the uterus, both ovaries, and

uterus

fallopian (uterine)

both _____ tubes.

When the uterus is removed through an incision in the abdominal wall, it is called an abdominal hysterectomy. When the ovaries and uterine tubes are also removed, it is called a total abdominal hysterectomy (TAH).

12-59 Oophoro/hyster/ectomy (o-of″ə-ro-his″tər-ek′tə-me) is removal of the

ovaries; uterus

_____ and the _____. If the uterus and the ovaries are removed, the fallopian tubes are also removed. In an oophorohysterectomy, it is understood that the fallopian tubes are removed also; however, if one wanted to include all these terms in one word, the word would be oophoro/salpingo/hyster/ectomy (o-of″ə-ro-sal-ping″go-his″tər-ek′tə-me).

12-60 Removal of the uterus is also commonly performed for large fibroids. Symptoms and treatment of fibroids vary widely. When a hyster/ectomy is performed, the uterus is

removed

_____.

In cases other than cancer, a hysterectomy is performed in one of three ways: abdominally, vaginally, or laparoscopically. A colpo/hyster/ectomy (kol″po-his″tər-ek′tə-me) is removal of the uterus by way of the vagina. In a colpohysterectomy, an abdominal incision is not required because the uterus is removed through the vagina. This is also called a _____

vaginal

hysterectomy.

In a few cases, the uterus can be removed laparoscopically. A laparo/hyster/ectomy (lap″ə-ro-his″tə-rek′tə-me) is removal of the uterus through a small opening in the

abdominal

_____ wall.

12-61 Salpingectomy (sal″pin-jek′tə-me) is surgical removal of one or both

uterine

_____ tubes. It is performed for removal of a tumor or cyst, or as a method of sterilization, and is included in a hysterectomy and oophorectomy.

A tubal ligation (lĭ-ga′shən) is one of several sterilization procedures in which both uterine tubes are constricted, severed, or crushed to prevent conception. The procedure originally involved the use of a ligature (a substance that tied or constricted), hence its name. This is now most often performed laparoscopically. Tubal ligation can be reversed in some cases by making a new opening to restore patency (condition of being open), but this is not always successful. Salpingostomy (sal″ping-gos′tə-me),

opening

making a new _____ into a uterine tube, may be performed also for the purpose of drainage if a uterine tube is obstructed by infection or scar tissue.

12-62 A common surgical procedure that is performed for either diagnosis or treatment is dilation and curettage (ku″rə-tahzh′) (D & C). In this procedure, the cervix is dilated to allow the insertion of a curet into the uterus. The curet is a surgical instrument shaped like a spoon or scoop and is used for scraping and removal of material from the endometrium. In this procedure, called D & C,

cervix
endometrium

what structure is dilated? _____. What structure is scraped? _____.

This surgical procedure is done to assess disease of the uterus, to correct heavy or prolonged vaginal bleeding, or to empty the uterus of residue after childbirth.

12-63 Cryo/therapy (kri″o-ther′ə-pe), also called cryosurgery (kri″o-sər′jər-e), is a treatment that uses a subfreezing temperature to destroy tissue. Cryosurgery and laser surgery are especially useful in the treatment of lesions of condyloma acuminatum, commonly called genital warts. In cryotherapy, cry(o) means cold, and -therapy is a suffix that means treatment. The literal interpretation of

cold

cryotherapy is treatment with the use of _____ temperatures.

To burn tissues by laser, hot metal, electricity, or another agent with the objective of destroying tissue is cauterization. The verb is cauterize (**kaw′tər-īz**). For example, tissue is cauterized in cauterization.

hysteropexy
(his′tər-o-pek″se)

12-64 Build a word that means surgical fixation of a displaced uterus by adding -*pexy* to the combining form that means abdominal wall: _____. A laparo/hystero/pexy (**lap″ə-ro-his′tər-o-pek-se**) is fixation of the uterus to the abdominal wall.

salpingorrhaphy
(sal″ping-gor′ə-fe)

12-65 Salpingopexy (**sal-ping′go-pek″se**) is surgical fixation of a fallopian tube. Write the term for suture of a fallopian tube: _____.

Exercise 7

Write a word in each blank to complete these sentences.

1. A pharmaceutical intervention for treating the symptoms of menopause is

   _____ replacement therapy.

2. Excision of the vulva is _____.

3. Suture of the vagina is _____.

4. Surgical fixation of an ovary is _____.

5. When the ovaries, uterus, and fallopian tubes are removed, this surgery is called a total abdominal

   _____.

6. Removal of the uterus through a small opening in the abdominal wall is

   _____.

7. Removal of a fallopian tube is _____.

8. The sterilization procedure in which both fallopian tubes are constricted, severed, or crushed is called tubal

   _____.

9. Forming a new opening into a fallopian tube is

   _____.

10. Dilation of the cervix and removal of material from the endometrium is called dilation and

    _____.

11. Treatment using subfreezing temperature to destroy tissue is

    _____.

12. Surgical fixation of the uterus to the abdominal wall is

    _____.

Male Reproductive System

ANATOMY AND PHYSIOLOGY

12-66 The male reproductive system produces, sustains, and transports spermatozoa; introduces them into the female vagina; and produces hormones. The testes are responsible for production of both spermatozoa and hormones. *Testes* is the plural form of *testis*, which means the same as testicle.

All other organs, ducts, and glands in this system transport and sustain the spermatozoa, the male sex cells, which is often shortened to *sperm* (singular, spermatozoon, or sperm).

The male gonads are the testes (**tes′tēz**), the primary organs of the male reproductive system. The _____ are the male gonads.

testes

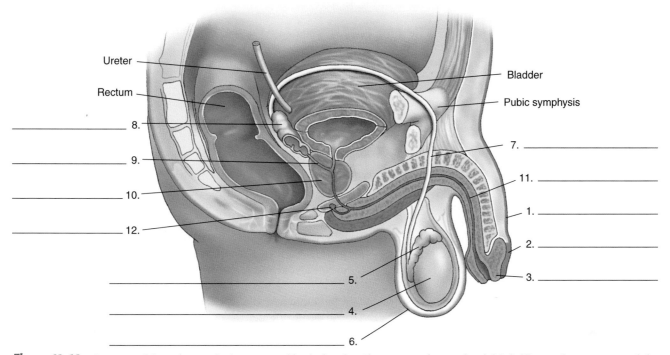

Ureter

Rectum

8.

9.

10.

12.

Bladder

Pubic symphysis

7.

11.

1.

2.

3.

5.

4.

6.

Figure 12-16 Structures of the male reproductive system, midsagittal section. The structures that are already labeled lie near, but are not part of, the male reproductive system.

12-67 Study Figure 12-16 and write the names of the structures in the blank lines as you read the following information. Label the penis on line l. A loose fold of skin, the prepuce (foreskin, line 2), covers the glans penis (line 3).

Figure 12-16 is a midsagittal section, so only one testis is shown. Label the testis (line 4). Sperm leave the testes through ducts that enter the epididymis (ep″ĭ-did′ə-mis), a tightly coiled comma-shaped organ located along the superior and posterior margins of the testes. Label the epididymis (line 5). The testes and epididymides are contained in a pouch of skin that is posterior to the penis. This pouch of skin is called the scrotum (skro′təm). Label the scrotum (line 6).

Each ductus deferens (line 7), also called the vas deferens, begins at the epididymis, continues upward, and then enters the abdominopelvic cavity. Each ductus deferens joins a duct from the seminal vesicle (line 8) to form a short ejaculatory (e-jak′u-lə-to″re) duct. Label the ejaculatory duct (line 9), which passes through the prostate (pros′tāt) gland and then empties into the urethra. Label the prostate (line 10) and the urethra (line 11). Paired bulbourethral glands contribute an alkaline mucuslike fluid to the semen. Label the bulbourethral gland (line 12). Ejaculation (e-jak″u-la′shən) is the expulsion of semen (se′mən) from the urethra.

Learn the following word parts that pertain to the male reproductive system.

Word Parts for the Male Reproductive System

Male Reproductive Structures		OTHER WORD PARTS	MEANING
WORD PARTS	MEANING	rect(o)	rectum
balan(o)	glans penis	semin(o)	semen
epididym(o)	epididymis	sperm(o), spermat(o)	spermatozoa
orchi(o), orchid(o),		urethr(o)	urethra
test(o), testicul(o)	testicle		
pen(o)	penis		
prostat(o)	prostate		
scrot(o)	scrotum		
vas(o)	vessel; ductus deferens		

12-68 The penis (pe′nis), the male organ for copulation, transfers sperm to the vagina. The combining form *pen(o)* means penis. *Pen/ile* means pertaining to the penis.

balan(o)

  The conical tip of the penis is the glans penis. Write the combining form that means glans penis: _____.

  Sexual intercourse refers to physical contact involving stimulation of the genitals between persons of the same or opposite gender. However, the medical definition of copulation (kop″u-la′shən), also called coitus* (ko′ĭ-tus), is sexual union between male and female during which the penis is inserted into the vagina.

coitus

  Write this word that means the same as copulation: _____.

12-69 In labeling Figure 12-16, you read that the scrotum is a pouch of loose skin that contains the two testes and their accessory organs. The combining form *scrot(o)* means scrotum. Use the suffix *-al* to write a term that means pertaining to the scrotum: _____.

scrotal (skro′təl)

  Four combining forms are used to write words about the testes: *orchi(o)*, *orchid(o)*, *test(o)*, and *testicul(o)*. *Testicul/ar* (tes-tik′u-lər) means pertaining to a _____, but most diagnostic and surgical terms will use either *orchi(o)* or *orchid(o)*. Practice in later frames will help you remember which combining form to use.

testicle or testis

  The combining form *epididym(o)* means epididymis.

12-70 Each testicle is suspended in the scrotum by the spermat/ic cord, which is made up of arteries, veins, lymphatic vessels, nerves, and the ductus deferens. *Spermatic* (spər-mat′ik) has two meanings, either pertaining to _____ or pertaining to semen.

sperm

12-71 The ductus deferens is a long duct that begins at the epididymis, enters the abdominal cavity, and connects with other structures of the internal reproductive tract. The combining form for ductus deferens is *vas(o)*, which also means vessel. It will mean the ductus deferens most of the time in this chapter.

  The combining form *prostat(o)* means the prostate. Using the suffix *-ic*, write a term that means pertaining to the prostate: _____.

prostatic (pros-tat′ik)

  The prostate, the seminal vessels, and the bulbourethral glands produce fluids that contribute to the semen and are necessary for the survival of the sperm. Semen is the secretion of the male reproductive organs that is discharged from the urethra during ejaculation. Combine *semin(o)* and *-al* to write a word that means pertaining to semen: _____.

seminal

Exercise 8

Write the meaning of the following combining forms.

1. epididym(o) _____

2. orchi(o)   _____

3. rect(o)   _____

4. urethr(o) _____

5. vas(o)   _____

Exercise 9

Write adjectives (words that mean pertaining to) for these structures.

1. penis   _____

2. prostate _____

3. scrotum _____

4. semen   _____ (or spermatic)

5. testicle _____

---

*Coitus (Latin: *coitio*, a coming together, meeting).

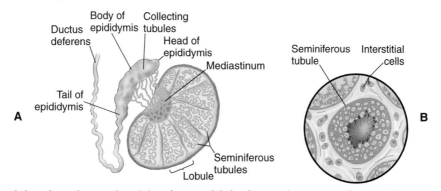

Figure 12-17 Sectional view of a testis. **A,** Each testis has about 250 lobules that contain as many as four seminiferous tubes where sperm are produced. **B,** Cross section of a seminiferous tube. The tubule is surrounded by interstitial cells, which are responsible for the production of testosterone.

Spermatogenesis

production
(or formation)

12-72 Each testis is capable of producing sperm and male hormones. Spermato/genesis (**sper″mə-to-jen′ə-sis**) is the _____ of mature, functional sperm capable of participating in conception, the union of a sperm with an ovum.

12-73 Sperm production requires a temperature slightly lower than normal body temperature. Because the scrotum is outside the body cavity, it provides the proper environment.

The testes are paired oval glands. In Figure 12-17, A, notice that a testis is divided into several compartments called lobules, and each lobule contains convoluted seminiferous tubules. Sperm are produced in these tubules. Lying just posterior to the testis is the epididymis, where sperm are stored until they are released. The duct leading from the epididymis is the vas

deferens

_____.

A cross section of a seminiferous (**sem″ĭ-nif′ər-əs**) tubule (Figure 12-17, B) shows that seminiferous tubules are surrounded by cells called interstitial cells of Leydig. These cells produce a major male sex hormone, testosterone (**tes-tos′tə-rōn**).

12-74 Sperm are produced within the seminiferous tubules. In the development of mature sperm, early spermatocytes (**sper′mə-to-sītz**) undergo a process called meiosis, which eventually results in mature, functional spermatozoa (Figure 12-18). Write the singular form of spermatozoa:

spermatozoon

_____.

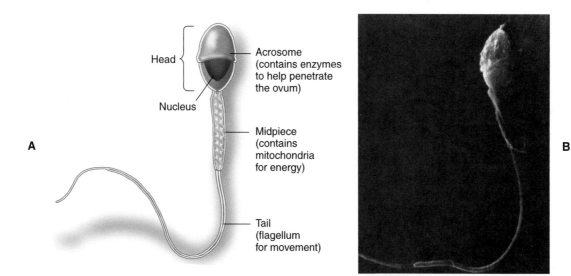

Figure 12-18 The human spermatozoon. **A,** A sperm in cross section. The nucleus contains the chromosomes and is located in the head. The tip of the head is covered by an acrosome, which contains enzymes that help the sperm penetrate the ovum. The midpiece contains mitochondria that provide energy, and the tail is a typical flagellum. **B,** Spermatozoon as seen using a scanning electron microscope.

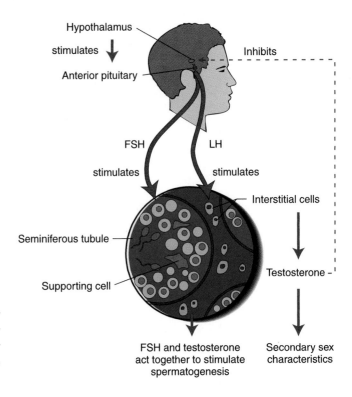

Figure 12-19   Hormonal control of the testes. The hypothalamus produces hormones that stimulate the anterior pituitary to produce follicle-stimulating hormone (FSH) and luteinizing hormone (LH). Luteinizing hormone stimulates the interstitial cells of the testes to secrete testosterone. Acting together, FSH and testosterone stimulate spermatogenesis.

testosterone

12-75 The hypothalamus, the pituitary gland, and the testes produce hormones that influence spermatogenesis (Figure 12-19).

FSH and testosterone produced by the testes stimulate spermatogenesis. LH acts on interstitial cells in the testes to produce testosterone. Testosterone also brings about male secondary sex characteristics—for example, enlarging of the sex organs, distribution of hair, deepening of the voice, and increased muscular development. Write the name of this hormone, which is often called the masculinizing hormone: _____.

seminal

12-76 Spermatogenesis begins at puberty and normally continues throughout life, showing a decline in later years. Semen, also called seminal fluid, is a mixture of sperm cells and secretions from the accessory glands (prostate, seminal vesicles, and bulbourethral glands). The combining form *semin(o)* means semen. Write the other name for semen that uses this combining form: _____ fluid.

There are usually millions of sperm each time semen is ejaculated, and although only one sperm fertilizes an ovum, it takes millions of sperm to ensure that fertilization will take place.

Exercise 10

Write a term in each blank.

1. The production of sperm is called _____.

2. The structure that is responsible for sperm production is the _____.

3. Sperm are produced within the _____ tubules.

4. The major male sex hormone produced by the testicles is _____.

5. Two important hormones that stimulate sperm production are follicle-stimulating hormone and

_____ hormone.

DIAGNOSTIC TESTS AND PROCEDURES

urethra

12-77 Three important parts of a routine examination of the male genitalia are inspection of the external genitalia, palpation for inguinal hernias, and the digital rectal examination.

The external genitalia are examined for the descent and size of the testicles, abnormalities of the scrotum and penis, and the presence of urethral discharge. <u>Urethr/al discharge</u> is a secretion from the _____. <u>Smears</u> of the secretions are stained and examined if gonorrhea is suspected, or material is collected for bacterial or fungal culture.

Lesions or ulcers on the penis may indicate a sexually transmitted disease such as genital herpes, which produces blisters, or a chancre, a lesion that indicates the first stage of syphilis. The <u>VDRL</u> test and the <u>RPR</u> are blood tests to detect and monitor syphilis.

hands

12-78 Remember from a previous chapter that <u>palpation</u> is a technique in which the examiner uses the _____ to feel the size and location of internal structures. An inguinal hernia is one in which a loop of intestine enters the inguinal canal, the passageway in the lower muscular layers of the abdominal wall that is a common site for hernias. An inguinal hernia in a male sometimes fills the entire scrotal sac.

rectum

12-79 The <u>digital rectal examination</u> is an assessment of the prostate gland and the _____. The examiner inserts a lubricated, gloved finger (a digit— hence, the name of the procedure) into the rectum, and the size and consistency of the prostate gland is assessed.

12-80 The <u>prostate-specific antigen</u> (PSA) <u>test</u> is a blood test used to screen for prostatic cancer and to monitor the patient's response to treatment. Elevated PSA levels are associated with prostatic cancer.

The antigen that is a tumor marker for prostatic cancer is called _____ specific antigen.

prostate

testicles

12-81 <u>Testicular self-examination</u> is a procedure recommended by the National Institutes of Health for detecting tumors or other abnormalities of the _____. The presence of swelling or a small lump on either testicle should be reported to one's physician.

12-82 <u>Needle biopsy of the prostate</u> is generally performed if cancer of the prostate is suspected. In a needle biopsy, a small amount of tissue is removed using a needle inserted from the outside. In this case, the needle is inserted through the rectal mucosa to the prostate. <u>Cyto/logy</u> is performed on the tissue, examining the cells for the presence of cancer cells. Cyto/logy is the study of

cells

_____.

12-83 The <u>sperm count</u> is a test for male fertility. In a sperm count, the number, appearance, and motility of the sperm are examined in a collected sample of semen. The test that evaluates the number and health of spermatozoa is called a _____ count.

sperm

Exercise 11

Match the diagnostic tests in the left column with their descriptions in the right column.

A. blood test for prostatic cancer
B. blood test for syphilis
C. removal of tissue for cytologic study
D. test of semen

_____ 1. needle biopsy

_____ 2. PSA

_____ 3. RPR

_____ 4. sperm count

PATHOLOGIES

testicular

12-84 Uro/logy (**u-rol´ə-je**) is the branch of medicine that specializes in the male and female urinary tract and also includes male reproductive structures.

Testicular cancer occurs most often in younger men, and prostatic cancer is common in older men. Which type of cancer is more common in younger men? _____ cancer.

Learn these word parts that are used to describe pathologies of the male reproductive system.

Word Parts Used to Describe Male Reproductive Pathologies

WORD PART	MEANING
crypt(o)	hidden
olig(o)	few
varic(o)	twisted and swollen

testicular

12-85 *Torsion* means twisting. Torsion of the testis, axial rotation of the spermatic cord, cuts off the blood supply to the testicle and can lead to loss of the testicle. Surgical correction within a few hours of the injury is required in most cases to save the testicle. Torsion of the testicle can also be called _____ torsion.

absence

living

12-86 Oligo/sperm/ia (**ol″ĭ-go-sper´me-ə**) means insufficient sperm in the semen. A/spermia (**ə-spər´me-ə**) or a/spermato/genesis (**a-sper″mə-to-jen´ə-sis**) is _____ of sperm. A/zoo/spermia (**a-zo″ə-spər´me-ə**) is absence of living sperm. Literal interpretation of the word parts of azoospermia is that *a-* means not, *zo(o)* means animal, and *spermia* means a condition of the sperm. But you need to remember that *azoospermia* means the absence of _____ sperm.

In addition to sufficient numbers, sperm must be actively motile and live long enough to reach the ovum. There are many causes of infertility besides insufficient sperm, and for this reason, it is best that the partners be treated together.

dysfunction

12-87 Erection is the condition of swelling, rigidity, and elevation of the penis, and to a lesser degree in the clitoris of the female, caused by sexual arousal. It can also occur during sleep. Erection is necessary for the introduction of the penis into the vagina and for the emission of semen. The inability to achieve penile erection, alternating periods of normal function and dysfunction, or inability to ejaculate after achieving an erection is called erectile dysfunction, also known as male impotence.

Poor health, certain drugs, fatigue, and vascular problems can cause sexual dysfunction. Males can often be treated by medications or changes in drugs that are causing erectile _____.

hidden

cryptorchidism

12-88 The production of sperm outside the body cavity is necessary for the production of viable sperm. The testes develop in the abdominal cavity of the fetus and normally descend through the inguinal canal into the scrotum shortly before birth (sometimes shortly after birth). This provides a temperature about 3°F below normal body temperature.

Crypt/orchid/ism (**krip-tor´kĭ-diz″əm**) is a developmental defect characterized by the failure of one or both testes to descend into the scrotum. The combining form *crypt(o)*, means hidden. The *o* in *crypt(o)* is usually omitted when joined to a combining form that begins with a vowel. Translated literally, *crypt/orchid/ism* means a condition of _____ testicle or testes.

Cryptorchidism is the same as undescended testicle. If the testes do not descend spontaneously or with hormonal injections, surgery is usually performed. Write the word that means the same as undescended testicle: _____.

pain

12-89 Test/algia (**tes-tal´jə**), orchi/algia (**or″ke-al´jə**), and orchid/algia (**or″kĭ-dal´jə**) mean testicular _____.

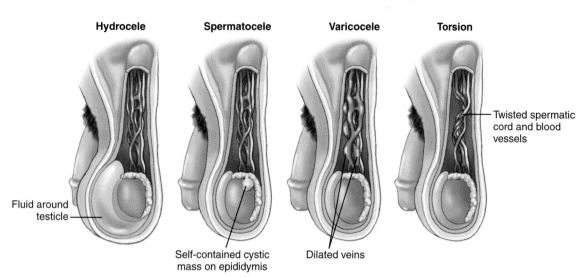

Hydrocele   **Spermatocele**   **Varicocele**   **Torsion**

Twisted spermatic cord and blood vessels

Fluid around testicle

Self-contained cystic mass on epididymis

Dilated veins

Figure 12-20   Comparison of four common problems that affect the testes and adjacent structures.

orchiopathy
(or″ke-op′ə-the)

Write a word using *orchi(o)* that means any disease of the testes:

_____.

Both *anorchidism* (**an-or′kĭ-diz″əm**) and *an/orchism* (**an-or′kiz-əm**) mean a congenital absence of the testis, which may occur unilaterally or bilaterally.

inflammation

Both *orchiditis* (**or″kĭ-di′tis**) and *orchitis* (**or-ki′tis**) mean_____ of a testis, marked by pain, swelling, and a feeling of weight.

12-90 Epididym/itis (**ep″ĭ-did″ə-mi′tis**) is inflammation of the

epididymis

_____.

Orchi/epididymitis (**or″ke-ep″ĭ-did″ĭ-mi′tis**) is inflammation of a testicle and its epididymis.

12-91 Several less severe problems occur within the scrotum, including hydrocele, spermatocele, and varicocele. You have learned that *-cele* means hernia, but in these three terms *-cele* is used to mean a swelling. See Figure 12-20 for these three disorders, as well as testicular torsion.

A hydro/cele (**hi′dro-sēl**) is a mass, usually filled with a straw-colored fluid. For this reason, its name incorporates the combining form *hydr(o)*, which means

water

_____. In this term, *hydr(o)* may help you remember that the swelling contains a straw-colored fluid. A hydrocele in the scrotum may be the result of orchitis, epididymitis, or venous or lymphatic obstruction.

sperm

A spermato/cele (**sper′mə-to-sēl**) is a mass that contains _____. This develops on the epididymis. A spermatocele is often painless and may need no intervention.

A varico/cele (**var′ĭ-ko-sēl**) is a cluster of dilated veins that occurs above the testis. The combining form *varic(o)* means twisted and swollen. In many cases, varicoceles are asymptomatic but may contribute to infertility.

12-92 Two disorders of the penis are phimosis* (**fi-mo′sis**) and balanitis (**bal″ə-ni′tis**). Phimosis occurs when the prepuce is constricted at the opening so that it cannot be retracted back over the glans penis. It is caused by inflammation or edema. It is sometimes accompanied by balan/itis (*balan[o]*, glans penis + *-itis*, inflammation), inflammation of the glans penis.

When the prepuce is constricted so that it cannot be retracted, the disorder is called

phimosis
balanitis

_____.

Inflammation of the glans penis is called _____.

---

*Phimosis (Greek: *phimgsis*, a muzzling or closure).

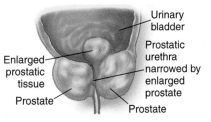

Figure 12-21   Benign prostatic hyperplasia. This nonmalignant enlargement of the prostate is common among men over 50 years of age. As the prostate enlarges, it extends upward into the bladder and inward, obstructing the outflow of urine from the bladder.

hyperplasia

prostatitis
(pros″tə-ti′tis)

without

prostate

12-93 It is unclear why the prostate is so often affected by benign and malignant neoplasms. Benign prostatic hyperplasia (hi″pər-pla′zhə) (BPH) is a common disorder, particularly in men over 50 years of age. Hyperplasia is an increase in the size of an organ resulting from an increase in the number of cells. The condition is not malignant; however, it is usually progressive and may lead to obstruction of the urethra and to interference with urination (Figure 12-21). The increase in the number of cells (hyperplasia) results in prostatic enlargement (hypertrophy). The common name of the disorder that is nonmalignant and results in an enlarged prostate is benign prostatic

_____.

Urinary frequency, pain, and urinary tract infections are characteristic of BPH. Inflammation of the prostate may also occur. Write a term that means inflammation of the prostate:

_____.

12-94 Prostatitis can occur in other situations besides BPH. It can be acute or chronic, bacterial or abacterial (a″bak-tēr′e-əl), and an exact cause may not be found. A/*bacterial* means

_____ bacteria.

12-95 Prostatic carcinoma usually occurs after 50 years of age and is the most common cancer among men, excluding skin cancer. Prostatic carcinoma is cancer of the

_____.

Exercise 12

Write a word in each blank to complete the sentences.

1. The branch of medicine that specializes in the male and female urinary tract and also includes male reproductive

   structures is _____.

2. Axial rotation of the spermatic cord is testicular _____.

3. Insufficient sperm in the semen is _____.

4. A developmental defect characterized by the failure of one or both testes to descend into the scrotum is

   _____.

5. Inflammation of the epididymis is _____.

6. A mass in the scrotum that contains straw-colored fluid is called _____.

7. A cluster of dilated veins above the testis is _____.

8. Tightness of the prepuce of the penis that prevents the retraction of the foreskin over the glans is

   _____.

9. Inflammation of the glans penis is _____.

10. A nonmalignant increase in the size of the prostate is benign prostatic _____.

SURGICAL AND THERAPEUTIC INTERVENTIONS

12-96 Testicular cancer is often curable. Some men choose semen storage as soon as possible after diagnosis. Semen storage is a special processing, freezing, and storage of sperm by a sperm bank for future use. Depending on the type of cancer, chemo/therapeutic agents may save the testis. Otherwise,

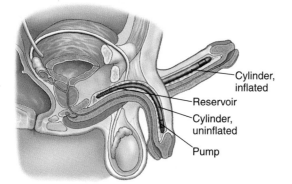

Cylinder,
inflated
Reservoir
Cylinder,
uninflated
Pump

Figure 12-22   A penile prosthesis. One of several types of prostheses, this self-contained type consists of a pump, a cylinder filled with fluid, and a reservoir, all in one unit. The patient squeezes the pump just below the head of the penis to fill the cylinder and achieve erection. When an erection is no longer desired, the patient presses a release valve located behind the pump.

excision	orchi/ectomy may be necessary. Orchi/ectomy is _____ of the testis. Removal of both testes results in infertility. Radiation therapy is sometimes used after surgery. Stem-cell transplantation is sometimes used after high-dose chemotherapy. In stem-cell transplantation, the patient's stem cells are removed from the bone marrow and preserved by freezing for later transplantation. **12-97** When torsion, twisting of the spermatic cord, has occurred, loss of blood supply to a testicle for more than a few hours will result in deterioration of the testicle. Surgical correction soon after the injury is important to prevent loss of the testicle. Write a term using *orchi(o)* that means surgical repair of a testicle: _____.
orchioplasty (or′ke-o-plas″te)	
	Orchio/tomy (or″ke-ot′ə-me) is incision (and drainage) of a testis. Orchio/rrhaphy (or″ke-or′ə-fe) is suture of a testicle. **12-98** Antiimpotence (an″ti-im′pə-təns) drugs, such as sildenafil (Viagra), are used to treat erectile dysfunction, particularly when the problem is inability to sustain an erection. Anti/impotence drugs act _____ impotence.
against	In some cases, treatment may include correction of the cause of the problem, such as restoration of the flow of blood to the penis or modification of medications that interfere with sexual activity. Surgical treatment includes injections and surgical implantation of a penile prosthesis (pros-the′sis). The term *prosthesis* means an artificial replacement for a body part (for example, an artificial arm or leg) or a device designed to improve function (for example, a hearing aid). The prosthesis that is designed to treat an
penile	erectile dysfunction is called a _____ prosthesis (Figure 12-22). **12-99** Orchio/pexy (or′ke-o-pek″se) is corrective surgery for cryptorchidism. Orchiopexy, sometimes called orchidopexy (or′kĭ-do-pek″se), is the attachment of the previously undescended testis to the wall of the scrotum. **12-100** A hydrocele in a newborn may resolve spontaneously. In an adult, a hydrocele may become large and uncomfortable and require surgical incision of the scrotum and removal of the hydrocele, because aspiration of the fluid with a needle is a temporary measure and may induce infection.
hydrocele	A hydrocel/ectomy (hi″dro-se-lek′tə-me) is surgical removal of a _____.
circumcision	**12-102** The tightness of the prepuce in phimosis can usually be corrected by circumcision (sər″kəm-sizh′ən). Circumcision is surgical removal of the end of the prepuce and is commonly performed on the male infant at birth. Write this term that means surgical removal of the end of the prepuce: _____.
urethra	**12-103** A transurethral resection prostatectomy (TURP) may be necessary to correct the enlarged prostate of BPH. A trans/urethral resection is a surgical procedure that is performed through the _____. In a TURP, small pieces of the enlarged prostate are excised.
	The inflammation of prostatitis is often the result of infection and is treated with antibiotics.

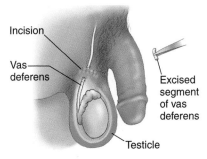

Figure 12-23   Vasectomy. This elective surgical procedure is performed as a permanent method of contraception (although it sometimes can be surgically reversed). It is usually performed under local anesthesia. A small incision is made in the scrotum, and a piece of the vas deferens is removed.

excision

excision

suture

incision

12-104 There are several treatments for prostatic (**pros-tat′ik**) carcinoma, including radiation, hormonal therapy, and prostatectomy (**pros″tə-tek′tə-me**). A prostat/ectomy is _____ of all or part of the prostate gland.

12-105 A vas/ectomy (**və-sek′tə-me**) is _____ of a portion of the vas deferens (Figure 12-23). Bilateral vasectomy results in sterility.
    Vaso/rrhaphy (**vas-or′ə-fe**) is _____ of the vas deferens. In a vasectomy it is necessary to incise the pouch that contains the testes.
    Vaso/tomy (**va-zot′ə-me**) is _____ of the vas deferens. A vasostomy (**vas-os′, va-zos′tə-me**) is surgical formation of a new opening into the vas deferens, but the term is sometimes used as a synonym for vasotomy.
    A vaso/vaso/stomy (**vas″o, va″zo-va-zos′tə-me**) can sometimes be used to correct an obstruction or to restore the severed ends of the vas deferens. The latter is used to reverse a vasectomy.

Exercise 13

Match the operations listed in the surgical schedule with their descriptions in the right column.

_____ 1. chemotherapy

_____ 2. circumcision

_____ 3. orchiectomy

_____ 4. orchiopexy

_____ 5. orchioplasty

_____ 6. penile prosthesis

_____ 7. TURP

_____ 8. vasectomy

A. chemical treatment for cancer
B. removal of small pieces of the prostate via the urethra
C. surgical repair of a testicle
D. surgical excision of a testicle
E. surgical fixation of a testicle
F. surgical implantation to correct erectile dysfunction
G. surgical removal of the end of the prepuce
H. surgical excision of a portion of the vas deferens

SELECTED ABBREVIATIONS

BPH	benign prostatic hyperplasia	**Pap**	Papanicolaou smear, stain, or test
Cx	cervix	**PID**	pelvic inflammatory disease
D & C	dilation and curettage	**PMS**	premenstrual syndrome
FSH	follicle-stimulating hormone	**PSA**	prostate-specific antigen
GU	genitourinary	**RPR**	rapid plasma reagin test (for syphilis)
Gyn	gynecology	**STD**	sexually transmitted disease
HCG	human chorionic gonadotropin	**TURP**	transurethral resection of the prostate
HRT	hormone replacement therapy	**VDRL**	Venereal Disease Research Laboratories
LH	luteinizing hormone		

CHAPTER 12 REVIEW

■ Basic Understanding

Labeling

I. Label the diagram with the following combining forms that correspond to numbered lines 1 through 5 (the first one is done as an example): cervic(o), colp(o), hyster(o), oophor(o), salping(o).

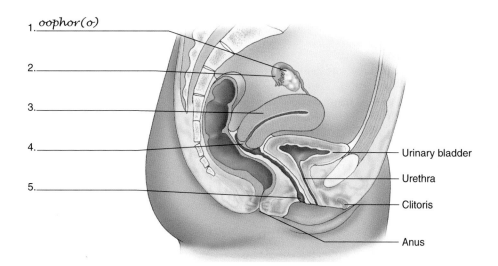

1. *oophor(o)*
2.
3.
4.
5.

Urinary bladder

Urethra

Clitoris

Anus

II. Label the diagram with the following combining forms that correspond to numbered lines 1 through 7 (the first one is done as an example): epididym(o), orchi(o), pen(o), prostat(o), scrot(o), urethr(o), vas(o).

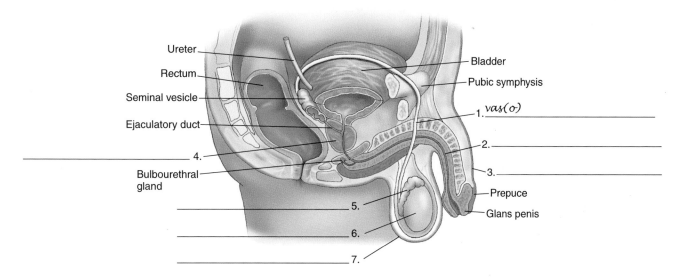

Ureter

Rectum

Seminal vesicle

Ejaculatory duct

4.

Bulbourethral gland

Bladder

Pubic symphysis

1. *vas(o)*
2.
3.

Prepuce

Glans penis

5.

6.

7.

Matching

III. Names of the three types of uterine tissue are in the left column. Match them with their locations in the uterus (A-C):

_____ 1. endometrium

_____ 2. myometrium

_____ 3. perimetrium

A. innermost
B. middle
C. outermost

IV. *Match terms on the left with descriptions in the right column. (Selections A-F may be used more than once.)*

_____ 1. ovary

_____ 2. ovum

_____ 3. sperm

_____ 4. testis

_____ 5. uterus

_____ 6. uterine tube

_____ 7. vagina

A. gonad
B. female sex cell
C. male sex cell
D. normal site of implantation
E. receives the sperm during intercourse
F. usual site of fertilization

Multiple Choice
V. *Circle one answer for each of the following questions.*

1. Which term means difficult or painful menstruation? (amenorrhea, dysmenorrhea, metrorrhagia, menorrhea)

2. Which of the following instruments is commonly used in a gynecologic examination? (curet, hysterosalpingograph, hysteroscope, speculum)

3. Which examination of the abdominal cavity uses an instrument that is inserted through one or more small incisions in the abdominal wall? (dilation and curettage, hysteroscopy, laparoscopy, ultrasonography)

4. Which term means inflammation of an ovary? (cervicitis, oophoritis, salpingitis, vulvitis)

5. Which term means the first occurrence of menstruation? (amenorrhea, dysmenorrhea, menarche, mittelschmerz)

6. Which term means surgical fixation of a prolapsed uterus? (cervicectomy, hysterectomy, hysteropexy, leiomyomectomy)

7. Which term means a white, viscid discharge from the vagina and uterine cavity? (leukorrhea, occult blood, Mittelschmerz, trichomoniasis)

8. Which term means a condition in which tissue that contains typical endometrial elements is present outside the uterus? (endometriosis, endometritis, hysteropathy, salpingopathy)

9. Which term means surgical repair of the vagina? (colpectomy, colpoplasty, colporrhaphy, oophorectomy)

10. Which term means absence of a testis? (anorchidism, aspermia, oligospermia, orchidectomy)

11. Which of the following result is expected following a bilateral vasectomy? (impotence, increased PSA, oligospermia, sterility)

12. What is surgically removed in a circumcision? (glans penis, prepuce, prostate, testes)

13. What is a term for undescended testicle? (cryptorchidism, orchidism, orchidorrhaphy, testalgia)

14. What is the term for twisting of the spermatic cord that results in cutting off the blood supply to the testicle? (hydrocele, spermatocele, torsion, varicocele)

15. Which term means testicular pain? (orchialgia, orchidism, orchiopathy, orchiotomy)

Fill in the Blanks
VI. *Write a word in each blank to complete this paragraph.*

The female reproductive cycle is composed of two cycles that occur simultaneously. The

(1) _____ cycle reflects the changes that occur in the ovaries. The changes in the

ovarian follicle are called follicle development, (2) _____, and the corpus luteal stage.

Two important hormones secreted by the follicles are (3) _____ and progesterone. The

(4) _____ cycle is also called the menstrual cycle. In this cycle, the endometrium

thickens and prepares for a developing embryo. If fertilization does not occur, the endometrial lining is shed, a process that

is called (5) _____.

Writing Terms

VII. *Write a term for each of the following:*

1. excision of the uterus _____

2. heavy or long menstrual periods _____

3. herniation of a fallopian tube _____

4. incision of the vas deferens _____

5. inflammation of the cervix uteri _____

6. inflammation of the vulva and vagina _____

7. insufficient sperm in the semen _____

8. surgical fixation of a fallopian tube _____

9. viewing the vagina and cervix with magnification _____

10. excision of the prostate _____

■ Greater Comprehension

Labeling

VIII. *The following diagrams represent displacements of the uterus. Label them as anteflexion, anteversion, retroflexion, or retroversion.*

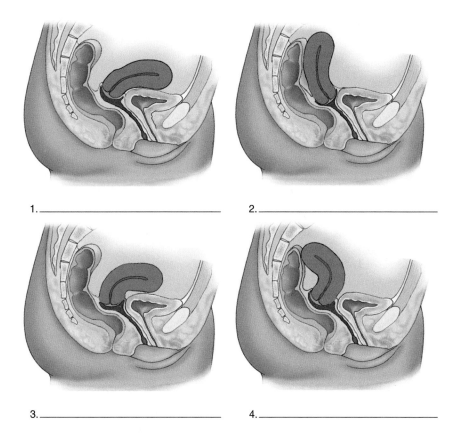

1._____   2._____

3._____   4._____

Health Report

IX. Read the following medical report and answer the questions.

MID-CITY MEDICAL CENTER

222 Medical Center Drive   Main City, US 63017-1000   Phone (555) 434-0000
                                                                                 Fax (555) 434-0001

HISTORY AND PHYSICAL

NAME OF PATIENT: Joan Martin (DOB 5-21-1972)   Date: 7/22/2003

HISTORY: Pt is a 31-year-old black female admitted with complaints of low back and pelvic pain. No history of uterine pathology. Pain is midline pelvic pain, as well as low back pain. Denies dysuria, urgency, or frequency of urination. No vaginal bleeding or other gynecologic history. Hysteroscopy showed no uterine pathology. Low grade temperature. Completed a 7-day cycle of Cipro with no relief. UA negative.

ALLERGIES: Penicillin.

MEDICAL HISTORY: Carcinoma of the right breast with lymphadenopathy. Lumpectomy. Left ovarian cyst with oophorectomy; D & C.

PHYSICAL EXAMINATION: Tender over mid-pelvis. Bowel sounds present. Temp. 99.8.

IMPRESSION: Endometritis.

PLAN: Triple IV antibiotics for 5 days; control pain; follow-up with Dr. Stevens in 7 days.

Emma Stevens, M.D.
Emma Stevens, M.D.

Circle the correct answer for each of these questions.

1. This patient's history indicates removal of which organ? (breast, ovary, uterus, vagina)
2. Hysteroscopy is direct visualization of which organ? (breast, ovary, uterus, vagina)
3. Endometritis is inflammation of which of the following? (inner lining of the uterus, lower part of the uterus, muscle of the uterus, outer layer of the uterus)

Write the meaning of this abbreviation:

4. D & C _____

Health Report

X. Read the following medical report and define the terms that are underlined.

CASE STUDY

Patient: A. M. Kinder (female, age 61)

Symptoms: Pelvic pressure.

History: 6 children; <u>ectopic pregnancy</u>; <u>vaginal hysterectomy</u> and bilateral <u>oophorosalpingectomy</u>.

Family History: Mother deceased at age 68 with history of carcinoma of the cervix with metastasis to the colon. Father age 85 with high blood pressure and <u>benign prostatic hyperplasia</u>.

Physical Exam: Bladder, rectum, and part of colon herniating into vagina, with vagina prolapsing.

Diagnosis: <u>Cystocele</u>, <u>rectocele</u>, and <u>vaginal prolapse</u>.

Plan: Surgery including cystocele and rectocele repairs; <u>perineoplasty</u>; <u>colpopexy</u>.

1. ectopic pregnancy _____

2. vaginal hysterectomy _____

3. oophorosalpingectomy _____

4. benign prostatic hyperplasia _____

5. cystocele _____

6. rectocele _____

7. vaginal prolapse _____

8. perineoplasty _____

9. colpopexy _____

Spelling

XI. *Circle all incorrectly spelled terms and write their correct spelling.*

colpectomy   displasia   ginecology   salpingorhaphy   seminiferous

Interpreting Abbreviations

XII. *Write the meanings of these abbreviations:*

1. BPH _____

2. FSH _____

3. HCG _____

4. Pap _____

5. VDRL _____

Pronunciation

XIII. *The pronunciation is shown for several medical words. Indicate which syllable has the primary accent by marking it with an '.*

1. perimetrium (per ĭ me tre əm)

2. perineum (per ĭ ne əm)

3. progesterone (pro jes tə rōn)

4. testicular (tes tik u lər)

5. spermatogenesis (sper mə to jen ə sis)

Categorizing Terms

XIV. Classify the terms in the left column (1-10) by selecting A, B, C, D, or E from the right column.

_____ 1. anorchidism

_____ 2. balanitis

_____ 3. colpodynia

_____ 4. curettage

_____ 5. hysterosalpingography

_____ 6. orchidalgia

_____ 7. scrotum

_____ 8. speculum

_____ 9. tubal ligation

_____ 10. vestibule

A. anatomy
B. diagnostic test or procedure
C. pathology
D. surgery
E. therapy

(Check your answers with the solutions in Appendix VI.)

LISTING OF MEDICAL TERMS

Use the practice CD to review the terms that have been presented. Look closely at the spelling of each term as it is pronounced and be sure you know the meaning of each term.

abdominal hysterectomy
adhesion
amenorrhea
anorchidism
anorchism
anovulation
anteflexion
anteversion
antiimpotence drug
antiinflammatory drug
aspermatogenesis
aspermia
azoospermia
balanitis
Bartholin's gland
bulbourethral gland
candidiasis
cauterization
cauterize
cervical biopsy
cervical polyp
cervicitis
cervix
cervix uteri
chancre
chemotherapeutic
chemotherapy
circumcision
climacteric
clitoris
coitus
colpectomy

colpitis
colpocervical
colpocystitis
colpodynia
colpohysterectomy
colpoplasty
colporrhagia
colporrhaphy
colposcope
colposcopy
computed tomography
conception
condyloma acuminatum
contraception
copulation
corpus luteum
cryosurgery
cryotherapy
cryptorchidism
cystocele
cytology
dilation and curettage
ductus deferens
dysmenorrhea
dysplasia
ectopic pregnancy
ejaculation
ejaculatory
endometrial biopsy
endometriosis
endometritis
endometrium

endoscope
epididymis
epididymitis
erectile dysfunction
erection
estrogen
fallopian tube
fimbria
fistula
follicle-stimulating
    hormone
fundus
genitalia
genitourinary
glans penis
gonad
gonadotropin
gonorrhea
graafian follicles
Gram stain
gynecologic
gynecology
human chorionic
    gonadotropin
hydrocele
hydrocelectomy
hyperplasia
hypertrophy
hypothalamus
hysterectomy
hysteropathy
hysteropexy

hysteroptosis
hysterosalpingogram
hysterosalpingography
hysteroscopy
inguinal hernia
interstitial cells of Leydig
labia majora
labia minora
laparohysterectomy
laparohysteropexy
laparoscope
laparoscopic hysterectomy
laparoscopy
leiomyoma
leukorrhea
luteinizing hormone
menarche
menopause
menorrhagia
menorrhea
menses
menstruation
metritis
metrorrhagia
mittelschmerz
mons pubis
myometritis
myometrium
oligospermia
oogenesis
oophoralgia
oophorectomy

oophoritis
oophorohysterectomy
oophoropathy
oophoropexy
oophorosalpingectomy
oophorosalpingitis
oophorosalpingohysterec–
   tomy
orchialgia
orchidalgia
orchiditis
orchidopexy
orchiectomy
orchiepididymitis
orchiopathy
orchiopexy
orchioplasty
orchiorrhaphy
orchiotomy
orchitis
ovarian
ovarian cyst
ovary
ovulation
ovum
palpation
Pap smear
Papanicoloau test
paraurethral gland

pelvic inflammatory
   disease
penile
penis
perimetrium
perineum
phimosis
pituitary gland
polycystic ovary syndrome
premenstrual syndrome
prepuce
progesterone
prostate
prostatectomy
prostate-specific antigen
prostatic
prostatic carcinoma
prostatitis
prosthesis
puberty
rapid plasma reagin test
rectocele
rectovaginal
rectum
retroflexion
retroversion
salpingectomy
salpingocele
salpingopexy

salpingorrhaphy
salpingostomy
scrotal
scrotum
semen
seminal vesicles
seminiferous tubule
sexually transmitted
   disease
speculum
spermatic
spermatocele
spermatogenesis
spermatozoon
symphysis pubis
syphilis
testalgia
testicular
testicular torsion
testis
testosterone
toxic shock syndrome
transurethral
   prostatectomy
trichomonas
tubal ligation
tubal pregnancy
ultrasonography
urethra

urethrovaginal
urogenital
urology
uterine
uterine fibroid
uterine tube
uterus
vagina
vaginal
vaginal hysterectomy
vaginal speculum
vaginectomy
vaginitis
varicocele
vas deferens
vasectomy
vasorrhaphy
vasostomy
vasotomy
vesicovaginal
vestibular
vestibule
visceral peritoneum
vulva
vulval
vulvar
vulvectomy
vulvitis
vulvovaginitis

español ENHANCING SPANISH COMMUNICATION

ENGLISH	SPANISH (PRONUNCIATION)
circumcision	circuncisión (ser-coon-se-se-ON)
conception	concepción (con-sep-se-ON)
condom	condón (con-DON)
erection	erección (ay-rec-se-ON)
hormone	hormona (or-MOH-nah)
impotency	impotencia (im-po-TEN-se-ah)
intercourse, sexual	cópula (CO-poo-lah)
masculine	masculino (mas-coo-LEE-no)
menopause	menopausia (may-no-PAH-oo-se-ah)
menstruation	menstruación (mens-troo-ah-se-ON)
ovarian	ovárico (o-VAH-re-co)
ovary	ovario (o-VAH-re-o)
penis	pene (PAY-nay)
prostate	próstata (PROS-ta-tah)
prostatic	prostático (pros-TAH-te-co)
prostatitis	prostatitis (pros-ta-TEE-tis)
sexual	sexual (sex-soo-AHL)
testicle	testículo (tes-TEE-coo-lo)
uterus	útero (OO-tay-ro)
vagina	vagina (vah-HEE-nah)

CHAPTER 13

Reproduction and Sexually Transmitted Diseases

LEARNING GOALS

In this chapter, you will learn to do the following:

Basic Understanding

1. Demonstrate a general understanding of fertilization, implantation, and growth of the embryo by selecting the correct terms to match descriptions.
2. Define or select the correct meanings of terms related to pregnancy, labor, and the newborn.
3. Match contraceptives with their characteristics.
4. Match sexually transmitted diseases with their characteristics.

Greater Comprehension

5. Use word parts from this chapter to determine the meaning of terms in a health care report.
6. Spell the terms accurately.
7. Pronounce the terms correctly.
8. Write the meanings of the abbreviations.
9. Categorize terms as anatomy, diagnostic test or procedure, pathology, surgery, or therapy.

THESE ARE THE MAJOR SECTIONS IN THIS CHAPTER:

- ❏ **Reproduction**
- ❏ **Pregnancy and Childbirth**
- ❏ **Diagnostic Tests and Procedures**
- ❏ **Pathologies of Pregnancy, Childbirth, and the Newborn**
- ❏ **Surgical and Therapeutic Interventions**
- ❏ **Sexually Transmitted Diseases**

FUNCTION FIRST

Sexual reproduction is the way in which genetic material is passed from one generation to the next. Sexually transmitted diseases are passed from one person to another by anal, oral, or vaginal intercourse, but some are transmitted by contaminated materials or may infect the fetus or the infant at birth.

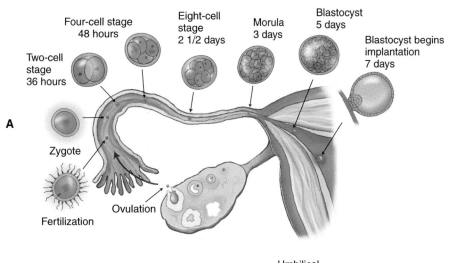

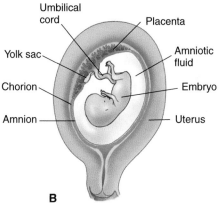

Figure 13-1 Fertilization, implantation, and growth of the embryo. **A,** A mature ovum is released in ovulation. The ovum is fertilized by a sperm, and the product of fertilization, the zygote, undergoes rapid cell division known by these stages: 2-cell stage, 4-cell stage, 8-cell stage, morula, and blastocyst. The blastocyst implants in the endometrium. **B,** The placenta and extraembryonic membranes (the amnion and the chorion) form and surround the embryo, providing nourishment and protection. The human embryonic stage begins about 2 weeks after conception and lasts until about the end of the eighth week, after which time the fetal stage begins.

Reproduction

gonad

13-1 The gonads (go′nadz), ovaries and testes, produce ova and sperm, as well as hormones necessary for proper functioning of the reproductive organs. Write this term that means an organ that produces ova or sperm: _____.

ovum

13-2 A gamete (gam′ēt) is a reproductive cell (ovum or spermatozoon), and the union of the ovum and sperm is necessary in sexual reproduction to initiate the development of a new individual. The ovum (o′vəm), also called the egg, lives only a few days, and the sperm have about the same time or less before they die after being discharged into the vagina. The gametes of reproduction are the _____ and the sperm.

uterus

13-3 Ovulation (ov″u-la′shən) is the release of an ovum from the ovary. Fertilization, or conception, is the union of the sperm cell nucleus with an egg cell nucleus. This usually occurs in the uterine tube.

The fertilized ovum undergoes a series of cell divisions as it moves along the uterine tube and then enters into the uterine cavity. About the seventh day after ovulation, the fertilized ovum attaches to the endometrium. This is called implantation.

The endo/metrium (endo-, inside + metr[o], uterine tissue + -ium, membrane) is the inner lining of the _____.

fetus

13-4 The product of fertilization is the zygote (zi′gōt), which undergoes rapid cell divisions. The zygote is known by different names at various stages. Some of these stages between fertilization and implantation are shown in Figure 13-1, A. It is usually at the beginning of the third week that the developing offspring is called an embryo. After the eighth week, it is called a fetus. The combining form fet(o) means fetus, so fet/al means pertaining to the _____.

outside

13-5 It is during the embryonic stage that all the organ systems form, making this the most critical time in development. This is also when the extraembryonic (eks″trə-em″bre-on′ik) membranes form. Knowing that *embryonic* refers to the embryo, *extra/embryonic* means _____ the embryo. Look at Figure 13-1, *B*, and locate two extraembryonic membranes, the amnion (am′ne-on) and the chorion (kor′e-on), that surround the embryo. The amnion and chorion are membranes that provide protection by surrounding the embryo with amniotic fluid. Although *amnion/ic* (am″ne-on′ik) has the same meaning as *amniotic* (am″ne-ot′ik), the latter is more commonly used.

Learn the following word parts and their meanings.

Principal Word Parts Pertaining to Reproduction

COMBINING FORMS	MEANING	SUFFIX	MEANING
amni(o)	amnion	-blast	embryonic or immature
chori(o)	chorion		
fet(o)	fetus		
gonad(o)	gonad		
o(o)	ovum		
spermat(o)	sperm		

ovum

13-6 The combining form *o(o)* means ovum. An ooblast (o′o-blast) is an immature _____. (The suffix *-blast* means embryonic or early form.)

sperm

13-7 Use *spermat(o)* to write terms about spermatozoa (sper″mə-to-zo′ə) or sperm. A spermato/blast (sper′mə-to-blast″) is an immature form of _____.

chorionic

amnion

13-8 Use *chori(o)* to write words about the chorion. You have already used a word that means pertaining to the chorion, which is _____.

Amnio/chorionic (am″ne-o-kor″e-on′ik) pertains to two membranes, the _____ and the chorion. *Amnio/chorial* (am″ne-o-kor′e-əl) is another word that means pertaining to the amnion and chorion.

progesterone

13-9 The placenta, formed in the embryonic stage, is a highly vascular structure that nourishes the fetus. Oxygen, nutrients, and antibodies diffuse from the mother to fetal blood vessels, and fetal wastes diffuse from the fetal blood into the maternal blood. *Maternal* means from the mother. Membranes normally keep the fetal and maternal blood from actually mixing.

The placenta also secretes large amounts of progesterone (pro-jes′tə-rōn), which is necessary for maintaining the uterus during pregnancy. The hormone that is responsible for maintaining the uterus throughout pregnancy is _____. Along with the placenta, the amnion and chorion are called the afterbirth and are shed shortly after birth.

Exercise 1

Write a word in each blank space to complete these sentences.

1. An organ that produces ova or sperm is called a _____.

2. An ovum or sperm is called a _____.

3. The product of fertilization is called a _____.

4. The release of an ovum from the ovary is called _____.

5. Another name for fertilization is _____.

6. Attachment of the fertilized ovum to the endometrium is called _____.

7. After the eighth week, the developing individual is called a _____.

8. Two extraembryonic membranes are the amnion and the _____.

9. An embryonic sperm is called a _____.

10. The placenta secretes large amounts of the hormone, _____, which is necessary for maintaining the uterus during pregnancy.

Pregnancy and Childbirth

parturition

13-10 Pregnancy is the process of growth and development of a new individual from conception through the embryonic and fetal periods to birth. The birth of the baby is parturition **(pahr″tu-rĭ′shən)**. Write this term that means childbirth: _____.

obstetrics (ob-stet′riks)

13-11 An obstetrician **(ob″stə-trĭ′shən)** specializes in _____, the medical specialty that is concerned with pregnancy and childbirth, and includes the time immediately after childbirth.

A nurse midwife has advanced education and clinical experience in obstetric care and care of the newborn. The nurse midwife manages care of women having a normal pregnancy, labor, and childbirth. A midwife is a person who assists women in childbirth.

Learn the meanings of the following terms.

Word Parts Pertaining to Pregnancy and Childbirth

COMBINING FORMS	MEANING		SUFFIXES	MEANING
nat(o)	birth		-cyesis	pregnancy
par(o)	bearing offspring		-gravida	pregnant female
			-para	woman who has given birth
PREFIX	MEANING		-tropin	that which stimulates
pseudo-	false			

before

13-12 Gestation **(jes-ta′shən)** is another name for pregnancy. This is also called the prenatal **(pre-na′təl)** period. Knowing that nat(o) means birth, pre/natal is that time _____ birth.

We saw in the previous section that the developing human individual is called an embryo at the beginning of the third week. By the end of the eighth week after fertilization, the developing individual is called a fetus, because by this time there are recognizable human features. Look at the timetable of prenatal development (Figure 13-2) and see the age when different features are present. Quickening, the first recognizable movements of the fetus in the uterus, occurs at about 18 to 20 weeks in a first pregnancy and slightly sooner in later pregnancies.

13-13 The average period of gestation is about 266 days from the date of fertilization, but it is clinically considered to last 280 days from the first day of the last menstrual period (LMP). The expected date of delivery (EDD) is usually calculated on the latter basis.

For convenience, pregnancy is discussed in terms of the first, second, and third trimester. A trimester is one of the three periods of approximately 3 months into which pregnancy is divided. The time from the first day of the last menstrual period to the end of 12 weeks is the first

trimester

_____.

pregnant

13-14 Gravid **(grav′id)** means pregnant, and gravida **(grav′ĭ-də)** refers to a pregnant female. If a female is gravid, she is _____.

second

The female may be identified more specifically as gravida I, if pregnant for the first time, or gravida II, if pregnant for the _____ time.

A designation for a female who has been pregnant three times is

gravida III

_____.

13-15 The suffix -gravida also refers to a pregnant female and is combined with various prefixes that designate the number of pregnancies. Because the prefix primi- means first, a primi/gravida

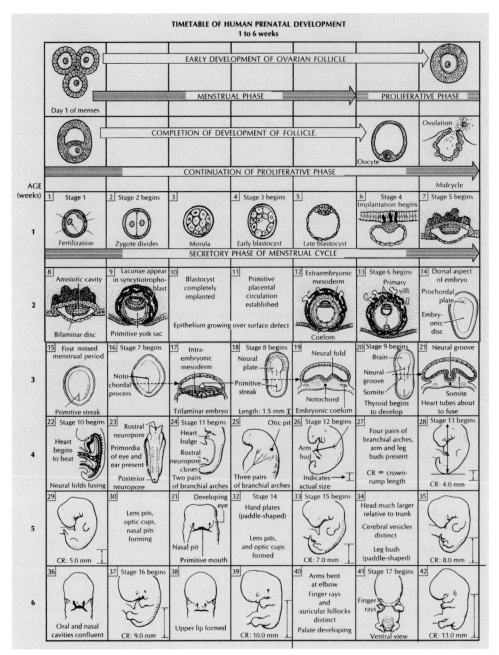

Figure 13-2   Timetable of prenatal development. Several significant events in the process of growth, maturation, differentiation, and development are shown in the timetable: three germ layers develop; heart begins beating; fingers, eyelids, toes, and external genitalia are visible, and face has human appearance.

first

(pri″mǐ-grav′ǐ-də) is a female during her _____ pregnancy. This is the same as gravida I.

The prefix *multi-* means many, and *multi/gravida* (mul″tǐ-grav′ǐ-də) means a female who has been pregnant more than one time.

13-16 A term that is used for a female who has produced viable offspring is *para*. A viable offspring is defined as one that has reached a stage of development that it can live outside the uterus and usually means a fetus that weighs at least 500 grams (just over 1 pound) and has reached a gestational age of 20 weeks (22 weeks after fertilization). The term is used with numerals to indicate the number of pregnancies carried to more than 20 weeks' gestation, such as para III, indicating three pregnancies, regardless of the number of offspring produced in a single pregnancy or the number of stillbirths after 20 weeks.

The combining form *par(o)* means producing or bearing viable offspring. *Par/ous* (par′əs) refers

offspring

to producing viable _____.

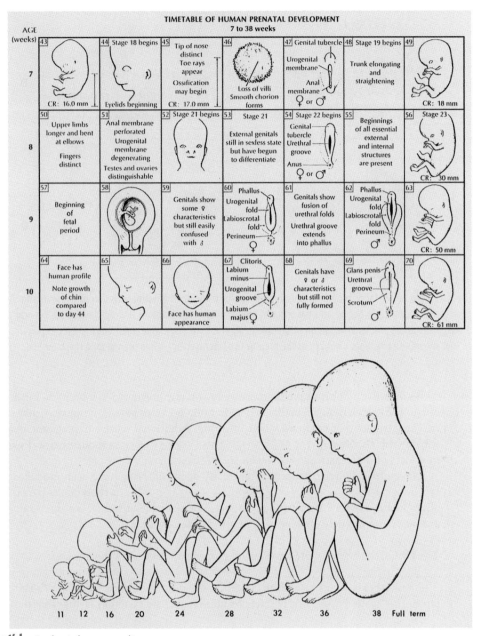

Figure 13-2, cont'd   For legend, see opposite page.

13-17 The suffix *-para* refers to a female who has given birth, specifically one who has produced viable offspring.

Determine the designation, para I, para II, or para III, for the following females. In each case, the pregnancies lasted more than 20 weeks.

What is the *para* designation for a female who has one living child and has had no other pregnancies? _____

para I

The para status of a female who has twins and has had no other pregnancies is para I. What is the para status of a female who has four children that resulted from three pregnancies and has had no additional pregnancies? _____

para III

13-18 A female who is designated as para I is also called a *primi/para* (**pri-mip′ə-rə**), which means that she has produced _____ viable offspring. (The number is implied from the prefix *primi-*, which means first.)

one

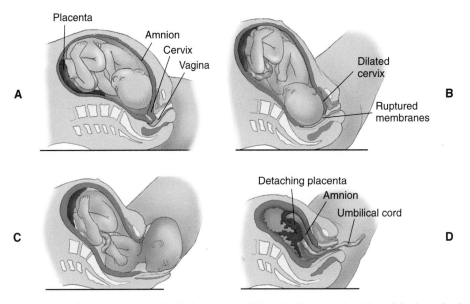

Figure 13-3   The fetus in utero before labor compared with three stages of labor. **A,** The normal position of the fetus shortly before labor begins. **B,** The first stage of labor (cervical dilatation) begins with the onset of regular uterine contractions and ends when the cervical opening is completely dilated. **C,** The second stage (expulsion) results in expulsion of the infant. **D,** The third stage (placental) ends when the placenta and membranes are expelled. A fourth stage (not shown) is sometimes identified as the hour or two after delivery, when uterine tone is established.

	Because the number or prefix indicates how many pregnancies, a multiple birth counts as just one in the calculation. Secundipara* (se″kən-dip′ə-rə), or para II, designates that a woman has had two pregnancies that produced viable offspring. Additional successful pregnancies are designated as
three	tripara (trip′ə-rə) for _____, and quadripara (kwod-rip′ə-rə) for four successful pregnancies. The prefix *quadri-* means four.
	The prefix *nulli-* refers to none. How many viable offspring have been produced by a nulli/para
zero	(nə-lip′ə-rə)? _____. This is the same as para 0. Translated literally, a multi/para (məl-tip′ə-rə) has produced many viable offspring, but the term is used to indicate a woman who has delivered more than one viable offspring.
	13-19 Using *-rrhexis,* write a new word that means rupture of the amnion:
amniorrhexis (am″ne-o-rek′sis)	_____. Amniorrhexis occurs before the child is born and sometimes is the mother's first sign of impending labor. The "water breaks" or the "bag of water breaks" are common sayings that mean amniorrhexis.
	13-20 Labor, the process by which the child is expelled from the uterus, is that time from the beginning of cervical dilation to the delivery of the placenta. Look closely at the term *dilation* and its three-syllable pronunciation: (di-la′shən). A synonym for dilation is dilatation (dil″ə-ta′shən). Cervical dilation is enlargement of the diameter of the opening of the uterine cervix in labor. The
uterus	uterine cervix is the neck of the _____.
	Dilatation is the condition of being dilated or stretched beyond the normal dimensions. Cervical dilatation is the dilation or stretching of the cervical opening. The shortening and thinning of the cervix during labor is called effacement (ə-fās′mənt). This term describes how the constrictive neck of the uterus is obliterated or effaced.
	Shortening and thinning of the cervix during labor is called
effacement	_____. When this occurs, the mucus plug that fills the cervical canal dislodges.

*Secundipara (Latin: *secundus,* following; *parere,* to bring forth).

cervical

expulsion

placenta

cesarean

after

before

parturition (childbirth)

birth

neonatologist
(ne″o-na-tol′ə-jist)

13-21 Labor may be divided into three (or sometimes four) stages: cervical dilatation, expulsion, placental, and postpartum (**pōst-pahr′təm**) stages (Figure 13-3). Not everyone recognizes the postpartum stage as a stage of labor, because it occurs after childbirth. The first stage (cervical dilatation) begins with the onset of regular uterine contractions and ends when the _____ opening is completely dilated.

The second stage (expulsion) extends from the end of the first stage until complete _____ of the infant. During this stage, the amniotic sac ruptures if that has not occurred already.

The third stage, the placental stage, extends from the expulsion of the child until what structure and the membranes are expelled? _____

The fourth stage (postpartum) is the hour or two after delivery, when uterine tone is established. Study Figure 13-3 and try to determine the stage of labor for each drawing. Notice how the fetal head turns in order to pass through the vaginal opening. The fourth and final stage of labor is not shown.

13-22 The events just described are the stages of a vaginal delivery. A cesarean (**sə-zar′e-ən**) section or cesarean birth is performed when abnormal fetal or maternal conditions make vaginal delivery hazardous. A cesarean section is a surgical procedure in which the abdomen and uterus are incised and the baby is removed from the uterus. Write this term that means removing the baby from the uterus after incision of the abdomen and uterus: _____ birth.

13-23 *Post/partum* means after childbirth because the prefix *post-* means _____.

You have learned that the prefixes *ante-* and *pre-* mean before. *Prenatal* and *ante/natal* (**an″te-na′təl**) both refer to the time _____ birth.

The prefix *ante-* is not always joined to the word, and sometimes there are two acceptable ways to write the same word. Either *antepartum* (**an″te-pahr′təm**) or *ante partum* is acceptable and means before _____.

13-24 *Postnatal* (**pōst-na′təl**) means the time after _____.

The prefix *neo-* means new. A neonate (**ne′o-nāt**) is a newborn child. *Neo/natal* (**ne″o-na′təl**) is a specific term that refers to the period covering the first 28 days after birth. *Neonatal* also means pertaining to the newborn child.

Neonatology (**ne″o-na-tol′ə-je**) is the branch of medicine that specializes in the care of the newborn. Write the term for a physician who specializes in neonatology: _____.

Exercise 2

Complete the table by writing a word part or its meaning in each blank.

COMBINING FORM	MEANING
1. _____	birth
2. _____	bearing offspring

PREFIX	MEANING
3. pseudo-	_____

SUFFIXES	MEANING
4. -cyesis	_____
5. -gravida	_____
6. -tropin	_____

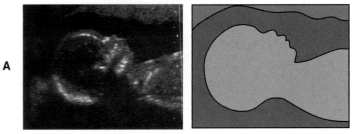

Figure 13-4 Ultrasound imaging of a fetus in the second trimester. **A**, sonogram, **B**, drawing.

DIAGNOSTIC TESTS AND PROCEDURES

stimulates

gonadotropin

measurement

fetus

amniocentesis

13-25 Within a few days after conception, the chorion starts producing a hormone, human chorionic gonadotropin (go′nə-do-tro″pin) (HCG). *Gonado/tropin* means a substance (hormone) that _____ the gonads. HCG is present in body fluids (urine, blood) of pregnant females, and blood or urine is tested to determine if pregnancy exists. HCG can be detected long before other signs of pregnancy appear. The hormone that is tested for in pregnancy tests is HCG, or human chorionic _____.

13-26 Literal translation of *pelvi/metry* (pel-vim′ə-tre) is _____ of the pelvis. This procedure is usually performed by the obstetrician during the first prenatal examination of a pregnant woman, or may be used if problems arise during labor. Clinical pelvimetry is vaginal palpation of specific bony landmarks and is used to estimate the size of the birth canal.

A cephalo/pelvic (sef″ə-lo-pel′vik) disproportion (CPD) is a condition in which a baby's head is too large or the mother's birth canal is too small to permit normal labor or birth. If the disproportion is too great, a cesarean delivery will be necessary. X-ray pelvimetry can be performed but is not generally used because of the risk of radiation exposure to the fetus.

13-27 Other diagnostic tools, such as sonography, provide a great deal of information about the fetus with less apparent risk. Fetal sonography is a noninvasive procedure that is used to assess structural abnormalities and monitor development of the _____ (Figure 13-4). The gender of the fetus can sometimes be determined by sonography.

13-28 Amnio/centesis (*amni(o)*, amnion + *-centesis*, surgical puncture) (am″ne-o-sen-te′sis) is a surgical procedure in which a needle is passed through the abdominal and uterine walls to obtain a small amount of amniotic fluid for laboratory analysis (Figure 13-5). The procedure is usually performed to aid in the assessment of fetal health and diagnosis of genetic defects or other abnormalities. Fetal cells in the fluid can be cultured (grown in the laboratory), and biochemical and cytologic studies may be performed. Write the name of this procedure in which a needle is passed trans/abdominally to collect amniotic fluid: _____.

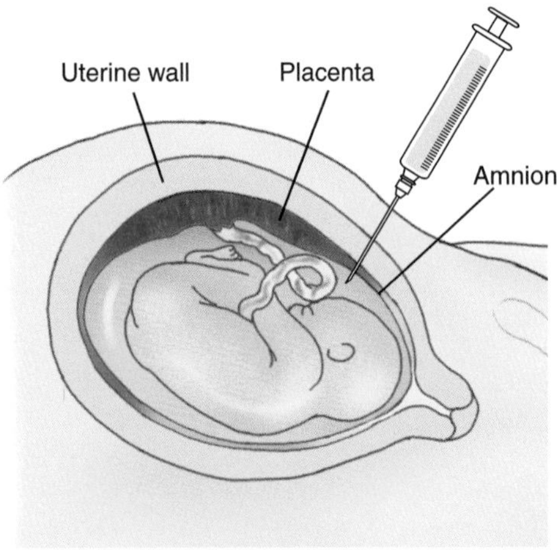

Uterine wall   Placenta

Amnion

Figure 13-5 Amniocentesis. Transabdominal puncture of the amniotic sac is done to remove fluid for diagnostic study.

chorionic

13-29 Chorionic villi (**vil′i**) are the tiny fingerlike projections of the chorion that infiltrate the endometrium and help form the placenta. Chorionic villus sampling is sampling of these villi (placental tissue) for prenatal diagnosis of potential genetic defects and is usually performed between the eighth and twelfth weeks of pregnancy. This test is called _____ villus sampling.

fetoscope

13-30 Looking again at the information in Figure 13-2, see how early the heart begins to beat. A feto/scope (**fe′to-skōp**) is a stethoscope for assessing the fetal heart rate (FHR) through the mother's abdomen. It may be used during prenatal visits to the doctor and during labor, when it also gives information about uterine contractions. Write the name of this special type of stethoscope that is used to monitor the fetal heartbeat: _____.

fetal

13-31 An electronic fetal monitor (EFM) may be used during labor to monitor the fetal heart and record the fetal heart rate and the maternal uterine contractions. The EFM may be applied either internally or externally. *EFM* means an electronic _____ monitor.

Exercise 3

Write a word in each blank to complete these sentences.

1. HCG is the hormone that is tested for in _____ tests.

2. An estimation of the size of the birth canal to determine if the baby's head is too large to permit normal birth is called

_____.

3. Surgical puncture of the amnion to obtain amniotic fluid for testing is _____.

4. A sampling of placental tissue early in pregnancy to determine potential genetic defects is called

_____ villus sampling.

5. A stethoscope for assessing the fetal heart rate is a _____.

PATHOLOGIES

ectopic

13-32 Whenever a fertilized ovum implants anywhere other than the uterus, this is an ectopic (**ek-top′ik**) pregnancy. The prefix *ecto-* means situated on or outside. The combining form *top(o)* refers to place. When *ecto-* and *top(o)* are combined, as in *ectopic*, it means outside the usual place. If the ovum implants in a fallopian tube, we call this a tubal pregnancy, or an _____ pregnancy.

outside

13-33 An ectopic pregnancy could also be called an extra/uterine (**eks″trə-u′tər-in**) pregnancy, because *extra-* means outside. *Extrauterine* means pertaining to _____ the uterus.

Ectopic pregnancy implantation sites include various places in the uterine tube, the ovary, the cervix, and the abdominal cavity. Sonography and radiography are important in diagnosing these abnormal pregnancies, and the products of fertilization are removed by surgery.

13-34 The prefix *pseudo-* means false and *-cyesis* means pregnancy. Pseudo/cyesis (**soo″do-si-e′sis**) is a term for false _____. This is also called pseudopregnancy (**soo″do-preg′nən-se**), in which certain signs and symptoms suggest pregnancy, such as the absence of menstruation. Pseudocyesis is the presence of one or more of these signs or symptoms when conception has not occurred. The condition may be psycho/genic (**si″ko-jen′ik**) or caused by a physical disorder.

Figure 13-6 Comparison of two complications of pregnancy. **A,** Abruptio placenta. Separation of the placenta implanted in a normal position in a pregnancy of 20 weeks or more or during labor before delivery of the fetus. This causes severe maternal hemorrhage that may be evident externally (as shown in this example), or the hemorrhage may be concealed within the uterus. **B,** Placenta previa. Abnormal implantation of the placenta too low in the uterus. Even slight dilation of the cervical opening can cause separation of an abnormally implanted placenta. This is the most common cause of painless bleeding in the third trimester.

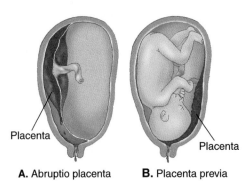

Placenta

Placenta

A. Abruptio placenta   **B.** Placenta previa

13-35 Pre/eclampsia (pre″e-klamp′se-ə) is one of several complications of pregnancy. This condition is characterized by the onset of acute high blood pressure after the twenty-fourth week of gestation. Protein/uria (pro″te-nu′re-ə), protein in the urine, and edema may also be present. Write the name of this complication of pregnancy characterized by acute high blood pressure:

preeclampsia

_____.
    Preeclampsia may progress to eclampsia (ə-klamp′se-ə), the gravest form of pregnancy-induced high blood pressure. The latter, characterized by seizures, coma, high blood pressure, proteinuria, and edema, leads to convulsions and death if untreated.

13-36 A second complication of pregnancy is abruptio placenta (ab-rup′she-o plə-sen′tə). This condition is a separation of the placenta from the uterine wall after 20 weeks or more or during labor and often results in severe hemorrhage. Fetal death results if there is complete separation of the placenta from the uterine wall, so cesarean sections are performed in severe cases.

abruptio

Labor and normal delivery may be possible if only partial separation exists. This complication of separation of the placenta from the uterine wall is called _____ placenta.

13-37 Placenta previa (pre′via) is a condition in which the placenta is implanted abnormally in the uterus so that it impinges on or covers the internal os (opening at the upper end) of the uterine cervix. This is one of the most common reasons for painless bleeding in the last trimester. Cesarean section is required if severe hemorrhage occurs. This condition in which the placenta is

previa

implanted abnormally in the uterus is called placenta _____.
Study Figure 13-6 and compare placenta previa with abruptio placenta, which was described in the previous frame.

13-38 Stillbirth is the birth of a fetus that dies before or during delivery. A fetus that would usually have been expected to live but dies before or during delivery is also called a

stillbirth

_____.

13-39 Abnormal or difficult labor is called dystocia.* Literal translation of dys/tocia (dis-to′shə) is

difficult

_____ labor. It may be caused by an obstruction or constriction of the birth passage or abnormal shape, size, position, or condition of the fetus.

13-40 One genetic disorder that can be detected by study of the amniotic fluid is Down syndrome. Patients with Down syndrome have an extra chromosome, usually number 21, and have moderate to severe mental retardation. This chromosomal aberration, also called trisomy 21 (tri- means three), is most often associated with late maternal age (Figure 13-7). The name

*Dystocia (dys- + Greek: tokos, birth).

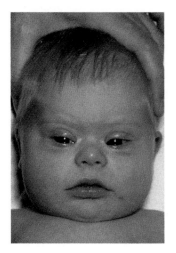

Figure 13-7   Typical facial characteristics of Down syndrome. This congenital condition, usually caused by an extra chromosome 21, is characterized by varying degrees of mental retardation and multiple defects. It can be diagnosed prenatally by amniocentesis. Infants with the syndrome generally have a small, flattened skull, flat-bridge nose, and eyes with the mongoloid slant shown here. Down syndrome was formerly called mongolism.

Down	of this genetic disorder, usually associated with trisomy of chromosome number 21, is _____ syndrome.

13-41 Another condition that may be diagnosed by means of amniocentesis is <u>hemolytic disease of the newborn</u>, an anemia of newborns characterized by premature destruction of red blood cells and resulting from maternal-fetal blood group incompatibility, specially involving the Rh factor and the ABO blood groups. In Rh incompatibility, the hemolytic reaction occurs because the mother is Rh negative and the infant is Rh positive. The name of the disease,

hemolytic

_____ disease of the newborn, describes the destruction of the red blood cells. This is also called <u>erythro/blast/osis fetalis</u> (ə-rith″ro-blas-to′sis fe-tă′lis). An erythro/blast (*erythr[o]*, red + *-blast*, embryonic form) is an immature form of a red blood cell that is present in the blood of newborns with this type of anemia.

The first pregnancy usually does not present a serious problem, and complications in a future pregnancy can generally be prevented by injection of the mother shortly after delivery with RhoGAM or a similar immune globulin (or abortion of an Rh positive fetus).

When hemolytic disease of the newborn is suspected, prenatal diagnosis of the disease is confirmed by high levels of bilirubin in the amniotic fluid, obtained by amniocentesis. Intra/uterine transfusion or immediate exchange transfusions after birth may be necessary. Intra/uterine transfusion is transfusion of the fetus while it is still within the uterus. Another name for hemolytic disease

erythroblastosis

of the newborn is _____ fetalis.

13-42 Fetal presentation describes the part of the fetus that is touched by the examining finger through the cervix or has entered the mother's lesser pelvis during labor. The normal fetal presentation is cephalic, which means that the top of the head, the brow, the face, or the chin presents itself at the cervical opening during labor. To help you remember cephalic presentation, remember the meaning of cephalic, which is pertaining to the

head

_____.

A <u>breech presentation</u> is one in which the buttocks, knees, or feet are presented. It occurs in approximately 3% of labors. Because the head is generally larger than the rest of the body, it may become trapped. If the buttocks or feet are felt by the examining finger during labor, it is called

breech

_____ presentation.

Shoulder presentation is one in which the long axis of the baby's body is across the long axis of the mother's body, and the shoulder is presented at the cervical opening. This type of presentation is also called <u>transverse presentation</u>. Vaginal delivery is impossible unless the baby turns spontaneously or is turned in utero. Compare the different types of presentations shown in Figure 13-8.

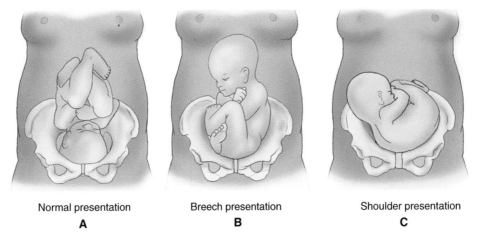

Normal presentation
A

Breech presentation
B

Shoulder presentation
C

Figure 13-8   Fetal presentation. **A,** Cephalic presentation, the normal presentation of the top of the head, the brow, the face, or the chin at the cervical opening. **B,** Breech presentation. **C,** Shoulder presentation.

Exercise 4

Match terms in the left column with their descriptions in the right column.

_____ 1. abruptio placentae

_____ 2. dystocia

_____ 3. ectopic pregnancy

_____ 4. placenta previa

_____ 5. pseudocyesis

A. abnormal or difficult labor
B. false pregnancy
C. fertilized egg implants outside the uterus
D. placenta covers the internal os of the cervix
E. separation of the placenta from the uterine wall

SURGICAL AND THERAPEUTIC INTERVENTIONS

amniotomy
(am″ne-ot′ə-me)

13-43 The word for deliberate rupture of the fetal membranes to induce labor is translated literally as incision of the amnion. Write this new term: _____.
   Oxytocin (ok″sĭ-to′sin) is a hormone that is produced by the pituitary gland and stimulates uterine contraction. Oxytocin is also used as a drug to induce or augment uterine contractions. Other drugs, uterine relaxants, slow or stop labor by slowing to stopping contractions of the

uterus

_____.

episiotomy

13-44 An episiotomy* (ə-piz″e-ot′o-me) facilitates delivery if the vaginal opening is too small. An episio/tomy is a surgical procedure in which an incision is made in the female perineum to enlarge her vaginal opening for delivery. The suffix -tomy will help you remember that an episiotomy involves an incision. Write this new term that means an incision that enlarges the vaginal opening to facilitate delivery: _____.

abdominal

13-45 A laparotomy (lap″ə-rot′ə-me) is necessary in cesarean sections and in all other abdominal surgeries that require opening of the abdominal cavity. Because lapar(o) means abdominal wall, laparo/tomy is incision of the _____ wall.

*Episiotomy (Greek: epision, pubic region + -tomy, incision).

If the abdominal wall is incised, it must be sutured (or stapled). Suturing of the abdominal wall is
_____.

laparorrhaphy
(lap″ə-ror′ə-fe)

13-46 A pregnant woman does not ovulate because high levels of estrogen and progesterone prevent ova from maturing. Knowledge of the interaction of hormones that prevent ovulation forms the basis of some types of contraception. Literal translation of *contra/ception* is
_____ conception. In other words, contraception is birth control, a process or technique for preventing pregnancy.

against

13-47 <u>Oral contraceptives</u>, <u>contraceptive implants</u>, <u>contraceptive patches</u>, and <u>injectable contraceptives</u> are methods that use hormones to prevent ovulation. Oral contraceptive is what is meant when someone says she is on the pill. The word *oral* in the name tells us that the medication is taken by _____.

mouth

13-48 An <u>intrauterine (in″trə-u′tər-in) device</u> (IUD) is inserted into the
_____ by the physician. It can be removed when the woman wishes to become pregnant.

uterus

13-49 Sometimes *sperm(i)* is used instead of *spermat(o)* to write words about sperm. A <u>spermi/cide</u> (**sper′mĭ-sīd**) is a chemical substance that kills _____.
Spermicides are placed in the vagina before intercourse to kill sperm but are not as effective as several other contraceptive methods. Spermicides are also used with other devices that are placed in the vagina to prevent sperm from reaching the uterus. Read about the different contraceptive methods in Table 13-1.
Abstinence is refraining from sexual intercourse and is the only means of contraception that is 100% effective.

sperm

13-50 <u>Tubal ligation</u> (**too′bəl lĭ-ga′shən**) and <u>vasectomy</u> (**və-sek′tə-me**) are sterilization procedures. Tubal ligation is constricting, severing, or crushing both fallopian
_____. Tubal ligation should be considered a permanent means of sterilization because it is not always reversible.
A vas/ectomy is bilateral excision of the vas deferens (**vas def′ər-enz**), the duct that transports sperm. It also should be considered a permanent means of sterilization because it is not always reversible. The surgical procedure in which the function of the vas deferens on each side of the testes is restored after a vasectomy is a <u>vaso/vaso/stomy</u> (**vas″o-, va″zo-va-zos′tə-me**). Notice that this term uses *vas(o)* twice. Write this term that means a surgical procedure that is used to reverse a vasectomy: _____.
Conception cannot occur after a <u>hysterectomy</u> (surgical removal of the uterus); however, the surgery is not done for the purpose of contraception.

tubes

vasovasostomy

13-51 Infertility is the condition of being unable to produce offspring. It may be present in one or both sex partners and may be temporary and reversible, as in the performance of a vasovasostomy. Administration of hormones, use of vaginal medications, surgery, and counseling are some of the treatments used in correcting infertility, depending on the cause. In/fertility is the condition of
_____ being able to produce offspring.
<u>In vitro fertilization</u> (IVF) may be successful when failure to conceive is caused by insufficient numbers of sperm. In vitro fertilization is a method of fertilizing the ova outside the body by collecting mature ova and placing them in a dish with spermatozoa. Fertilized ova are then placed in the uterus for implantation.

not

13-52 Termination of pregnancy before the fetus is capable of survival outside the uterus is an <u>abortion</u>. In lay language, a spontaneous or natural loss of the fetus is called a miscarriage, and *abortion* most often refers to a deliberate interruption of pregnancy. In the medical sense, both spontaneous loss and deliberate interruption of pregnancy are called abortion. A miscarriage is a spontaneous _____.

abortion

TABLE 13-1 Selected Contraceptive Methods*

Method	Action
100% Effective	
Abstinence	Refraining from sexual intercourse.
Very Effective	
Injectable contraceptive	Hormonal injection on a specific schedule prevents ovulation.
Implant (Norplant)	Capsules surgically implanted under the skin slowly release a hormone that blocks the release of ova.
Contraceptive patch	Transdermal patch worn on the skin.
Effective	
Intrauterine device	Small plastic or metal device placed in the uterus. Cause of effectiveness is not known but may prevent fertilization or implantation. Some release hormones.
Oral contraceptives	Hormones, usually progestin and estrogen, which prevent ovulation.
Less Effective	
Douche	Washing out of the vagina immediately after intercourse.
Spermicides	Vaginal foams, creams, jellies that are inserted into the vagina before intercourse to destroy the sperm.
Coitus interruptus	Withdrawal of the penis before ejaculation.
Diaphragm with spermicide	Soft rubber cup that covers the uterine cervix and prevents sperm from reaching the egg.
Condom	Thin sheath (usually latex) worn over the penis or in the vagina to collect semen.
Cervical cap with spermicide	Similar to diaphragm, but smaller, and covers cervix closely.
Sponge with spermicide	Acts as barrier to the sperm and releases spermicide.
Calendar or rhythm method	Determine fertile period and practice abstinence (voluntarily avoiding sexual intercourse) during "unsafe" days.
Basal body temperature (BBT)	Ovulation is determined by drop and subsequent rise in BBT; abstinence is practiced during fertile periods.
Cervical mucus	Ovulation is determined by observing the changes in the cervical mucus; abstinence is practiced during fertile period.
Symptothermal	Combination of observing symptoms and increase in body temperature (cervical mucus and BBT); abstinence is practiced on fertile days.

*Tubal ligation and vasectomy are not included here because they are forms of sterilization, often permanent.

Exercise 5

Match the contraceptive methods in the left column with their descriptions in the right column.

_____ 1. coitus interruptus

_____ 2. condom

_____ 3. diaphragm

_____ 4. Norplant

_____ 5. spermicide

A. rubber cup that covers the uterine cervix
B. thin sheath that collects semen
C. substance placed in the vagina to destroy the sperm
D. surgically implanted capsules that prevent ovulation
E. withdrawal of the penis before ejaculation

Write a word in each blank to complete these sentences.

1. Bilateral excision of the vas deferens is a _____.

2. Constricting, severing, or crushing the fallopian tubes is called a tubal _____.

3. In vitro _____ is a method of fertilizing the ova outside the body, then placing them in the uterus for implantation.

4. Termination of pregnancy before the fetus is capable of survival outside the uterus is an _____.

5. A surgical procedure to enlarge the vaginal opening for delivery is an _____.

Sexually Transmitted Diseases

sexually

13-53 Sexually transmitted diseases (STDs) are usually caused by infectious organisms that have been passed from one person to another through anal, oral, or vaginal intercourse. Some of the organisms that cause STDs are transmitted only through sexual intercourse, but others are transmitted also by infected blood or needles, by intrauterine transmission to the fetus, or by infection of the infant during birth. STDs were formerly called venereal (və-nēr′e-əl) diseases (VDs), named for Venus, goddess of love. These diseases are now called _____ transmitted diseases.

within

13-54 Different STDs are caused by specific types of viruses, bacteria, protozoa, fungi, and parasites. Without treatment, they can contribute to infertility, ectopic pregnancy, cancer, and death. One sexually transmitted disease, gonorrhea, was discussed in Chapter 11, the Urinary System. Gonorrhea (*gon[o]*, genitals + *-rrhea*, discharge) (**gon″o-re′ə**) is caused by the gono/coccus (**gon″o-kok′əs**), a gram-negative intracellular diplococcus (Figure 13-9). Intra/cellular means that the bacteria are located _____ the cells (in this case, white blood cells).
 Gonorrhea causes a heavy urethral discharge in males, but females may be asymptomatic. The disease can usually be treated with penicillin or with another antibiotic in penicillin-sensitive persons.

gonococcus

13-55 Many of the words in the medical dictionary that begin with *gon(o)* pertain to the gono/coccus, the type of bacteria that causes gonorrhea.
 Write the name of the microorganism that causes gonorrhea: _____.

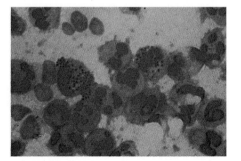

Figure 13-9   Gram-negative intracellular diplococci. The presence of gram-negative intracellular diplococci in a urethral smear is usually indicative of gonorrhea in males. The same finding in females is considered presumptive and is generally followed by culture to confirm the diagnosis. Note also the presence of many extracellular diplococci.

The gonococcus that causes gonorrhea, *Neisseria gonorrhoeae,* is a bacterium. Gram stain is a special staining technique that serves as a primary means of identifying and classifying bacteria. The presence of gram-negative intracellular diplococci is generally followed by a bacterial culture to confirm that the organisms are gonococci. This technique of growing microorganisms, done for the purpose of identifying the pathogen, is called _____.

culturing

13-56 The origin of syphilis (**sif′ĭ-lis**) is not clear, but the disease occurred throughout Europe shortly after the return of Christopher Columbus and his crew from the New World in 1493. Write the name of this sexually transmitted disease, being careful of its spelling:

syphilis

_____.

The first stage of syphilis is characterized by swollen lymph nodes and the appearance of a painless sore called a chancre (**shang′kər**). Do not confuse *chancre* with the word *canker* (**kang′kər**), which is an ulceration of the mouth or lips. The painless sore of syphilis that occurs usually on the genitals is called a _____.

chancre

Material from a chancre may be examined for the spirochete that causes syphilis (see Figure 7-10). Syphilis can be spread to another person through sexual contact.

13-57 If not treated with penicillin or another antibiotic, the second stage of syphilis occurs 2 weeks to 6 months after the chancre disappears. Blood tests for syphilis (Venereal Disease Research Laboratories [VDRL] or rapid plasma reagin [RPR]) are generally positive at this time but should be confirmed by additional tests. The disease becomes systemic as organisms spread throughout the body and a generalized rash appears. It can affect many organs. The outward sign that is characteristic for the second stage of syphilis is the _____. The second stage lasts 2 to 6 weeks and is followed by a fairly asymptomatic latent stage. Transmission of the disease can occur by blood transfer to another person during the latent stage.

rash

Only about one third of untreated individuals progress to the third stage, which has irreversible complications, including changes in the cardiovascular and nervous system and soft rubbery tumors, called gummas (**gum′əz**), on any part of the body.

13-58 Before the problems of the third stage of syphilis were recognized, some "psychotic" patients in mental hospitals may have been suffering from neuro/syphilis (**noor″o-sif′ĭ-lis**), a complication of late syphilis. Fever therapy (such as intentional infection with malaria, a disease characterized by chills and fever) was used to treat mental illness in past times. Syphilitic patients who were infected with malaria developed high fever and improved. The organisms that cause syphilis, like many others, are adversely affected by high temperatures (sometimes a rise of as little as only 1 or 2°F).

13-59 Congenital syphilis is acquired by the fetus in utero. The bacteria that cause syphilis can cross the placenta of an infected female and cause congenital _____.
Infants who are born with congenital syphilis may have severe physical and mental defects and die within a few weeks after birth.

syphilis

Several of the organisms that cause STDs can cross the placenta and infect the fetus, sometimes causing physical and mental defects or stillbirth. Others may infect the infant during childbirth. In the latter cases, a cesarean section is usually performed when the mother is known to be infected.

The stages of syphilis and information about additional STDs are summarized in Table 13-2.

13-60 Chlamydial (**klə-mid′e-əl**) infection, chlamyd/iosis (**klə-mid″e-o′sis**), is a treatable bacterial disease transmitted by intimate sexual contact and is the most common sexually transmitted disease in the United States. Antibiotics are used to treat chlamydiosis. Undetected and untreated cases can progress to scarring and ulcerations of the epididymis in males or the uterine tubes in females, causing infertility.

Read and answer questions about the characteristics of sexually transmitted diseases using the information in Table 13-2.

13-61 Chancroid is another STD caused by a bacterium. As shown in the table, the major characteristic of chancroid (**shang′kroid**) is _____ of the genitals.
Unlike the painless chancre of syphilis, the ulceration of chancroid is painful. Like other sexually transmitted diseases that are caused by bacteria, it can be treated with an antibiotic.

ulceration

TABLE 13-2 Sexually Transmitted Diseases and Their Causes

Disease of the Genitals*	Causative Agent	Characteristics
Bacterial		
Gonorrhea	*Neisseria gonorrhoeae*	Males: Urethral discharge, dysuria Females: Often asymptomatic
Syphilis	*Treponema pallidum* (a spirochete)	Primary stage: Painless chancre Secondary stage: Rash Late: Only about one third of untreated cases progress to syphilitic involvement of the viscera, the cardiovascular system, and the central nervous system
Chlamydial infection	*Chlamydia trachomatis*	Males: Urethritis, dysuria, and frequent urination Females: mild symptoms to none. One of the most common STDs in North America, often the cause of pelvic inflammatory disease, and a common cause of sterility
Chancroid (nonsyphilitic venereal ulcer)	*Haemophilus ducreyi*	Painful ulceration of the genitals
Nonspecific genital infection	Various organisms, not all of which are bacteria	Males: Nongonococcal urethritis Females: Pelvic inflammatory disease, cervicitis
Viral		
acquired immunodeficiency syndrome	Human immunodeficiency virus	A fatal late stage of infection with HIV that involves profound immunosuppression. To be diagnosed as having AIDS, one must be infected with HIV and have a clinical disease that indicates cellular immunodeficiency or have a specified level of CD4 and T-lymphocytes (T4). Characterized by opportunistic infections and malignant neoplasms that rarely afflict healthy individuals, especially Kaposi's sarcoma. Transmitted by infected body fluids (sexual contact, blood and blood products, breast milk)
Herpes genitalis (genital herpes)	Herpes simplex virus type 2 (HSV-2)	Blisters and ulceration of the genitalia, fever, and dysuria
Condyloma acuminatum (genital warts)	Human papillomavirus (HPV)	Genital and anal warts
Hepatitis B	Hepatitis B virus (HBV)	Disease varies from mild symptoms to serious complications. Transmitted by contaminated blood or needles and sexual contact. (Hepatitis B vaccine is available for those at high risk. HBIG, hepatitis B immune globulin, provides postexposure passive immunity.)
Hepatitis C	Hepatitis C virus (HCV)	Symptoms are generally mild. About 50% of the patients progress to chronic hepatitis. Transmitted mainly by blood products, sharing needles or straws for inhaling cocaine. Transmitted less commonly by sexual intercourse.
Hepatitis D	Hepatitis D virus (HDV)	Occurs only in patients infected with HBV. Usually develops into a chronic state. Transmitted through sexual contact and needle sharing. Prevention of hepatitis B with vaccine prevents hepatitis D.
Protozoal		
Trichomoniasis	*Trichomonas vaginalis*	Females: Frothy discharge of varying severity Males: Often asymptomatic
Fungal		
Candidiasis	*Candida albicans*	Vulvovaginitis: White patches, cheeselike discharge
Parasitic		
Pubic lice	*Phthirus pubis*	Severe itching and erythema

*Although diseases of the genitals are given emphasis here, many of the organisms can infect other organs.

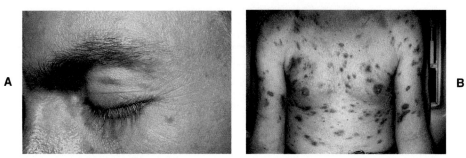

Figure 13-10   Kaposi's sarcoma. **A,** An early lesion of Kaposi's sarcoma. **B,** Advanced lesions of Kaposi's sarcoma. Note widespread hemorrhagic plaques and nodules.

gonorrhea

13-62 Nonspecific genital infections are caused by a variety of microorganisms. Non/gonococcal urethritis (u″rə-thri′tis) is inflammation of the urethra by an organism other than the gonococcus, the bacteria that causes _____.

immunodeficiency

13-63 Four general types of viral STDs are acquired immunodeficiency (im″u-no-də-fish′ən-se) syndrome, genital herpes, genital warts, and several types of hepatitis (hep″ə-ti′tis).
      The abbreviation *AIDS* means acquired _____ syndrome. As a result of the deficiency of antibodies, the immune response does not adequately protect the person from malignancies or opportunistic infections, infections that are caused by normally nonpathogenic organisms in someone whose resistance is decreased.
      AIDS is caused by the human immunodeficiency virus (HIV) and is spread by sexual intercourse or exposure to contaminated blood, semen, breast milk, or other body fluids of infected persons. The virus has a long incubation period (time between exposure and the onset of symptoms), and the disease we recognize as AIDS is the late, fatal stage of infection. Some persons with AIDS are susceptible to opportunistic infections and malignant neoplasms (tumors), especially Kaposi's sarcoma (sahr-ko′mə) (Figure 13-10).

genital

13-64 *Herpes genitalis* (hər′pēz jen-ĭ-tal′is), a viral infection caused by the herpes simplex virus (HSV-2), is also known as _____ herpes. Painful genital blisters and ulceration are characteristic of this disease. Anti/viral agents may lessen the severity and duration of the symptoms.
      Active infection during pregnancy can lead to spontaneous abortion, stillbirth, or congenital birth defects. Delivery of the infant is often by cesarean section to prevent infection of the infant at the time of delivery.

warts

13-65 Looking at Table 13-2, you see that *Condyloma acuminatum* (kon″də-lo′mə ə-ku″mĭ-nāt′əm) is commonly called genital _____, which also describes its major characteristic. Persons who have had genital warts are at greater risk of genital malignancy, especially cervical cancer.
      Treatment to destroy the genital warts includes destruction with acid, laser, or cryo/therapy (*cry[o]*, cold + *-therapy*, treatment). Cryo/therapy is destruction of the lesions using very

cold

_____ temperatures.

liver

13-66 Viral hepatitis is an inflammatory condition of the _____ caused by one of the hepatitis viruses, A, B, C, D, or E. Hepatitis A and E are not considered sexually transmitted diseases because transmission is generally through direct contact with contaminated food or water.

blood

      Hepatitis B is transmitted by sexual contact, _____ products, and contaminated needles. Hepatitis B vaccine is available, required by various educational institutions, and recommended for health care workers and others at greater than usual risk.
      Hepatitis C is primarily transmitted by blood products, shared needles, or shared straws for inhaling cocaine. It is transmitted less commonly by sexual intercourse. This type of hepatitis has a high likelihood of progressing to chronic hepatitis.

hepatitis	Hepatitis D occurs only in patients who are infected with _____ B. It is transmitted by sexual contact and needle sharing. Hepatitis B, C, and D are caused by hepatitis viruses B, C, and D, respectively.
Trichomonas	**13-67** Trichomon/iasis (**trik″o-mo-ni′ə-sis**) is an infection caused by _____ *vaginalis*, a protozoon. Diagnosis is by microscopic examination of fresh urethral or vaginal secretions (see Figure 7-12). Symptoms of trichomoniasis are a frothy discharge with a bad odor in females; symptoms are minor or absent in males.
vulva	**13-68** Candid/iasis (**kan″dĭ-di′ə-sis**) is a fungal infection that is not limited to the genitals but can cause *vulvo/vaginitis* (**vul″vo-vaj″ĭ-ni′tis**), which means inflammation of the _____ and the vagina. The infection is usually caused by *Candida albicans*, a yeast-type fungus (see Figure 7-11, A), and sometimes occurs after administration of antibiotics for a bacterial infection or when immunity is suppressed.
mouth	The fungus can be seen microscopically in urethral or vaginal secretions and can be treated with oral and topical anti/fungal medications. Oral medications are taken by _____ and topical ones are applied directly to the affected area. *C. albicans* is also called *Monilia* (**mo-nil′e-ə**), and the infection is sometimes called moniliasis (**mon-ĭ-li′ə-sis**).
itching	**13-69** Pubic (**pu′bik**) lice are external parasites and are sometimes included with STDs because they can be transmitted by sexual contact. They are also transmitted by close contact with contaminated objects, such as linens. They are commonly called crab lice and primarily infest the pubic region but are also found in armpits, beards, eyebrows, and eyelashes. Observe in Table 13-2 that characteristic symptoms of pubic lice are severe _____ and redness. The use of topical agents and particular attention to hygiene is used in treating lice.

Exercise 7

Match sexually transmitted diseases in the left column with their characteristics in the right column.

_____ 1. AIDS

_____ 2. genital herpes

_____ 3. gonorrhea

_____ 4. hepatitis B

_____ 5. syphilis

A. fatal late stage of infection with HIV
B. blisters and ulcerations of the genitals
C. caused by gram-negative intracellular diplococci
D. caused by HB virus
E. one sign is a painless chancre

SELECTED ABBREVIATIONS

AIDS	acquired immunodeficiency syndrome	**HDV**	hepatitis D virus
BBT	basal body temperature	**HIV**	human immunodeficiency virus
CPD	cephalopelvic disproportion	**HPV**	human papillomavirus
CS or C-section	cesarean section	**HSV-2**	herpes simplex virus type 2 (genital herpes)
EDD	expected delivery date	**IUD**	intrauterine device
EFM	electronic fetal monitor	**IVF**	in vitro fertilization
FHR	fetal heart rate	**LMP**	last menstrual period
G	gravida (pregnant)	**OB**	obstetrics
GC	gonococcus	**RPR**	rapid plasma reagin
HBV	hepatitis B virus	**STD**	sexually transmitted disease
HCG	human chorionic gonadotropin	**VD**	venereal disease
HCV	hepatitis C virus	**VDRL**	Venereal Disease Research Laboratories

CHAPTER 13 REVIEW

■ Basic Understanding

Labeling

I. Label the following structures in the drawing: amnion, amniotic fluid, chorion, placenta, umbilical cord, uterus.

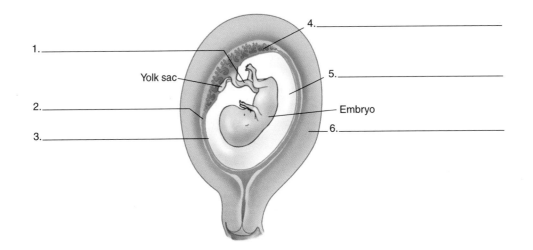

Matching

II. Match terms in the left column with their descriptions in the right column.

_____ 1. gamete

_____ 2. gonad

_____ 3. placenta

_____ 4. progesterone

_____ 5. zygote

A. afterbirth
B. important hormone of pregnancy
C. ovary or testis
D. ovum or spermatozoon
E. product of fertilization

III. Match the following pathologies of pregnancy with their descriptions.

_____ 1. abruptio placentae

_____ 2. ectopic pregnancy

_____ 3. placenta previa

_____ 4. preeclampsia

_____ 5. pseudocyesis

A. abnormal implantation of the placenta in the uterus
B. onset of acute high blood pressure after the twenty-fourth week
C. false pregnancy
D. implantation of a fertilized ovum outside the uterus
E. premature separation of the placenta from the uterine wall

Multiple Choice

IV. Circle the correct answer in each of the following.

1. Which of the following is the hormone tested for in a pregnancy test? (CPD, EFM, HCG, LMP)

2. Which of the following is estimation of the size of the birth canal? (amniocentesis, cephalopelvic disproportion, chorionic villus sampling, pelvimetry)

3. Which term means abnormal or difficult labor? (abortion, dystocia, eclampsia, stillbirth)

4. Which of the following is a genetic disorder in which the fetus has an extra chromosome? (Down syndrome, erythroblastosis fetalis, hemolytic anemia, implantation)

5. Which term means the same as pregnancy? (embryonic, gestation, ovulation, parturition)

6. Which of the following is the normal presentation of the fetus during labor? (breech, cephalic, shoulder, transverse)

7. Which contraceptive acts by killing the sperm? (hormonal implant, intrauterine device, oral contraceptive, spermicide)

8. Which of the following is a primipara? (para I, para II, para III, para IV)

9. Which of the following is the common name for *Condyloma acuminatum*? (genital herpes, genital warts, moniliasis, venereal ulcer)

10. Which of the following sexually transmitted diseases is caused by a fungus? (candidiasis, chancroid, chlamydiosis, trichomoniasis)

Writing Terms

V. *Write a term for each of the following.*

1. a newborn _____

2. a woman who has produced many viable offspring _____

3. an embryonic form of spermatozoa _____

4. attachment of a fertilized ovum to the endometrium _____

5. deliberate rupture of the fetal membranes to induce labor _____

6. incision made to enlarge the vaginal opening for delivery _____

7. painless sore of syphilis _____

8. pertaining to the amnion and the chorion _____

9. pertaining to the fetus _____

10. release of an ovum from the ovary _____

■ Greater Comprehension

Health Care Report

VI. *Answer the questions after reading the following report.*

PHYSICIAN'S LABORATORY

222 Medical Center Drive   Main City, US 11111   Phone: 555 222-0000

LABORATORY REPORT

Date of Report: 2/2/2005
NAME OF PATIENT: Esra Esselman
SS # 498-04-0003
SPECIMEN RECEIVED 1/27/2005: Vaginal swab
FINDINGS: Gram stain of the material showed the presence of both intracellular and extracellular gram-negative diplococci. *Neisseria gonorrhoeae* grown in culture.

---

1. What type of specimen was received by the laboratory? Describe it. _____

_____

2. What is meant by intracellular and extracellular diplococci? _____

_____

3. What is the name of the sexually transmitted disease that is implied? _____

4. What is the name of the organism that causes this disease? _____

5. Describe how this disease is usually treated. _____

Spelling
VII. Circle all incorrectly spelled terms and write their correct spellings.

amniosentesis   antenatal   contraseptive   extraembryonic   parturition

Interpreting Abbreviations
VIII. Write the meanings of these abbreviations.

1. AIDS _____

2. CPD _____

3. FHR _____

4. GC _____

5. IUD _____

Pronunciation
IX. The pronunciation is shown for several medical words. Indicate which syllable has the primary accent by marking it with an '.

1. amnion (am ne on)

2. chancre (shang kər)

3. gamete (gam ēt)

4. immunodeficiency (im u no də fish ən se)

5. secundipara (se kən dip ə rə)

Categorizing Terms
X. Classify the terms in the left column by selecting A, B, C, D, or E.

_____ 1. cesarean section
_____ 2. antifungals
_____ 3. antivirals
_____ 4. chorion
_____ 5. episiotomy
_____ 6. fetoscope use
_____ 7. hepatitis C
_____ 8. laparorrhaphy
_____ 9. preeclampsia
_____ 10. trichomoniasis

A. anatomy
B. diagnostic test or procedure
C. pathology
D. surgery
E. therapy

(Check your answers with the solutions in Appendix VI.)

LISTING OF MEDICAL TERMS

Use the practice CD to review the terms that have been presented. Look closely at the spelling of each term as it is pronounced and be sure you know the meaning of each term.

abortion	condom	human chorionic	preeclampsia
abruptio placentae	condyloma acuminatum	gonadotropin	prenatal
acquired	contraceptive	implantation	primigravida
immunodeficiency	cryotherapy	internal os	primipara
syndrome	diaphragm	intrauterine device	progesterone
amniocentesis	dilatation	intrauterine transfusion	pseudocyesis
amniochorial	Down syndrome	Kaposi's sarcoma	pseudopregnancy
amniochorionic	dystocia	laparorrhaphy	pubic lice
amnion	dysuria	laparotomy	quadripara
amnionic	eclampsia	*Monilia*	quickening
amniorrhexis	ectopic pregnancy	moniliasis	secundipara
amniotic	effacement	neonatal	spermatoblast
amniotomy	endometrium	neonate	spermatozoon
antenatal	episiotomy	neonatologist	spermicide
antepartum	erythroblastosis fetalis	neonatology	stethoscope
bilirubin	extraembryonic	neurosyphilis	stillbirth
breech presentation	extrauterine	nongonococcal urethritis	symptothermal
candidiasis	fetal	nullipara	syphilis
cephalopelvic	fetoscope	obstetrician	transabdominal
disproportion	fetus	obstetrics	transverse presentation
cesarean section	gamete	ooblast	trichomoniasis
chancre	genital herpes	ovulation	trimester
chancroid	genital warts	ovum	tripara
chlamydial	gestation	oxytocin	tubal ligation
chlamydiosis	gonad	parous	tubal pregnancy
chorion	gonococcus	parturition	vasectomy
chorionic	gonorrhea	pelvimetry	vasovasostomy
chorionic villi	gravid	placenta	venereal
chorionic villus sampling	gravida	placenta previa	viral hepatitis
coitus interruptus	herpes genitalis	postnatal	vulvovaginitis
conception	herpes simplex virus	postpartum	zygote

español ENHANCING SPANISH COMMUNICATION

ENGLISH	SPANISH (PRONUNCIATION)
birth	nacimiento (nah-se-me-EN-to)
childbirth	parto (PAR-to)
contraception	contracepción (con-trah-cep-se-ON)
cream	crema (CRAY-mah)
diaphragm	diafragma (de-ah-FRAHG-mah)
foam	espuma (es-POO-mah)
newborn	recién nacida (ray-se-EN nah-SEE-dah)
parturition	parto (PAR-to)
pregnancy	embarazo (em-bah-RAH-so)
pregnant	embarazada (em-bah-rah-SAH-dah)
reproduction	reproducción (ray-pro-dooc-se-ON)
rhythm method	método de ritmo (MAY-to-do day REET-mo)

Musculoskeletal System

LEARNING GOALS

In this chapter, you will learn to do the following:

Basic Understanding

1. Identify the major bones of the body and write their combining forms.
2. Match bones, muscles, and supporting structures with their functions.
3. Differentiate the different types of body movements.
4. Match types of fractures with their descriptions.
5. List and describe the functions of the three types of muscle tissue.
6. Write the meanings of the word parts and use them to build and analyze terms.

Greater Comprehension

7. Use word parts from this chapter to determine the meanings of terms in a health care report.
8. Spell the terms accurately.
9. Pronounce the terms correctly.
10. Write the meanings of the abbreviations.
11. Categorize terms as anatomy, diagnostic test or procedure, pathology, surgery, or therapy.

THESE ARE THE MAJOR SECTIONS IN THIS CHAPTER:

❑ **Anatomy and Physiology**
Characteristics of Bone
Bones of the Skeleton
Axial Skeleton
Appendicular Skeleton
Joints, Tendons, and Ligaments
Muscles
❑ **Diagnostic Tests and Procedures**

❑ **Pathologies**
Stress and Trauma Injuries
Infections
Tumors and Malignancies
Metabolic Disturbances
Congenital Defects
Arthritis and Connective Tissue Diseases
Muscular Disorders
❑ **Surgical and Therapeutic Interventions**

FUNCTION FIRST

The most widely known function of the skeletal system is that of support, providing form and shape for the body. Additional functions are protection of soft body parts, movement, blood cell formation, and storage. Bones provide a place for muscles and supporting structures to attach. Muscles function in the movement of body parts by contraction and relaxation of muscle fibers.

ANATOMY AND PHYSIOLOGY

muscles

14-1 *Musculo/skeletal* (mus″ku-lo-skel′ə-təl) means pertaining to the _____ and the skeleton. Because of the close association of the body's skeleton and muscles, the two systems are often referred to as one, as in musculoskeletal disorders. The muscular system is also closely associated with the nervous system, because a muscle fiber must first be stimulated by a nerve impulse before it can contract.

Cells of the musculo/skeletal system are derived from ancestral cells that mature and then begin to function as bone cells, muscle cells, and so on. This is not unlike cells of other body systems.

■ Characteristics of Bone

yellow

14-2 Bone marrow is the soft tissue that fills the cavities of the bones. Red bone marrow functions in the formation of red blood cells, white blood cells, and platelets. In addition, bones store and release minerals, especially calcium, and are essential parts of mineral balance in the body. Fat is stored in the yellow bone marrow. The two types of bone marrow are red and _____ marrow.

calcium

14-3 The intercellular substance of bone contains an abundance of mineral salts, primarily calcium phosphate and calcium carbonate, which gives bone its unique hardness. Most of the calcium in our bodies is stored in the skeleton. The endocrine system controls the release of calcium from the bone when the level of _____ in the blood is decreased.

compact

14-4 Bones may be classified as long, short, flat, or irregular. Examples of long bones are those in the arm, leg, and thigh. Bones of the wrist are examples of short bones. Most of the bones of the skull are flat bones, and bones of the spine are classified as irregular bones.

The general features of a long bone are shown in Figure 14-1, A. The drawing shows that some parts of bone are hard and compact (compact bone), whereas other parts are spongy (spongy bone). Which type of bony tissue do you suspect serves as protection and support, compact or spongy? _____

The chief characteristic of bone is its rigid nature, but it is important to remember that bone contains living cells and is richly supplied with blood vessels and nerves.

diaphysis (di-af′ə-sis)

epiphysis (ə-pif′ə-sis)

14-5 Answer these questions as you look at Figure 14-1. The long shaft of the long bone is called the _____. This long shaft is thick, compact bone that surrounds yellow marrow in adults.

At each end of the diaphysis, there is an expanded portion called the _____. The epiphysis is spongy bone that is covered by a thin layer of compact bone. The two ends are covered by articular cartilage (kahr′tǐ-ləj) to provide smooth surfaces for movement of the joints. Except in the areas where there is articular cartilage, the bone is covered with a tough membrane called periosteum (per″e-os′te-əm). Analyzing the word parts of peri/ost/eum will help you remember its meaning. The prefix *peri-* means around, *oste(o)* means

bone

_____, and *-ium* means membrane. (In writing periosteum, an *i* is omitted to facilitate pronunciation.)

Bone is richly supplied with blood vessels. Like other body tissues, bone requires oxygen and nutrients and produces wastes, the end products of metabolism.

14-6 Note that bone has four types of tissue: compact bone, spongy bone, the medullary cavity containing the yellow marrow, and the periosteum.

The type of bone tissue that lies just beneath the periosteum is called

compact

_____ bone. It has a system of small canals (haversian canals) that run parallel to the bone's long axis and contain blood vessels (Figure 14-1, B). The canals are surrounded by concentric rings characteristic of mature bone.

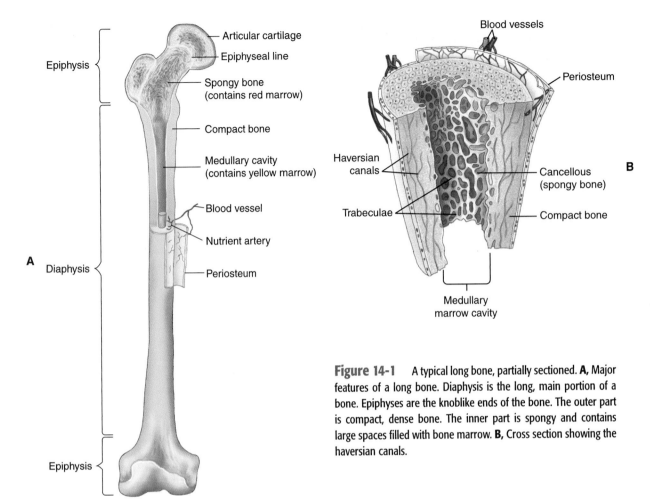

Figure 14-1 A typical long bone, partially sectioned. **A,** Major features of a long bone. Diaphysis is the long, main portion of a bone. Epiphyses are the knoblike ends of the bone. The outer part is compact, dense bone. The inner part is spongy and contains large spaces filled with bone marrow. **B,** Cross section showing the haversian canals.

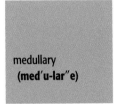

medullary
(med′u-lar″e)

Spongy bone is lighter than compact bone and contains a large spongy meshwork called trabeculae **(trə-bĕ′ku-le)**. Spongy bone is found largely in the epiphyses (plural form of epiphysis) and inner portions of long bones and is filled with red and yellow marrow.

The _____ cavity contains yellow marrow. The periosteum is composed of fibrous tissue that covers the bone.

Learn the following word parts.

General Word Parts for Describing Bone

WORD PARTS	MEANINGS
blast(o), -blast	embryonic form
myel(o)	bone marrow or spinal cord
oste(o)	bone

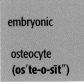

embryonic

osteocyte
(os′te-o-sīt″)

14-7 The combining form *blast(o)* and its corresponding suffix *-blast* mean embryonic or early form. An osteo/blast **(os′te-o-blast″)** is an _____ bone cell. With growth, osteoblasts develop into mature bone cells. Use *oste(o)* to write a word that literally means a bone cell: _____. Osteocytes are mature bone cells that become embedded in the calcified intercellular substance of bone.

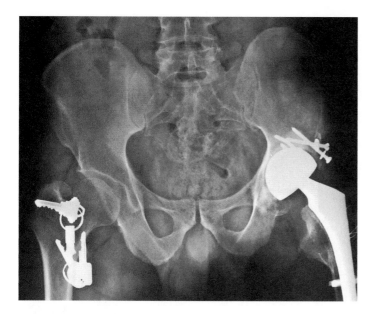

Figure 14-2   X-ray film of the pelvis. Keys were left in the pocket of a lightweight hospital robe during the examination, so radiography had to be repeated. Note also the metal fixation devices in the hip. Metal objects are radiopaque. Bones appear white, and soft tissue appears gray.

14-8 Calcium in bone is radiopaque (**ra″de-o-pāk′**); hence bones can block x-rays so that they do not reach image receptors. Bones are represented by white areas in an x-ray image (Figure 14-2). Unimpeded x-rays expose image receptors and cause a black or dark area in the image.

14-9 Calci/fication (**kal″sĭ-fĭ-ka′shən**) is the process by which organic tissue becomes hardened by

calcium

deposit of what substance in tissue? _____

Normally calcium is deposited in bone in large amounts to give bone its hardness. Calcification in soft tissue is abnormal.

14-10 Osteo/genesis (**os″te-o-jen′ə-sis**) or ossification (**os″ĭ-fĭ-ka′shən**) is the formation of bone substance. Human embryos contain no bone but do contain cartilage, a more flexible tissue that is shaped like bone. Osteo/genesis is the process whereby cartilage is used as a model to form what

bone

kind of tissue? _____

The Latin term for bone, *os* (plural, *ossa*), is often used in the naming of bones. For example, os coccygis is the formal name for the coccyx, or the tailbone. *Os* and *ossa* are not word parts but instead are Latin terms that mean bone and are commonly used in naming them.

myel(o)

14-11 The combining form for bone marrow is _____. This combining form also means the spinal cord.

The cells of red marrow are responsible for producing new blood cells. An embryonic bone mar

myeloblast
(**mi′ə-lo-blast**)

row cell is called a _____.

Myeloblasts mature into myelocytes (**mi′ə-lo-sītz**), which mature into leukocytes that are normally found in blood.

Exercise 1

Write a word in each blank to complete these sentences.

1. The soft tissue that fills the cavities of the bones is bone _____.

2. The long shaft of a long bone is called the diaphysis, and the expanded portions at the ends are called the

    _____.

3. Most of the bone is covered with a tough membrane called _____.

4. An osteoblast is an embryonic form of a _____ cell.

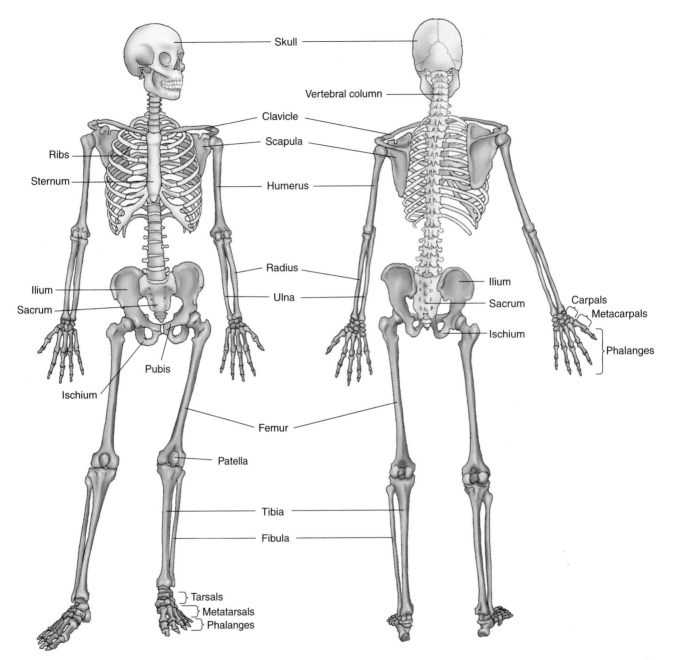

Figure 14-3   Anterior and posterior views of the human skeleton with major bones identified. The bones are grouped in two divisions. The axial skeleton forms the vertical axis of the body and is shown here as bone colored. The appendicular skeleton includes the free appendages and their attachments and is shown in blue.

■ *Bones of the Skeleton*

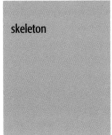

skeleton

14-12 The human skeleton* is the bony framework of the body. *Skeletal* means pertaining to the _____. The skeletal system consists of the bones and the cartilages, ligaments, and tendons that are associated with the bones. Bones and muscles work together to enable us to bend our arms and legs, turn our heads, or perform other voluntary movements.

14-13 The adult human skeleton usually consists of 206 named bones. There are also a few others that vary in number from one individual to another, so they are not counted with the other 206 bones. The major bones are identified in Figure 14-3. Study the names of the bones and their locations.

*Skeleton (Greek: a dried body or a mummy).

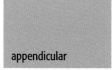

appendicular

Note that the skeleton is divided into the axial (**ak′se-əl**) skeleton and the appendicular (**ap″en-dik′u-lər**) skeleton. The division of the skeleton that forms the vertical axis of the body is the axial skeleton. The free appendages and their attachments are called the

_____ skeleton.

Exercise 2

Write a word in each blank to complete these sentences.

1. The bony framework of the body is the _____ .

2. A term that means pertaining to the skeleton is _____ .

3. The division of the skeleton that forms the vertical axis of the body is the _____ skeleton.

4. Bones of the extremities and their attachments to the axial skeleton are called the _____ skeleton.

■ *Axial Skeleton*

axial

14-14 The skull, spinal column, sternum, and ribs make up the

_____ skeleton. It consists of 80 major bones. These bones form the vertical axis to which the appendicular skeleton attaches. Learn the word parts associated with bones of the axial skeleton.

Word Parts for Bones of the Axial Skeleton

Combining Forms	Bone	Common Name
cost(o)	costae	ribs
crani(o)	cranium	skull
rach(i), rachi(o), spin(o)	vertebral or spinal column	spine (backbone)
spondyl(o), vertebr(o)	vertebrae	bones of the spine
stern(o)	sternum	breastbone

Types of Vertebrae (Uppermost to Lowermost)

Combining Forms	Meaning
cervic(o)	cervical
thorac(o)	thoracic
lumb(o)	lumbar
sacr(o)	sacral
coccyg(o)	coccygeal

skull

cranial (**kra′ne-əl**)

14-15 The cranium serves as protection for the brain and forms the framework of the face. The common name for the cranium is the _____ . It is composed of three types of bones: cranial bones; facial* bones; and the six auditory ossicles (**os′ĭ-kəlz**), three tiny bones in each middle ear cavity (Figure 14-4).

You learned that *crani(o)* means cranium or skull. The cranium is the major portion of the skull, that which encloses and protects the brain. Write a word that means pertaining to the skull:

_____ .

The bones that make up the skull are listed in Table 14-1. The opening at the base of the skull through which the spinal cord passes is called the foramen magnum (**fo-ra′mən mag′nəm**).

*Facial (Latin: *facialis*, from *facies*, face).

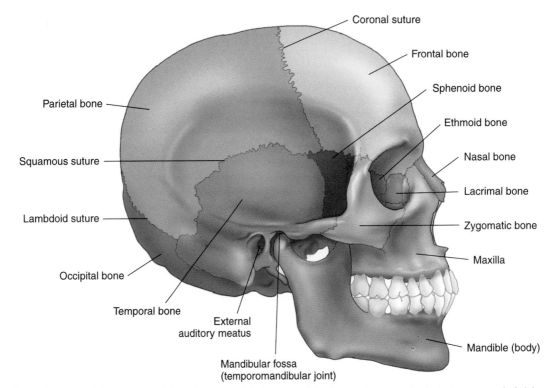

Figure 14-4 Major bones of the skull, lateral view. The cranium, that portion of the skull that encloses the brain, is composed of eight cranial bones (parietal, temporal, frontal, occipital, ethmoid, and sphenoid). Sutures are immovable fibrous joints between many of the cranial bones. The 14 facial bones (not all are shown) form the basic framework and shape of the face. The auditory ossicles (not shown) are three tiny bones in each middle ear cavity. The external auditory meatus is the external opening of the ear.

TABLE 14-1 Named Bones of the Skull

Cranial Bones	Facial Bones	Auditory Ossicles
Parietal (2)	Maxilla (2)	Malleus (2)
Temporal (2)	Zygomatic (2)	Incus (2)
Frontal (1)	Mandible (1)	Stapes (2)
Occipital (1)	Nasal (2)	
Ethmoid (1)	Palatine (2)	
Sphenoid (1)	Inferior nasal concha (2)	
	Lacrimal (2)	
	Vomer (1)	

spine

14-16 The vertebral or spinal column is attached at the base of the skull. The vertebral column is commonly called the backbone or the _____, and extends from the base of the skull to the pelvis. It encloses and protects the spinal cord, supports the head, and serves as a place of attachment for the ribs and muscles of the back.

spinal (spi′nəl)

The combining forms *rach(i)*, *rachi(o)*, and *spin(o)* mean spine. Combine *spin(o)* and *-al* to write a word that means pertaining to the spine: _____. Most medical terms pertaining to the spine use *rach(i)* and *rachi(o)*. *Rachi(o)* is more commonly used than *rach(i)*.

14-17 The vertebral column is composed of 26 vertebrae. Vertebrae (**vər′tə-bre**) is the plural form of vertebra (**vər′tə-brə**). *Inter/vertebral* (**in″tər-ver′tə-brəl**) means between two adjoining

vertebrae

_____. Cushions of cartilage between adjoining vertebrae are called intervertebral disks. These layers of cartilage absorb shock.

The vertebrae are named and numbered from the top downward (Figure 14-5). The combining form *cervic(o)* means neck. There are seven cervical (**sər′vĭ-kəl**) vertebrae located in the region

neck

called the _____.

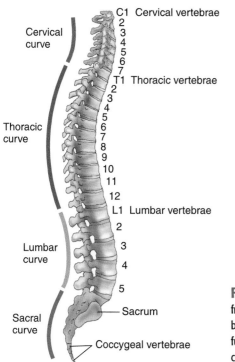

C1 Cervical vertebrae
2
3
4
5
6
7
T1 Thoracic vertebrae
2
3
4
5
6
7
8
9
10
11
12
L1 Lumbar vertebrae
2
3
4
5

Cervical curve

Thoracic curve

Lumbar curve

Sacral curve

Sacrum

Coccygeal vertebrae

Figure 14-5   The vertebral column with normal curvatures noted. The vertebrae are numbered from above downward. There are seven cervical vertebrae in the neck region, twelve thoracic vertebrae behind the chest cavity, five lumbar vertebrae supporting the lower back, five sacral vertebrae fused into one bone called the sacrum, and four coccygeal vertebrae fused into one bone called the coccyx.

chest	**14-18** *Thorac/ic* refers to the _____. The twelve thoracic vertebrae are part of the posterior wall of the chest. The combining form *lumb(o)* means the lower back. The five lumb/ar **(lum′bahr)** vertebrae are just below the thoracic vertebrae. In what part of the body are lumbar vertebrae located? lower
back	_____ *Thoraco/lumbar* **(thor″ə-ko-lum′bər)** means pertaining to two particular types of vertebrae. To what types of vertebrae does *thoracolumbar* refer? thoracic and
lumbar	_____
	14-19 Use *sacr(o)* to write words about the sacrum, the triangular bone below the lumbar vertebrae. In adults, five vertebrae fuse to form the sacrum. Which vertebrae are fused into one bone, the
sacral **(sa′krəl)**	sacrum? _____ vertebrae
	14-20 The combining form *coccyg(o)* means coccyx, or the tailbone. In adults, the coccyx **(kok′siks)** is the bone at the base of the vertebral column. It is formed by four fused vertebrae.
coccygeal **(kok-sij′e-əl)**	Which vertebrae fuse to form the coccyx? _____ vertebrae
breastbone	**14-21** Locate the elongated flattened sternum **(stər′nəm)** in Figure 14-3. The common name of the sternum is the _____.
sternum	The combining form that means sternum is *stern(o)*. *Stern/al* **(ster′nəl)** pertains to the _____. *Intra/sternal* means within the sternum.
	The prefix *infra-* means situated below. *Infrasternal* **(in″frə-stər′nəl)** means beneath the sternum. If *infra/sternal* means beneath the sternum, form a new word using *retro-* that means situated or
retrosternal **(ret″ro-ster′nəl)**	occurring behind the breastbone: _____.
	Supra/sternal **(soo″prə-ster′nəl)** means above the sternum. Using the prefix *sub-*, write the word
substernal **(səb-stər′nəl)**	that means below the sternum: _____.
	14-22 The sternum is one of the bones that make up the thoracic cage, which protects the heart, lungs, and great vessels and also plays a role in breathing. *Thoracic* means pertaining to the
thorax (chest)	_____. Attached to the sternum are the ribs, which support the chest wall and protect the lungs and heart. See the thoracic cage in Figure 14-6 and note the 12 pairs of ribs, which are numbered from

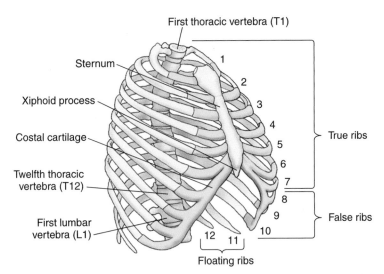

Figure 14-6   The thoracic cage. The ribs exist in pairs, twelve on each side of the chest, and are numbered from the top rib, beginning with *one*. The upper seven pairs join directly with the sternum by a strip of cartilage and are called *true ribs*. The remaining five pairs are referred to as *false ribs* because they do not attach directly to the sternum. The last two pairs of false ribs, called *floating ribs,* are attached only on the posterior aspect.

Labels in figure: First thoracic vertebra (T1); Sternum; Xiphoid process; Costal cartilage; Twelfth thoracic vertebra (T12); First lumbar vertebra (L1); True ribs; False ribs; Floating ribs; 1, 2, 3, 4, 5, 6, 7, 8, 9, 10, 11, 12

true	the top rib, beginning with one. Note that the first seven ribs on each side join directly with the sternum by a strip of cartilage and are called _____ ribs.
	Also note the xiphoid (**zif′oid, zi′foid**) process, the smallest and lowermost part of the sternum, which is often used as a point of reference when examining the chest.
	14-23 The combining form *cost(o)* means ribs. Another term for a rib is *costa* (**kos′tə**), and the plural is *costae* (**kos′te**). *Cost/al* (**kos′təl**) means pertaining to the ribs. The location of sub/cost/al (**səb-kos′təl**) is below a rib. Write a term using *supra-* that means above or upon a rib:
supracostal (soo″prə-kos′təl)	_____. *Infra/cost/al* (**in″frə-kos′təl**) means below a rib.
ribs	*Inter/costal* (**in″tər-kos′təl**) is a term that means between the _____. Intercostal muscles lie between the ribs and draw adjacent ribs together to increase the volume of the thorax in breathing.
sternum	**14-24** *Sterno/cost/al* (**stər″no-kos′təl**) pertains to the _____ and the ribs.
	Both *vertebr(o)* and *spondyl(o)* are combining forms that mean vertebrae. *Vertebro/costal* (**vər″tə-bro-kos′təl**) and *costo/vertebral* (**kos″to-vər′tə-brəl**) both mean pertaining to a vertebra and a rib.
sternum	**14-25** Two other terms, *vertebrosternal* (**vər″tə-bro-stər′nəl**) and *sternovertebral* (**stər″no-vər′tə-brəl**), can also be reversed in this way. These terms mean pertaining to the vertebrae and the _____.

Exercise 3

Write a word in each blank to complete these sentences.

1. The axial skeleton is composed of the skull, the spinal column, the _____, and the ribs.

2. The combining form *crani(o)* means the _____ or the skull.

3. The combining form that means rib is _____.

4. The combining forms *rach(i)* and *rachi(o)* mean _____.

5. The combining form that means the breastbone is _____.

6. The spine is composed of 26 bones that are called _____.

7. The uppermost vertebrae are located within the neck and are called _____ vertebrae.

8. The coccyx is formed by four fused _____ vertebrae.

■ *Appendicular Skeleton*

appendicular	**14-26** Bones of the extremities, the shoulder girdle, and the pelvic girdle compose the appendicular skeleton. In other words, the appendicular skeleton includes the bones of the limbs and their attachments to the axial skeleton. The shoulder girdle includes the clavicle and the scapula, and the pelvic girdle includes the bones of the pelvis. The major division of the skeleton that attaches to the axial skeleton is called the _____ skeleton. Learn the following word parts for the names of the bones of the appendicular skeleton.

Word Parts for Bones of the Appendicular Skeleton

COMBINING FORMS	BONE	COMMON NAME
clavicul(o)	clavicle	collarbone
scapul(o)	scapula	shoulder blade

Bones of the Pelvic Girdle*

COMBINING FORMS	BONE
ili(o)	ilium
ischi(o)	ischium
pub(o)	pubis

Bones of the Upper Extremities

COMBINING FORMS	BONE	COMMON NAME
carp(o)	carpus	wrist
humer(o)	humerus	upper arm bone
phalang(o)	phalanx (plural, phalanges)	finger
radi(o)	radius (sometimes, radiant energy)	bone of the forearm

Bones of the Upper Extremities

COMBINING FORMS	BONE	COMMON NAME
uln(o)	ulna	bone of the forearm

Bones of the Lower Extremities†

COMBINING FORMS	BONE	COMMON NAME
calcane(o)	calcaneus	heel bone
femor(o)	femur	thigh bone
fibul(o)	fibula	calf bone
tibi(o)	tibia	shin bone
patell(o)	patella	kneecap
phalang(o)	phalanx (plural, phalanges)	toe
tars(o)	tarsus (sometimes, edge of eyelid)	ankle

*These bones fuse to form the pelvic bone.
†The prefix *meta-* means change or next.

collarbone	**14-27** Locate the clavicle (**klav′ĭ-kəl**) in Figure 14-3. The clavicle is also known as the _____. *Infra/clavicul/ar* (**in″frə-klə-vik′u-lər**) means below the clavicle. The clavicles are long, curved horizontal bones that attach to the sternum and either the left or right scapula. The scapula (**skap′u-lə**) is a large triangular bone that is commonly called the shoulder blade. *Infra/scapul/ar* (**in″frə-skap′u-lər**) means below the
scapula	_____.
forearm carpals (**kahr′pəlz**)	**14-28** Each scapula is joined to the upper arm bone, the humerus (**hu′mər-əs**), by muscles and tendons. The ulna (**ul′nə**) and the radius (**ra′de-əs**) are bones of the _____. The wrist is composed of eight carpal bones, also called _____. Bones of the hand are meta/carpals (*meta-*, next), and bones of the fingers are phalanges (**fə-lan′jēz**).
pubis (**pu′bis**)	**14-29** Three types of pelvic bones are shown in Figure 14-3: the ilium (**il′e-əm**), the ischium (**is′ke-əm**), and the _____.
femur (**fe′mər**)	**14-30** The thighbone, the longest bone of the leg, is called the _____. The patella is the kneecap, and the two bones of the lower leg are the tibia (**tib′e-ə**) and the fibula (**fib′u-lə**). The ankle is composed of seven tarsal bones, also called the
tarsals (**tahr′səlz**)	_____. Bones of the feet are metatarsals. Like bones of the fingers, those of the toes are called phalanges.
	14-31 Many of the 126 bones that make up the appendicular skeleton are small and are found in the hands and feet, but several of the remaining bones in this part of the skeleton are the longest bones in the body. Bones of the appendicular skeleton are designed for movement.

Studying the individual bones of the appendicular skeleton, the combining form *clavicul(o)* means the clavicle. *Sterno/clavicul/ar* (**stər″no-klə-vik′u-lər**) pertains to the sternum and the

_____.

Costo/clavicul/ar (**kos″to-klə-vik′u-lər**) means pertaining to or involving the

_____ and the clavicle.

14-32 The combining form *scapul(o)* means scapula (shoulder blade). *Scapul/ar* (**skap′u-lər**) means pertaining to the scapula. Write a term that means between the two shoulder blades:

_____.

Scapulo/clavicul/ar (**skap″u-lo-klə-vik′u-lər**) means pertaining to the scapula and the clavicle. The clavicles and the two scapulae form the shoulder girdle, the connection between the arms and the axial skeleton.

14-33 Both the clavicle and the upper arm bone are attached to the scapula. The upper arm bone is the humerus and has the combining form *humer(o)*. *Humer/al* (**hu′mər-əl**) pertains to the

_____.

Humero/scapul/ar (**hu″mər-o-skap′u-lər**) means pertaining to the humerus and the

_____.

14-34 The bones of the forearm, the portion of the arm between the elbow and the wrist, are the ulna and the _____, and their combining forms are *uln(o)* and *radi(o)*, respectively. Also remember that *radi(o)* will sometimes refer to radiant energy, as you learned earlier. Use a combining form with radial to write a word that means pertaining to both the ulna and the radius: _____.

14-35 Use another combining form with radial to write a word that means pertaining to the humerus and the radius: _____.

Humeroulnar (**hu″mər-o-ul′nər**) means pertaining to the humerus and the ulna.

14-36 The combining form *carp(o)* means the carpus, or wrist. Observe in Figure 14-7 that the wrist consists of eight small bones, arranged in two transverse rows. *Carp/al* (**kahr′pəl**) pertains to the _____. Bones of the wrist are called carpals. Therefore *carpals* is a word that means the same as carp/al bones.

14-37 The metacarpals (**met″ə-kahr′pəlz**) connect the wrist bones (carpals) to the phalanges. You learned that *meta-* is a prefix that means a change or next, as in a series. The meta/carpals lie _____ to the carpals. The five metacarpals constitute the palm. The proximal ends of the metacarpals join with the distal row of what type of bones?

_____

14-38 The distal ends of the metacarpals join with the phalanges (**fə-lan′jēz**). The combining form *phalang(o)* means phalanges. The phalanges are bones of the _____, as well as bones of the toes. *Carpo/phalang/eal* (**kahr″po-fə-lan′je-əl**) pertains to the carpus and the _____—in this case, the fingers.

See Figure 14-7 to observe that there are three phalanges in each finger (a proximal, middle, and distal phalanx) but not in the thumb.

14-39 The pelvic girdle consists of two hipbones. Each of these bones consists of three separate bones in the newborn, but eventually the three fuse to form one bone. Names of the three bones are the ilium (**il′e-əm**), the ischium (**is′ke-əm**), and the _____. Their combining forms are *ili(o)*, *ischi(o)*, and *pub(o)*, respectively. The ilium is the largest of the three bones. The ischium is the posterior part of the pelvic girdle, and the pubis is the anterior part of the pelvic girdle.

Ili/ac (**il′e-ak**), *ischi/al* (**is′ke-əl**), and *pub/ic* (**pu′bik**) mean pertaining to the ilium, the _____, and the pubis, respectively.

---

clavicle

ribs

interscapular
(in″tər-skap′u-lər)

humerus

scapula

radius

ulnoradial
(ul″no-ra′de-əl)

humeroradial
(hu″mər-o-ra′de-əl)

carpus

next

carpal

fingers

phalanges

pubis

ischium

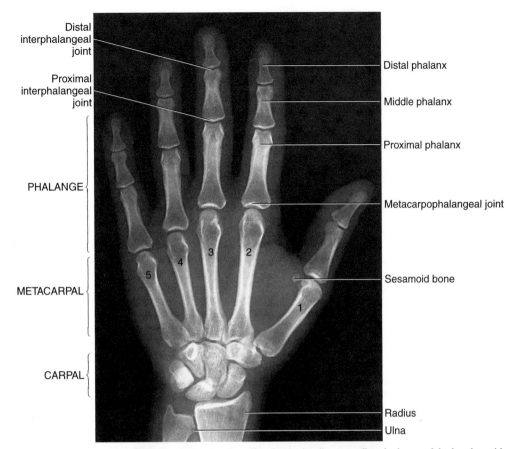

Distal interphalangeal joint

Proximal interphalangeal joint

PHALANGE

METACARPAL

CARPAL

Distal phalanx

Middle phalanx

Proximal phalanx

Metacarpophalangeal joint

Sesamoid bone

Radius
Ulna

5 4 3 2 1

Figure 14-7   Radiograph of the human hand, posteroanterior view. The ulna and radius, as well as the bones of the hand, are identified. Eight small carpal bones make up the wrist. The palm of the hand contains five metacarpal bones, which are numbered *1* to *5* starting on the thumb side. There are three phalanges in each finger (a proximal, middle, and distal phalanx) except the thumb, which has two. The sesamoid bone is a small, round bone embedded in the tendon that provides added strength for the thumb.

14-40 Locate these three bones that are fused to form each of the hipbones. The hipbones unite with the sacrum and coccyx to form the pelvis (Figure 14-8). Also compare the male pelvis with the female pelvis.

ilium
ischium

Ilio/pubic (il″e-o-pu′bik) pertains to the _____ and the pubis.

Ischio/pubic (is″ke-o-pu′bik) means pertaining to the _____ and the pubis.

Ischio/coccyg/eal (is″ke-o-kok-sij′e-əl) is pertaining to the ischium and the

coccyx

_____.

beneath

14-41 *Sub/pubic* (səb-pu′bik) means a location _____ the pubis. *Supra/pubic* (soo″prə-pu′bik) means above the pubis.

The hairs growing over the pubic region are called pubes (pu′bēz). This term is also used to denote the pubic region. The pubic region or the hairs that grow in this region are called the

pubes

_____.

The pubic symphysis is the inter/pubic (in″tər-pu′bik) joint where the two pubic bones meet.

14-42 The lower extremities, like the two upper extremities, are composed of sixty bones. The femur, or the thigh bone, is the longest and heaviest bone in the body (Figure 14-9). The combining form *femor(o)* means femur. *Femor/al* pertains to the _____.

Ilio/femor/al (il″e-o-fem′or-əl) means pertaining to the ilium and the

femur

_____.

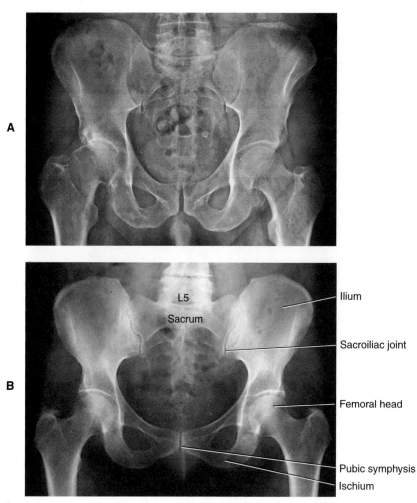

A

B

L5
Sacrum

Ilium

Sacroiliac joint

Femoral head

Pubic symphysis
Ischium

Figure 14-8   Radiographs comparing the male pelvis with that of the female, anterior views. **A,** Male pelvis. Bones of the male are generally larger and heavier. The pelvic outlet, the space surrounded by the lower pelvic bones, is heart shaped. **B,** Female pelvis. The pelvic outlet is larger and more oval than that of the male. The size and shape of the female pelvis varies and is important in childbirth. L5 is the fifth lumbar vertebra. The pubic symphysis is the joint where the two pubic bones are joined.

pubis	*Pubo/femor/al* (**pu″bo-fem′ə-rəl**) means pertaining to the _____ and the femur. Use pubofemoral as a model to write a word that means pertaining to the ischium and the femur: _____.
ischiofemoral (is″ke-o-fem′o-rəl)	
	14-43 The patella (**pə-tel′ə**), or kneecap, is anterior to the knee joint. The combining form *patell(o)* means patella. *Patello/femoral* (**pə-tel″o-fem′ə-rəl**) pertains to the
patella	_____ and the femur.
below	*Infra/patell/ar* (**in″frə-pə-tel′ər**) means _____ the patella.
	14-44 The lower leg is composed of two bones, the tibia and the fibula. The tibia, or shinbone, is the larger of the two bones. The combining form *tibi(o)* means tibia; the combining form *fibul(o)* means fibula.
fibula	*Fibul/ar* (**fib′u-lər**) means pertaining to the _____.
	14-45 The foot is composed of the ankle, instep, and toes. The ankle, or tarsus, consists of a group of seven short bones that resemble the bones of the wrist but are larger. The combining form *tars(o)* means the tarsus. In addition, *tars(o)* means the edge of the eyelid. This is because a second meaning of tarsus is a curved plate of dense white fibrous tissue forming the supporting structure of the eyelid.

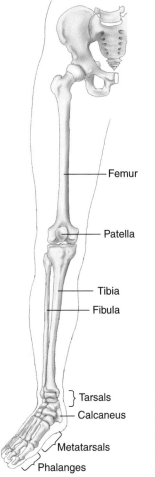

- Femur
- Patella
- Tibia
- Fibula
- } Tarsals
- Calcaneus
- Metatarsals
- Phalanges

Figure 14-9 Right lower extremity, anterior view. The lower extremity consists of the bones of the thigh, leg, foot, and patella (kneecap). The lower leg has two bones, the tibia and the fibula. The foot is composed of the ankle, instep, and five toes. The ankle has seven bones, the calcaneus (heel bone) being the largest. The instep has five metatarsals, numbered *1* through *5* starting on the medial side. There are three phalanges in each of the toes, except in the great (or big) toe, which has only two.

tarsus (or ankle)

It is not always obvious, when looking at a word containing *tars(o)*, which meaning is intended. Words used in the following frames refer to the ankle, but one should be aware that a second meaning of tarsus is the edge of the eyelid.

Tars/al (**tahr′səl**) means pertaining to the _____. One of the tarsal bones is the calcaneus, or heel bone.

calcaneus

14-46 The combining form *calcane(o)* refers to the calcaneus. *Calcane/al* (**kal-ka′ne-əl**) pertains to the calcaneus.

Calcaneo/plantar (**kal-ka″ne-o-plan′tər**) pertains to the _____ and the sole. *Plantar* is a word that means concerning the sole.

tibia

Calcaneo/tibial (**kal-ka″ne-o-tib′e-əl**) means pertaining to the calcaneus and the

_____.

Calcaneo/fibular (**kal-ka″ne-o-fib′u-lər**) means pertaining to the calcaneus and the fibula.

distal

14-47 The bones between the tarsus and the toes are the metatarsals (**met″ə-tahr′səlz**). Which end of the metatarsals joins with the toes? _____

phalang(o)

14-48 Bones of the toes are phalanges. Finger bones are also called phalanges. What is the combining form for phalanges? _____

There are two bones in the great toe and three in each of the lesser toes.

carpus

Carpo/ped/al (**kahr″po-ped′əl**) pertains to the _____ and the foot. A carpopedal spasm, for example, is involuntary contraction of the muscles of the hands and feet.

Exercise 4

Write a combining form for each of the following bones of the appendicular skeleton.

1. ankle _____
2. calf bone _____
3. collarbone _____
4. fingers or toes _____
5. heel bone _____
6. kneecap _____
7. shinbone _____
8. shoulder blade _____
9. thighbone _____
10. upper arm bone _____
11. wrist _____

Exercise 5

1. List three bones that fuse to form the pelvic bone.

_____

2. Write the names of the two bones of the forearm.

_____

■ *Joints, Tendons, and Ligaments*

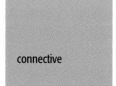

connective

14-49 Connective tissues, characterized by an abundance of intercellular material with relatively few cells, support and bind other body tissue and parts. Bone is the most rigid of all the connective tissues. The joints, tendons, and ligaments are also connective tissues. Tissue that supports and binds other body tissue and parts is called _____ tissue. Learn the following word parts for the joints, tendons, and ligaments.

Word Parts for Joints and Tendons

COMBINING FORMS	MEANINGS
arthr(o), articul(o)	joint; articulation
burs(o)	bursa
chondr(o)	cartilage
synov(o), synovi(o)	synovial membrane
ten(o), tend(o), tendin(o)	tendon

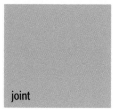

joint

14-50 A joint, or articulation (**ahr-tik″u-la′shən**), is a place of union between two or more bones. You are familiar with many joints—for example, the ankle, wrist, and knee. Joints are classified according to their structure and the amount of movement they allow. Joints are immovable, slightly movable, and freely movable. Table 14-2 shows examples of the three types.
    Two combining forms that mean joint are *articul(o)* and *arthr(o)*. Most terms use *arthr(o)*, but *articul/ar* (**ahr-tik′u-lər**) means pertaining to a _____.

TABLE 14-2 Types of Movement in Joints

Type of Movement	Examples
Immovable: Bones come in close contact and are separated only by a thin layer of fibrous connective tissue	Sutures in the skull
Slightly movable: Bones are connected by cartilage and joint, which allows slight movement only	Symphysis pubis, joints that connect the ribs to the sternum
Freely movable: Ends of the opposing bones are covered with articular cartilage and separated by a space called the joint cavity; these joints are sometimes called synovial joints	Shoulder, wrist, knee, elbow

14-51 Most joints in the adult body are freely movable joints, also called synovial (**sǐ-no′ve-əl**) joints. The combining forms *synov(o)* and *synovi(o)* mean synovial joint. The knee is an example of a synovial joint. The tibio/femoral (**tib″e-o-fem′ə-rəl**) or knee joint is the largest joint of the body.

Articular cartilage covers the ends of the opposing bones in a synovial joint, and they are separated by a space called the joint cavity that is filled with synovial fluid for lubrication (Figure 14-10).

The articular cartilage provides protection and support for the joint. Some joints also have pads and cushions that help stabilize the joint and act as shock absorbers. Bursae are fluid-filled sacs that help reduce friction. The combining form *burs(o)* means a bursa. Note the location of the bursa in Figure 14-10. Bursae are commonly located between the skin and underlying bone or between tendons and ligaments.

14-52 Tendons are bands of strong, fibrous tissue that attach the muscles to the bones (Figure 14-11). Ligaments connect bones or cartilage and serve to support and strengthen joints. What type of connective tissue attaches the muscles to the bones? _____

What type of connective tissue connects bones or cartilage? _____

tendons
ligaments

14-53 The temporomandibular (**tem″pə-ro-mən-dib′u-lər**) joint is one of a pair of joints connecting the mandible of the jaw to the temporal bone of the skull. It is abbreviated TMJ.

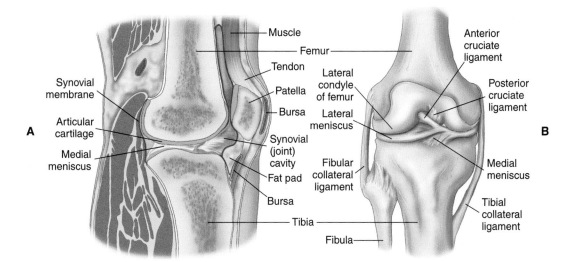

Figure 14-10 The knee joint. **A,** Lateral view, sagittal section. The hinged joint at the knee is a synovial joint. The ends of the opposing bones are covered by articular cartilage. The synovial membrane secretes synovial fluid into the joint cavity for lubrication. Menisci and bursae are special structures that act as protective cushions. **B,** Anterior view. Twelve ligaments, flexible bands of fibrous tissue, bind the structures of the knee to provide strength. Note how the anterior and posterior cruciate ligaments cross each other, a characteristic from which their name is derived (Latin: *crux*, cross, and *ligare*, to bind).

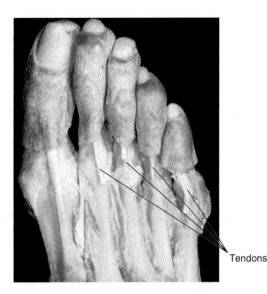

Figure 14-11 Tendons. Strong and flexible bands of dense fibrous connective tissue attach muscles to bones.

Tendons

	14-54 Embryos contain a great deal of translucent, elastic tissue that, for the most part, is transformed into bone as the embryo matures. This elastic tissue is cartilage. Not all cartilage becomes bone, as evidenced by cartilage found in several parts of the adult body, such as the nose and ear. The combining form *chondr(o)* means cartilage. Use *-al* to write a term that means pertaining to cartilage:
chondr/al **(kon′drəl)**	_____. *Chondr/oid* **(kon′droid)** means resembling cartilage.
vertebrae	**14-55** *Vertebro/chondral* **(vər″tə-bro-kon′drəl)** means pertaining to the _____ and the adjacent cartilage.
ribs	*Chondro/costal* **(kon″dro-kos′təl)** pertains to what structures and their associated cartilage? _____.
	14-56 Perichondrium **(per″ĭ-kon′dre-əm)** is the membrane around the surface of cartilage. *Peri/chondrial* **(per″ĭ-kon′dre-əl)** means pertaining to or composed of perichondrium, the membrane
cartilage	around the _____, or concerning the perichondrium.

Exercise 6

Write a word in each blank to complete these sentences.

1. Tissue that supports and binds other body tissue and parts is _____ tissue.

2. Another name for a joint is an _____.

3. Freely movable joints are filled with a fluid for lubrication and are called _____ joints.

4. Articular cartilage provides protection and support for the _____.

5. Fluid-filled sacs that help reduce friction in a joint are called _____.

6. Tissues that attach muscles to bones are _____.

7. Connective tissue that connects bones or cartilages and serves to support and strengthen joints is called a _____.

8. The membrane around the surface of cartilage is called the _____.

Word Parts for Describing Muscle

COMBINING FORMS	MEANING
fasci(o)	fascia
muscul(o), my(o)*	muscle

*My(o) (Greek: *myos*, of muscle).

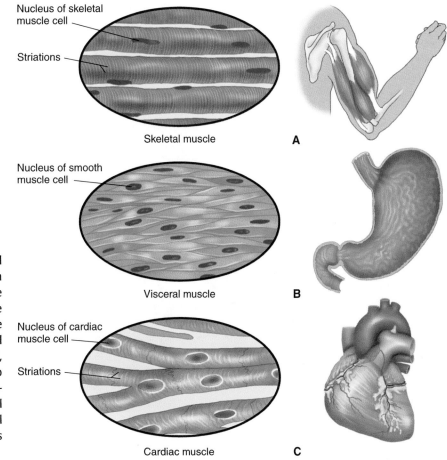

Nucleus of skeletal
muscle cell

Striations

Skeletal muscle   **A**

Nucleus of smooth
muscle cell

Visceral muscle   **B**

Nucleus of cardiac
muscle cell

Striations

Cardiac muscle   **C**

Figure 14-12 Types of muscle. **A,** Skeletal muscle cells (fibers) are long and cylindrical with alternating light and dark bands that give the cell a striated appearance. Skeletal muscles are also known as voluntary muscles because we have conscious control over them. **B,** Visceral muscle cells are elongated, spindle shaped, and involuntary. Visceral muscle is also called smooth muscle because it lacks striations. **C,** Cardiac muscle cells are cylindrical and are striated but are shorter than skeletal muscle cells and are involuntary. These cells branch and interconnect.

■ *Muscles*

14-57 Muscle is a type of tissue that is composed of fibers or cells that are able to contract, causing movement of body parts and organs. Before a skeletal muscle contracts, it receives an impulse from a nerve cell. The muscle exerts force on tendons, which in turn pull on bones, producing movement. You learned in the previous section that tendons attach a muscle to a

bone

_____.

14-58 You know that *my(o)* and *muscul(o)* mean muscle. *Muscul/ar* means pertaining to

muscle
embryonic

_____.

A myo/blast **(mi′o-blast)** is an _____ cell that develops into muscle fiber.

There are three types of muscle tissue in the body: skeletal, visceral, and cardiac. Skeletal muscle, with the primary function of movement of the body and its parts, is voluntarily controlled by the nervous system. Visceral muscle, located in the walls of organs and blood vessels, is involuntary.

not

In/voluntary means it is _____ voluntary, or not under our conscious control. (Visceral muscle is controlled by the autonomic nervous system described in Chapter 15.) The combining form *viscer(o)* means viscera, the internal organs enclosed within a body cavity, including the abdominal, thoracic, pelvic, and endocrine organs.

Cardiac muscle, myocardium, is also involuntary. Myo/cardium is

heart

_____ muscle. Characteristics of the three types of muscle tissue are shown in Figure 14-12.

14-59 Skeletal muscle makes up more than 600 muscles that are attached to and control the movement of the bones of the skeleton. The major muscles are shown in Figure 14-13.

Most skeletal muscles have names that describe some feature of the muscle, sometimes with several features combined in one name. Muscle features such as size, shape, direction of fibers,

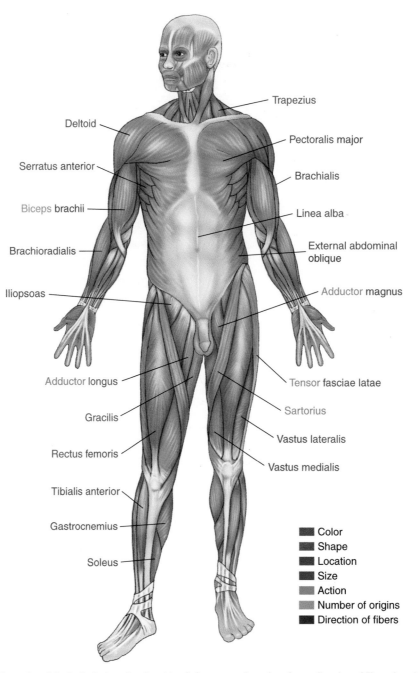

Figure 14-13   Major skeletal muscles of the body. **A,** Anterior view. Muscle features such as size, shape, direction of fibers, location, number of attachments, origin, and action are often used in naming muscles. This is demonstrated by the use of color-coding of the names on the anterior view.

Continued

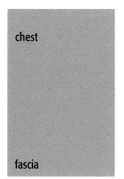

chest

location and number of attachments, origin, and action are often used in naming muscles. The name *pectoralis major* tells us it is a large muscle of the _____; *major* indicates the large size of the muscle. The names of the muscles in the anterior view have been color coded to indicate the origin of their names. For practice, color code as many muscles shown in the posterior view as you can, using terms you have learned and a medical dictionary.

14-60 A fibrous membrane called fascia **(fash′e-ə)** covers, supports, and separates muscles. The combining form for fascia is *fasci(o)*. *Fascial* means pertaining to a _____.

fascia

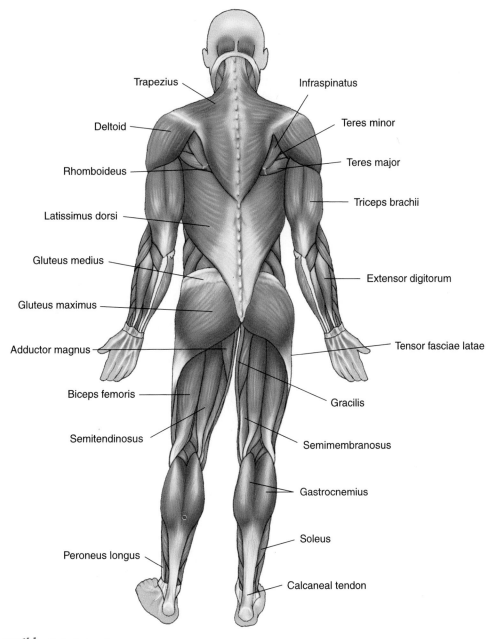

Trapezius

Deltoid

Rhomboideus

Latissimus dorsi

Gluteus medius

Gluteus maximus

Adductor magnus

Biceps femoris

Semitendinosus

Peroneus longus

Infraspinatus

Teres minor

Teres major

Triceps brachii

Extensor digitorum

Tensor fasciae latae

Gracilis

Semimembranosus

Gastrocnemius

Soleus

Calcaneal tendon

Figure 14-13—cont'd   B, Posterior view.

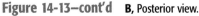

Most skeletal muscles are attached to bones by tendons that span joints. When the muscle contracts, one bone moves relative to the other bone, and muscles sometimes work in groups to perform a particular movement. Muscles are arranged in antagonistic pairs. This means that when one muscle of the pair is contracted, the other is relaxed. For example, the biceps brachii muscle on the anterior arm bends the forearm at the elbow. The triceps brachii muscle on the posterior arm straightens the forearm at the elbow. When the former muscle contracts, the other is

relaxed

_____.

14-61 There are several commonly used terms to describe different types of movement brought about by muscular activity (Figure 14-14). Use the information to write the answers in the following blanks.

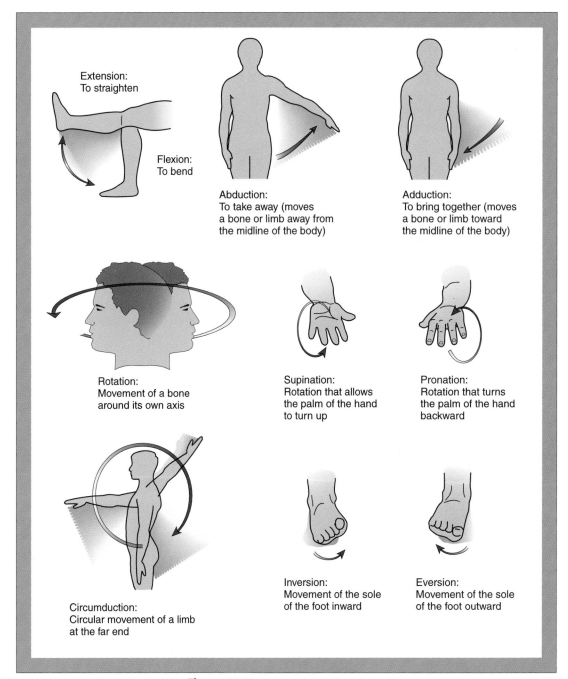

Figure 14-14 Types of muscular actions.

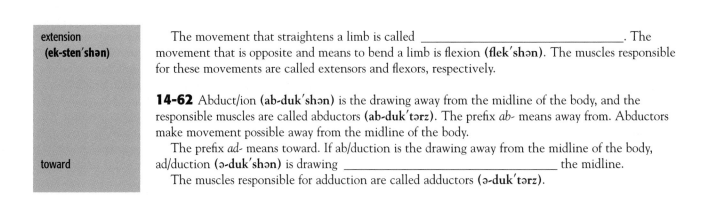

extension
(ek-sten′shən)

The movement that straightens a limb is called _____. The movement that is opposite and means to bend a limb is flexion **(flek′shən)**. The muscles responsible for these movements are called extensors and flexors, respectively.

14-62 Abduct/ion **(ab-duk′shən)** is the drawing away from the midline of the body, and the responsible muscles are called abductors **(ab-duk′tərz)**. The prefix *ab-* means away from. Abductors make movement possible away from the midline of the body.

The prefix *ad-* means toward. If ab/duction is the drawing away from the midline of the body, ad/duction **(ə-duk′shən)** is drawing _____ the midline.

toward

The muscles responsible for adduction are called adductors **(ə-duk′tərz)**.

14-63 Rotation is the movement of a bone around its own axis, and the muscle that is responsible for rotation is called a rotator.

supination
(soo″pĭ-na′shən)

    The rotation that allows the palm of the hand to turn up is called

_____.

    The rotation that turns the palm of the hand backward is called

pronation
(pro-na′shən)

_____.

circumduction
(sər″kəm-duk′shən)

14-64 A circular movement of a limb at the far end is _____.

inversion
(in-vər′zhən)

    Movement of the sole of the foot inward is _____, and the opposite movement is eversion (e-ver′zhən).

Exercise 7

Match the types of body movements in 1 through 5 with their meanings (A through I). Not all selections will be used.

_____ 1. adduction

_____ 2. circumduction

_____ 3. eversion

_____ 4. flexion

_____ 5. supination

A. circular movement of a limb at the far end
B. drawing toward the midline of the body
C. movement of a bone around an axis
D. movement that allows turning the sole inward
E. movement that allows turning the sole outward
F. movement that bends a limb
G. movement that straightens a limb
H. rotation that turns the palm of the hand up
I. rotation that turns the palm of the hand down

DIAGNOSTIC TESTS AND PROCEDURES

14-65 Initial examination for musculoskeletal problems may include testing for range of motion (ROM), muscle strength, and reflexes. Range of motion is the maximum amount of movement that a healthy joint is capable of and is measured in degrees of a circle. Range-of-motion exercises are also used to increase muscle strength and joint mobility. ROM means range of

motion

_____.

    Muscle strength can be graded by asking the patient to apply resistance to the force exerted by the examiner (for example, the examiner tries to pull the bent arm down while the patient tries to raise it).

    Reflex action is the immediate and involuntary functioning or movement of an organ or body part in response to a particular stimulus. The reflex hammer is a mallet with a rubber head that is used to tap tendons, nerves, or muscles to test reflex reactions. This instrument for testing reflex

hammer

reactions is called a reflex _____.

14-66 Electro/myo/graphy (e-lek″tro-mi-og′rə-fe) is used to record the response of a muscle to

electrical

_____ stimulation. This is particularly useful in studying nerve damage and certain other disorders. Electromyography is abbreviated EMG. The resulting record is called an electromyogram (e-lek″tro-mi′o-gram).

14-67 Diagnostic studies of the bones and connective tissues include radiologic studies, bone scans, laboratory tests, and a few invasive procedures. Standard x-rays provide information about the joints and bone density or congenital deformities or fractures. Bone density testing, also called bone densito/metry (den″sĭ-tom′ə-tre), is any one of several methods of determining

measures

bone mass with a machine that _____ how well the rays penetrate the bone. This is helpful in diagnosing osteoporosis and determining the effectiveness of therapy.

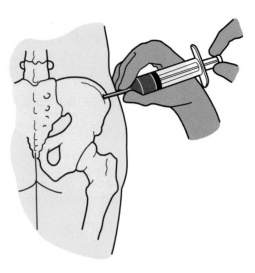

Figure 14-15   Bone marrow aspiration from the posterior iliac crest.

tomography

14-68 Bone tumors may be discovered in a routine radiologic examination. <u>Computed tomography</u> (CT), magnetic resonance imaging (MRI), bone scans, and biopsy are used to distinguish between benign and malignant tumors. Computed _____ produces an image of a cross section of tissue. <u>Magnetic resonance imaging</u> is used to view soft tissue (for example, to visualize a cartilage tear). A <u>bone scan</u> is often useful in demonstrating malignant bone tumors, which appear as areas of increased uptake of radioactive material.

marrow

14-69 A <u>bone marrow examination</u> may include <u>biopsy of the bone</u>, as well as aspiration of bone marrow for microscopic study. These studies may be performed for other reasons, such as hemato/logic (he″mə-to-loj′ik) evaluation. Bone marrow studies are used to diagnose leukemia, identify tumors or other disorders of the bone marrow, and determine the extent of myelosuppression. Myelo/suppression is inhibition of the bone _____.
    The posterior iliac crest is generally the preferred site for <u>bone marrow aspiration</u> (Figure 14-15). In adults, the anterior iliac crest or the sternum may also be used.

vertebrae

14-70 A <u>lumbar puncture</u> is performed for various therapeutic and diagnostic procedures. Diagnostic purposes include obtaining cerebrospinal fluid, measuring its pressure, or injecting substances for radiographic studies of the nervous system. Therapeutic indications include removing blood or pus, injecting drugs, and introducing an anesthetic for spinal anesthesia (Figure 14-16).
    The lumbar puncture is so named because the needle is inserted between two _____, usually the second and third or the third and fourth lumbar vertebrae.

joint

within

14-71 <u>Arthro/graphy</u> (ahr-throg′rə-fe) is radiographic visualization of the inside of a _____. This is usually done by an intraarticular injection of a radiopaque substance. Both *intraarticular* and *intra-articular* mean _____ the joint.
    The radiographic record produced after introduction of opaque contrast material into a joint is an <u>arthrogram</u> (ahr′thro-gram).

arthroscopy
(ahr-thros′kə-pe)

14-72 An <u>arthro/scope</u> (ahr′thro-skōp) is a fiberoptic instrument used for direct visualization of the interior of a joint. The process is called _____.

    This procedure permits biopsy of cartilage or damaged synovial membrane, diagnosis of a torn cartilage, and, in some instances, removal of loose bodies in the joint space (Figure 14-17).

puncture

14-73 <u>Arthro/centesis</u> (ahr″thro-sen-te′sis) is surgical _____ of a joint with a needle. This is performed to obtain samples of synovial fluid for diagnostic purposes, to remove excess fluid from joints to relieve pain, or to instill medications.

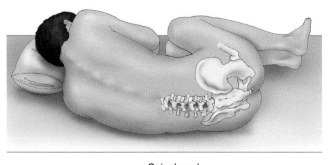

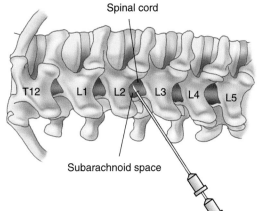

Spinal cord

T12   L1   L2   L3   L4   L5

Subarachnoid space

Figure 14-16   Lumbar puncture. The patient is generally positioned in the flexed lateral (fetal) position. The needle is inserted between the second and third or the third and fourth lumbar vertebrae. Cerebrospinal fluid can be removed, or its pressure can be measured, and drugs can be introduced as done for spinal anesthesia.

14-74 Table 14-3 lists several important laboratory tests that are used to assess musculoskeletal disorders. Use the material in the table to complete the next several blanks. In an <u>anti/nuclear antibody</u> (an″te-, an″ti-noo′kle-ər an′tĭ-bod″e) test, serum is tested for

antibodies   _____ that react with nuclear material. The ANA test is used primarily to diagnose systemic lupus erythematosus (described in Arthritis and Connective Tissue Diseases, later in this chapter), although a positive result may indicate other autoimmune diseases, such as rheumatoid arthritis or other connective tissue diseases.

erythrocyte   **14-75** <u>ESR</u> means _____ sedimentation rate. This is the rate at which red blood cells (erythrocytes) settle out in a tube of blood that has been treated to prevent clotting. Elevated levels are found in any inflammatory process, especially rheumatoid arthritis.

rheumatoid   **14-76** <u>RF</u> means the _____ factor. This test is positive in most patients with rheumatoid arthritis.

decreased   **14-77** The levels of <u>serum calcium</u> and <u>serum phosphorus</u> are _____ in osteomalacia (os″te-o-mə-la′shə), a disorder characterized by excessive loss of calcium from the bone.

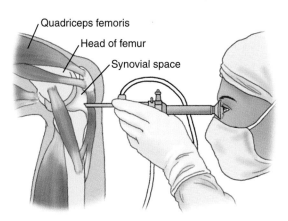

Quadriceps femoris

Head of femur

Synovial space

Figure 14-17   Arthroscopy of the knee. The examination of the interior of a joint is performed by inserting a specially designed endoscope through a small incision. This procedure also permits biopsy of cartilage or damaged synovial membrane, diagnosis of a torn meniscus, and, in some instances, removal of loose bodies in the joint space.

TABLE 14-3 Abnormal Findings in Laboratory Testing for Musculoskeletal Disorders

Test	Associated Musculoskeletal Disorders
Antinuclear antibody (ANA)	Serum is tested for antinuclear antibodies. Finding is positive in most patients with systemic lupus erythematosus, sometimes positive with scleroderma or rheumatoid arthritis.
Erythrocyte sedimentation rate (ESR)	Blood test shows elevated levels with any inflammatory process, especially rheumatoid arthritis and osteomyelitis.
Rheumatoid factor (RF) test	Blood test is positive in most patients with rheumatoid arthritis; sometimes there are lower levels in other connective tissue diseases.
Serum calcium	Decreased in osteomalacia; increased in some bone tumors.
Serum creatine phosphokinase (CPK)	Elevated levels are found in skeletal muscle disorders and myocardial infarction (death of heart muscle).
Serum phosphorus	Decreased in osteomalacia; increased in certain bone tumors.
Serum uric acid	Elevated levels are usually found in patients with gout.
Urine calcium	Sometimes detected in metastatic bone disease.

creatine	**14-78** _CPK_ means _____ phosphokinase. Increased serum levels of CPK are found in skeletal muscle disorders and myocardial infarction (death of a portion of cardiac muscle, commonly called a heart attack).
gout (**gout**)	**14-79** Elevated levels of <u>serum uric acid</u> are usually found in patients with a condition called _____, a disease associated with an inborn error of uric acid metabolism that can result in painful swelling of joints.
calcium	**14-80** _Calci/uria_ (**kal″se-u′re-ə**) means _____ in the urine. Although calcium may be present in normal urine in minute amounts, it is not readily detectable. (Urinary excretion of calcium is affected by several things, including diet.) <u>Hyper/calciuria</u> (**hi″pər-kal″se-u′re-ə**) is often seen in metastatic bone disease, in which there is rapid bone destruction.

Exercise 8

Write a word in each blank to complete these sentences.

1. _BDT_ means _____ density testing.

2. _EMG_ is the abbreviation for _____.

3. _ROM_ means range of _____.

4. _ESR_ means _____ sedimentation rate.

5. _RF_ means _____ factor.

6. Arthrography is radiographic visualization of the inside of a _____.

7. A fiberoptic instrument that is used for direct visualization of the inside of a joint is an

_____.

8. Surgical puncture of a joint is _____.

PATHOLOGIES

connective

14-81 Although injury is a primary cause of problems of the musculoskeletal system, the bones, muscles, and associated tissue are subject to various pathologies, including infections, metabolic disturbances, congenital disorders, and connective tissue diseases. You learned earlier that bone, cartilage, ligaments, and tendons are called _____ tissue because they support and bind other tissues.

Word Parts to Describe Musculoskeletal Disorders

Combining Forms	Meanings		Suffixes	Meanings
ankyl(o)	stiff		-asthenia	weakness
troph(o)	nutrition		-sarcoma	malignant tumor from connective tissue

■ Stress and Trauma Injuries

strain

14-82 Common musculoskeletal injuries include simple muscle strains, sprains, dislocations, and fractures. A <u>strain</u> is damage, usually muscular, that results from excessive physical effort.

A <u>sprain</u> is a traumatic injury to the tendons, muscles, or ligaments around a joint, characterized by pain, swelling, and discoloration of the skin over the joint. Radiography is often needed to rule out fractures. Strains and sprains are common traumatic injuries that cause much discomfort and can interfere with normal activities.

If a muscle in the arm is very sore but shows no swelling or discoloration of the skin after many hours playing games at the computer, is this more likely to be a strain or a sprain?

_____

pain

14-83 <u>My/algia</u> (mi-al′jə) is muscular _____. Another word that means the same as myalgia is <u>myodynia</u> (mi″o-din′e-ə).

A <u>muscle cramp</u> is a painful, involuntary muscle spasm, often caused by inflammation of the muscle, but it can be a symptom of electrolyte imbalance. An example of the latter is <u>tetany</u> (tet′ə-ne), a condition characterized by cramps, convulsions, twitching of the muscles, and sharp flexion of the wrists and ankle joints. It is caused by an imbalance in calcium metabolism.

14-84 A break in a bone is called a <u>fracture</u>. Fractures are classified as complete fractures, with the break across the entire width of the bone so it is divided into two sections, or incomplete fractures. They are also described by the extent of associated soft tissue damage as simple or compound.

The bone protrudes through the skin in a <u>compound fracture</u>, also called an open fracture. If a bone is fractured but does not protrude through the skin, it is called a simple or <u>closed fracture</u> (Figure 14-18). Which type of fracture is a broken bone that causes an external wound?

compound (or open)

_____.

An incomplete fracture in which the bone is bent and fractured on one side only, as in Figure 14-18, is called a <u>greenstick fracture</u> and is seen principally in children.

14-85 Figure 14-19 illustrates four types of fractures. In an <u>impacted fracture</u>, one bone fragment is firmly driven into the fractured end of another fragment.

Notice the many fragments of bone present in the <u>comminuted</u> (kom′ĭ-nōōt′əd) fracture. In which type of fracture is the bone twisted apart? _____ The

spiral

bone is also displaced in the example. Displacement of a bone from a joint is also called a <u>dislocation</u> (Figure 14-20). Dislocations and fractures are usually evident on x-ray images of the affected bones.

The example of a <u>transverse fracture</u>, one in which the break is at right angles to the axis of the bone, also shows displacement. It will be helpful to remember that <i>trans-</i> in transverse means

across

_____.

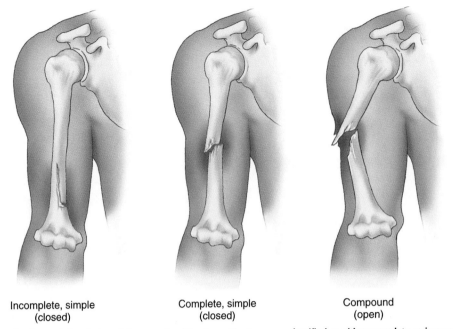

Incomplete, simple
(closed)

Complete, simple
(closed)

Compound
(open)

Figure 14-18   Classification and description of the severity of fractures. Fractures are classified as either complete or incomplete and are described as either open or closed.

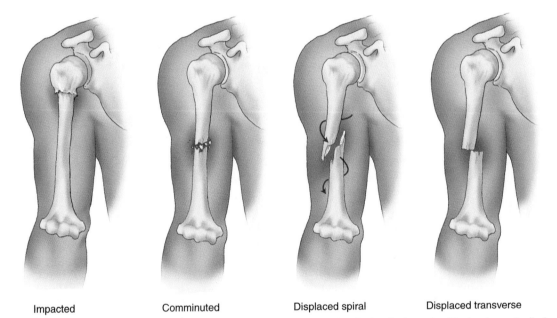

Impacted   Comminuted   Displaced spiral   Displaced transverse

Figure 14-19   Common types of fractures. The spiral and transverse fractures are also displaced. The ends of broken bones in displaced fractures often pierce the surrounding skin, resulting in open fractures; however, these two examples are closed fractures.

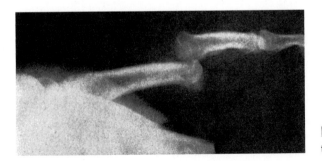

Figure 14-20   Radiograph demonstrating an interphalangeal dislocation of the finger.

14-86 Treatments for dislocations and fractures are included later in this chapter, but immobilization of fractures by use of a cast is common. Muscle shrinks when a limb is immobilized for a long period. The term *atrophy* means a decrease in size of an organ or tissue. This type of atrophy is called disuse _____. Atrophy is noticeable in these cases, because the limb has decreased in size.

atrophy

14-87 Carpal tunnel syndrome (CTS) is an example of trauma that results from prolonged, repetitive movements. CTS is a condition in which the median nerve in the wrist becomes compressed, causing pain and discomfort. Excessive hand exercise, a potential occupational hazard, can lead to a chronic condition of CTS. Carpal in its name will help you remember that CTS is a condition of the _____. Surgery to relieve the pressure on the nerve may be necessary.

wrist

14-88 Rotator cuff injury may occur as a result of repetitive motions, injury, or the degenerative processes of aging. The rotator cuff is a structure of muscles and tendons that stabilizes and allows range of motion in the shoulder joint and, as the name implies, _____ of the humerus.

rotation

14-89 Inflammation of a bursa is called _____. This condition can result from repetitive motion, as well as trauma, infection, or other disorders of the musculoskeletal system.

bursitis (bər-si′tis)

Both *tendin/itis* (ten″dĭ-ni′tis) and *tendon/itis* (ten″də-ni′tis) mean inflammation of a _____.

tendon

Bursitis and tendinitis can be related to overuse, repetitive motion, or irritation, and symptoms usually disappear with rest.

14-90 Tenodynia (ten″o-din′e-ə) may be caused by tendonitis. *Teno/dynia* means _____ in a tendon and is the same as tenalgia (te-nal′jə).

pain

Using *synov(o)*, write a word that means inflammation of a synovial joint: _____.

synovitis (sin″o-vi′tis)

14-91 Common symptoms of persons with musculoskeletal disorders include pain, weakness, deformity, limitation of movement, stiffness, and joint crepitus (krep′ĭ-təs), the crackling sound produced when a bone rubs against another bone or roughened cartilage.

Both *rachio/dynia* (ra″ke-o-din′e-ə) and *rachialgia* (ra″ke-al′jə) mean a painful condition of the _____. Spondyl/algia (spon″dĭ-lal′jə) is pain in a vertebra.

spine

Sacro/dynia (sa″kro-din′e-ə) is pain of the sacrum. Using a different suffix, write another word that means pain in the ischium: _____. Ischio/dynia (is″ke-o-din′e-ə) is also pain in the _____.

ischialgia (is″ke-al′jə)
ischium
sternum
pain

Stern/algia (stər-nal′jə) is pain in the _____.
Tibi/algia (tib″e-al′jə) is _____ of the tibia.

14-92 Calcaneo/dynia (kal-ka″ne-o-din′e-ə) is a painful heel. Write a word that means inflammation of the heel bone: _____.

**calcaneitis
(kal-ka″ne-i′tis)**

14-93 The knee is subject to many injuries, particularly tearing of the cartilage. Chondr/itis (kon-dri′tis), inflammation of the cartilage, can cause chondro/dynia (kon″dro-din′e-ə), pain of the cartilage. Use a different suffix to write another term that means painful cartilage: _____.

**chondralgia
(kon-dral′jə)
bone**

Osteo/chondr/itis (os″te-o-kon-dri′tis) is inflammation of cartilage and _____.

14-94 Arthro/chondr/itis (ahr″thro-kon-dri′tis) is inflammation of an articular _____.

**cartilage
chondropathy
(kon-drop′ə-the)**

Write a word that means any disease of a cartilage: _____.

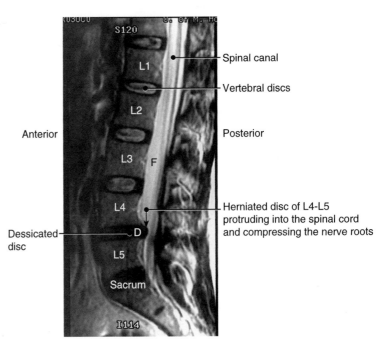

Figure 14-21   A lumbar MRI scan of a herniated disk.

14-95 An abnormal condition characterized by facial pain and by mandibular dysfunction, apparently caused by a defective or dislocated temporomandibular joint (TMJ), is called <u>TMJ pain dysfunction syndrome</u> or is sometimes shortened to TMJ disorder.

Some indications of this disorder are clicking of the joint when the jaw moves, limitation of jaw movement, and temporomandibular dislocation. TMJ is an abbreviation for the

temporomandibular _____ joint.

14-96 Low back pain that radiates down the buttock and below the knee, resulting from pressure on spinal nerve roots, is the most common symptom of a <u>herniated disk</u>, rupture of an intervertebral disk, the tough fibrous cushion between two vertebral bodies. This condition can result from repeated stress or injury to the spine, as well as natural degeneration with aging.

This is also called a slipped disk, but a more appropriate name is a

herniated _____ disk (Figure 14-21).

14-97 Feet absorb considerable shock while running and walking, activities that can bring about a variety of disorders, particularly when structural weaknesses and other problems exist or improperly fitted shoes are worn.

<u>Tars/optosis</u> **(tahr″sop-to′sis)** is prolapse of the _____. This is

tarsus commonly called flatfoot.

Hallux means the great toe. <u>Hallux valgus</u> **(hal′əks val′gəs)** is a deformity of the foot, sometimes called a <u>bunion</u>. The great toe deviates laterally at the metatarso/phalang/eal (MTP) joint (Figure 14-22, *A*). The correct name for bunion is _____ valgus.

hallux A <u>hammertoe</u> is a toe that is permanently flexed at the midphalangeal joint, producing a clawlike appearance. This common abnormality often occurs simultaneously with hallux valgus (Figure 14-22, *B*). Hammertoe may be present in more than one digit, but the second toe is most often affected. Corns (hard masses of epithelial cells overlying a bony prominence) may develop on the dorsal side, and calluses (thickening of the outer layers of the skin at points of friction or pressure) may appear on the plantar surface.

14-98 In <u>Morton's neur/oma</u> **(noo-ro′mə)** a small, painful

tumor _____ grows in a digital nerve of the foot. Surgical removal of the neuroma is generally indicated if the pain persists and interferes with walking.

<u>Tarsal tunnel syndrome</u> is the ankle version of the carpal tunnel syndrome. Treatment is similar to that for carpal tunnel syndrome.

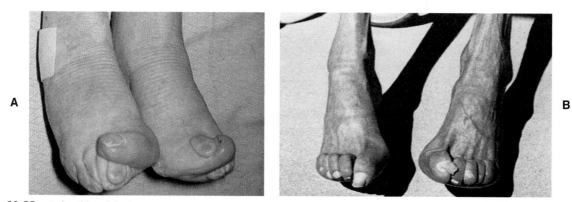

Figure 14-22   Deformities of the feet. **A,** Hallux valgus. The great toe rides over the second toe in this example. **B,** Hammertoe. The toes are permanently flexed. Hallux valgus is also present.

14-99 The cause of some musculoskeletal disorders is not known, such as <u>Dupuytren's contracture</u>, a thickening and tightening of the palmar fascia, causing the fourth or fifth finger to bend into the palm and resist extension.

■ Infections

bone

pain

marrow

myocellulitis

14-100 <u>Oste/itis</u> (os″te-i′tis) is inflammation of a _____. It may be caused by infection, as well as degeneration or trauma. Osteitis results in <u>oste/algia</u> (os″te-al′jə), also called <u>osteo/dynia</u> (os″te-o-din′e-ə), which means bone

_____.

    <u>Osteo/mye/litis</u> (os″te-o-mi″ə-li′tis) is an infection of the bone and bone marrow caused by infectious microorganisms that are introduced by trauma or surgery, by extension from a nearby infection, or via the bloodstream. Staphylococci are common causes of osteomyelitis.

14-101 Sometimes it is difficult to know if *myel(o)* in a word refers to bone marrow or the spinal cord, and in some words it can refer to either. For example, <u>*myel/itis*</u> (mi″ə-li′tis) means inflammation of either the bone _____ or the spinal cord.

14-102 <u>Cellul/itis</u> (sel″u-li′tis) is an acute, spreading, swollen, pus-forming inflammation of the deep subcutaneous tissues. It may be associated with abscess formation. If the muscle is also involved, it is called <u>myocellulitis</u> (mi″o-sel″u-li′tis).
    You learned earlier that *cellul(o)* means small cell, but that may not be helpful in remembering this term. Write the term that means an acute, pus-forming inflammation of the tissues and muscle: _____.

■ Tumors and Malignancies

muscular

14-103 A <u>ganglion</u> (gang′gle-on) is a round, cystlike lesion that often occurs over a wrist joint or a tendon. A ganglion is usually painless and may disappear, then recur. Fluid can often be removed with a needle (aspirated), but excision will more likely resolve the problem.

14-104 A <u>myo/fibr/oma</u> (mi″o-fi-bro′mə) is a tumor composed of _____ and fibrous tissue.

14-105 Malignant bone tumors may be primary (originating in the bone) or secondary (originating in other tissue and metastasizing to the bone). The latter greatly outnumber primary bone tumors.

marrow

bone

Multiple myel/oma (mi″ə-lo′mə) is a malignant neoplasm of the bone
_____ that disrupts and destroys bone marrow function.
Osteo/sarcoma (os″te-o-sahr-ko′mə) is an extremely malignant primary
_____ tumor. The suffix -sarcoma means a malignant tumor from connective tissue.

cartilage
fibrous

14-106 Three other types of primary bone tumors are chondrosarcoma, fibrosarcoma, and Ewing's sarcoma. A chondro/sarcoma (kon″dro-sahr-ko′mə) is derived from _____, spreads to the bone, and destroys it.
A fibro/sarcoma (fi″bro-sahr-ko′mə) arises from _____ tissues. Ewing's sarcoma is an extremely malignant bone tumor.

white

14-107 Leukemia is a broad term given to a group of malignant diseases that are characterized by replacement of bone marrow with proliferating immature leukocytes and abnormal numbers of immature leukocytes in the blood circulation. Leukemia is classified according to the predominant type of proliferating leukocytes. It is also classified as acute or chronic. Leuk/emia received its name from the large number of _____ blood cells in the circulation.

■ Metabolic Disturbances

hard

14-108 There is a delicate balance between bone destruction and bone formation. Excessive formation can lead to abnormal hardness and unusual heaviness of bone, called osteo/sclerosis (os″te-o-sklə-ro′sis).
Despite its density, osteosclerotic bone is brittle and subject to fracture. Literal interpretation of osteosclerotic is pertaining to bone that is _____.

destruction

Softening and destruction of bone is called osteo/lysis (os″te-ol′ĭ-sis). Paget's disease (named for Sir James Paget, an English surgeon) is a skeletal disease in which osteolysis is usually evident. Osteo/lysis is _____ of bone.

calcium

14-109 Vitamin D aids in the absorption of calcium from the intestinal tract. A deficiency of vitamin D results in insufficient calcium absorption and calci/penia (kal″sĭ-pe′ne-ə), a deficiency of _____ in the body.
Remember that de- means down or from. De/calci/fication (de-kal″sĭ-fi-ka′shən) is loss of calcium from bone or teeth.

osteopenia

14-110 Osteo/penia (os″te-o-pe′ne-ə) is not a disease but a condition that is common to metabolic bone disease. Osteopenia is a reduced bone mass, usually the result of synthesis not compensating for the rate of destruction of bone. Write this term that means a reduced bone mass:
_____.

osteoporosis

14-111 Osteo/porosis (os″te-o-pə-ro′sis) is a metabolic disease in which reduction in the amount of bone mass leads to subsequent fractures. It occurs most commonly in postmenopausal women, sedentary individuals, and patients on long-term steroid therapy. The bones appear thin and fragile, and fractures are common (Figure 14-23). This metabolic bone disease in which there is a reduction in bone mass and increased porosity is called
_____.
It may cause pain, especially in the lower back, and loss of height, and spinal deformities are common. Figure 14-24 shows the effect of the disease on height and shape of the spine with advancing years.

softening

14-112 Translated literally, osteo/malacia (os″te-o-mə-la′shə) means abnormal _____ of bone. It is a reversible metabolic disease in which there is a defect in the mineralization of bone, resulting from inadequate phosphorus and calcium. The deficiency may be caused by a diet lacking phosphorus and calcium or vitamin D, which is necessary for bone formation. Other causes include malabsorption or a lack of exposure to sunlight, which is necessary for the body to synthesize vitamin D. Osteomalacia is the adult equivalent of rickets in children.

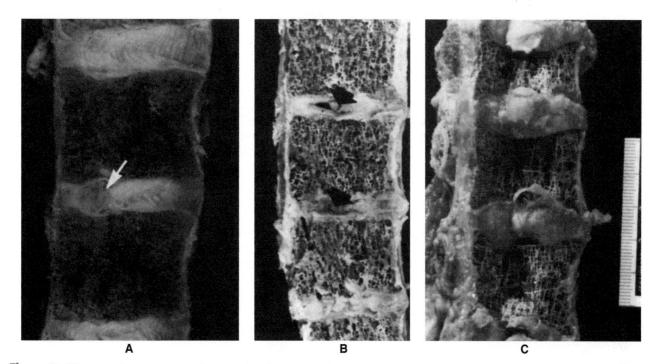

Figure 14-23   Normal versus osteoporotic vertebral bodies. **A,** Normal vertebral bodies. **B,** Vertebrae showing moderate osteoporosis. **C,** Vertebrae showing severe osteoporosis. The vertebral bodies are sectioned to show internal structure. *A* shows well-formed, normal vertebrae and disks. The *white arrow* points to a small focus of degeneration. In *B* the overall shape of the vertebrae is preserved, but osteoporosis is already well developed. The disks show severe degeneration *(black arrows)*. Notice in *C,* severe osteoporosis, how the vertebrae have been compressed by the bulging disks.

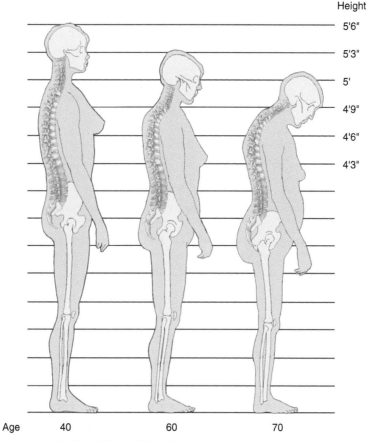

Figure 14-24   The effects of osteoporosis on height and shape of the spine. Compare the normal spine at age 40 with the changes that have occurred by ages 60 and 70. These changes can cause a loss of as much as 6 inches or more in height and can result in the so-called dowager's hump *(far right)* in the upper thoracic vertebrae.

rickets osteomalacia	Insufficient calcium for bone mineralization during the growing years causes rickets (**rik'əts**). Skeletal deformities of rickets are much more severe than those of osteomalacia in adults. In children, the disorder takes the form of _____. In adults, the disorder is called _____.
Paget's	**14-113** <u>Osteitis deformans</u> (**os″te-i′tis de-for′manz**), also called <u>Paget's disease</u>, is a disorder characterized by excessive bone destruction and unorganized bone repair. The disease was thought to be an infectious inflammatory process and was named osteitis deformans. The other name for osteitis deformans is _____ disease.

■ *Congenital Defects*

two skull	**14-114** The skeletal system is affected by several developmental defects, including malformations of the spine. <u>Spina bifida</u> (**spi′nə bif′ĭ-də, bi′fə-də**) is a congenital abnormality characterized by defective closure of the bones of the spine. It can be so extensive that it allows herniation of the spinal cord, or it might be evident only on radiologic examination. Perhaps it will be helpful if you remember that the prefix *bi-* in bi/fida means _____. A <u>cranio/cele</u> (**kra′ne-o-sēl″**) is a hernial protrusion of the brain through a defect in the _____. This is the same as an <u>encephalocele</u>.
spine	**14-115** Literal translation of <u>rachi/schisis</u> (**ra-kis′kĭ-sis**) is split _____. This is congenital fissure (split) of one or more vertebrae.
split	**14-116** <u>Sterno/schisis</u> (*stern[o]*, sternum + *-schisis*, split) means _____ sternum. In sternoschisis (**stər-nos′kĭ-sis**), there is congenital fissure of the sternum. The suffix *-schisis* means split.*
scoliosis	**14-117** Scoliosis (**sko″le-o′sis**) is lateral curvature of the spine, a fairly common abnormality of childhood, especially in females. Write this term that means lateral curvature of the spine: _____. Causes include congenital malformations of the spine, poliomyelitis, spastic paralysis, and unequal leg lengths. <u>Lordosis</u> (**lor-do′sis**) is the anterior concavity of the lumbar and cervical spine as viewed from the side. The term *lordosis* is often used to mean an abnormal increase in this curvature. <u>*Kyphosis*</u> (**ki-fo′sis**) refers to the convexity in the curvature of the thoracic spine as viewed from the side, but it usually means an abnormally increased convexity. Compare these abnormal curvatures of the spine (Figure 14-25).
muscular	**14-118** The suffix *-trophy* means nutrition. Dystrophy is any abnormal condition caused by defective nutrition, often entailing a developmental change in muscles. <u>Muscular dystrophy</u> is a group of inherited diseases that are characterized by weakness and atrophy of muscle without involvement of the nervous system. In all forms of muscular dystrophy, there is progressive disability and loss of strength. The name of this disease, the cause of which is unknown but appears to be an inborn error of metabolism, is _____ dystrophy.
many	**14-119** An <u>anomaly</u>† (**ə-nom′ə-le**) is a deviation from what is regarded as normal, especially as a result of congenital defects. Each hand and foot normally has five digits. <u>Poly/dactyl/ism</u> (**pol″e-dak′təl-iz-əm**) or <u>poly/dactyly</u> (**pol″e-dak′tə-le**) is the presence of _____ digits on the hands or feet. In either of these terms, it is understood that the number of digits is greater than the expected number of five.

---

*-Schisis (Greek: *schizein*, split).
†Anomaly (Greek: *anomalos*, irregular).

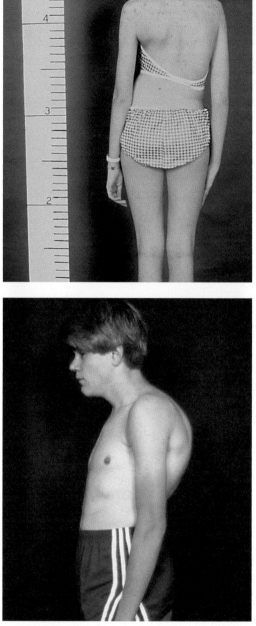

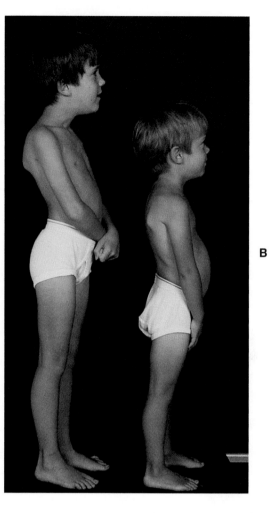

Figure 14-25   Three abnormal curvatures of the spine. **A,** Scoliosis, lateral curvature of the spine. **B,** Lordosis, abnormal anterior concavity of the lumbar spine. **C,** Severe kyphosis of the thoracic spine.

syndactyly

Syndactyly (**sin-dak′tə-le**) is a congenital anomaly of the hand or foot, marked by persistence of the webbing between adjacent digits, so they are more or less completely attached. It can be so severe that there is complete union of the digits and fusion of the bones. Write this term that means a congenital anomaly marked by webbing between adjacent digits: _____. This is also called syndactylism (**sin-dak′tə-liz-əm**). Compare polydactyly and syndactyly in Figure 14-26.

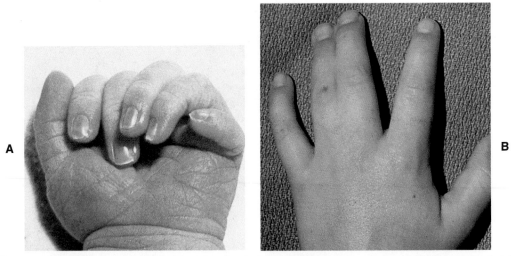

Figure 14-26   Comparison of the fingers in polydactyly and syndactyly. **A,** Polydactyly. Note the presence of six fingers. **B,** Syndactyly. Note the webbing of the third and fourth phalanges.

■ *Arthritis and Connective Tissue Diseases*

joints	**14-120** <u>Arthr/itis</u> is any inflammatory condition of the _____, characterized by pain, heat, swelling, redness, and limitation of movement. Write a word that
arthropathy (ahr-throp′ə-the)	means any disease of the joints: _____. An <u>osteo/arthro/pathy</u> (os″te-o-ahr-throp′ə-the) is a disease of the bones and joints.
arthrodynia (ahr″thro-din′e-ə)	**14-121** <u>Arthr/algia</u> (ahr-thral′jə) means pain in a joint. Write another word that means pain in a joint, using a different suffix: _____.
hardening	Many forms of arthritis are accompanied by pain and stiffness in adjacent parts. <u>Spondyl/arthritis</u> (spon″dəl-ahr-thri′tis) is accompanied by <u>dors/algia</u> (dor-sal′jə), pain in the back. <u>Arthro/scler/osis</u> (ahr″thro-sklə-ro′sis) is _____ of the joints.
	14-122 <u>Osteo/arthritis</u> (os″te-o-ahr-thri′tis), also called <u>degenerative joint disease</u> (DJD), is a form of arthritis in which one or many joints undergo degenerative changes, particularly loss of articular cartilage. This is the most common type of arthritis and is often classified as a connective tissue disease. <u>Connective tissue diseases</u> are a group of acquired disorders that have immunologic and inflammatory changes in small blood vessels and connective tissue.
cartilage	Hips, knees, the vertebral column, and the hands are primarily affected because they are used most often and bear the stress of body weight. This disease is characterized by progressive deterioration and loss of articular _____.
	Possible causes of DJD include the wear and tear effects of aging, genetics, mechanical stress (abuse or overuse of certain joints), and certain metabolic diseases such as diabetes mellitus. Routine x-rays are usually helpful in confirming the diagnosis. CT and MRI may be used to determine the extent of vertebral involvement.
	14-123 <u>Rheumatoid arthritis</u> (RA) is the second most commonly occurring connective tissue disease. It is also the most destructive to joints. It is a chronic, progressive, systemic inflammatory process that affects primarily synovial joints.
	RA affects females more often than males, and people with a family history of RA two or three times more often than the rest of the population. It is believed to be an <u>autoimmune disease</u>—that is, one that is characterized by an alteration of the immune system, resulting in the production of antibodies against the body's own cells. You have learned that the combining form *aut(o)* means self. An alteration in the immune system, resulting in the production of antibodies against the
autoimmune	body's own cells, is called an _____ disease.

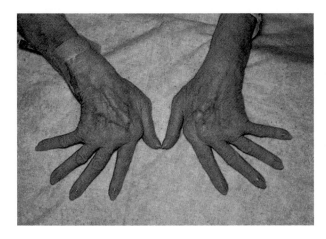

Figure 14-27 Hand deformities characteristic of chronic rheumatoid arthritis. There is marked deformity of the metacarpophalangeal joints, causing deviation of the fingers to the ulnar side of the hand.

Fever and fatigue are common findings in rheumatoid arthritis. As the disease worsens, the joints become progressively inflamed and painful. Joint deformity is common (Figure 14-27).

14-124 Lupus erythematosus (**loo′pəs er″ə-them″ə-to′sis**), systemic scleroderma (**sklēr″o-der′mə**), and Sjögren's (**shər′grenz**) syndrome are also autoimmune diseases that involve connective tissue. Lupus erythematosus is named for the characteristic butterfly rash that appears across the bridge of the nose in some cases (see Figure 7-14). There are two classifications of lupus: cutaneous or discoid* lupus erythematosus (DLE) and systemic lupus erythematosus (SLE). The discoid type affects only the skin. The systemic type can cause major body organs and systems to fail and is potentially fatal. Prolonged exposure to sunlight and other forms of ultraviolet lighting aggravates the skin rash. The name of this autoimmune disease is _____ erythematosus.

14-125 Systemic scleroderma (**sklēr″o-der′mə**), also called systemic sclerosis (**sklə-ro′sis**), is another connective tissue disease. Translated literally, *sclero/derma* means hardening of the _____. Associated with a high mortality rate, systemic sclerosis is characterized by inflammation, fibrosis, and sclerosis of the skin and vital organs. The cause is unknown, but autoimmunity is suspected.

14-126 Sjögren's syndrome is an immunologic disorder characterized by deficient fluid production, which leads to dry eyes, dry mouth, and dryness of other mucous membranes. This disorder primarily affects women over 40 years of age.

14-127 Gout is a systemic disease associated with an inborn error of uric acid metabolism. Urate crystals deposit in the joints, myocardium, kidneys, and ears, causing inflammation. The disease can cause painful swelling of a joint, accompanied by chills and fever. Males are affected more often than females, and diet and medication are critical in the management of this disease called _____.

14-128 The literal interpretation of polyarthritis (**pol″e-ahr-thri′tis**) is inflammation of _____ joints; however, this term means inflammation of more than one joint. The inflammation may migrate from one joint to the other or several joints may be affected simultaneously.

14-129 Spondylo/arthro/pathy (**spon″də-lo-ahr-throp′ə-the**) is a term that means any one of a group of inflammatory disorders that affect the joints and spine.

lupus

skin

gout

many

---

*Discoid (Greek: *diskos*, flat plate).

spine	**14-130** The combining form *ankyl(o)* means stiff. <u>Ankylosing spondylitis</u> causes inflammation and stiffening of the _____. *Ankylosis* (**ang″kə-lo′sis**) means stiffening of a joint.
Lyme	**14-131** <u>Lyme disease</u> is an infection caused by the bite of an infected deer tick. Symptoms in the early stages of the disease are a circular rash, ill feeling, fever, headache, and muscle and joint aches. Prompt antibiotic treatment is effective. Without treatment, a small percentage of infected persons will develop arthritis, as well as heart and neurologic problems. This disease, called _____ disease, is named for the place where it was originally described, Lyme, Connecticut.

■ *Muscular Disorders*

many myopathy (**mi-op′ə-the**) muscle	**14-132** <u>Polymyositis</u> (**pol″e-mi″o-si′tis**) is an inflammatory myo/pathy that involves _____ muscles, which leads to atrophy (**at′rə-fe**) of the muscle. Weight loss, fatigue, and gradual weakness of the muscles are characteristic. A disease of the muscles is called a _____.
	14-133 <u>Myo/fascial</u> (**mi″o-fash′e-əl**) pertains to a _____ and its fascia. <u>Myofascial pain syndrome</u> is pain in one region of the body, often diagnosed by palpation of a "trigger point" that causes pain and twitching of a muscle some distance away from the point of palpation. *Myo/fascial* means pertaining to a muscle and its fascia.
fatigue	**14-134** <u>Chronic fatigue syndrome</u> is a disorder characterized by disabling fatigue accompanied by a variety of associated complaints, including muscle and joint pain and headache. This disabling disorder that is named for its chief symptom is called chronic _____ syndrome.
muscles	**14-135** <u>Poly/my/algia</u> (**pol″e-mi-al′jə**) means pain of many _____. Polymyalgia rheumatica (**roo-mat′ik-ə**) is a chronic, inflammatory disease that primarily affects the arteries in muscles. The major symptoms are stiffness, weakness, and aching, most commonly in the shoulder or pelvic girdle.
joints	**14-136** <u>Fibro/my/algia</u> (**fi″bro-mi-al′jə**), also called <u>fibromyalgia syndrome</u>, is characterized by widespread non/articular pain of the torso, extremities, and the face. It may be attributable to deep sleep deprivation. *Non/articular* means that the _____ are not involved in this chronic disorder.
softening	**14-137** <u>Atrophy</u> of muscle tissue occurs as one ages, but the rate is slowed by exercise. Therapeutic exercise that increases muscle strength and tone is helpful with balance in walking and provides support for the joints as one ages. <u>Myo/lysis</u> (**mi-ol′ĭ-sis**) means disintegration or degeneration of muscle, and myo/malacia (**mi″o-mə-la′shə**) is abnormal _____ of muscular tissue.
myasthenia	**14-138** <u>My/asthenia</u> (**mi″əs-the′ne-ə**) is a term specifically applied to muscle weakness. The suffix *-asthenia* means weakness. Write this new word that means muscle weakness: _____. <u>Myasthenia gravis</u> is a disease of unknown cause, characterized by fatigue and muscle weakness resulting from a defect in the conduction of nerve impulses. It may be restricted to one muscle group or become generalized. The disorder may affect any muscles of the body but especially those of the eye, face, lips, tongue, neck, and throat.
muscle	**14-139** A <u>myo/cele</u> (**mi′o-sēl**) is herniation of a _____ through its ruptured sheath.
muscle	**14-140** <u>Myo/fibr/osis</u> (**mi″o-fi-bro′sis**) is a condition in which _____ tissue is replaced by fibrous tissue.

Exercise 9

Match the terms in the left column (1-6) with their meanings in the right column (A-I). Not all choices will be used.

_____ 1. comminuted fracture
_____ 2. compound fracture
_____ 3. dislocation
_____ 4. greenstick fracture
_____ 5. sprain
_____ 6. strain

A. bone is shattered, producing numerous fragments
B. broken bone is at right angle to the axis of the bone
C. broken bone protrudes through the skin
D. displacement of a bone from a joint
E. incomplete fracture in which the bone is fractured on one side only
F. muscular damage that results from excessive physical effort
G. one bone fragment is firmly driven into another fragment
H. painful, involuntary muscle spasm
I. injury to the tendons, muscles, or ligaments around a joint

Exercise 10

Write a word in each blank space to complete these sentences.

1. A condition in which the median nerve in the wrist becomes compressed, causing pain, is

   _____ tunnel syndrome.

2. Inflammation of a bursa is _____.

3. Inflammation of an articular cartilage is _____.

4. TMJ disorder is a dysfunction of the _____ joint.

5. Another name for flatfoot is _____.

6. An osteosarcoma is a malignant bone _____.

7. A metabolic disease in which there is a defect in the mineralization of bone, resulting from inadequate phosphorus and

   calcium is _____.

8. A congenital abnormality characterized by defective closure of the spine is called spina

   _____.

9. Degenerative joint disease is also called _____.

10. A disease of the nervous system that is characterized by fatigue and muscle weakness is called

    _____ gravis.

SURGICAL AND THERAPEUTIC INTERVENTIONS

reduction

14-141 Orthopedics (or″tho-pe′diks) is the branch of medicine that specializes in the prevention and correction of disorders of the musculoskeletal system. Orthopedic surgeons, also called orthopedists, restore fractures to their normal positions by <u>reduction</u>, pulling the broken fragments into alignment. A cast immobilizes a broken bone until it heals. Pulling a fracture (fx) into alignment is called _____.

A fracture is usually restored to its normal position by manipulation without surgery. This is called <u>closed reduction</u>. Management usually involves immobilization with a <u>splint</u>, <u>bandage</u>, <u>cast</u>, or <u>traction</u>. Traction is the use of a pulling force to a part of the body to produce alignment and rest, while decreasing muscle spasm and correcting or preventing deformity.

14-142 If a fracture must be exposed by surgery before the broken ends can be aligned, it is an <u>open reduction</u>. The fracture shown in Figure 14-28 was corrected by surgery that included <u>internal</u>

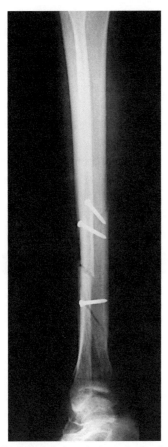

Figure 14-28   A lateral view of a lower leg break after reduction and internal fixation using screws.

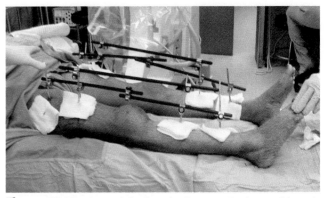

Figure 14-29   External fixation of a fracture. The fractured bone is held together by pins that are attached to a compression device. The pins are removed when the fracture is healed.

fixation to stabilize the alignment. Internal fixation uses pins, rods, plates, screws or other materials to immobilize the fracture. After healing, the fixation devices may be removed or left in place.

External fixation may be used in both open and closed reductions. This method uses metal pins attached to a compression device outside the skin surface (Figure 14-29).

After a bone is broken, the body begins the healing process to repair the injury. Electrical bone stimulation, bone grafting, and ultrasound treatment may be used when healing is slow or does not occur.

14-143 Persons with osteoporosis are predisposed to fractures. Calcium therapy, vitamin D, and osteo/porotics (os″te-o-pə-rot′ikz) are used to treat osteoporosis. Estrogen therapy, begun soon after the start of menopause, may help in the prevention and maintenance of osteoporosis, but there is not agreement on its value versus its risks. Osteoporotics are medications that are used to treat

osteoporosis

_____. Read more about hormone replacement therapy (HRT) for women at high risk for osteoporosis in Chapter 12.

14-144 Excision of a bone (or a portion of it) is oste/ectomy (os″te-ek′tə-me). (One e is often dropped, and this is written ostectomy [os-tek′tə-me].) Write the name of the instrument used to cut bone: _____.

osteotome
(os′te-o-tōm″)
bone

Osteo/plasty (os′te-o-plas″te) means surgical repair of a _____.

14-145 Cranio/plasty (kra′ne-o-plas″te) is plastic surgery, or surgical repair, of the

skull

_____.

craniotome
(kra′ne-o-tōm″)
sternotomy
(stər-not′ə-me)

coccygectomy
(kok″sĭ-jek′tə-me)

phalangectomy
(fal″ən-jek′tə-me)

tendon
incision

tenorrhaphy
(tə-nor′ə-fe)
bursectomy
(bər-sek′tə-me)
muscle

Crani/ectomy (**kra″ne-ek′tə-me**) means excision of a segment of the skull. Incision into the cranium is cranio/tomy (**kra″ne-ot′ə-me**). Write the name of the instrument used in performing craniotomy: _____.

14-146 Incision of the sternum is _____. This is a common incision of open-heart surgery.

Excision of a rib is costectomy (**kos-tek′tə-me**), and excision of a vertebra is vertebrectomy (**ver″tə-brek′tə-me**).

Write a word that means excision of the coccyx: _____.

14-147 _Carp/ectomy_ (**kahr-pek′tə-me**) is excision of one or more of the bones of the wrist. Write a word that means excision of a bone of a finger or toe: _____.

14-148 Tendons may become damaged when a person suffers a deep wound. _Tendo/plasty_ (**ten′do-plas″te**) is surgical repair of a _____.

Teno/tomy (**tə-not′ə-me**) is _____ of a tendon.

Write a word using _ten(o)_ and _-rrhaphy_ that means union of a divided tendon by a suture (suture of a tendon): _____.

14-149 Write a word that means excision of a bursa: _____.

Myo/plasty (**mi′o-plas″te**) is surgical repair of muscle. _Teno/myo/plasty_ (**ten″o-mi′o-plas″te**) is surgical repair of a tendon and _____.

Myorrhaphy (**mi-or′ə-fe**) means suture of a torn or cut muscle.

Learn the two suffixes in the box below that are used to write surgical terms pertaining to the musculoskeletal system.

Word Parts That Pertain to Orthopedics

SUFFIX	MEANING
-clasia	break
-desis	binding; fusion

binding or fusion

laminectomy

vertebroplasty

14-150 Analyze spondylo/syn/desis: _spondyl(o)_ means vertebra; _syn-_ means joined (or together); and _-desis_ means _____.

Spondylosyndesis (**spon″də-lo-sin-de′sis**) is spinal fusion. It is fixation of an unstable segment of the spine, generally accomplished by surgical fusion with a bone graft or a synthetic device.

14-151 _Muscle relaxants_ are prescribed to relieve muscle spasms, such as the spasms that accompany a herniated disk. If bed rest and other treatments do not alleviate the problem, a _lamin/ectomy_ (**lam″ĭ-nek′tə-me**) may be indicated. This is surgical removal of the bony posterior arch of a vertebra to permit surgical access to the disk so that the herniated material can be removed. Write this term that means the surgical removal of the bony arch of a vertebra:

_____.

Complete excision of an intervertebral disk is a _disk/ectomy_ (**dis-kek′tə-me**).

14-152 Vertebral fractures can sometimes be repaired by _vertebro/plasty_ (**vər′tə-bro-plas″te**). In this procedure, a plasticlike substance is injected on each side of the fractured vertebra to hold the fragments in position while the bone heals. The name of the procedure used to assist the healing of a fractured vertebra is called _____.

excision

14-153 A <u>partial fasciectomy</u> (**fas″e-ek′tə-me**) is generally performed to relieve Dupytren's contracture when function becomes impaired. A partial fasci/ectomy is

_____ of fascia.

bunion

14-154 Numerous surgeries are performed to straighten the toes, remove bunions, and correct various deformities of the feet. A <u>bunion/ectomy</u> (**bun″yən-ek′tə-me**) is excision of a

_____. Surgical repair to straighten the great toe is usually done at the same time.

Surgery may be performed to correct the alignment in hammertoe also.

arthrotomy
(**ahr-throt′ə-me**)

14-155 Write a word that means incision of a joint, using _arthr(o)_ and the suffix that means incision: _____.

<u>Arthr/ectomy</u> (**ahr-threk′tə-me**) is excision of a joint.

repair

14-156 <u>Arthro/plasty</u> (**ahr′thro-plas″te**) is surgical _____ of a joint. When other measures are inadequate to provide pain control for degenerative joint disease, surgery may be indicated, often total joint replacement (TJR).

Replacement of hips, knees, elbows, wrists, shoulders, and joints of the fingers and toes are common. Total knee replacement is the surgical insertion of a hinged device to relieve pain and restore motion to a knee that is severely affected by arthritis or injury.

chondroplasty
(**kon′dro-plas″te**)

14-157 Surgical repair of damaged cartilage is _____. This may be necessary if the cartilage becomes torn or displaced.

<u>_Chondrectomy_</u> (**kon-drek′tə-me**) means surgical removal of cartilage.

arthrocentesis
(**ahr″thro-sen-te′sis**)
arthrodesis
(**ahr″thro-de′sis**)

14-158 Sometimes, excessive fluid accumulates in a synovial joint after injury and must be extracted with a needle. Write a word that means surgical puncture of a joint:

_____.

The suffix _-desis_ means binding or fusion. Use this suffix with _arthr(o)_ to form a word that literally means fusion of a joint: _____.

<u>Arthrodesis</u> is a surgical procedure that is used to immobilize a joint. It is artificial ankylosis. Fusing the bones together stabilizes painful joints that have become unable to bear weight. Thus a stiff but stable and painless joint results.

joint

14-159 <u>Arthro/clasia</u> (**ahr″thro-kla′zhə**) is artificial breaking of an ankylosed

_____ to provide movement. Arthroclasia is a surgical procedure that is used to break adhesions of an ankylosed joint. Another term that means operative loosening of adhesions in an ankylosed joint is formed by combining the word part for joint and the suffix that means dissolving or destruction. Use these word parts to write the new term:

arthrolysis
(**ahr-throl′ə-sis**)

_____.

inflammation

14-160 Many drugs are available to treat different forms of arthritis and other connective tissue diseases. <u>Antiinflammatories</u> (**an″te-in-flam′ə-to″rēz**) are generally used to reduce inflammation and pain, especially drugs classified as <u>nonsteroidal antiinflammatory drugs</u> (NSAIDs). These drugs primarily reduce _____ that leads to pain. Two examples are aspirin and ibuprofen.

<u>COX-2 inhibitors</u> (for example, Celebrex) are also commonly used to reduce the inflammation of arthritis, and are less likely to cause stomach distress and ulcers. (See the pharmacology appendix for more information.)

<u>Anti/arthritics</u> (**an″te-ahr-thrit′ikz**) are various forms of therapy that relieve the symptoms of arthritis.

DMARDs, <u>disease-modifying antirheumatic drugs</u>, may actually modify the course of inflammatory conditions, such as rheumatoid arthritis, slowing progression of the disease. They tend to be slower acting than NSAIDs and may be prescribed with antiinflammatories.

myelosuppressive
(mi″ə-lo-sə-pres′iv)

14-161 Cancer treatment often induces <u>myelosuppression</u>. Write a word that is an adjective that means inhibiting bone marrow activity: _____. (Drugs that inhibit bone marrow are called myelosuppressive agents or simply myelosuppressives.)

<u>Bone marrow transplants</u> are used to stimulate the production of normal blood cells. The patient's bone marrow is first destroyed with radiation and chemotherapy. Healthy bone marrow cells (stem cells) are transfused into the patient's blood; they migrate to the spongy bone and multiply into cancer-free bone marrow cells. (Cord blood, collected immediately after birth, is rich in stem cells and may be an alternative to bone marrow transplants.)

Exercise 11

Match the surgical terms in the left column with their meanings in the right column.

_____ 1. closed reduction

_____ 2. internal fixation

_____ 3. open reduction

_____ 4. osteectomy

_____ 5. osteoplasty

A. excision of a bone
B. exposing a broken bone by surgery and aligning it
C. pulling a broken bone into alignment without surgery
D. surgery that uses pins or other materials to immobilize a broken bone
E. surgical repair of a bone

Exercise 12

Write terms for the following meanings:

1. breaking an ankylosed joint _____

2. excision of a rib _____

3. incision of a joint _____

4. inhibiting bone marrow activity _____

5. medications that reduce inflammation _____

6. spinal fusion _____

7. surgical puncture of a synovial joint _____

8. surgical removal of cartilage _____

9. surgical repair of the skull _____

10. suture of a torn or cut muscle _____

SELECTED ABBREVIATIONS

ANA	antinuclear antibody	**L-l, L-2, etc.**	lumbar vertebrae
Ca	calcium	**LE**	lupus erythematosus
C-l, C-2, etc.	cervical vertebrae	**MTP**	metatarsophalangeal
CPK	creatine phosphokinase	**NSAID**	nonsteroidal antiinflammatory drug
CTS	carpal tunnel syndrome	**RA**	rheumatoid arthritis
DJD	degenerative joint disease	**RF**	rheumatoid factor
DLE	discoid lupus erythematosus	**ROM**	range of motion
DMARDs	disease-modifying antirheumatic drugs	**SLE**	systemic lupus erythematosus
EMG	electromyography	**T-l, T-2, etc.**	thoracic vertebrae
ESR	erythrocyte sedimentation rate	**TJR**	total joint replacement
fx	fracture	**TMJ**	temporomandibular joint
lig	ligament		

CHAPTER 14 REVIEW

■ Basic Understanding

Labeling
I. Label the diagram with the combining forms for the bones that are indicated. For example, number 1 is clavicul(o).

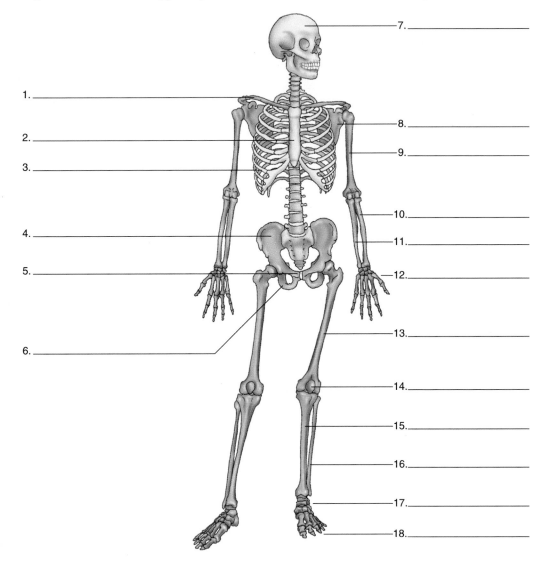

7._____

1._____

2._____

3._____

8._____

9._____

4._____

10._____

11._____

5._____

12._____

6._____

13._____

14._____

15._____

16._____

17._____

18._____

Matching
II. Match the following connective tissues with their descriptions.

_____ 1. bone

_____ 2. bursa

_____ 3. cartilage

_____ 4. joint

_____ 5. ligament

_____ 6. synovial membrane

_____ 7. tendon

A. connects bones or cartilages
B. fluid-filled sac that helps reduce friction
C. fluid-secreting tissue lining the joint
D. place of union between two or more bones
E. provides protection and support for a joint
F. strong, fibrous tissue that attaches muscles to bones
G. the most rigid connective tissue

III. *Match the types of body movements in 1 through 10 with their meanings (A-J).*

_____ 1. abduction

_____ 2. adduction

_____ 3. circumduction

_____ 4. eversion

_____ 5. extension

_____ 6. flexion

_____ 7. inversion

_____ 8. pronation

_____ 9. rotation

_____ 10. supination

A. circular movement of a limb at the far end
B. movement of a bone around an axis
C. movement of the sole of the foot inward
D. movement of the sole of the foot outward
E. rotation that allows the palm of the hand to turn up
F. rotation that turns the palm of the hand backward (down)
G. to bend
H. to bring together
I. to straighten
J. to take away

IV. *Match the types of fractures in 1 through 5 with their meanings (A-E).*

_____ 1. comminuted

_____ 2. greenstick

_____ 3. impacted

_____ 4. spiral

_____ 5. transverse

A. a break in which there are many bone fragments
B. bone is bent and fractured on one side only
C. bone is twisted apart
D. break is at right angles to the axis of the bone
E. one bone fragment is firmly driven into another

V. *Match the bones in 1 through 10 with their common names (A-J).*

_____ 1. carpal

_____ 2. clavicle

_____ 3. coccyx

_____ 4. femur

_____ 5. patella

_____ 6. pelvis

_____ 7. phalanges

_____ 8. scapula

_____ 9. sternum

_____ 10. tarsal

A. ankle bone
B. bones of the fingers and toes
C. breastbone
D. collarbone
E. hip bone
F. kneecap
G. shoulder blade
H. tailbone
I. thigh bone
J. wrist bone

Sequencing

VI. *The five types of vertebrae are listed. Indicate their position by numbering them from uppermost (1) to the lowest (5):*

_____ cervical

_____ coccygeal

_____ lumbar

_____ sacral

_____ thoracic

Listing

VII. List five functions of the skeletal system.

1. _____

2. _____

3. _____

4. _____

5. _____

VIII. List the three types of muscle and describe their functions.

1. _____

2. _____

3. _____

Multiple Choice

IX. Circle the correct answers in the following multiple choice questions.

1. Which term means congenital fissure of the breastbone? (costectomy, rachischisis, spondylosyndesis, sternoschisis)

2. Which term means pertaining to two bones of the forearm? (carpopedal, carpophalangeal, humeroulnar, ulnoradial)

3. Which term means any disease of the joints? (arthropathy, bursopathy, chondropathy, osteopathy)

4. Which of the following is the record produced in a procedure that records the response of a muscle to electrical stimulation? (arthrocentesis, electromyogram, myograph, range-of-motion reading)

5. Which of the following means loss of calcium from bone? (calcification, calciuria, decalcification, osteogenesis)

6. What is the term for the presence of extra fingers or toes? (carpopedal disease, Paget's disease, phalangitis, polydactylism)

7. What is the name of the soft tissue that fills the cavity of a bone? (bone marrow, diaphysis, epiphysis, periosteum)

8. Which term means the process of using a fiberoptic instrument to view the interior of a joint? (arthrogram, arthrography, arthroscope, arthroscopy)

9. Which of the following pathologies means flatfoot? (Dupuytren's contracture, hallux valgus, tarsal tunnel syndrome, tarsoptosis)

10. Which term means a reversible metabolic disease in which there is a defect in the bone, resulting from inadequate phosphorus and calcium? (osteitis deformans, osteolysis, osteomalacia, osteoporosis)

Writing Terms

X. Write a term for each of the following meanings:

1. aligning a broken bone   _____

2. between the ribs   _____

3. degenerative joint disease _____

4. excision of the tailbone   _____

5. herniation of a muscle   _____

6. inflammation of a bone   _____

7. lateral curvature of the spine   _____

8. pertaining to a muscle and its fascia   _____

9. pertaining to the joints   _____

10. surgical puncture of a joint   _____

■ Greater Comprehension

Health Care Report
XI. Answer the questions after reading the following health care report.

MID-CITY MEDICAL CENTER

222 Medical Center Drive   Main City, USA 63017-1000   Phone: (555) 434-0000
                                                                       Fax (555) 434-0001

PREOPERATIVE HISTORY AND PHYSICAL

PT. NAME: Thomas Shaw   **ID NO:** 22222222   **ROOM NO:** 444
ATTENDING PHYSICIAN: John T. Riley, M.D.
DATE OF ADMISSION: 2/11/2005
HISTORY OF PRESENT ILLNESS: 40-year-old male who fell yesterday injuring left leg; radiologic findings showed comminuted proximal rt. femur fracture
MEDICATIONS: Insulin, Neurontin, Effexor, Paxil
ALLERGIES: Penicillin
SURGICAL HISTORY: Laminectomy, rt. knee arthroscopy
MEDICAL HISTORY: Insulin-dependent diabetes mellitus, neuropathy, herniated disk, arthralgias, depression
REVIEW OF SYSTEMS: No significant findings, except for the following:
   MUSCULOSKELETAL: left thigh with edema, sensation intact left foot, able to move left ankle and toes
   HEMATOLOGIC: blood sugar 120
FAMILY HISTORY: Diabetes mellitus—father; osteoporosis—mother
SOCIAL HISTORY: Divorced; lives alone

MR: aba   *Michael Rawlings, M.D.*
DATE: 2/11/05   Michael Rawlings, M.D.
T: 2/12/05

---

1. Describe the meaning of a comminuted proximal rt. femur fracture.

2. Describe the two procedures mentioned in the patient's surgical history.

3. What is meant by a *herniated disk?*

4. What is meant by the term *arthralgias?*

5. Describe the mother's medical history.

XII. Read the following report and define the terms that are indicated.

MID-CITY MEDICAL CENTER

222 Medical Center Drive   Main City, USA 63017-1000   Phone: (555) 434-0000
                                                                       Fax (555) 434-0001

DIAGNOSIS RECORD/DISCHARGE SUMMARY

PATIENT: Martha Watkins
FINAL DIAGNOSIS: <u>Osteoarthritis</u> of the right knee
SECONDARY DIAGNOSIS: <u>Rheumatoid arthritis</u>; <u>degenerative joint disease left knee</u>
COMPLICATIONS: Postoperative deep vein thrombosis—right lower extremity
PRINCIPAL OPERATION/PROCEDURE(S)/TREATMENT RENDERED: <u>Right total knee arthroplasty</u>, posterior stabilized, cemented.
DISCHARGE INSTRUCTIONS: Up ad lib with full weight bearing to <u>right lower extremity</u>. Ambulate with wheeled walker. Home health for physical and occupational therapy 3x week, and nursing visits to monitor incision and medication. Patient to change dry dressing to incision daily.
MEDICATIONS: Coumadin 5 mg daily
DIET: Regular
FOLLOW-UP: Patient to make appointment with Dr. Withers for staple removal in 10 days
DATE ADMITTED: 1/31/2005
DATE DISCHARGED: 2/05/2005
SURGEON: Dr. John Withers

Define:

1. osteoarthritis

_____

2. rheumatoid arthritis

_____

3. degenerative joint disease left knee

_____

4. right total knee arthroplasty

_____

5. right lower extremity

_____

Spelling
XIII. Circle all incorrectly spelled terms and write their correct spelling.

adductor   anomaly   femural   fissure   ileofemoral

Interpreting Abbreviations

XIV. *Write the meanings of these abbreviations.*

1. ANA _____

2. DJD _____

3. EMG _____

4. ROM _____

5. SLE _____

Pronunciation

XV. *The pronunciation is shown for several medical words. Indicate which syllable has the primary accent by marking it with an '.*

1. arthroclasia (ahr thro kla zhə)

2. chondrosarcoma (kon dro sahr ko mə)

3. lumbar (lum bahr)

4. myasthenia (mi əs the ne ə)

5. sternocostal (stər no kos təl)

Categorizing Terms

XVI. *Classify the terms in the left column (1-10) by selecting A, B, C, D, or E.*

_____ 1. antiarthritics   A. anatomy

_____ 2. atrophy   B. diagnostic test or procedure

                      C. pathology

_____ 3. bone densitometry   D. surgery

_____ 4. calcaneofibular   E. therapy

_____ 5. epiphysis

_____ 6. fibromyalgia

_____ 7. infrapatellar

_____ 8. reflex hammer

_____ 9. vertebroplasty

_____ 10. xiphoid process

(Check your answers with the solutions in Appendix VI.)

LISTING OF MEDICAL TERMS

Use the practice CD to review the terms that have been presented. Look closely at the spelling of each term as it is pronounced and be sure you know the meaning of each term.

abduction
abductor
adduction
adductor
ankylosed
ankylosing spondylitis
ankylosis
anomaly
antiarthritic
antiinflammatory
antinuclear antibody test
appendicular
arthralgia
arthrectomy
arthritis
arthrocentesis
arthrochondritis
arthroclasia
arthrodesis
arthrodynia
arthrogram
arthrography
arthrolysis
arthropathy
arthroplasty
arthrosclerosis
arthroscope
arthroscopy
arthrotomy
articular
articulation
aspiration
atrophy
auditory ossicle
autoimmune
autoimmune disease
autonomic nervous system
axial
bone densitometry
bone density
bone grafting
bone marrow
bunionectomy

bursa
bursectomy
bursitis
calcaneal
calcaneitis
calcaneodynia
calcaneofibular
calcaneoplantar
calcaneotibial
calcaneus
calcification
calcipenia
calciuria
callus
cardiac muscle
carpal
carpal tunnel syndrome
carpals
carpectomy
carpopedal
carpophalangeal
carpus
cartilage
cellulitis
cerebrospinal fluid
cervical
chondral
chondralgia
chondrectomy
chondritis
chondrocostal
chondrodynia
chondroid
chondropathy
chondroplasty
chondrosarcoma
circumduction
clavicle
coccygeal
coccygectomy
coccyx
comminuted fracture
compound fracture

connective tissue
costa
costal
costectomy
costoclavicular
costovertebral
COX-2 inhibitors
craniectomy
craniocele
cranioplasty
craniotome
craniotomy
cranium
creatine phosphokinase
cutaneous lupus
    erythematosus
decalcification
degenerative joint disease
diaphysis
discoid lupus
    erythematosus
diskectomy
dislocation
dorsalgia
Dupuytren's contracture
dystrophy
electromyogram
electromyography
encephalocele
epiphysis
erythrocyte sedimentation
    rate
eversion
Ewing's sarcoma
extension
extensor
external fixation
facial
fascia
fascial
fasciectomy
femoral
femur

fibromyalgia
fibrosarcoma
fibula
fibular
fissure
flexion
flexor
fracture
ganglion
gout
greenstick fracture
hallux valgus
hammertoe
haversian canals
herniated disk
humeral
humeroradial
humeroscapular
humeroulnar
humerus
hypercalciuria
iliac
iliofemoral
iliopubic
ilium
impacted fracture
infraclavicular
infracostal
infrapatellar
infrascapular
infrasternal
intercostal
internal fixation
interscapular
intraarticular
inversion
involuntary muscle
ischial
ischialgia
ischiococcygeal
ischiodynia
ischiofemoral
ischiopubic

ischium
joint crepitus
kyphosis
laminectomy
leukemia
leukocyte
ligament
lordosis
lumbar
lumbar puncture
lupus erythematosus
Lyme disease
mandible
mandibular
medullary cavity
metacarpal
metatarsal
metatarsophalangeal
midphalangeal
Morton's neuroma
multiple myeloma
multiple sclerosis
muscle relaxants
muscular
muscular dystrophy
musculoskeletal
myalgia
myasthenia
myasthenia gravis
myelitis
myeloblast
myelocyte
myelography
myelosuppression
myelosuppressive
myoblast
myocardium
myocele
myocellulitis
myodynia
myofascial
myofibroma
myofibrosis
myolysis
myomalacia
myopathy
myoplasty
myorrhaphy

nonarticular
nonsteroidal
    antiinflammatory
open fracture
orthopedics
orthopedist
ossification
ostealgia
ostectomy
osteectomy
osteitis
osteitis deformans
osteoarthritis
osteoarthropathy
osteoblast
osteochondritis
osteocyte
osteodynia
osteogenesis
osteolysis
osteomalacia
osteomyelitis
osteopenia
osteoplasty
osteoporosis
osteoporotics
osteosarcoma
osteosclerosis
osteosclerotic
osteotome
Paget's disease
patella
patellofemoral
pelvic
pelvic girdle
perichondrial
perichondrium
periosteum
phalangectomy
phalanges
plantar
polyarthritis
polydactylism
polymyalgia
polymyalgia rheumatica
polymyositis
pronation
pubes

pubic
pubic symphysis
pubis
pubofemoral
rachialgia
rachiodynia
rachischisis
radiopaque
radius
reduction
reflex hammer
retrosternal
rheumatoid arthritis
rheumatoid factor
rickets
rotation
rotator cuff
sacral
sacrodynia
sacrum
scapula
scapular
scapuloclavicular
scleroderma
scoliosis
shoulder girdle
simple fracture
Sjögren's syndrome
skeletal muscle
spina bifida
spinal fusion
spondylalgia
spondylarthritis
spondylarthropathy
spondylosyndesis
sprain
sternal
sternalgia
sternoclavicular
sternocostal
sternoschisis
sternotomy
sternovertebral
sternum
strain
subcostal
subpubic
substernal

supination
supracostal
suprapubic
suprasternal
syndactylism
syndactyly
synovial
synovitis
systemic lupus
    erythematosus
systemic sclerosis
tarsal
tarsal tunnel syndrome
tarsoptosis
tarsus
temporal
temporomandibular
tenalgia
tendinitis
tendon
tendonitis
tendoplasty
tenodynia
tenomyoplasty
tenorrhaphy
tenotomy
tetany
thoracic
tibia
tibialgia
tibiofemoral
trabeculae
traction
transverse fracture
ulna
ulnoradial
vertebra
vertebrectomy
vertebrochondral
vertebrocostal
vertebroplasty
vertebrosternal
viscera
visceral muscle
xiphoid process

ENGLISH	SPANISH (PRONUNCIATION)
ankle	tobillo (to-BEEL-lyo)
arm	brazo (BRAH-so)
back	espalda (es-PAHL-dah)
bones	huesos (oo-AY-sos)
calcium	calcio (CAHL-se-o)
cartilage	cartílago (car-TEE-lah-go)
cheek	mejilla (may-HEEL-lyah)
chew, to	masticar (mas-te-CAR)
collarbone	clavícula (clah-VEE-coo-lah)
cranium	cráneo (CRAH-nay-o)
elbow	codo (CO-do)
extremity	extremidad (ex-tray-me-DAHD)
face	cara (CAH-rah)
finger	dedo (DAY-do)
foot (plural feet)	pie (PE-ay, PE-ays)
forearm	antebrazo (an-tay-BRAH-so)
fracture	fractura (frac-TOO-rah)
head	cabeza (cah-BAY-sah)
heel	talón (tah-LON)
hip	cadera (cah-DAY-rah)
jaw	mandíbula (man-DEE-boo-lah)
joint	articulacíon (ar-te-coo-lah-se-ON), coyuntura (co-yoon-TOO-rah)
knee	rodilla (ro-DEEL-lyah)
kneecap	rótula (RO-too-lah)
ligament	ligamento (le-gah-MEN-to)
movement	movimiento (mo-ve-me-EN-to)
neck	cuello (coo-EL-lyo)
nutrition	nutrición (noo-tre-se-ON)
phalanges	falanges (fah-LAHN-hays)
phosphorus	fósforo (FOS-fo-ro)
reduction	reducción (ray-dooc-se-ON)
rib	costilla (cos-TEEL-lyah)
sacrum	hueso sacro (oo-AY-so SAH-cro)
shoulder	hombro (OM-bro)
shoulder blade	espaldilla (es-pal-DEEL-lyah)
skeleton	esqueleto (es-kay-LAY-to)
skull	cráneo (CRAH-nay-o)
spinal column	columna vertebral (co-LOOM-nah ver-tay-BRAHL)
spine	espinazo (es-pe-NAH-so)
spiral	espiral (es-pe-RAHL)
sprain, to	torcer (tor-SERR)
sternum	esternón (es-ter-NON)
stiff	tieso (te-AY-so)
support	sustento (sus-TEN-to)
temple	sien (se-AYN)
tendon	tendón (ten-DON)
thigh	muslo (MOOS-lo)
thumb	pulgar (pool-GAR)
toe	dedo del pie (DAY-do del pe-AY)
vertebral column	columna vertebral (co-LOOM-nah ver-tay-BRAHL)
weakness	debilidad (day-be-le-DAHD)
wrist	muñeca (moo-NYAY-cah)

CHAPTER 15

Nervous System and Psychological Disorders

LEARNING GOALS

In this chapter, you will learn to do the following:

Basic Understanding
1. Match the major divisions of the nervous system with their functions.
2. Match the structures of the nervous system with their descriptions.
3. Identify the stimulus for each of the five types of receptors.
4. Use the word parts to build and analyze terms.
5. Match several disorders of the nervous system with their characteristics.

Greater Comprehension
6. Use word parts from this chapter to determine the meanings of terms in a health care report.
7. Spell the terms accurately.
8. Pronounce the terms correctly.
9. Write the meanings of the abbreviations.
10. Categorize terms as anatomy, diagnostic test or procedure, pathology, surgery, or therapy.

THESE ARE THE MAJOR SECTIONS IN THIS CHAPTER:

❏ **Anatomy and Physiology**
  Organization of the Nervous System
  Central Nervous System
  Peripheral Nervous System and the Sense Organs
❏ **Diagnostic Tests and Procedures**
❏ **Pathologies**
  Headaches
  Trauma

Paralysis
Congenital Disorders
Infections
Tumors
Seizure Disorders
Degenerative Disorders
Eye and Ear Disorders
Psychological Disorders
❏ **Surgical and Therapeutic Interventions**

FUNCTION FIRST

The nervous system is the body's control center and communications network. It stimulates movement, senses changes both within and outside the body, and provides us with thought, learning, and memory. With the help of the hormonal system, the nervous system maintains homeostasis, a dynamic equilibrium of the internal environment of the body.

ANATOMY AND PHYSIOLOGY

nerve

15-1 The nervous system is the network of structures that activates, coordinates, and controls all functions of the body. The terms *nervous* and *neur/al* (**noor′əl**) mean pertaining to a _____ or the nerves, but the nervous system includes the brain and spinal cord, as well as the nerves.

15-2 The nervous system is the body's most organized and complex system. It affects both psychological and physiologic functions. In addition to being the center of thinking and judgment, the nervous system influences other body systems. For example, damage to the spinal nerves that supply nerve impulses to the diaphragm may result in respiratory arrest.

The various activities of the nervous system can be grouped as sensory, integrative, and motor functions. Sensory receptors detect changes that occur inside and outside the body. For example, receptors monitor external changes such as light or room temperature. They also monitor changes within the body such as body temperature and blood pressure. The gathering of this type of information is the

sensory

_____ function of the nervous system.

15-3 Integrative functions create sensations, produce thoughts and memory, and make decisions based on sensory input. The nervous system responds to sensory input and integration by sending signals to muscles or glands and causing an effect. Responding and causing an effect in muscles or glands is the motor function of the nervous system.

The activities of the nervous system include sensory receptors that detect change, integrative functions that produce thoughts and memory and help us make decisions, and

motor

_____ functions that enable us to respond to a stimulus.

■ *Organization of the Nervous System*

central
peripheral

15-4 The two principal divisions of the nervous system are the central nervous system (CNS) and the peripheral (**pə-rif′ər-əl**) nervous system (PNS). *CNS* is an abbreviation for _____ nervous system.

PNS means _____ nervous system.

brain

15-5 Looking at Figure 15-1, you see that the CNS is composed of the _____ and the spinal cord. This part of the system is the control center.

The second division of the nervous system is the PNS, the various nerves and nerve masses that connect the brain and the spinal cord with receptors, muscles, and glands. Observing the diagram, you see that the PNS is divided into a sensory or afferent (**af′ər-ənt**) system and a motor or

efferent (**ef′ər-ənt**)

_____ system.

Which system conveys information from the CNS to muscles and glands?

efferent

_____

nerve

15-6 The nervous system is composed of two types of cells: neurons (**noor′onz**) and neuroglia (**noŏ-rog′le-ə**). Both types of cells that compose nervous tissue are named using *neur(o)*, which means _____.

Neurons conduct impulses either to or from the central nervous system. Neuroglia, or glia* cells, provide special support and protection. If a neuron is destroyed, it cannot replace itself. On the other hand, neuroglia are far more numerous and, because they can reproduce, are the only source of primary malignant brain tumors, those originating in the brain.

Learn the following word parts.

---

*Glia (Greek: *glia*, glue).`

Word Parts That Pertain to Cells of the Nervous System

COMBINING FORM	MEANING
dendr(o)	tree
nerv(o), neur(o)	nerve
gli(o)	neuroglia or a sticky substance

15-7 The neuron, or nerve cell, is the basic unit of the nervous system. Neurons carry out the function of the nervous system by conducting nerve impulses. Each neuron has a cell body, a single axon (ak′son), and one or more dendrites (den′drīts) (Figure 15-2).

The axon and dendrites are cytoplasmic projections, or processes, that project from the cell body. They are sometimes called nerve fibers. An axon carries impulses away from the cell body. Dendrites transmit impulses to the cell body. Which type of cytoplasmic projection carries a nervous impulse away from the cell body? _____

axon

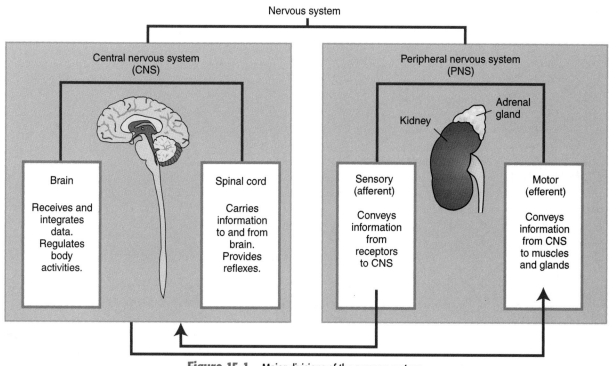

Figure 15-1   Major divisions of the nervous system.

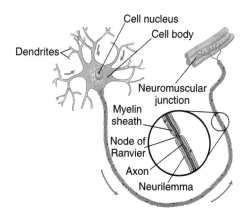

Figure 15-2   Structure of a typical neuron. The basic parts of a neuron are the cell body, a single axon, and several dendrites. *Arrows* indicate the direction that an impulse travels to or from the cell body. The axon is surrounded by a segmented myelin sheath with neurilemma that forms a tight covering over each segment. The unmyelinated regions between the myelin segments are called the nodes of Ranvier. A myelinated nerve fiber is capable of conducting an impulse many times faster than if it were not myelinated.

The combining form *dendr(o)* means tree. Which type of cytoplasmic projection has numerous branches? _____

15-8 Many axons are surrounded by a white lipid covering called a myelin sheath. The myelinated axons appear whitish and are called white matter. Those that are not myelinated appear grayish and are called _____ matter.

In a myelinated fiber, the nerve impulse "jumps" from one node of Ranvier (see Figure 15-2) to the next and results in a faster rate of conduction than in an unmyelinated nerve fiber. If the myelin sheath becomes damaged, as it does in diseases such as multiple sclerosis, conduction of the impulse is impaired.

The region of communication between one neuron and another is called the synapse **(sin′aps)**. An axon terminates in several short branches that together form a synaptic bulb. The synaptic bulb releases a neurotransmitter that either inhibits or enhances a nervous impulse. A neuro/transmitter is a chemical that transmits a _____ impulse that either inhibits or enhances a reaction.

15-9 Some of the best known neurotransmitters are acetylcholine (ACh) **(as″ə-təl-, as″ə-tēl-ko′lēn)**, epinephrine **(ep″ĭ-nef′rin)**, dopamine **(do′pə-mēn)**, serotonin **(ser″o-to′nin)**, and endorphins **(en-dor′finz, en′dor-finz)**. To prevent prolonged reactions, a neurotransmitter is quickly inactivated by an enzyme.

Disorders involving neurotransmitters have been implicated in the origin of various psychological disorders. The substances released at the synapse that either enhance or inhibit a nervous impulse are called _____.

15-10 *Neuro/muscul/ar* **(noor″o-mus′ku-lər)** means concerning both _____ and muscles. A neuro/muscular junction is the area of contact between a neuron and adjoining skeletal muscle. When a nerve impulse reaches the neuromuscular junction, acetylcholine is released, which leads to contraction of the muscle. Acetylcholine acts rapidly on muscle tissue, and most of it is then promptly inactivated by an enzyme, acetylcholinester/ase **(as″ə-təl-, as″ə-tēl-ko″lĭ-nes′tə-rās)**. The latter ends in the suffix *-ase*, meaning _____, which should help you distinguish between these two terms.

Certain drugs can block transmission of impulses to the skeletal muscle. The transmission is blocked at the neuromuscular junction.

15-11 Conduction of nervous impulses is often described as a reflex arc. A reflex is an automatic, involuntary response to some change, either inside or outside the body. Reflexes help maintain homeostasis by making constant adjustments to our blood pressure, breathing rate, and pulse. A common reflex is that of quickly removing your hand from a hot object.

A deep tendon reflex (DTR) is one way of assessing the reflex arc. For example, a sharp tap on the tendon just below the kneecap normally causes extension of the leg at the knee. This is called the patellar **(pə-tel′ər)** response or knee jerk response. A normal response indicates an intact reflex arc between the nervous system and the muscles that are involved in the response. Other areas are also assessed for reflex activities. An automatic, involuntary response to some change, either inside or outside the body, is called a _____.

15-12 The reflex arc involves two types of neurons: a sensory neuron and a motor neuron. Sensory neurons transmit nerve impulses toward the spinal cord and the brain. Motor neurons transmit nerve impulses from the brain and the spinal cord (Figure 15-3).

Notice that the _____ neuron causes the muscle to contract.

Margin answer column (left):

dendrite

gray

nervous

neurotransmitters

nerves

enzyme

reflex

motor

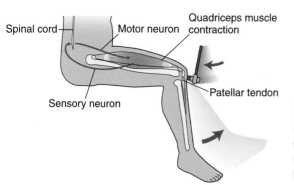

Spinal cord
Motor neuron
Quadriceps muscle contraction
Patellar tendon
Sensory neuron

Figure 15-3   Conceptual drawing of the reflex arc. A receptor detects the stimulus, the tap on the patellar tendon with the reflex hammer. The sensory neuron transmits the nerve impulse to the spinal cord. The motor neuron conducts a nervous impulse that causes the quadriceps muscle to contract. Extension of the leg at the knee is the normal patellar response, also called knee jerk.

Exercise 1

1. List four functions of the nervous system:

_____.

2. The various activities of the nervous system can be grouped as detecting changes, producing thoughts and making decisions, and causing an effect in muscles or glands. What are the names of these three activities?

_____, _____, and

_____ functions

3. Name the two principal divisions of the nervous system: _____ and

_____.

4. Name the two types of cells of the nervous system: _____ and

_____.

5. Name the two types of cytoplasmic projections of a basic nerve cell: _____ and

_____.

■ Central Nervous System

brain

15-13 The central nervous system consists of the _____ and spinal cord. The brain, a soft mass of tissue weighing approximately 1360 grams (3 pounds) in the average adult, receives thousands of bits of information and integrates all the data to determine the appropriate response. The brain is surrounded by the cranium (**kra′ne-əm**) (skull), and the spinal cord is protected by the vertebrae. In addition to the skull and vertebrae, the brain and spinal cord are protected by three membranes called meninges (**mə-nin′jēz**) and circulating cerebrospinal fluid. The singular form of meninges is meninx (**me′ninks**).
   Learn the following word parts.

Word Parts Pertaining to the Central Nervous System

COMBINING FORM	MEANING	COMBINING FORM	MEANING
cerebell(o)	cerebellum	mening(i), mening(o)	meninges
cerebr(o), encephal(o)	brain (cerebr[o] sometimes means cerebrum)	arachn(o)	spider or arachnoid (a meningeal membrane)
myel(o)	spinal cord (sometimes, bone marrow)		

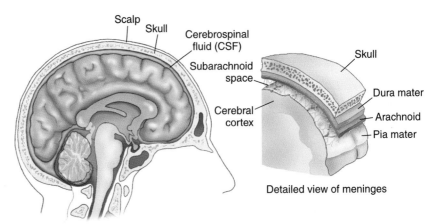

Figure 15-4   The brain and its protective coverings, the meninges. The tough outer membrane, the dura mater, lies just inside the skull. The thread-like strands of the middle layer, the arachnoid, resemble a cobweb. The pia mater is the innermost meningeal layer and is so tightly bound to the brain that it cannot be removed without damaging the surface.

15-14 The meninges (singular, meninx) enclose the brain and the spinal cord (Figure 15-4). The tough outer layer, the dura mater* (**doo′rə ma′tər**), lies just inside the cranial bones and lines the vertebral canal. The middle layer is the arachnoid (**ə-rak′noid**), a thin layer with numerous thread-like strands that attach it to the innermost layer. The combining form *arachn(o)* means either the arachnoid membrane or spider. The innermost layer, the pia mater† (**pi′ə ma′tər, pe′ə mah′tər**), is thin and delicate and is tightly attached to the surface of the brain and spinal cord.

dura
pia

The outer layer is the_____ mater. The middle layer is the arachnoid, and the innermost layer is the _____ mater.

meninges

15-15 The combining form *mening(o)* means the _____.
Meningeal (**mə-nin′je-əl**) means pertaining to the meninges.

below (or beneath)

15-16 *Sub/dural* (**səb-doo′rəl**) means _____ the dura mater, so it refers to the area between the dura mater and the arachnoid. The potential space between these two membranes is the subdural space.

cerebrum

15-17 The cerebrum is the largest and uppermost portion of the brain, and the combining form *cerebr(o)* means either the cerebrum or the brain in general. It is concerned with interpretation of impulses and all voluntary muscle activities. It is the center of higher mental faculties. *Cerebr/al* (**sə-re′brəl, ser′ə-brəl**) means pertaining to the _____.

cranium

Both *craniocerebral* (**kra″ne-o-ser′ə-brəl**) and *cerebrocranial* (**ser″ə-bro-kra′ne-əl**) mean pertaining to the _____ and the cerebrum.

15-18 The brain is that part of the CNS contained within the skull. A longitudinal fissure almost completely divides it into two cerebral hemispheres (*hemi-* means half). The surface of each hemisphere is covered with a convoluted layer of gray matter called the cerebral cortex. Division of the cortex into lobes provides useful reference points (Figure 15-5).

frontal

The lobe that is located near the front of the cerebrum is called the _____ lobe.

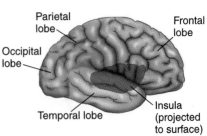

Figure 15-5   Lateral view of the cerebrum. The surface of the cerebrum is marked by convolutions. The pia mater closely follows the convolutions and goes deep into the grooves (sulci). Each cerebral hemisphere is divided into five lobes: the frontal lobe, the parietal lobe, the occipital lobe, the temporal lobe, and an insula that is covered by parts of the other lobes.

---

*Dura mater (Latin: *durus*, hard; *mater*, mother).
†Pia mater (Latin: *pia*, tender; *mater*, mother).

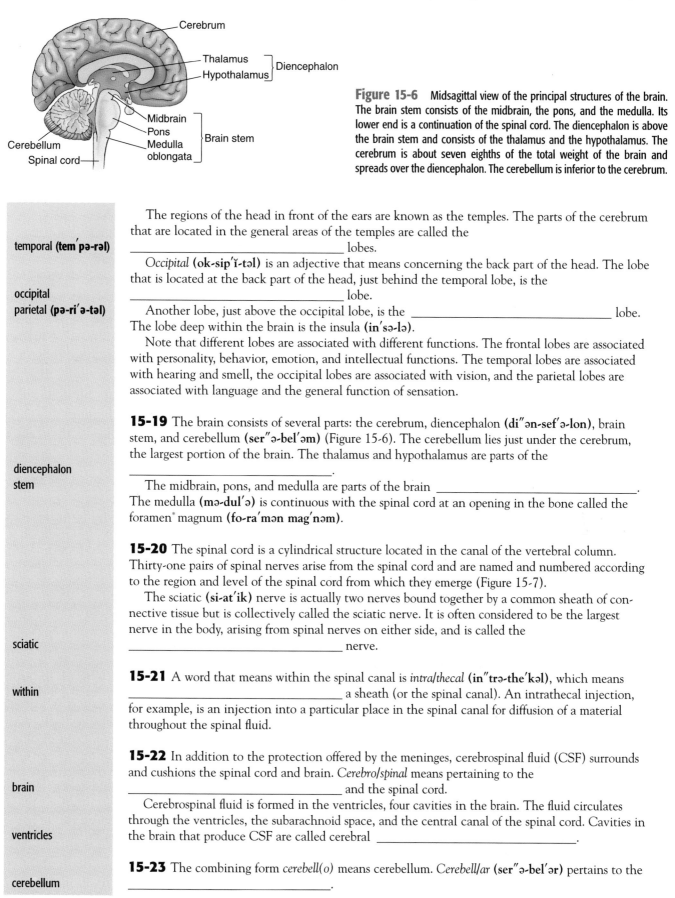

Figure 15-6 Midsagittal view of the principal structures of the brain. The brain stem consists of the midbrain, the pons, and the medulla. Its lower end is a continuation of the spinal cord. The diencephalon is above the brain stem and consists of the thalamus and the hypothalamus. The cerebrum is about seven eighths of the total weight of the brain and spreads over the diencephalon. The cerebellum is inferior to the cerebrum.

temporal (**tem′pə-rəl**)

occipital
parietal (**pə-ri′ə-təl**)

The regions of the head in front of the ears are known as the temples. The parts of the cerebrum that are located in the general areas of the temples are called the
_____ lobes.

    Occipital (**ok-sip′ĭ-təl**) is an adjective that means concerning the back part of the head. The lobe that is located at the back part of the head, just behind the temporal lobe, is the
_____ lobe.

    Another lobe, just above the occipital lobe, is the _____ lobe. The lobe deep within the brain is the insula (**in′sə-lə**).

    Note that different lobes are associated with different functions. The frontal lobes are associated with personality, behavior, emotion, and intellectual functions. The temporal lobes are associated with hearing and smell, the occipital lobes are associated with vision, and the parietal lobes are associated with language and the general function of sensation.

diencephalon
stem

15-19 The brain consists of several parts: the cerebrum, diencephalon (**di″ən-sef′ə-lon**), brain stem, and cerebellum (**ser″ə-bel′əm**) (Figure 15-6). The cerebellum lies just under the cerebrum, the largest portion of the brain. The thalamus and hypothalamus are parts of the
_____.

    The midbrain, pons, and medulla are parts of the brain _____.
The medulla (**mə-dul′ə**) is continuous with the spinal cord at an opening in the bone called the foramen* magnum (**fo-ra′mən mag′nəm**).

15-20 The spinal cord is a cylindrical structure located in the canal of the vertebral column. Thirty-one pairs of spinal nerves arise from the spinal cord and are named and numbered according to the region and level of the spinal cord from which they emerge (Figure 15-7).

sciatic

    The sciatic (**si-at′ik**) nerve is actually two nerves bound together by a common sheath of connective tissue but is collectively called the sciatic nerve. It is often considered to be the largest nerve in the body, arising from spinal nerves on either side, and is called the
_____ nerve.

within

15-21 A word that means within the spinal canal is *intra/thecal* (**in″trə-the′kəl**), which means _____ a sheath (or the spinal canal). An intrathecal injection, for example, is an injection into a particular place in the spinal canal for diffusion of a material throughout the spinal fluid.

brain

15-22 In addition to the protection offered by the meninges, cerebrospinal fluid (CSF) surrounds and cushions the spinal cord and brain. *Cerebro/spinal* means pertaining to the
_____ and the spinal cord.

    Cerebrospinal fluid is formed in the ventricles, four cavities in the brain. The fluid circulates through the ventricles, the subarachnoid space, and the central canal of the spinal cord. Cavities in the brain that produce CSF are called cerebral _____.

ventricles

15-23 The combining form *cerebell(o)* means cerebellum. *Cerebell/ar* (**ser″ə-bel′ər**) pertains to the _____.

cerebellum

*Foramina (Latin: hole).

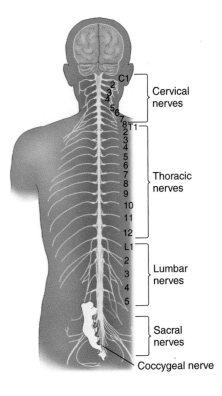

Figure 15-7   The spinal cord and nerves emerging from it. The spinal cord, about 44 cm (16 to 18 inches) long, extends from the medulla to the second lumbar vertebra. It ends at the cauda equina (meaning horse's tail), a group of nerves that arise from the lower portion of the cord and hang like wisps of coarse hair. There are 31 pairs of spinal nerves: 8 cervical, 12 thoracic, 5 lumbar, 5 sacral, and 1 coccygeal. The sciatic nerve, actually two nerves bound together by a common sheath of connective tissue, is often considered to be the largest nerve in the body. It supplies the entire musculature of the leg and foot. Irritation or injury to this nerve causes pain, often from the thigh down its branches into the toes. Neuralgia along the course of the sciatic nerve is called sciatica.

Exercise 2

Write words in the blanks to complete the following:

1. List the three types of meninges: _____, _____, and

_____.

2. The combining form for cerebellum is _____.

3. The combining form for cerebrum or brain is _____.

4. The combining form for meninges is _____.

5. The combining form for spinal cord is _____.

■ *Peripheral Nervous System and the Sense Organs*

15-24 The peripheral nervous system is that portion of the nervous system that is outside the central nervous system. The PNS consists of the nerves that branch out from the brain and spinal cord to form the communication network between the central nervous system and the rest of the body. It is further divided into the sensory (afferent) and motor (efferent) systems. Special sense organs have receptors that detect sensations, and then sensory neurons transmit the information to the CNS. Motor neurons carry impulses that initiate muscle contraction.

Peripheral means located away from the center. The PNS is located away from the nervous system control center, the CNS or the _____ nervous system.

central

15-25 Receptors are sensory nerve endings that respond to various kinds of stimulation. The awareness that results from the stimulation is what we know as sensation. The major senses are sight, hearing, smell, taste, and touch. Receptors are _____ nerve endings.

sensory

Touch is subdivided into several sensations that we receive through the skin: touch, pressure, pain, heat, and cold. The skin contains numerous sense receptors for these sensations. Hair has no receptors, but the movement of hair can be detected by receptors near the hair follicle. The skin and many tissues have pain receptors.

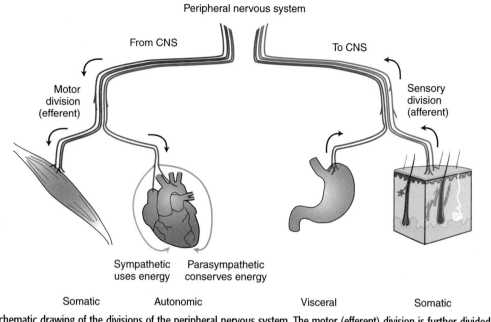

Figure 15-8 Schematic drawing of the divisions of the peripheral nervous system. The motor (efferent) division is further divided into the somatic and autonomic systems. The sensory (afferent) division is further subdivided into the visceral and somatic systems.

The PNS consists of nerves that connect with somatic (so-mat′ik) tissues (skin and muscles that are involved in conscious activities) and also nerves that link the CNS to autonomic (aw″to-nom′ik) tissues (the visceral organs, such as the stomach and heart, which function without conscious effort). These further divisions of the PNS are illustrated in Figure 15-8.

The autonomic system regulates and coordinates visceral activities without our conscious effort. This helps maintain a stable internal environment. The autonomic system has two divisions, the sympathetic and parasympathetic nervous systems.

15-26 Sympathetic (sim″pə-thet′ik) and parasympathetic (par″ə-sim″pə-thet′ik) systems are divisions of the _____ nervous system. In general, impulses transmitted by the nerve fibers of one division stimulate an organ, whereas impulses from the other division decrease or halt organ activity.

autonomic

Activation of the sympathetic division causes a series of physiologic responses called the fight-or-flight response. These responses increase the heart and breathing rates and prepare the body for fighting off danger. When danger is past, which system would counteract these responses? _____ system

parasympathetic

15-27 Sympathetic and parasympathetic nerve fibers, like other axons of the nervous system, release neurotransmitters and are classified on the basis of the substance produced. Cholinergic (ko″lin-ər′jik) fibers release acetylcholine. Adrenergic (ad″ren-ər′jik) fibers release epinephrine (ep″ĭ-nef′rin). (Epinephrine is also called adrenaline; hence the term *adren/ergic*.)
Cholinergic fibers release _____.
Adrenergic fibers release _____.

acetylcholine
epinephrine

15-28 Special sense organs—the eyes, ears, skin, mouth, and nose—have receptors that enable us to see, hear, feel, taste, and smell. The receptors that detect changes in our environment can be grouped into five types: chemoreceptors (ke″mo-re-sep′tərz), mechanoreceptors (mek″ə-no-re-sep′torz), photoreceptors (fo″to-re-sep′torz), thermoreceptors (thər″mo-re-sep′torz), and nociceptors (no″sĭ-sep′tərz). Review the combining forms used to name the receptors on p. 432.
Chemo/receptors are nerve endings adapted for excitation by what type of substances? _____

chemical

Taste buds contain chemoreceptors for sweet, sour, bitter, and salty tastes. Receptors that are stimulated by chemical stimuli are called _____. The nose and tongue have chemo/receptors, which detect chemicals.

chemoreceptors

Word Parts for the Types of Receptors

Combining Form	Meaning	Combining Form	Meaning
chem(o)	chemical	phot(o)	light
mechan(o)	mechanical	therm(o)	heat
noc(i)	cause harm, injury, or pain		

light

heat

eye

outside

15-29 Mechano/receptors that are sensitive to mechanical changes in touch or pressure are widely distributed in the skin. Mechanoreceptors for hearing are located within the ear.

The eyes contain photoreceptors that detect _____.

Thermoreceptors are located immediately under the skin and are widely distributed throughout the body. Thermo/receptors detect changes in temperature. There are cold receptors and, as the name implies, _____ receptors.

The sense of pain is initiated by special receptors, nociceptors, that are widely distributed throughout the skin and the internal organs.

15-30 The sense organs contain the receptors that help us detect changes in our environment.

The eyes are the paired organs of sight. Having earlier learned the meaning of *ophthalm(o)* and *ocul(o)*, both *ophthalm/ic* and *ocul/ar* mean pertaining to the _____, because *ocul(o)* and *ophthalm(o)* mean eye.

Intra/ocular (in″trǝ-ok′u-lǝr), *interocular* (in″tǝr-ok′u-lǝr), and *extra/ocular* (eks″trǝ-ok′u-lǝr) mean within, between, and _____ the eye, respectively.

15-31 The structures of the eye and ear are shown in Figure 15-9, A. Although it is probably not necessary to memorize the structures that make up these two sense organs, it is important to recognize names associated with them.

Eyelids open and close the eye and keep foreign objects from entering the eye. The eyelids, as well as the anterior portion of the sclera, are lined with a mucous membrane called conjunctiva (kǝn-jǝnk′ti-vǝ).

15-32 The eyeball, or globe, is composed of three layers (Figure 15-9, B). The tough outer layer is composed of the sclera (the white, opaque membrane covering most of the eyeball) and the transparent cornea. The cornea is the convex, transparent structure at the front of the eyeball that helps focus light rays entering the eye. The combining form *kerat(o)* means the cornea, but it also means hard, like horn.

The lens of the eye is located posterior to the pupil and is responsible for focusing the light rays so they form a perfect image on the retina. The iris is the pigmented portion that accounts for blue, brown, gray, green, and combinations of these colors in eyes. The retina, the innermost layer of the eye, contains photoreceptors (rods and cones) that receive images of external objects. The retina is continuous with the optic nerve, which carries the nervous impulse to the cerebrum and enables vision. Examine the appearance of the optic nerve and retina in Figure 15-10.

Learn the following word parts.

Word Parts Pertaining to the Eye

Structures Combining Form	Meaning	Functions Combining Form	Meaning
ir(o), irid(o)	iris	dacry(o), lacrim(o)	tear
kerat(o)	cornea; hard, horny	opt(o), optic(o)	vision
ocul(o), ophthalm(o)	eye		

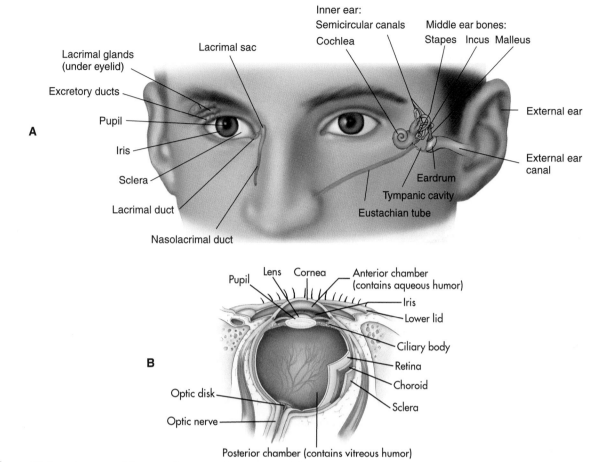

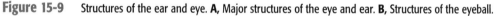

Figure 15-9   Structures of the ear and eye. **A,** Major structures of the eye and ear. **B,** Structures of the eyeball.

crying	**15-33** The combining forms *dacry(o)* and *lacrim(o)* mean tear, as in crying. The lacrim/al gland produces fluid (tears) that keeps the eye moist. (Refer again to Figure 15-9.) If more lacrimal **(lak′rĭ-məl)** fluid is produced than can be removed, we say that the person is _____. (This is also called tearing.) *Lacrim/ation* **(lak″rĭ-ma′shən)** refers to crying, the production and discharge of tears.
lacrimal	**15-34** Tears produced by the _____ gland wash over the eyeball and are drained through small openings in the inner corner of the eye. Tears pass through these openings into small ducts that lead to the lacrimal sac. From here they pass into the large nasolacrimal duct that ends in the nasal cavity. *Naso/lacrimal* pertains to the
nose	_____ and the lacrimal apparatus. Another name for the lacrimal sac is dacryo/cyst **(dak′re-o-sist″)**.

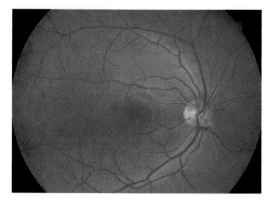

Figure 15-10   Ophthalmoscopic view of the interior of the eye. A normal retina and optic nerve are shown. The normal retina and blood vessel walls are mainly transparent. Note that the branching points of the blood vessels "point" toward the optic nerve.

Word Parts Pertaining to the Ear

COMBINING FORM	MEANING
audi(o)	hearing
ot(o)	ear

external

15-35 The ears have receptors that detect touch, pain, heat, and cold, but the mechanoreceptors that enable us to hear usually come to mind when we think of the ear as a sense organ. We depend on our ears not only for hearing but also for the sense of equilibrium, both functions of mechanoreceptors.

Anatomically, the ear is divided into the external ear, middle ear, and inner ear. (Refer again to Figure 15-9.) The part of the ear that is visible is the _____ ear. With the function of collecting sound waves and directing them into the ear, the outer (external) ear ends at the tympanic membrane (eardrum).

The middle ear is an air-filled cavity and has three tiny bones. When the eardrum vibrates, these bones transmit the vibrations to fluids in the inner ear. The inner ear contains the cochlea (**kok′le-ə**) and the semicircular canals. The cochlea contains receptors that enable us to hear. The semicircular canals enable us to maintain a sense of balance.

hearing

15-36 *Audi/ble* pertains to _____. *Audio/logy* is the science of hearing, particularly the study of impaired hearing that cannot be improved by medication or surgery. An audiologist (**aw″de-ol′ə-jist**) is a person skilled in audiology.

15-37 The nose is responsible for the sense of smell, and this sense is intricately linked with chemoreceptors in the tongue that enable us to experience different tastes of food and other substances.

smell

The term *olfaction* (**ol-fak′shən**) means the sense of smell, and *olfactory* (**ol′fak′tə-re**) means pertaining to the sense of _____. Anosmia* (**an-oz′me-ə**) is loss or impairment of the sense of smell, and hyperosmia (**hi″pər-oz′me-ə**) is an abnormally increased sensitivity to odors.

Exercise 3

Write words in the blanks to complete these sentences.

1. The peripheral nervous system is divided into the afferent or _____ system and the motor system.

2. The organs that have receptors that detect sensations are called _____ organs.

3. Cholinergic nerve fibers release _____.

4. Adrenergic nerve fibers release _____.

5. Nerve endings that are stimulated by chemical stimuli are called _____.

6. Nerve endings that detect light are called _____.

7. Nerve endings that detect changes in temperature are called _____.

8. Nerve endings that detect pain are called _____.

9. The _____ gland produces tears.

10. The science of hearing is _____.

*Anosmia (Greek: *a*, without; *osme*, smell).

DIAGNOSTIC TESTS AND PROCEDURES

consciousness

15-38 A change in the level of consciousness may be the first indication of a decline in central nervous system function. The <u>levels of consciousness</u> include alert wakefulness (normal); response to stimuli, although it may be slow; drowsiness; stupor (patient is vaguely aware of the environment); and coma (patient does not appear to be aware of the environment). The various stages of response of the mind to stimuli are called the levels of _____.

Memory, another means of assessing neurologic function, is classified as <u>long-term, recent, and immediate memory</u>. Loss of memory is often an early sign of neurologic problems.

15-39 <u>Deep tendon reflex</u> (DTR) and <u>superficial reflex</u> are used to assess neurologic and muscular damage. A deep tendon reflex, a brisk contraction of a muscle in response to a sharp tap by a finger or rubber hammer on a tendon, is often helpful in diagnosing stroke. A superficial reflex is evaluated by stimulation of the skin, such as stroking the sole of the foot to evaluate the response.

tendon

The two types of reflex that are easily tested are the deep _____ reflex and the superficial reflex.

15-40 Certain illnesses may require <u>chemical analysis and microscopic examination of the cerebrospinal fluid</u>. Only a few cells are normally present, and a large number of leukocytes may indicate infection. <u>Bacterial and fungal cultures</u> of the CSF are done if indicated.

Cerebrospinal fluid is obtained by <u>spinal puncture</u> (usually a lumbar puncture) and is performed for diagnostic purposes, as well as to introduce substances into the spinal canal.

lumbar

The <u>lumbar puncture</u> is the introduction of a hollow needle into the subarachnoid space of the _____ part of the spinal canal (see Figure 14-16). It is performed not only for diagnostic purposes but also for the injection of an anesthetic solution for spinal anesthesia or contrast media for imaging procedures.

15-41 You are probably familiar with the term *electrocardiography*, which means the process of recording the electrical activity of the heart. <u>Electro/encephalo/graphy</u> (e-lek″tro-ən-sef″ə-log′rə-fe) is the process of recording the electrical activity of the _____ **brain** and is abbreviated EEG. An <u>electroencephalograph</u> (e-lek″tro-ən-sef′ə-lo-graf″) is the **instrument** _____ used in electroencephalography.

Electrodes are attached to various areas of the patient's head using a special gel (Figure 15-11). During neurosurgery, the electrodes can be applied directly to the brain. Electroencephalography is used to diagnose several disorders, including seizures, lesions, and impaired consciousness.

15-42 Although the legal definition of brain death varies from state to state, it is generally defined as an irreversible form of unconsciousness characterized by a complete loss of brain function while

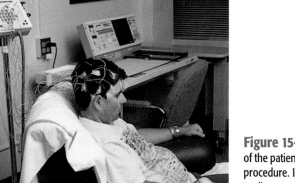

Figure 15-11 Electroencephalography. Electrodes are attached to various areas of the patient's head. The patient generally remains quiet with closed eyes during the procedure. In certain cases, prescribed activities may be requested. The test is used to diagnose epilepsy, brain stem disorders, lesions, and impaired consciousness.

record

the heart continues to beat. A diagnosis of brain death may require a demonstration that electrical activity of the brain is absent. An <u>electro/encephalo/gram</u> (e-lek″tro-en-sef′ə-lo-gram″) is the _____ produced by the electrical activity of the brain.

15-43 A number of radiographic examinations are available to assess the nervous system. Plain x-ray studies of the skull and spine are often helpful in diagnosing fractures, abnormal curvatures, or other bony abnormalities.

Computed tomography (CT) and magnetic resonance imaging (MRI) are used to assess structural changes of the brain and spinal cord. CT is particularly helpful in detecting intracranial bleeding, lesions, and cerebral edema (see Figure 3-6). MRIs and CTs provide information about the structure of tissue.

brain

Echo/encephalo/graphy uses ultrasonic waves beamed through the head to record structural aspects of the _____. The record produced is an echo/encephalo/gram (ek″o-en-sef′ə-lo-gram″).

15-44 <u>Positron emission tomography</u> (PET) is a computerized nuclear medicine technique that uses radioactive substances to assess the function of various body structures, particularly the brain. The patient inhales or is injected with radioactive material. The radioactivity is short lived, so that patients are exposed to only very small amounts of radiation. PET and other nuclear medicine imaging techniques provide information about function.

function

An important advantage of positron emission tomography is that it assesses _____, whereas most radiographic imaging studies of the brain assess structure.

brain

15-45 <u>Encephalo/graphy</u> (en-sef″ə-log′rə-fe) is radiography of the _____. It is accomplished by withdrawal and replacement of the cerebrospinal fluid by a gas. Because of the risks involved, it is generally used only when results of CT and MRI are not definitive.

myelography (mi″ə-log′rə-fe)

15-46 Write a word that means radiography of the spinal cord (after injection of a contrast medium): _____.

myelogram (mi′ə-lo-gram)

Myelography can be useful in studying spinal lesions, spinal injuries, or disk disease. It is often supplemented by CT. The record produced in myelography is a _____.

brain

15-47 <u>Cerebral angio/graphy</u> is used to visualize the blood vessels of the _____ after injection of a radiopaque contrast medium. Although it is not used as often as less invasive tests, such as CT, it can be used to diagnose abnormalities of blood vessels, such as aneurysms (an′u-rizmz), a ballooning out of the wall of a vessel (Figure 15-12).

15-48 <u>Brain scans</u> are used to assess aneurysms, as well as to locate abscesses, tumors, or hematomas. In this diagnostic test, a radioisotope that is selective for certain types of abnormal brain tissue is injected intravenously. Imaging with a gamma camera demonstrates the area of accumulation of the radioisotope.

radioisotope

In a brain scan, imaging is accomplished using a _____.

15-49 <u>Dacryo/cysto/graphy</u> (dak″re-o-sis-tog′rə-fe) is radiography of the _____ sac. This procedure may be used to diagnose narrowing or obstruction of the lacrimal sac.

lacrimal

15-50 You learned earlier that <u>ophthalmo/scopy</u> (of″thəl-mos′kə-pe) is visual examination of the eye. The instrument is an _____.

ophthalmoscope (of-thal′mə-skōp)

instrument

An <u>ophthalmo/meter</u> is an _____ for measuring the eye.

15-51 The ear is examined in <u>oto/scopy</u> (o-tos′kə-pe) (see Figure 3-4). The instrument used in otoscopy is an _____.

otoscope (o′to-skōp)

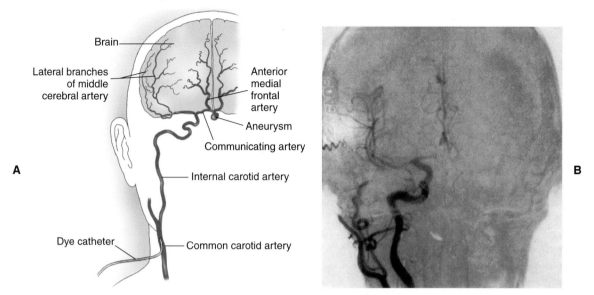

Figure 15-12 Cerebral aneurysm. **A,** Diagram of an aneurysm and the major cerebral arteries visible in cerebral angiography. **B,** A cerebral angiogram. Cerebral angiography is used to study intracranial circulation and is especially helpful in visualizing aneurysms and vascular occlusions. A contrast medium is used that outlines the vessels of the brain.

---

hearing	An <u>audio/meter</u> **(aw″de-om′ə-tər)** is a device for measuring _____. The record produced is an audiogram **(aw′de-o-gram″)**.

15-52 Sleep studies are not invasive and are used to diagnose sleep apnea **(ap′ne-ə)**, a sleep disorder characterized by short periods in which respiration is absent. These tests are performed in a sleep laboratory where the patient is monitored electronically while sleeping.

Tests that consist of electronic monitoring of a sleeping person to diagnose sleep apnea are called

sleep _____ studies.

Exercise 4

Match diagnostic procedures in the left column with their descriptions in the right column.

_____ 1. brain scan

_____ 2. cerebral angiography

_____ 3. dacryocystography

_____ 4. deep tendon reflex

_____ 5. echoencephalography

_____ 6. electroencephalography

_____ 7. myelography

A. brisk muscular contraction in response to stimuli
B. imaging of the brain using radioisotopes
C. radiography of the lacrimal sac
D. radiography of the spinal cord
E. recording the electrical activity of the brain
F. use of ultrasound to study brain structure
G. visualization of blood vessels of the brain

PATHOLOGIES

15-53 The nervous system is a complicated body system, and many of its functions are not well understood, particularly in the realm of psychological disorders. Disturbances of the central nervous system vary from acute to chronic, short term to long term, and minor to life threatening. Pathologies include trauma, congenital disorders, infections, tumors, degenerative disorders, diseases of the sense organs, and psychological disturbances.

Some disorders of the nervous system do not fit into the categories presented here. For example, the learning disorder <u>dyslexia</u> (**dis-lek′se-ə**) is an impairment of the ability to read and results from a variety of pathologic conditions, some of which are associated with the nervous system. The prefix *dys-* means _____, and *lexis* is a Greek term meaning word. Dyslexic persons often reverse letters and words, cannot adequately distinguish the letter sequences in written words, and have difficulty determining right from left. Dyslexia is unrelated to intelligence, and the exact cause is not known.

difficult

Learn the meanings of the following word parts.

Additional Word Parts Pertaining to Nervous System Pathologies

COMBINING FORM	MEANING	SUFFIXES	MEANING
pseud(o)	false	-asthenia	weakness
		-esthesia	sensitivity to pain

15-54 Pain, which is caused by stimulation of the sensory nerve endings, is the most common symptom for which patients seek medical advice. You have learned that *-algia* means _____.

pain

<u>Algesia</u> (**al-je′ze-ə**) is a word that refers to sensitivity to pain and is also used as a suffix. <u>Hyper/algesia</u> (**hi″pər-al-je′ze-ə**) is _____ sensitivity to pain.

increased

Literal interpretation of <u>hyp/algesia</u> (**hi″pal-je′ze-ə**) or <u>hypo/algesia</u> (**hi″po-al-je′ze-ə**) is _____ sensitivity to pain. Either term means a decrease in sensation in response to stimulation of the sensory nerves.

decreased

Paresthesia (**par″əs-the′zhə**) is a subjective sensation, experienced as numbness, tingling, or a "pins and needles" feeling, often in the absence of an external stimulus.

<u>Pseud/esthesia</u> (**sood″əs-the′zhə**) is an imaginary or false sensation. The prefix *pseudo-* means false. Pseud/esthesia is a sensation occurring in the absence of the appropriate stimulus, and its cause is not well understood. (Pseudesthesia is also called pseudoesthesia. Two spellings are accepted for many terms in which *pseud[o]* is joined to a combining form that begins with a vowel.)

Pseudesthesia can occur in a lost arm or leg after amputation. This imaginary or false sensation is termed _____.

pseudesthesia

15-55 Using *-algia*, write a word that means pain of a nerve: _____. <u>Poly/neur/algia</u> (**pol″e-noo-ral′jə**) is a type of neuralgia that affects many nerves simultaneously.

neuralgia (noo-ral′jə)

A <u>poly/neuro/pathy</u> (**pol″e-noo-rop′ə-the**) is a condition in which many peripheral nerves are affected. <u>Poly/neur/itis</u> (**pol″e-noo-ri′tis**) is an example of a polyneuropathy. *Polyneuritis* means inflammation of many nerves (simultaneously). Damage to cranial or peripheral nerves can lead to various neuropathies that may be evidenced by tingling, burning, or decreased sensitivity in an extremity.

<u>Neuro/scler/osis</u> (**noor″o-sklə-ro′sis**) is _____ of nervous tissue.

hardening

15-56 <u>Sciatica</u> (**si-at′ĭ-kə**) is inflammation of the sciatic nerve, usually marked by pain and tenderness along the course of the nerve through the thigh and leg. This may arise from problems in the lower back as a result of a herniated intervertebral disk or arthritis and is accompanied by lower back pain (LBP). Write this term that means inflammation of the sciatic nerve: _____.

sciatica

■ Headaches

15-57 A headache is pain in the head from any cause and is a symptom. Most headaches do not indicate serious disease. <u>Cephal/algia</u> (**sef″ə-lal′jə**), often shortened to ceph/algia (**sə-fal′jə**), is a synonym for _____.

headache

The most common types of headaches are pain related to the eyes, ears, teeth, and paranasal structures (for example, a sinus headache). Other kinds of headaches include tension headaches (muscle contraction headaches), cluster headaches, and migraine headaches (Figure 15-13).

15-58 <u>Tension headaches</u> result from the long-sustained contraction of skeletal muscles around the scalp, face, neck, and upper back. This is the primary source of many headaches associated with excessive emotional tension, anxiety, and depression. Also called muscle contraction headaches,

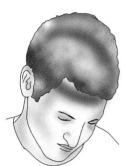

Muscle contraction
headache

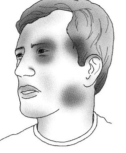

Cluster headache

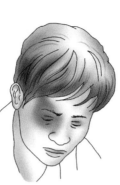

Migraine headache

Figure 15-13   Three types of headaches. Shaded areas show regions of most intense pain.

tension

side

light

_____ headaches result from long-sustained contraction of skeletal muscles of the head and upper back.

15-59 <u>Cluster headaches</u> are characterized by intense unilateral pain. *Uni/lateral* means occurring on one _____ only. They are very painful, occur in clusters, and fortunately do not last long.

15-60 A <u>migraine headache</u> is a vascular disorder characterized by recurrent throbbing headaches, often accompanied by loss of appetite, photophobia, and nausea with or without vomiting. Photophobia is sensitivity of the eyes to light. Translated literally, <u>*photo/phobia*</u> means an abnormal fear of _____ .

Migraine headaches occur more often in females than in males and sometimes begin in childhood. The classic migraine begins with an aura of depression, irritability, restlessness, and perhaps loss of appetite. There may also be transient neurologic disturbances, including visual problems (flashes of light, distorted or double vision, seeing spots), dizziness, and nausea. The headache increases in severity until it becomes intense and may last a few hours or up to several days if not treated.

■ *Trauma*

speech

concussion

semicoma
(sem″e-ko′mə)

15-61 <u>Craniocerebral trauma</u> is commonly called head trauma or head injury. It is a traumatic insult to the brain caused by an external physical force that may produce a diminished or altered state of consciousness. It may result in impairment of cognitive abilities (perception, reasoning, judgment, and memory) or physical functions and may be temporary or permanent. Skull fractures, gunshot wounds, and knife injuries are examples of open head traumas. Blunt trauma as seen in motor vehicle accidents can lead to concussions (**kən-kush′ənz**), contusions (bruises), or tearing of the brain.

An abnormal condition in which language function is absent or disordered because of an injury to certain areas of the cerebral cortex can result in a/phasia (**ə-fa′zhə**) or dys/phasia (**dis-fa′zhə**). Literal translation of a/phasia is absence of _____ .

Difficult, poorly articulated speech, usually caused by damage to a central or peripheral motor nerve, is called dys/arthria* (**dis-ahr′thre-ə**).

15-62 Consciousness is responsiveness of the mind to the impressions made by the senses. A <u>cerebral concussion</u> usually causes loss of consciousness. A concussion is an injury resulting from impact with an object. A blow to the head can cause a cerebral _____ .

A person who is responsive to impressions made by the senses is said to be conscious. A person who is <u>semi/conscious</u> (**sem″e-kon′shəs**) is only partially aware of his or her surroundings.

A <u>coma</u> is a profound unconsciousness from which the patient cannot be aroused. Using semiconscious as a model, write a word that means a partial or mild coma from which the patient can be aroused: _____ .

*Dysarthria (*dys-*, difficult + Greek: *arthroun*, to articulate).

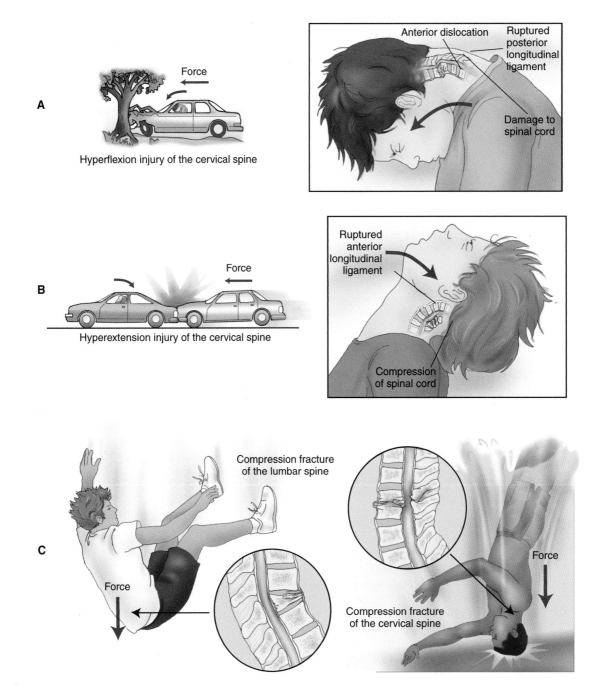

Figure 15-14   Closed spinal cord injuries. Fractures and dislocations to the vertebral column can result in injury to the spinal cord. These types of vertebral injuries occur most often at points where a relatively mobile portion of the spine meets a relatively fixed segment. **A,** Hyperflexion of the cervical vertebrae. **B,** Hyperextension of the cervical vertebrae. **C,** Vertical compression of the cervical spine and the lumbar spine.

brain

15-63 Head injuries can also result in a <u>spinal cord injury</u> (SCI). An <u>encephalo/myelo/pathy</u> (en-sef″ə-lo-mi″əl-op′ə-the) is any disease involving the _____ and the spinal cord.

Forceful injuries to the vertebral column can damage the spinal cord and lead to neurologic problems. Injuries to the vertebral column that can result in damage to the spinal cord include excessive rotation, hyperextension, hyperflexion, and vertical compression (Figure 15-14).

15-64 Three types of <u>hemat/omas</u> associated with head injuries are shown in Figure 15-15. You learned earlier that a hematoma is a collection of blood in the tissues of the skin or in an organ.

Because *epi-* means above or on, *epi/dural* means situated on or outside the dura mater.

epidural
(ep″ĭ-doo′rəl)

Accumulation of blood in the epidural space is an _____ <u>hematoma</u>. This hematoma compresses the dura mater and thus compresses the brain.

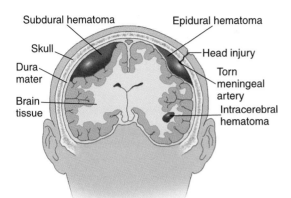

Figure 15-15   Three types of hematomas associated with head injuries: subdural hematoma, epidural hematoma, and intracerebral hematoma.

within

Accumulation of blood between the dura mater and the arachnoid is called a <u>subdural hematoma</u>. The acute form is often the result of a tear in the arachnoid associated with a head injury.

Notice that bleeding occurs _____ the brain in an <u>intra/cerebral</u> (in″trə-ser′ə-brəl) <u>hematoma</u>. Fortunately this type of hematoma is less common than a subdural or epidural hematoma. Intracerebral hematomas have a high mortality rate because of the damage they cause to brain tissue.

15-65 In a <u>cerebro/vascular</u> (ser″ə-bro-vas′ku-lər) <u>accident</u> (CVA, stroke, or stroke syndrome), normal blood supply to the brain has been disrupted. CVA results in insufficient oxygen to brain tissue, caused by hemorrhage, occlusion (closing), or constriction of the blood vessels that normally supply oxygen to the brain.

A <u>cerebral aneurysm</u> (sə-re′brəl, ser′ə-brəl an′u-rizm) is an abnormal, localized dilation of a cerebral artery. The aneurysm may rupture to produce a <u>cerebral hemorrhage</u>. <u>Hemorrhagic strokes</u> are caused by the rupture of a cerebral artery.

brain

<u>Embolic strokes</u> are caused by a <u>cerebral embolus</u> (sə-re′brəl, ser′ə-brəl em′bo-ləs), a plug of matter (usually a blood clot) brought by the blood to the _____. A cerebral embolus is one cause of a CVA.

artery

<u>Thrombotic strokes</u> are caused by plaque deposits that build up on the interior of a cerebral _____. Both embolic and thrombotic strokes are commonly preceded by warning signs, such as a transient ischemic attack (TIA), caused by a brief interruption in cerebral blood flow. The term *ischemic* pertains to deficient blood circulation (in this case, in the brain). TIA symptoms often include disturbance of normal vision, dizziness, weakness, and numbness. A transient ischemic attack is important because it may be a warning sign of an impending

stroke (CVA)

_____. The types of stroke are shown in Figure 15-16.

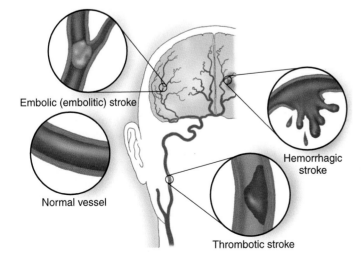

Embolic (embolitic) stroke

Normal vessel

Hemorrhagic stroke

Thrombotic stroke

Figure 15-16   Types of stroke. A cerebrovascular accident, commonly referred to as a stroke, is a disruption in the normal blood supply to the brain. An embolic stroke is caused by an embolus or a group of emboli that break off from one area of the body, often the heart, and travel to the cerebral arteries. Thrombotic strokes are caused by plaque deposits that build up on the interior of a cerebral artery, gradually occluding it. Hemorrhagic strokes are caused by rupture of a cerebral arterial wall.

disease	**15-66** The peripheral nerves are subject to many types of trauma. A peripheral neuropathy (noŏ-rop′ə-the) is any _____ of the peripheral nerves. Those of the extremities are commonly affected. An example is <u>wristdrop</u>, in which nerve damage results in the hand remaining in a flexed position at the wrist, and it cannot be extended. Write the term that means wristdrop by combining *carp(o)* and *-ptosis*: _____.
carpoptosis (kahr″pop-to′sis)	

Exercise 5

Match terms in the left column with their meanings in the right column.

_____ 1. encephalomyelopathy

_____ 2. hypalgesia

_____ 3. hyperalgesia

_____ 4. neurosclerosis

_____ 5. polyneuritis

_____ 6. pseudesthesia

A. any disease involving the brain and spinal cord
B. decreased response to stimulation of the sensory nerves
C. hardening of nervous tissue
D. imaginary or false sensation
E. increased sensitivity to pain
F. inflammation of many nerves simultaneously

■ *Paralysis*

paralysis	**15-67** <u>Paralysis</u> is the loss of muscle function, loss of sensation, or both and is a sign of an underlying problem. Paralysis may be caused by trauma, disease, or poisoning. Injury to different areas of the spinal cord results in different types of paralysis. Remembering that *-plegia* means paralysis, in <u>hemi/plegia</u> (hem″e-ple′jə) there is _____ of one half of the body (only one side).
	Paralysis of both sides of the body is <u>di/plegia</u> (di-ple′je-ə). In diplegia there is paralysis of similar parts on both sides of the body.
four	<u>Quadri/plegia</u> (kwod″rĭ-ple′jə) is paralysis of all _____ extremities.
paralysis	**15-68** In <u>para/plegia</u> (par″ə-ple′jə), the upper limbs are not affected. Para/plegia is _____ of the lower portion of the body and both legs. The prefix *para-* means near, beside, or abnormal. Some interpretation is needed in the term *paraplegia*. <u>Mono/plegia</u> (mon″o-ple′jə) is paralysis of one limb.
facial	**15-69** Facial paralysis, or <u>Bell's palsy</u>, is a neuropathy that drastically affects the body image. The cause is unknown; the onset is acute and is characterized by a drawing sensation and paralysis of all facial muscles on the affected side. Bell's palsy is acute paralysis of a cranial nerve affecting one side of the face and is also called _____ paralysis.

■ *Congenital Disorders*

meninges	**15-70** Congenital defects of the nervous system may be obvious at birth and may vary from minor to severe. An abnormal protrusion near the spine may be a <u>meningocele</u> (mə-ning′go-sēl″) or <u>meningo/myelo/cele</u> (mə-ning″go-mi′ə-lo-sēl″). A meningo/cele is hernial protrusion of _____ through a defect in the skull or vertebral column (Figure 15-17).
meninges	A meningo/myelo/cele is hernial protrusion of parts of the _____ and spinal cord through a defect in the vertebral column. Both these congenital defects are generally repaired by surgery.

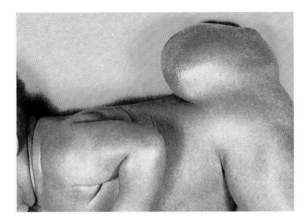

Figure 15-17   Meningocele. The spinal meninges have formed a hernial cyst that is filled with cerebrospinal fluid and is protruding through a defect in the vertebral column.

palsy

15-71 Cerebral palsy (**pawl′ze**) is a motor function disorder caused by a permanent, nonprogressive brain defect present at birth or occurring shortly thereafter. It may result in spastic paralysis in various forms, seizures, and varying degrees of impaired speech, vision, and hearing. It is often associated with asphyxia during birth. This congenital defect is called cerebral _____.

Huntington's

15-72 Huntington's disease, also called Huntington's chorea (**kə-re′ə**), is a hereditary disorder that affects both genders equally. Symptoms begin between 30 and 50 years of age. The two main symptoms are progressive mental status changes leading to dementia and rapid, jerky movements in the trunk, facial muscles, and extremities. Neurotransmitters have been implicated in the symptoms of this inherited disorder called _____ disease.

anotia (an-o′shə)

15-73 One developmental defect that is not life threatening but life altering is absence of one or both ears. Combine an- + ot(o) + -ia to write a word that means absence of the ear: _____.

Anotia is absence of one or both external ears. It is generally accompanied by lack of an internal ear also. Cosmetic reconstructive surgery is generally performed while the child is still young, but this does not, of course, correct the deafness.

■ Infections

brain

15-74 Infections of the CNS include encephalomyelitis (**en-sef″ə-lo-mi″ə-li′tis**), meningitis (**men″in-ji′tis**), and encephalitis (**en-sef″ə-li′tis**). Encephalomyelitis is inflammation of the _____ and spinal cord.

meninges

15-75 Mening/itis is inflammation of the _____ of the brain and the spinal cord. Although other infectious organisms can invade the nervous system, bacterial or viral organisms are most often responsible for meningitis.

brain

15-76 Encephal/itis is inflammation of the brain tissue. It is most often caused by a virus, usually having gained access to the bloodstream from a viral infection elsewhere in the body. Encephalo/meningitis (**en-sef″ə-lo-men″in-ji′tis**) is inflammation of the _____ and its coverings.

cerebellitis
(ser″ə-bel-i′tis)

15-77 If the inflammation is confined to the cerebellum, this condition (inflammation of the cerebellum) is _____.

ventricle

You learned in another chapter that the combining form ventricul(o) means ventricle. The word part can refer to a ventricle in either the brain or the heart. Ventricul/itis (**ven-trik″u-li′tis**) is inflammation of a _____. Although it is not obvious, ventriculitis refers especially to inflammation of a ventricle of the brain.

15-78 Four other diseases caused by infectious microorganisms that have a devastating effect on the central nervous system are tetanus (**tet′ə-nəs**), botulism (**boch′ə-liz-əm**), poliomyelitis (**po″le-o-mi″ə-li′tis**), and rabies (**ra′bēz, ra′be-ēz**).

Tetanus, also known as lockjaw, is caused by a bacterium and is easily preventable through immunization. The infection is commonly transmitted through a wound contaminated with the bacteria. The bacterial toxin attacks the nervous system and results in muscle rigidity and spasms. Taking its name from the "locked jaw" rigidity that results, this disease is known as

_____.

tetanus

15-79 Botulism is caused by a type of bacteria that is toxic to nervous tissue and causes paralysis of both voluntary and involuntary motor activity. Most cases are caused by eating improperly canned foods. Symptoms usually appear 12 to 36 hours after eating contaminated food in this neurotoxic disease, called _____.

botulism

15-80 Poliomyelitis is an acute viral disease that attacks the gray matter of the spinal cord and parts of the brain. It can be asymptomatic, mild, or paralytic. This disease is rarely seen in North America because it can be prevented by immunization. It is informally called polio.*

15-81 Rabies is an acute, often fatal, disease of the central nervous system transmitted to humans by infected animals. After introduction of the virus into the human body, often by an animal bite, the virus travels along nerve pathways to the brain and later to other organs. Without medical intervention and possibly the use of vaccine, coma and death are likely.

A nontechnical term for rabies that is obsolete is hydrophobia (**hi″dro-fo′be-ə**). Literal translation of hydro/phobia is abnormal fear of _____. The name *hydrophobia* was given after observation that rabid animals avoid water. Infected animals avoid water because paralysis prevents them from being able to swallow.

water

■ *Tumors*

15-82 Primary brain tumors arise within the brain structures and rarely spread outside the brain. Glia cells are the only source of primary malignant brain tumors. The tumors are called gliomas (**gli-o′məz**). A gli/oma is a primary tumor of the brain and is composed of which type of nerve cell?

_____

neuroglia

A meningi/oma (**mə-nin″je-o′mə**) is a tumor of the meninges that grows slowly and may invade the skull. Tumors within the skull can invade and compress brain tissue, which generally leads to increased intracranial pressure (ICP), headaches, and many neurologic problems, such as a neuro/genic (**noor″o-jen′ik**) bladder, a dysfunction of the urinary bladder caused by a lesion, such as a tumor, of the nervous system. Normal control of urination and emptying of the bladder is usually absent.

15-83 You know that *crani(o)* means the cranium, or skull, so *intra/cranial* means _____ the skull. Brain tumors can become quite large and occupy considerable intracranial space, as shown in Figure 15-18.

within

15-84 Disorders such as brain tumors that interfere with the flow of CSF cause fluid accumulation in the skull, called hydrocephalus (**hi″dro-sef′ə-ləs**). Translated literally, *hydro/cephalus* means _____ in the _____. Hydrocephalus is a pathologic condition characterized by an abnormal accumulation of CSF within the skull and is usually accompanied by increased intracranial pressure. When this happens in an infant, before the cranial bones fuse, the cranium enlarges. In an older child or adult, the pressure damages the soft brain tissue.

water; head

*Polio (Greek: *polios*, gray).

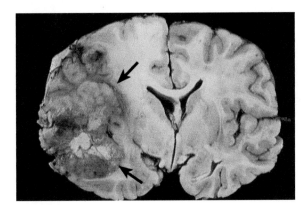

Figure 15-18 A primary brain tumor. This autopsy specimen of the brain shows a large tumor *(arrows)*. This patient had multiple distant metastases in the lung and spine.

tumor	**15-85** A <u>neur/oma</u> (noo-ro′mə) is a benign _____ composed chiefly of neurons and nerve fibers. Although they are benign, they can be painful (for example, a Morton's neuroma that occurs in the foot) or can compress brain tissue (for example, an acoustic neuroma).

■ *Seizure Disorders*

	15-86 A <u>seizure</u> is an abnormal, sudden, excessive discharge of electrical activity within the brain. Seizures are also known as <u>convulsions</u>. This abnormal activity is assessed in electroencephalography. A seizure may be recurrent, as in a seizure disorder, or transient and acute, as after a concussion. A concussion is damage to the brain caused by a violent jarring or shaking.
seizure	Remember that the suffix *-lepsy* means _____. Epilepsy (ep′ĭ-lep″se) is a group of chronic neurologic disorders characterized by recurrent episodes of convulsive seizures, sensory disturbances, loss of consciousness, or all of these. Anti/convulsants are
seizures (or convulsions)	medications used to prevent or reduce the severity of _____.
	15-87 <u>Narcolepsy</u> (nahr′ko-lep″se) is uncontrollable, brief episodes of sleep and uses the combining form *narc(o)*, which means stupor. In narcolepsy, the person cannot prevent a sudden attack of sleep while performing daytime activities. Its cause is unknown, and no pathologic lesions are found in the brain. The person may experience momentary loss of muscle tone. Visual or auditory hallucinations often occur at the onset of sleep. Stimulant drugs are often prescribed to prevent the sudden attacks of sleep at inappropriate times. The name of this disorder is
narcolepsy	_____.

■ *Degenerative Disorders*

	15-88 Degenerative disorders are those in which there is deterioration of structure or function of tissue. Included in this section are neurologic disorders that affect motor ability or nerve transmission (Parkinson's disease, multiple sclerosis, amyotrophic lateral sclerosis [a-mi″o-trof′ik lat′ər-əl sklə-ro′sis], myasthenia gravis [mi″əs-the′ne-ə gră′vis]) and mental deterioration (dementia, Alzheimer's [awltz′hi-mərz] disease).
	<u>Parkinson's disease</u> is a slowly progressing, debilitating, neurologic disease that affects motor ability. It is characterized by muscle rigidity, bradykinesia (brad″e-kĭ-ne′zhə), and tremor (trem′ər, tre′mər). The suffix *-kinesia* means movement. *Brady/kinesia* means _____
slow	movement, or slowness of all voluntary movement or speech. Tremor is rhythmic, purposeless, quivering involuntary movement. A characteristic posture and masklike facial expression are often seen.
	Parkinson's disease occurs most often in people over 50 years of age and results from widespread degeneration of a part of the brain that produces dopamine. The cause is not known, but treatment usually includes the administration of dopaminergics, precursors to dopamine.

15-89 <u>Multiple sclerosis</u> (MS) is a progressive degenerative disease that affects the myelin sheath and conduction pathways of the central nervous system. One of the earliest signs is <u>paresthesia</u>, abnormal sensations in the extremities or on one side of the face. The disease is characterized by periods of remission and exacerbation (flare). Disability increases as the disease progresses and the periods of exacerbation become more frequent.

In multiple sclerosis, the myelin sheath deteriorates and is replaced by scar tissue that interferes with normal transmission of the nerve impulse. This disease that is named for the multiple areas of
sclerosis   sclerotic tissue that replace the myelin sheath is multiple _____.

15-90 <u>Amyotrophic lateral sclerosis</u> (ALS) is also called Lou Gehrig's disease. It is characterized by atrophy (wasting) of the hands, forearms, and legs. The disease results in paralysis and death. The cause of the disease is unknown. Analyzing the parts of *a/myo/trophic*, *a-* means without, *my(o)*
muscle   means _____, and *-trophic* means nutrition.

This rare degenerative disease of the motor neurons, characterized by weakness and atrophy of
amyotrophic   the muscles, is ALS, which means _____ lateral sclerosis.

15-91 <u>My/asthenia gravis</u>, meaning grave muscle weakness, is a chronic neuromuscular disease characterized by great muscular weakness and fatigue. The suffix *-asthenia* means weakness, so
muscle   *my/asthenia* means weakness of the _____.

This degenerative condition results from a defect in the conduction of nerve impulses at the neuromuscular junction. Characterized by chronic fatigue and muscle weakness, it is called
myasthenia   _____ gravis.

15-92 <u>Dementia</u> (**də-men′shə**) is a progressive mental disorder of the brain characterized by confusion, disorientation, deterioration of memory and intellectual abilities, and personality disintegration. Dementia occurs most often in older adults. Dementia caused by drug intoxication, insulin shock, hydrocephalus, or certain other causes may be reversed by treating the underlying cause. Organic forms of dementia, such as Alzheimer's disease, are generally considered incurable.

<u>Alzheimer's disease</u> is chronic, progressive mental deterioration that is sometimes called dementia, Alzheimer's type. This accounts for more than half of the persons with dementia who are older than 65 years of age. It is less common in people in their 40s and 50s. Although the exact cause is not known, both chemical and structural changes occur in the brain.

Alzheimer's disease is characterized by confusion, memory failure, disorientation, inability to carry out purposeful activities, and speech and gait disturbances. It involves irreversible loss of memory. The patient becomes increasingly mentally impaired, severe physical deterioration takes place, and
Alzheimer's   death occurs. This type of dementia is called _____ disease.

■ *Eye and Ear Disorders*

15-93 We depend on the sense organs to detect sensations. Disorders of the eyes and ears can interfere with this ability; hence the inclusion of the eyes and ears in this chapter. The more common problems of the eyes and ears are injury and infection. The eyes are protected by the bony orbit, but more than a million eye injuries occur each year by blunt objects, penetration of the eyeball, or chemicals.

15-94 <u>Blephar/optosis</u> (**blef″ə-rop-to′sis**), also called <u>ptosis</u> (**to′sis**), is an abnormal condition in which one or both upper eyelids droop (Figure 15-19). It may be congenital or acquired as a result of weakness of the muscle (as in aging) or paralysis of the nerve.
eyelid   <u>Blephar/itis</u> (**blef″ə-ri′tis**) is inflammation of the _____ and is characterized by swelling and redness. Its causes include allergies, irritants, and infection. Crying can cause <u>blephar/edema</u> (**blef″ər-ĭ-de′mə**), swelling of the eyelid, and transient blephar/itis, but the crusts of dried mucus on the lids that are characteristic of true blepharitis are absent.

Blepharitis may be accompanied by <u>conjunctivitis</u> (**kən-junk″tĭ-vi′tis**), inflammation of the conjunctiva. Write this term that means inflammation of the conjunctiva,
conjunctivitis   _____.

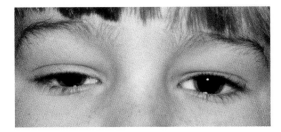

keratitis (ker″ə-ti′tis)

15-95 A hordeolum (**hor-de′o-ləm**), also called sty or stye, is an infection of a sebaceous gland in the lid margin. It usually affects only one eye at a time.

<u>Iritis</u> (**i-ri′tis**) is inflammation of the iris.

Write a term that means inflammation of the cornea: _____.
Treatment of keratitis is important to avoid corneal scarring or perforation.

Dry eyes are caused by a variety of conditions and disorders caused by decreased tear secretion or increased evaporation of moisture from the eye, as in an extremely dry or windy environment.

Inflammation of the external eye is a common condition because it is sensitive to many external irritants, including cosmetics, dust, and fumes. In addition, microorganisms can cause infection.

softening

hemorrhage
pain

15-96 Several terms are used to describe various eye conditions, such as <u>ophthalmo/malacia</u> (**of-thal″mo-mə-la′shə**), which is abnormal _____ of the eyeball. *Ophthalmo/plegia* (**of-thal″mo-ple′jə**) means paralysis of the eye.

<u>Ophthalmo/rrhagia</u> (**of-thal″mo-ra′je-ə**) is _____ from the eye.

<u>Ophthalm/algia</u> (**of″thəl-mal′jə**) means _____ in the eye. This can lead to excessive lacrimation.

cataract

15-97 A <u>cataract</u> (**kat′ə-rakt**) is an abnormal progressive condition of the lens of the eye, characterized by loss of transparency. Write the name of this abnormal opacity of the lens of the eye, being careful with its spelling: _____.

15-98 <u>Glaucoma</u> (**glaw-, glou-ko′mə**) is an abnormal condition of increased pressure within the eye. Prolonged pressure can damage the retina and optic nerve. Several drugs or laser surgery may be used to relieve the increased pressure.

retina

15-99 Any disease of the retina is a <u>retino/pathy</u> (**ret″ĭ-nop′ə-the**). A <u>detached retina</u> is separation of the retina from the back of the eye (Figure 15-20). Although it can be caused by severe trauma, most cases are associated with internal changes within the eye. Retinal detachment requires surgical treatment to avoid deterioration that can lead to blindness in the affected eye. This disorder is called detached _____.

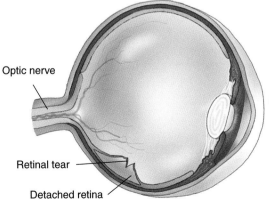

Optic nerve

Retinal tear

Detached retina

Figure 15-20   Retinal detachment. The onset of separation of the retina from the back of the eye is usually sudden and painless. The person may experience bright flashes of light or floating dark spots in the affected eye. Sometimes there is loss of visual field, as though a curtain is being pulled over part of the visual field. Retinal detachments are usually visible using ophthalmoscopy.

Macular degeneration is a progressive deterioration of the macula lutea of the retina, an oval yellow spot at the optical center of the retina, and can result in severe visual acuity problems.

15-100 Concretions (calculi) can form in the lacrimal passages. A dacryo/lith (dak′re-o-lith″) is a lacrimal _____, or a tear stone. Dacryo/lith/iasis (dak″re-o-lĭ-thi′ə-sis) is the presence of lacrimal calculi.

calculus

15-101 Dacryo/cyst/itis (dak″re-o-sis-ti′tis) is inflammation of the _____ sac.
Dacryo/sinus/itis (dak″re-o-si″nəs-i′tis) is inflammation of the lacrimal sac and the sinus.
A rhino/dacryo/lith (ri″no-dak′re-o-lith″) is a tear stone in the _____ duct.

lacrimal

nasal

15-102 Dipl/opia (dĭ-plo′pe-ə) means double _____.
Three common irregularities in vision are explained in Figure 15-21. These are refractive disorders, because light rays are not focused appropriately on the retina.
Another name for nearsightedness is _____. Farsightedness is the same as hyperopia (hi″pər-o′pe-ə). Uneven focusing of the image, resulting from distortion of the curvature of the lens or cornea, is astigmatism (ə-stig′mə-tiz-əm).
Presby/opia* (pres″be-o′pe-ə) is hyperopia and impairment of vision due to advancing years or to old age.

vision

myopia (mi-o′pe-ə)

15-103 Ear trauma can occur from a blow by a blunt object. The eardrum can be damaged by a penetrating injury, rupture, or perforation by shock waves from an explosion, deep sea diving, trauma, or acute middle ear infections, as seen in Figure 15-22.

15-104 Write a word that means inflammation of the ear: _____.
Otitis may produce ot/algia (o-tal′je-ə), pain in the ear, which is also called earache.
Otitis media (o-ti′tis me′de-ə) is _____ of the middle ear.
The middle ear is separated from the external ear by the eardrum. Mastoid/itis (mas″toid-i′tis) is an infection of one of the mastoid bones, usually an extension of a middle ear infection. It is difficult to treat and can result in hearing loss. Antibiotic therapy is aimed at treating middle-ear infections before they progress to mastoiditis.

otitis (o-ti′tis)

inflammation

15-105 A discharge from the ear may accompany otitis. Write a word that means discharge from the ear: _____.
Otorrhea may contain blood, pus, or even spinal fluid. Ear infections are just one cause of otorrhea.

otorrhea (o″to-re′ə)

15-106 Oto/sclerosis (o″to-sklə-ro′sis) means _____ of the ear. This condition is caused by formation of spongy bone around structures of the middle and inner ear, and it leads to hearing impairment.

hardening

15-107 Tinnitus† (tin′ĭ-təs, tĭ-ni′təs), noise in the ears, is one of the most common complaints of persons with ear or hearing disorders. The noise includes ringing, buzzing, roaring, or clicking. It may be a sign of something as simple as accumulation of earwax or cerumen‡ (sə-roo′mən) or as serious as Meniere's (mĕ-nyārz′) disease. The latter is a chronic disease of the inner ear with recurrent episodes of hearing loss, tinnitus, and vertigo (vər′tĭ-go). Vertigo is also called dizziness.
Ringing in the ears is called _____.

tinnitus

---

*Presbyopia (Greek: presbys, old man; -opia, vision).
†Tinnitus (Latin: tinnire, to tinkle).
‡Cerumen (Latin: cera, wax).

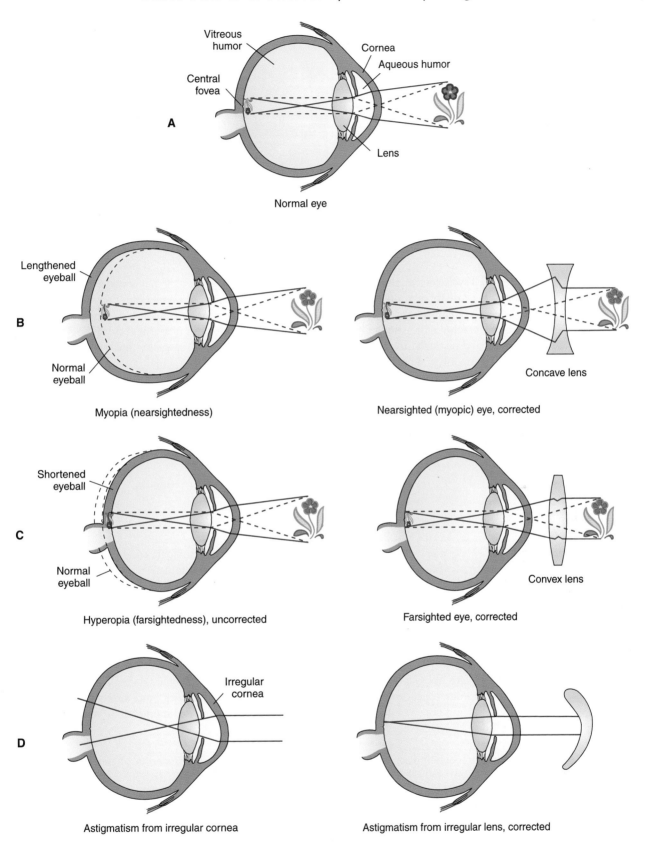

Figure 15-21 Normal and abnormal refraction in the eyeball. **A,** In the normal eye, a clear image is formed when light rays from an object are bent properly and converge on the center of the retina. **B,** In myopia (nearsightedness), the image is focused in front of the retina and is corrected by use of a concave lens. **C,** In hyperopia (farsightedness), the image is focused behind the retina and is corrected using a convex lens. **D,** In astigmatism, the curvature of the cornea or lens is uneven and results in the image being focused at two different points on the retina. A cylindrical lens is used to correct astigmatism.

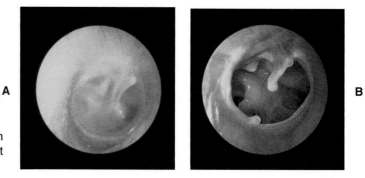

Figure 15-22   Comparison of the appearance of a normal eardrum and a perforated eardrum. **A,** Otoscopic view of a normal intact eardrum. **B,** Otoscopic view of a perforated eardrum.

■ *Psychological Disorders*

psychiatry

15-108 Psychological disorders are unlike most diseases or disorders that confront health professionals because there often is no change in the body structure, and sometimes not even detectable changes in chemistry, thus making the abnormalities difficult to demonstrate and treat in the usual sense. A psychologist is not a physician but one who is trained in methods of psychological analysis, therapy, and research. You learned in Chapter 2 that the medical specialty that deals with the diagnosis, treatment, and prevention of mental illness is _____.

Learn the meanings of the following combining forms related to psychology.

Additional Word Parts Pertaining to Psychology

Combining Forms	Meanings	Prefix	Meaning
ment(o), psych(o)	mind	idio-	individual
phren(o)	mind or diaphragm		
pyr(o)	fire		
schist(o), schiz(o)	split		

mind

15-109 Only a few psychological disorders have observable pathologic conditions of the brain. Some examples of observable pathologic conditions are mental retardation, dementia, and Alzheimer's disease.

<u>Mental retardation</u> is a disorder characterized by subaverage general intelligence with deficits or impairments in the ability to learn and to adapt socially. Mental retardation is abnormally low intellectual functioning of the _____, or deficient intellectual development.

autism

15-110 Signs of psychological disorders can appear in a very young child. Such is the case with mental retardation, autism (**aw′tiz-əm**), and attention deficit disorder. <u>Autism</u> is characterized by withdrawal and impaired development in social interaction and communication. Write the name of this disorder that may be characterized by extreme withdrawal: _____.

Attention deficit disorder and attention deficit hyperactivity disorder are abbreviated ADD and ADHD. These are characterized by short attention span, poor concentration, and, in ADHD, hyperactivity. Hyperactivity is also called <u>hyper/kinesia</u>. Translated literally, hyper/kinesia or <u>hyper/kinesis</u> is above normal _____.

movement

mind

15-111 <u>Anxiety disorders</u> are characterized by anticipation of impending danger and dread, the source of which is largely unknown or unrecognized. An anxiety attack is an acute, psycho/biological reaction that usually includes several of the following: restlessness, tension, tachycardia, and breathing difficulty. A psycho/biological response involves both the _____ and the physical body.

15-112 <u>Phobias</u> are obsessive, irrational, and intense fears of an object, an activity, or a physical situation. The suffix *-phobia* means abnormal _____. Phobias range from abnormal fear of public places, <u>agoraphobia</u> (**ag″ə-rə-fo′be-ə**), to abnormal fear of animals, <u>zoophobia</u> (**zo″o-fo′be-ə**), and even include an abnormal fear of acquiring a phobia, <u>phobophobia</u> (**fo″bo-fo′be-ə**).

fear

Write a word that means an irrational fear of heights by using the combining form for extremity and *-phobia*: _____.

acrophobia
(ak″ro-fo′be-ə)

<u>Claustro/phobia</u> (**klaws″tro-fo′be-ə**) is a morbid _____ of closed places. (A claustrum is a barrier.)
An abnormal fear of fire is pyro/phobia (**pi″ro-fo′be-ə**).

fear

15-113 An <u>obsession</u> is a persistent thought or idea that occupies the mind and cannot be erased by logic or reasoning. A <u>compulsion</u> is an irresistible, repetitive impulse to act contrary to one's ordinary standards. An <u>obsessive-compulsive disorder</u> is a pattern of persistent behaviors that involve compulsion to act on an obsession.

obsession

Write the term that means a persistent thought or idea that cannot be erased by logic or reasoning: _____.

15-114 <u>Posttraumatic stress disorder</u> is characterized by an acute emotional response _____ a traumatic event or situation involving severe environmental stress, such as military combat.

after

15-115 A <u>panic disorder</u> or <u>panic attack</u> is an episode of acute anxiety that occurs unpredictably with feelings of intense apprehension or terror, accompanied by dyspnea (difficult breathing), dizziness, sweating, trembling, and chest pain.

When these signs and symptoms occur unpredictably with feelings of extreme apprehension, the disorder is called a _____ attack.

panic

15-116 A <u>mania</u> is an unstable emotional state that includes excessive excitement, elation, ideas, and psychomotor activities. In an extreme manic episode, a delusion of grandeur may occur. The suffix *-mania* is used to write terms pertaining to excessive preoccupation. <u>Megalo/mania</u> (**meg″ə-lo-ma′ne-ə**) is an abnormal mental state in which one believes oneself to be a person of great importance, power, fame, or wealth. You learned earlier that *-mania* means excessive preoccupation; therefore the literal translation of megalo/mania is excessive _____ with greatness.

preoccupation

A <u>bipolar disorder</u> is a major mental disorder characterized by the occurrence of manic episodes and major depressive episodes. The term *bipolar* in the name indicates that the disorder has two distinct aspects. Megalomania may occur in an extreme manic episode of bipolar disorder.

15-117 The combining form *pyr(o)* means fire. <u>Pyro/mania</u> (**pi″ro-ma′ne-ə**) is excessive preoccupation with _____. A <u>pyro/maniac</u> has an obsessive preoccupation with fires. The combining form *pyr(o)* means fire. Pyro/mania is a compulsion to set fires or watch fires.

fire

<u>Klepto/mania</u>* (**klep″to-ma′ne-ə**) is characterized by an abnormal, uncontrollable, and recurrent urge to steal.

15-118 The suffix *-asthenia* means weakness. <u>Neur/asthenia</u> (**noor″əs-the′ne-ə**) is a nervous disorder (neurosis) characterized by _____ and sometimes nervous exhaustion. It is often associated with a depressed state and is believed by some to be psychosomatic. You learned in Chapter 6 that psychosomatic disorders are emotional states that influence the physical body's functioning.

weakness

---

*Kleptomania (Greek: *kleptein*, to steal; *mania*, madness).

split

against

Pseudo/mania (soo″do-ma′ne-ə) is a false or pretended mental disorder. Pseudo/plegia (soo″do-ple′jə) is hysterical paralysis. There is loss of muscle power without real paralysis.

15-119 Schizo/phrenia (skiz″o-fre′ne-ə, skit″so-fre′ne-ə) is any of a large group of psychotic disorders characterized by gross distortion of reality, hallucinations, disturbances of language and communication, and disorganized or catatonic behavior (psychologically induced immobility with muscular rigidity that is interrupted by agitation). Notice the two pronunciations of the term *schizophrenia*. The combining form *schiz(o)* means _____.

A psychotic disorder, or psychosis, is any major mental disorder characterized by a gross impairment in reality testing. Translated literally, *schizo/phrenia* means split mind and relates to the splitting off of a part of the psyche; the part that is expressed may be contrary to the original personality of the person.

15-120 A number of personality disorders exist with which you may already be familiar. These include antisocial behavior, paranoia, and others. Anti/social behavior is acting _____ the rights of others.

Paranoia (par″ə-noi′ah) is characterized by persistent delusions of persecution, mistrust, and combativeness. Additional information about psychological disorders can be found in the *Diagnostic and Statistical Manual of Mental Disorders (DSM)*.

Exercise 6

Write a term in each blank to complete these sentences.

1. Bleeding occurs within the brain in an _____ hematoma.

2. Accumulation of blood between the dura mater and the arachnoid is a _____ hematoma.

3. Another name for a stroke is a _____ accident.

4. Paralysis of all four extremities is called _____.

5. Hernial protrusion of the meninges through a defect in the skull or vertebral column is a

    _____.

6. Inflammation of the brain and spinal cord is called _____.

7. Gliomas are primary malignant _____ tumors.

8. Hydrocephalus is an abnormal accumulation of cerebrospinal fluid within the _____.

9. A group of chronic neurologic disorders often characterized by recurrent episodes of convulsive seizures is known as

    _____.

10. A progressive degenerative disease that affects the myelin sheath and conduction pathways of the central nervous

    system is called multiple _____.

11. A chronic neuromuscular disease characterized by great muscular weakness and fatigue is

    _____ gravis.

12. Dacryolithiasis is the presence of _____ calculi.

13. A term for nearsightedness is _____.

14. Inflammation of the middle ear is _____ media.

15. An obsessive, irrational, and intense fear of an object, an activity, or a physical situation is called a

    _____.

SURGICAL AND THERAPEUTIC INTERVENTIONS

sensitive

15-121 Pain management may be for a short time (for example, after surgery) or longer (chronic pain) and may include drug therapy and nondrug treatments. *An/algesic* (**an″al-je′zik**) means relieving pain or not _____ to pain. Agents that relieve pain without causing loss of consciousness are also called <u>analgesics</u>. Three well-known analgesics that are used for mild to moderate pain are aspirin, ibuprofen (Advil), and acetaminophen (Tylenol).

<u>Opioid analgesics</u> act on the central nervous system, are more often used for severe pain, and may alter the patient's perception and produce tolerance or dependency. Some examples are codeine and morphine.

nerve

15-122 <u>Nerve blocks</u> are used to reduce pain by temporarily or permanently blocking transmission of _____ impulses. <u>Nerve block anesthesia</u> is produced by injecting an anesthetic along the course of a nerve to inhibit the conduction of impulses to and from the area supplied by the nerve.

<u>Sympathectomy</u> (**sim″pə-thek′tə-me**) is a surgical procedure in which one or more sympathetic nerves are severed. This surgery has special uses, including alleviation of pain.

15-123 A <u>vago/tomy</u> (**va-got′ə-me**) is severing of various branches of the vagus nerve and is done to reduce the amount of acid secreted in the stomach. This is done to prevent the reoccurrence of an ulcer. Write this term that means severing of the vagus nerve:

vagotomy

_____.

15-124 <u>Epidural anesthesia</u> is injection of an anesthetic into the epidural space, which contains spinal fluid and spinal nerves. Epidurals, most commonly performed in the lumbar area, can be tailored to numb an area of the body from the lower extremities to the upper abdomen. They are often used in labor and childbirth.

15-125 <u>Neuro/tripsy</u> (**noor″o-trip′se**) is surgical crushing of a nerve.

Write a term that means excision of a nerve: _____.

neurectomy
(noo-rek′to-me)

15-126 <u>Trans/cutane/ous electrical nerve stimulation</u> (TENS) is a method of pain control by the application of electric impulses to the nerve endings. Pain signals to the brain are blocked by electric impulses generated by a stimulator that is attached to electrodes placed on the skin. Literal translation of transcutaneous is across or performed through the

skin

_____.

destruction

15-127 <u>Neuro/lysis</u> (**noo-rol′ĭ-sis**) is _____ of nerves. *Neurolysis* has several meanings, but all of them have to do with nervous tissue. The word is used to mean release of a nerve sheath by cutting it longitudinally, loosening of adhesions surrounding a nerve, or disintegration of nerve tissue.

neuroplasty
(noor′o-plas″te)

Write a word that means surgical repair of a nerve: _____.
<u>Neuro/rrhaphy</u> (**noo-ror′ə-fe**) specifically means suture of a nerve.

15-128 Use *cerebr(o)* to write a word that means incision of the brain:

cerebrotomy
(ser″ə-brot′ə-me)

_____.

Any surgical opening into the skull is a craniotomy (**kra″ne-ot′ə-me**), performed to gain access to the brain, relieve intracranial pressure, or control bleeding inside the skull. Surgical removal of a portion of the skull in order to perform surgery on the brain is a <u>craniectomy</u> (**kra″ne-ek′tə-me**). This type of surgery may be necessary to repair the brain or its vessels, remove a brain tumor, or repair an aneurysm.

excision

An <u>aneurysm/ectomy</u> (**an″u-riz-mek′to-me**) is _____ of an aneurysm. <u>Cranio/plasty</u> (**kra′ne-o-plas″te**) is surgical repair of the skull after surgery or injury to the skull.

Gamma knife stereotaxic radiosurgery (ster″e-o-tak′sik ra″de-o-sər′jər-e) is used to treat deep intracranial brain tumors with a focused beam of gamma radiation without surgical incision. In naming this procedure, *knife* was used because gamma radiation replaces the surgical knife that was used in the past.

15-129 A cerebrospinal fluid (CSF) shunt may be used to relieve hydrocephalus. This type of shunt is a tube that is placed in the brain to relieve the pressure of the fluid that accumulates. This treatment is called a CSF_____.

shunt

15-130 In addition to analgesics and anesthetics, many drugs act on the central nervous system, including hypnotics, anticonvulsants, and antipyretics.

Hypnotics* are drugs often used as sedatives to produce a calming effect. Functional activity, irritability, and excitement are decreased by sedatives.

Anti/convulsants act _____ convulsion, anti/pyretics are used to decrease fever, and antiparkinsonian drugs are used to treat Parkinson's disease.

against

15-131 Both *anti-* and *contra-* mean against. A contra/indication (kon″trə-in″dĭ-ka′shən) is any condition that renders a particular treatment improper or undesirable. *Contra-* means _____.

against

15-132 If a cerebral embolus is caused by a blood clot, a thrombo/lytic (throm″bo-lit′ik) may be used. Thrombolytics _____ blood clots.

dissolve

15-133 A blepharo/plasty (blef′ə-ro-plas″te) is just one of many types of eye surgery. Blepharoplasty is the use of plastic surgery to restore or repair the _____. If vision is adversely affected by sagging of the eyelids, it can be corrected by plastic surgery. If appearance is affected, this procedure can be done for cosmetic reasons. Write the name of this surgery: _____.

eyelid

blepharoplasty

15-134 Cataracts are usually treated with removal of the cataract. To prevent the need for a special contact lens or glasses, an intraocular lens (IOL) is sometimes surgically implanted when the cataract is removed. An intra/ocular lens is implanted _____ the eye.

Corneal grafting may be necessary to improve vision in cases of corneal scarring or perforation. The cornea was one of the first organs transplanted, and rejection of the transplanted tissue is uncommon.

within

15-135 Corrective glasses or contact lenses can often correct uncomplicated problems with vision, such as nearsightedness and farsightedness. Radial keratotomy (ker″ə-tot′ə-me) often reduces or eliminates the need for further correction in many persons with myopia, hyperopia, and astigmatism. Kerato/tomy is incision of the _____. The excimer laser is used in this type of corneal surgery and creates minimal damage to adjacent cells.

cornea

15-136 Dacryocyst/itis usually responds to systemic administration of antibiotics but rarely may require a dacryo/cysto/rhino/stomy (dak″re-o-sis″to-ri-nos′tə-me), surgical creation of a passageway between the lacrimal sac and the _____.

Dacryo/cysto/tomy (dak″re-o-sis-tot′ə-me) means incision of the lacrimal sac.

nose

*Hypnotics (Greek: *hypnos,* sleep).

<table>
<tr><td>mind</td><td>

15-137 Psycho/analysis (si"ko-ə-nal′ĭ-sis) is a method of diagnosing and treating disorders of the _____. This is accomplished by ascertaining and studying the facts of the patient's mental life.

Psycho/therapy (si"ko-ther′ə-pe) is treatment of disorders of the mind by psychological means rather than by physical means.

</td></tr>
<tr><td>mind</td><td>

15-138 Psycho/pharmacology (si"ko-fahr"mə-kol′ə-je) is the study of the action of drugs on functions of the _____.

Anti/depressants are medications that prevent or relieve depression. Anti/anxiety drugs are used to relieve feelings of anxiety. Anti/psychotics are medications that are used to treat the symptoms of severe psychiatric disorders. Tranquilizers are prescribed to calm anxious or agitated persons, ideally without decreasing their consciousness. Narcotic drugs produce stupor or sleep.

</td></tr>
</table>

Exercise 7

Match terms in the left column with descriptions in the right column.

_____ 1. analgesics

_____ 2. epidural

_____ 3. neurotripsy

_____ 4. TENS

_____ 5. vagotomy

A. application of electric impulses to the nerve endings
B. injection of anesthesia to produce numbness in the lower part of the body
C. act on CNS to relieve pain without causing loss of consciousness
D. severing of branches of the vagus nerve
E. surgical crushing of a nerve

Exercise 8

Write a term for each of the following:

1. agents used to dissolve blood clots   _____

2. excision of an aneurysm   _____

3. surgical removal of a portion of the skull _____

4. suture of a nerve   _____

5. surgical repair of the eyelid   _____

SELECTED ABBREVIATIONS

ACh	acetylcholine		**EEG**	electroencephalogram
ADD	attention deficit disorder		**ICP**	intracranial pressure
ADHD	attention deficit hyperactivity disorder		**MS**	multiple sclerosis
ALS	amyotrophic lateral sclerosis		**OCD**	obsessive-compulsive disorder
CNS	central nervous system		**PET**	positron emission tomography
CSF	cerebrospinal fluid		**PNS**	peripheral nervous system
CVA	cerebrovascular accident, costovertebral angle		**SCI**	spinal cord injury
DSM	*Diagnostic and Statistical Manual of Mental Disorders*		**TENS**	transcutaneous electrical nerve stimulation
DTR	deep tendon reflex		**TIA**	transient ischemic attack

Chapter 15 Review

■ Basic Understanding

Matching

I. Assign structures in the left column to the correct division of the nervous system by choosing either A or B.

_____ 1. brain   A. central nervous system
_____ 2. chemoreceptors   B. peripheral nervous system
_____ 3. pain receptors
_____ 4. sense organs
_____ 5. spinal cord

II. Match the types of receptors in the left column with the appropriate stimuli in the right column.

_____ 1. chemoreceptors   A. change in chemical concentration of substances
_____ 2. mechanoreceptors   B. changes in temperature
                                  C. light
_____ 3. nociceptors   D. movement in fluids or changes in pressure
_____ 4. photoreceptors   E. tissue damage
_____ 5. thermoreceptors

Multiple Choice

III. Circle the correct answer for each of the following:

1. Which of the following is the outermost meningeal membrane? (arachnoid, dura mater, epidural, pia mater)

2. Which of the following is chronic, progressive mental deterioration that involves irreversible loss of memory, disorientation, and speech and gait disturbances? (Alzheimer's disease, Lou Gehrig's disease, Meniere's syndrome, multiple sclerosis)

3. Which term means paralysis of the lower portion of the body and both legs? (diplegia, hemiplegia, paraplegia, quadriplegia)

4. Which of the following is the correct name for a stroke? (cerebrovascular accident, craniocerebral trauma, monoplegia, polyneuropathy)

5. Which of the following is the record produced in radiography of the spinal cord after injection of a contrast medium? (encephalogram, encephalography, myelogram, myelography)

6. Which term means a morbid fear of closed places? (acrophobia, agoraphobia, claustrophobia, zoophobia)

7. Which of the following means hernial protrusion of the meninges through a defect in the vertebral column? (meningitis, meningocele, myelocele, myelomalacia)

8. What is the term for any condition that renders a particular treatment improper or undesirable? (anotia, anticonvulsant, antipyretic, contraindication)

9. Which term means incision of the lacrimal sac? (cholecystotomy, cystolithectomy, dacryocystotomy, dacryolithiasis)

10. What does *algesia* mean? (oversensitivity to pain, pain, sensitivity to pain, undersensitivity to pain)

Fill in the Blanks

IV. *Write the appropriate word in each blank.*

Three membranes collectively known as (1) _____ cover the brain and spinal cord.

The largest and uppermost portion of the brain is the (2) _____. A fluid called

(3) _____ fluid surrounds and cushions the brain and spinal cord.

    The nervous system is composed of two types of cells. The basic unit of the nervous system is called a

(4) _____. The other type of cell that serves as support is a

(5) _____ cell.

    A cytoplasmic projection that carries impulses away from the cell body of the neuron is called an

(6) _____. Another type of cytoplasmic process that carries an impulse to the cell body is a

(7) _____.

Writing Terms

V. *Write one term for each of the following meanings.*

1. absence of one or both ears   _____

2. hardening of nervous tissue   _____

3. inflammation of the brain and spinal cord   _____

4. inflammation of the cornea   _____

5. nearsightedness   _____

6. partially aware of one's surroundings   _____

7. radiography of the spinal cord   _____

8. recording the electrical activity of the brain   _____

9. presence of lacrimal calculi   _____

10. uncontrollable, brief episodes of sleep   _____

■ Greater Comprehension

Health Care Report

VI. Read the following health care report. Then answer the questions that follow the report.

MID-CITY MEDICAL CENTER

222 Medical Center Drive   Main City, US 63017-1000   Phone: (555) 434-0000
                                                                      Fax (555) 434-0001

HISTORY AND PHYSICAL

PATIENT'S NAME: Emma Lang   **DATE OF ADMISSION:** 12/04/2004
ADMITTING COMPLAINT: Multiple sclerosis
HISTORY OF ADMITTING COMPLAINT: Diagnosis of multiple sclerosis was made in 1996 by MRI scan. Family has
   noted progressive confusion over last 3-4 months, especially in the morning, and anorexia. She frequently chokes on
   liquids and has difficulty understanding speech, weakness in both arms and legs, and severe spasticity. She seldom
   speaks. She is catheterized 3-4 times per day due to urinary retention.
ALLERGIES: None.
PHYSICAL EXAMINATION:
   Cardiovascular, Pulmonary and Gastrointestinal: No unusual findings.
   General: Disoriented to time, place, and person. Carries out simple commands.
   Neurological: Eyes and ears appear normal. Muscle power is decreased in both arms. Tone is increased in right leg.
      Apparently, there are no signs of vertigo or tinnitus.
   Genitourinary: No unusual findings.
FAMILY HISTORY: Mother had Alzheimer's disease.
IMPRESSION: Progressive neurologic disorder with dementia, ophthalmoplegia, dysarthria, neurogenic bladder, and
      dysphasia.

MEF:aba   *Milton Freeberger, M.D.*
Date: 12-6/2004   Milton Freeberger, M.D.

Match terms in the left column with their meanings in the right column.

_____ 1. diplopia   A. difficulty in language function
                                B. dizziness
_____ 2. dysphasia   C. double vision
_____ 3. ophthalmoplegia   D. paralysis of the eyes
                                E. ringing in the ears
_____ 4. tinnitus

_____ 5. vertigo

Circle one answer for each of the following questions.

6. Which type of disorder is multiple sclerosis? (congenital, degenerative, infectious, traumatic)

7. Which of the following is a progressive mental disorder characterized by confusion, disorientation, and personality disintegration? (dementia, dysphasia, multiple sclerosis, neurogenic bladder)

8. Which term in the report means difficult and poorly articulated speech? (Alzheimer's, depression, dysarthria, paranoia)

Health Care Report

VII. Read the following report and define the terms that are underlined.

MID-CITY MEDICAL CENTER

222 Medical Center Drive	Main City, US 63017-1000	Phone: (555) 434-0000 Fax (555) 434-0001

REHABILITATION CONSULTATION

NAME: Richard Mann   **DATE:** 04/16/2004

Richard Mann is a 69-year-old left-handed gentleman who is seen for management of ambulatory dysfunction secondary to <u>Parkinson's disease</u>. He has a history of diplopia, secondary to <u>meningioma</u>. He has also been diagnosed with an additional problem of <u>peripheral neuropathy</u>. He is able to ambulate with a wheeled walker with standby assist. He requires moderate assist for transfers. He has persistent problem with diplopia. He has no apparent problem with focal weakness.

GENERAL APPEARANCE:

   HEENT: Left <u>ptosis</u> with extraocular movements. Flat facies present. Mild decrease in left corneal reflex.

   Neck, lungs, heart, and extremities: No abnormal findings.

   Neurologic: Decreased muscle mass and moderate <u>bradykinesia</u>. Resting tremor, right upper extremity. Bilateral arm strength decreased. Bilateral lower extremity strength good. Both great toes were nonreactive to Babinski testing. No report of vertigo. Good gag response bilaterally. Mr. Mann was alert and oriented to person, place, and time. He did exhibit short-term memory and short attention span. He had trouble maintaining balance without use of a walker.

IMPRESSION: Parkinson's disease, ambulatory dysfunction, peripheral neuropathy.

PLAN: Mr. Mann will benefit from a rehabilitation program that will offer intensive physical therapy to maintain range of motion, build strength and balance, and optimize his mobility. Occupational therapy will optimize strength, dexterity, and self-care skills. Speech therapy will optimize communication skills, swallowing, and speech.

MW:aba   *Michael Wilson, MD*
04/17/2004   Michael Wilson, M.D.

---

1. Parkinson's disease: _____

2. meningioma: _____

3. peripheral neuropathy: _____

4. ptosis: _____

5. bradykinesia: _____

Spelling

VIII. Circle all incorrectly spelled terms and write their correct spelling.

acetylcoline   Alzheimer's   cerebrul   iritis   ophthalmoscopy

Interpreting Abbreviations
IX. Write the meanings of the following abbreviations.

1. ADHD _____

2. ALS _____

3. CSF _____

4. DTR _____

5. SCI _____

Pronunciation
X. Pronunciation is shown for several terms. Mark the primary accent in each term with an '.

1. arachnoid (ə rak noid)

2. cerebrotomy (ser ə brot ə me)

3. efferent (ef ər ənt)

4. glioma (gli o mə)

5. kleptomania (klep to ma ne ə)

Categorizing Terms
XI. Classify the terms in the left column by selecting A, B, C, D, or E.

_____ 1. arachnoid
_____ 2. audiometer
_____ 3. botulism
_____ 4. carpoptosis
_____ 5. cerebral angiography
_____ 6. cochlea
_____ 7. myelogram
_____ 8. opioid analgesics
_____ 9. sciatica
_____ 10. sympathectomy

A. anatomy
B. diagnostic test or procedure
C. pathology
D. surgery
E. therapy

(Check your answers with the solutions in Appendix VI.)

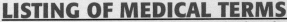

LISTING OF MEDICAL TERMS

Use the practice CD to review the terms that have been presented. Look closely at the spelling of each term as it is pronounced and be sure you know the meaning of each term.

acetylcholine	cataract	craniotomy	foramen magnum
acetylcholinesterase	central nervous system	cranium	frontal lobe
acrophobia	cephalalgia	dacryocyst	glaucoma
adrenaline	cephalgia	dacryocystitis	glia cell
adrenergic	cerebellar	dacryocystography	glioma
afferent	cerebellitis	dacryocystorhinostomy	hematoma
agoraphobia	cerebellum	dacryocystotomy	hemiplegia
algesia	cerebral	dacryolith	hemorrhagic stroke
Alzheimer's disease	cerebral aneurysm	dacryolithiasis	homeostasis
amyotrophic lateral	cerebral angiography	dacryosinusitis	hordeolum
sclerosis	cerebral concussion	dementia	Huntington's chorea
analgesic	cerebral cortex	dendrite	hydrocephalus
anesthesia	cerebral embolus	diencephalon	hydrophobia
anesthetic	cerebral hemisphere	diplegia	hypalgesia
aneurysm	cerebral hemorrhage	diplopia	hyperkinesia
aneurysmectomy	cerebral palsy	dopamine	hyperkinesis
anosmia	cerebral ventricle	dura mater	hyperopia
anotia	cerebrocranial	dysarthria	hyperosmia
antianxiety	cerebrospinal fluid	dyslexia	hypnotic
anticonvulsant	cerebrotomy	dyslexic	hypoalgesia
antidepressant	cerebrovascular accident	dysphasia	hypothalamus
antipsychotic	cerebrum	echoencephalogram	integrative
antipyretic	cerumen	echoencephalograph	interocular
arachnoid	chemoreceptor	echoencephalography	intracerebral
astigmatism	cholinergic	efferent	intracranial
audible	claustrophobia	electroencephalogram	intraocular
audiogram	cochlea	electroencephalograph	intrathecal
audiologist	coma	electroencephalography	involuntary
audiology	concussion	encephalitis	iris
audiometer	conjunctiva	encephalography	iritis
autism	conjunctivitis	encephalomeningitis	keratitis
autonomic	contraindication	encephalomyelopathy	kleptomania
axon	contusion	endorphin	lacrimal gland
blepharedema	convulsion	epidural anesthesia	lacrimal sac
blepharoplasty	cornea	epidural hematoma	lacrimation
blepharoptosis	corneal	epilepsy	lumbar puncture
botulism	craniectomy	epinephrine	mania
brain stem	craniocerebral	excimer laser	mastoiditis
carpoptosis	cranioplasty	extraocular	mechanoreceptor

medulla
megalomania
Meniere's disease
meningeal
meninges
meningioma
meningitis
meningocele
meningomyelocele
mental retardation
midbrain
monoplegia
motor neuron
multiple sclerosis
myasthenia gravis
myelin sheath
myelinated
myelogram
myelography
myopia
narcolepsy
nasolacrimal duct
neural
neuralgia
neurasthenia
neurectomy
neuroglia
neurolysis
neuroma
neuromuscular
neuron
neuropathy
neuroplasty
neurorrhaphy
neurosclerosis

neurotransmitter
neurotripsy
nociceptor
node of Ranvier
occipital lobe
ocular
olfaction
olfactory
ophthalmalgia
ophthalmic
ophthalmomalacia
ophthalmometer
ophthalmoplegia
ophthalmorrhagia
ophthalmoscope
ophthalmoscopy
opioid analgesics
otalgia
otitis
otitis media
otorrhea
otosclerosis
otoscope
otoscopy
palsy
paranasal
paranoia
paraplegia
parasympathetic
paresthesia
parietal lobe
Parkinson's disease
patellar response
peripheral nervous system
phobophobia

photoreceptor
pia mater
poliomyelitis
polyneuralgia
polyneuritis
polyneuropathy
pons
positron emission
    tomography
presbyopia
pseudesthesia
pseudoesthesia
pseudomania
pseudoplegia
psychiatry
psychoanalysis
psychologist
psychopharmacology
psychosis
psychotherapy
ptosis
pyromania
pyromaniac
quadriplegia
rabies
radial keratotomy
receptor
reflex arc
retina
retinal detachment
retinopathy
rhinodacryolith
schizophrenia
sciatic nerve
sciatica

sclera
semicircular canals
semiconscious
sensory
sensory neuron
serotonin
shunt
sleep apnea
somatic
stereotaxic radiosurgery
stye
subarachnoid space
subdural hematoma
subdural space
sympathectomy
sympathetic
synapse
synaptic bulb
temporal lobe
tetanus
thalamus
thermoreceptor
thrombolytic
thrombotic stroke
tinnitus
transient ischemic attack
tympanic membrane
unmyelinated
vagotomy
ventricle
ventriculitis
vertigo
zoophobia

españ* ENHANCING SPANISH COMMUNICATION

ENGLISH	SPANISH (PRONUNCIATION)
adrenaline	adrenalina (ah-dray-nah-LEE-nah)
anxiety	ansiedad (an-se-ay-DAHD)
brain	cerebro (say-RAY-bro)
concussion	concusión (con-coo-se-ON)
conscious	consciente (cons-se-EN-tay)
consciousness	conciencia (con-se-EN-se-ah)
convulsion	convulsión (con-vool-se-ON)
cranium	cráneo (CRAH-nay-o)
dizziness	vértigo (VERR-te-go)
ear	oreja (o-RAY-hah)
epilepsy	epilepsia (ay-pe-LEP-se-ah)
eye	ojo (O-ho)
eyeball	globo del ojo (GLO-bo del O-ho)
eyebrow	ceja (SAY-hah)
eyelash	pestaña (pes-TAH-nyah)
fainting	languidez (lan-gee-DES), desmayo (des-MAH-yo)
fatigue	fatiga (fah-TEE-gah)
fear	miedo (me-AY-do)
fiber	fibra (FEE-brah)
fire	fuego (foo-AY-go)
gray	gris (grees)
headache	dolor de cabeza (do-LOR day cah-BAY-sa)
heat	calor (cah-LOR)
light	luz (loos)
lobe	lóbulo (LO-boo-lo)
neck	cuello (coo-EL-lyo)
nerve	nervio (NERR-ve-o)
nervous	nervioso (ner-ve-O-so)
neurology	neurología (nay-oo-ro-lo-HEE-ah)
optic	óptico (OP-te-co)
painful	doloroso (do-lo-RO-so)
paralysis	parálisis (pah-RAH-le-sis)
psychiatry	psiquiatría (se-ke-ah-TREE-ah)
psychology	psicología (se-co-lo-HEE-ah)
seizure	ataque (ah-TAH-kay)
sensation	sensación (sen-sah-se-ON)
sleep	sueño (soo-AY-nyo)
spasm	espasmo (es-PAHS-mo)
spinal column	columna vertebral (co-LOOM-nah ver-tay-BRAHL)
stroke	ataque de apoplejía (ah-TAH-kay de ah-po-play-HEE-ah)
tear	lágrima (LAH-gre-mah)
trauma	daño (DAH-nyo)
vision	visión (ve-se-ON)
white	blanco (BLAHN-co)

CHAPTER 16

Integumentary System

FUNCTION FIRST

The skin (integument) is the external covering of the body, and it acts as a barrier to disease-causing organisms. It also helps regulate the temperature of the body, provides information about the environment through receptors, helps eliminate waste through perspiration, and is involved in the synthesis of vitamin D.

ANATOMY AND PHYSIOLOGY

■ *The Skin*

16-1 The term *integument* (in-teg′u-mənt) means a covering or skin. The integumentary (in-teg-u-men′tar-e) system is the skin and its glands, hair, nails, and other structures that are derived from it. Because it is on the outside of our bodies, we are more familiar with the skin than with any other organ. Write the name of this body system that includes the skin and other structures derived from it: _____ system.

integumentary

Modified skin continues into various parts of the body, for example, the mucous membrane that lines the mouth, the nose, the intestines, and other cavities or canals that open to the outside. The skin that is studied in this chapter is the body covering, the integument.

Learn the following word parts and their meanings.

Word Parts Pertaining to the Anatomy and Physiology of the Skin

Word Parts Pertaining to Skin Layers

WORD PART	MEANING
cutane(o), derm(o), dermat(o)	skin
adip(o), lip(o)	fat
kerat(o)	horny or cornea
-derm	skin or germ layer

Accessory Skin Structures and Substances

COMBINING FORM	MEANING
hidr(o)	sweat
onych(o), ungu(o)	nail
pil(o), trich(o)	hair
seb(o)	sebum

Other Word Parts

COMBINING FORM	MEANING
axill(o)	axilla (armpit)

16-2 The skin consists of two main parts: the epidermis (ep″ĭ-dər′mis) and the dermis (dər′mis) (Figure 16-1). Remembering that *epi-* means above or on, where is the epi/dermis located? _____ the dermis.

above

16-3 The epidermis consists of four to five layers. The palms and soles have the greatest number of layers. The outermost layer of epidermis consists of cells that are nonliving and are constantly being shed and replaced. These cells contain keratin (ker′ə-tin), a waterproofing protein that hardens over several days. Keratin is a scleroprotein (sklēr″o-pro′tēn). The combining form scler(o) means _____, which helps to describe the scaly, or horny, nature of keratin.

hard

16-4 The combining form kerat(o) means horny or the cornea—the convex, transparent structure at the front of the eye. When kerat(o) is used in discussions regarding the skin, it means hard or horny.

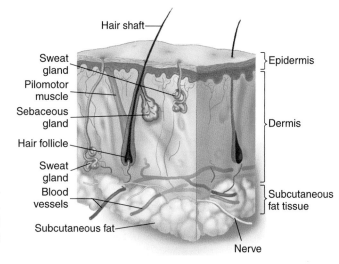

Figure 16-1 The skin. The epidermis, the thin outer layer, is composed of four to five layers. Underneath the epidermis is the thicker dermis, composed of connective tissue containing lymphatics, nerves, blood vessels, hair follicles, sebaceous glands, and sweat glands. Beneath the dermis is a layer of subcutaneous adipose tissue.

horny

Kerato/genesis (**ker″ə-to-jen′ə-sis**) is the formation of keratin, a
_____ material.

16-5 The dermis, also called the corium (**kor′e-əm**), is the thicker layer of the skin. It is a noncellular connective tissue that is composed of collagen and elastic fibers that provide strength and flexibility. The dermis contains numerous blood vessels, nerves, and glands. Hair follicles also are embedded in this layer. Which layer of the skin is thicker, the epidermis or the dermis?

dermis

_____.

The upper region of the dermis has many finger-like projections. The ridges marking the outermost layer of the skin are caused by the size and arrangement of these projections. The ridge patterns on the fingertips and thumbs (fingerprints) are different for each person.

16-6 Locate the subcutaneous (**sub″ku-ta′ne-əs**) adipose (**ad′ĭ-pōs**) tissue in Figure 16-1. Sub/cutaneous means _____ the skin.

below

The subcutaneous adipose layer lies just under the dermis. It serves as a cushion against shock and insulates the body. The combining form adip(o) means fat. Adipose means pertaining to

fat

_____.

Both the dermis and the subcutaneous fat layer become thinner as a result of decreased blood flow that occurs with aging. Decreased tone and elasticity lead to wrinkles, and thin, transparent skin is more susceptible to injury.

16-7 The skin is derived from a tissue layer called ectoderm (**ek′to-dərm**) that forms during embryonic development. Sense receptors of the skin, as well as other parts of the nervous system, are also derived from ectoderm.

Soon after fertilization, the fertilized egg undergoes cell division, producing a ball of cells that eventually differentiates into three distinct layers: endoderm (**en′do-dərm**), mesoderm (**mez′o-dərm**), and ectoderm. The suffix -*derm* means either skin or a germ layer. Here it is used to refer to a germ layer, a primary layer of cells of the developing embryo from which various organ systems develop.

ectoderm

Endo/derm, meso/derm, and ectoderm are the innermost, middle, and outermost germ layers, respectively. Skin is derived from which germ layer? _____

16-8 Remembering that derm(a) and dermat(o) mean skin, a dermato/logist (**dər″mə-tol′o-jist**) is a physician who specializes in the skin. Another combining form, cutane(o), also means skin.

dermatology
(**dər″mə-tol′o-je**)

Which specialty is practiced by a dermatologist? _____.

Accessory Skin Structures

16-9 The accessory skin structures include hair, nails, sebaceous (**sə-ba′shəs**) glands, and sweat glands. They are embedded in the dermis.

Hair protects the scalp from injury, eyebrows and eyelashes protect the eyes, and hair in the nostrils and external ear canal protects these structures from dust and insects. The differing distribution of hair in male and female individuals is controlled by hormones. At puberty, hair develops in the armpit and pubic regions and, in the male, on the face and other parts of the body. Two combining

trich(o)

forms that mean hair are pil(o) and _____.

16-10 The combining form *axill(o)* means axilla (**ak-sil′ə**) or armpit. Hair develops in the axill/ary region at puberty. The axillary (**ak′sĭ-lar″e**) region is the area of the

armpit
axillary

_____.

Write the word that means pertaining to the armpit: _____.

16-11 Observe the structure of a hair in Figure 16-2. The hair root is embedded in the dermis and is the portion of the hair below the surface. The shaft protrudes above the surface of the skin, or

epidermis

above what layer? _____

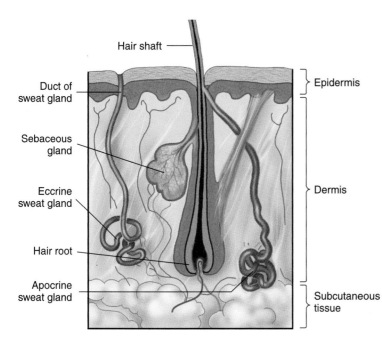

Hair shaft

Duct of
sweat gland

Sebaceous
gland

Eccrine
sweat gland

Hair root

Apocrine
sweat gland

Epidermis

Dermis

Subcutaneous
tissue

Figure 16-2   The structure of hair and associated glands. The hair shaft extends beyond the surface of the epidermis, and the root is the portion of the hair that is below the surface of the skin. Straight hair occurs when the hair shaft is round; wavy, if it is oval; curly or kinky, if it is flat. Hair can be cut without pain because it contains no nerves. The cuticle is the outermost covering and is the part that wears away at the tip of the shaft, resulting in split ends. Two types of glands (sebaceous glands and apocrine sweat glands) have ducts that open into hair follicles, and their secretions are transported to the skin surface. Stimulation of the eccrine sweat glands causes perspiration through ducts that open onto the surface of the skin. This is the single most important factor in the regulation of body temperature.

The arrector pili (ə-rek′tər pi′li) muscles contract under stresses of cold or fright, straighten the hair follicles, and raise the hairs, producing goose bumps or gooseflesh. Observing Figure 16-2, the name of the two glands that are directly connected with the hair follicle are the apocrine (ap′o-krin) sweat gland and the _____ gland.

sebaceous

16-12 Most sebaceous glands are structurally associated with hair follicles, but those of the eyelids, nipple, and genitalia are freestanding. Sebaceous glands are found in all areas of the body that have hair. Sebum (se′bəm), the oily material secreted by the sebaceous gland, keeps hair and skin soft and pliable and also inhibits growth of bacteria on the skin. Write the combining form that means sebum, the oily material for which sebaceous glands are named:
_____.

seb(o)

16-13 Another type of gland found in the skin is a sweat* gland or sudoriferous (soo″do-rif′ər-əs) gland. Another name for a sudoriferous gland is a _____ gland. Sweat glands are found in most parts of the skin, being most numerous in the palms and soles.

sweat

Look again at Figure 16-2 and study the two types of sweat glands. Those that are associated with the hair follicles interact with bacteria on the skin to produce a characteristic body odor. Sweat glands that are not associated with hair follicles open to the surface of the skin through pores. When stimulated by temperature increases or emotional stress, these glands produce perspiration that evaporates on the skin surface and has a cooling effect.

16-14 Perspiration, or sweat, is the substance produced by the sweat glands. Sweat is a mixture of water, salt, and other waste products. Although elimination of waste is a function of the sweat glands, their principal function is to help regulate body temperature. As sweat evaporates on the skin surface, the skin is cooled and the body temperature is decreased. The principal function of sweat glands is to help regulate body _____.

temperature

16-15 Use hidr(o) to write terms pertaining to sweat. Do not confuse hidr(o) and hydr(o). The combining form hydr(o) means _____, whereas hidr(o) means sweat or perspiration.

water

*Sweat (Latin: sudor).

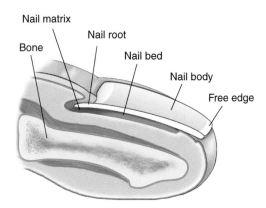

Nail matrix
Nail root
Bone
Nail bed
Nail body
Free edge

Figure 16-3   Structures of the nail. Each nail has a free edge, a nail body (the visible part), and a nail root, which is covered with skin. The nail bed is thickened to form the nail matrix, which is responsible for growth of the nail. The matrix is under the part of the nail body that appears as a whitish, crescent-shaped area called the lunula. Nails appear pinkish because of the rich supply of blood vessels in the underlying dermis.

16-16 Fingernails and toenails, modifications of the horny epidermal (ep″ĭ-dər′məl) cells, are composed of keratin. (See the fingernail components in Figure 16-3. The cuticle is not shown in the illustration.)

Nails are thin plates of dead epidermis that contain a very hard type of keratin, which protects the fingers and toes and helps us pick up small objects. The nail matrix is responsible for growth of the nail and appears as a whitish, crescent-shaped area called the lunula (loo′nu-lə). Nails appear pink because of the rich supply of blood vessels in the underlying dermis.

Onycho/phagia (on″ĭ-ko-fa′jə) is the habit of nail biting. An onycho/phag/ist (on″ĭ-kof′ə-jist) habitually bites the _____ .

nails

nail

16-17 Another combining form, ungu(o), also means nail. It is used to write an adjective, ungual (ung′gwəl), which means pertaining to the _____ .

Exercise 1

Write the meaning of the following word parts:

1. adip(o)   _____

2. axill(o)   _____

3. cutane(o) _____

4. hidr(o)   _____

5. kerat(o) _____

6. onych(o) _____

7. pil(o)   _____

8. seb(o)   _____

9. trich(o) _____

10. ungu(o) _____

11. Name the two layers of the skin: _____ and _____.

12. Name the germ layer from which the skin is derived: _____.

13. Write the name of the oily material secreted by sebaceous glands: _____.

14. Write another term for a sweat gland: _____.

15. Write an adjective that means pertaining to the nail: _____.

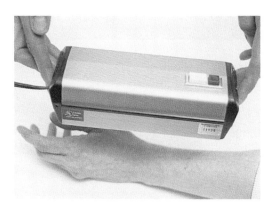

Figure 16-4   A Wood's lamp. This type of lamp is used extensively to help diagnose certain bacterial and fungal infections. The light causes hairs infected with certain microorganisms to become fluorescent.

DIAGNOSTIC TESTS AND PROCEDURES

16-18 Diagnostic tests are generally performed when inspection of the skin is not sufficient to diagnose a suspected condition. Biopsies (bx) are performed to remove samples of lesions if malignancy is suspected. Laboratory cultures are performed to identify the cause of an infection, and skin tests are used to determine the existence of allergies.

Of the diagnostic tests just described, which term means the removal of a small piece of living

biopsy

tissue? _____.

16-19 A skin biopsy may involve removal of part of a lesion, or either a punch biopsy or a shaved specimen. In a punch biopsy, an instrument called a punch is used to remove a small amount of material (at least to the level of the dermis) for microscopic study. A shaved specimen is performed on superficial lesions, using a razor blade to obtain the specimen. Material may also be obtained by curettage (ku″rə-tahzh′), the scraping of material from a lesion using an instrument called a curet (ku-ret′).

Write the name of the procedure that uses a curet to scrape material from a lesion for testing:

curettage

_____.

16-20 Tissue or fluids (obtained by needle aspiration) can be examined microscopically, and bacterial and fungal cultures may be done in an effort to grow the causative organisms in an artificial culture medium to establish the cause of an infection. Special microscopic studies can demonstrate the presence of fungal or bacterial infections and the presence of certain parasites, such as lice. Fungal

fungi

or bacterial infections are those caused by _____ or bacteria.

Some fungi are fluorescent when viewed with a Wood's lamp, an ultraviolet (UV) light that is also called a black lamp (Figure 16-4).

16-21 A skin test is one that is performed to determine the reaction of the body to a substance by observing the results of injecting the substance or applying it to the skin. When it is done to determine if an allergy to a particular substance exists, it is called an allergy test. A tuberculosis (TB) skin test is performed to test for TB infection, but the results can be positive for past as well as current TB infections.

A TB skin test is performed to detect TB infection, and an

allergy

_____ skin test is performed to detect allergic reactions.

16-22 A sweat test is specifically performed to diagnose cystic fibrosis (fi-bro′sis), a congenital disorder that causes abnormally thick secretions of mucus, particularly in the lungs. Increased levels of sodium and chloride are present in the sweat of individuals who have cystic fibrosis, and

sweat

_____ tests are used to diagnose the disorder.

Exercise 2

Write an answer in each blank in the following sentences.

1. The test in which a sample of living tissue is removed for diagnostic purposes is called a _____.

2. Fluids can be removed from a wound by _____ aspiration.

3. A _____ test is one that is done to determine the reaction to a substance by observing the results of injecting the substance or applying it to the skin.

4. A _____ test demonstrates increased levels of sodium and chloride in cystic fibrosis.

✚ PATHOLOGIES

16-23 An important characteristic of skin is its ability to communicate information to the trained observer. Normal skin has an even tone that is free of lesions, bruises, or signs of inflammation (pain, heat, or redness).

You learned that *ex-* means out, without, or away from. Ex/foliation (eks-fo″le-a′shən) is a falling _____ of tissue in scales or layers. Induration (in″du-ra′shən) is hardening of a tissue, especially the skin, and is usually caused by edema and inflammation.

away

Learn the following word parts and their meanings.

Word Parts Pertaining to Skin Pathologies and Treatments

COMBINING FORM	MEANING	COMBINING FORM	MEANING
cry(o)	cold	rhytid(o)	wrinkle
heli(o)	sun	seps(o), sept(o)*	infection
erythemat(o)	erythema or redness	xer(o)	dry
follicul(o)	follicle		
ichthy(o)	fish	**SUFFIX**	
necr(o)	dead or death	-phoresis	transmission

*Sometimes sept(o) means septum.

16-24 The skin is a reflection of the general health of a person. It can be excessively red in high blood pressure and other conditions involving dilation of the blood vessels. How might the skin appear in anemia? _____

pale

Severe heart or lung disease may cause cyanosis (si″ə-no′sis), in which the skin would appear _____. Unusually yellow skin suggests the presence of greater than the normal amount of bile pigment in the blood (jaundice).

bluish

16-25 A partial or total absence of pigment in the skin, hair, and eyes is called albinism (al′bǐ-niz-əm). Albinism is present at birth (see Figure 4-4). There is an absence of normal pigmentation caused by a defect in melanin precursors. In albinism, lack of pigmentation is implied by albin(o), which means _____. Sometimes the skin and eyes appear pinkish. An albin/o (al-bi′no) is a person affected with albinism.

white

16-26 Ichthy/osis (ik″the-o′sis) is a condition in which the skin is dry and scaly, resembling fish skin. The combining form *ichthy(o)* means fish. Ichthy/oid (ik′the-oid) means resembling a fish.

Some forms of ichthyosis, but not all, are hereditary. Ichthyosis is any of several generalized skin disorders marked by dryness and scaliness, resembling _____ skin.

fish

16-27 A mild, nonhereditary form of ichthyosis is called xero/derma (zēr″o-der′mə). Xero/derma literally means dry skin. Write the name of this mild form of ichthyosis, characterized by roughness and dryness of the skin: _____.

xeroderma

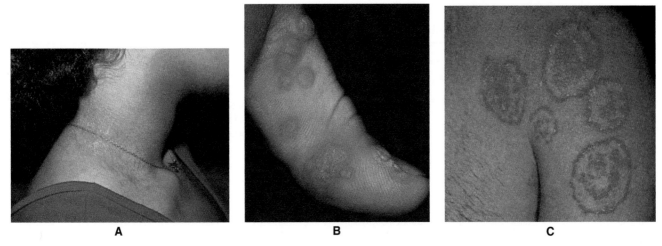

Figure 16-5   Three types of dermatitis. **A,** Nickel dermatitis is a type of contact dermatitis. **B,** A verruca, commonly called a wart, has a rough surface and is caused by a virus. **C,** Ringworm, a superficial fungal infection of the nonhairy skin of the body, which is named for circular lesions.

xerosis (zēr-o′sis)	**16-28** Using *-osis*, write a word that means any dry condition: _____. This word may refer to abnormal dryness, as of the eye, skin, or mouth, but it is sometimes used to mean excessive dryness of the skin. Dry skin is vulnerable to scaling, thinning, and injury.
pediculosis	**16-29** The skin can serve as a host to several parasitic diseases. Pediculosis (pə-dik″u-lo′sis) refers to infestation by human lice and is named for a genus of sucking lice, *Pediculus*. There are head lice, body lice, and pubic lice. Write the name of this disease that means infestation with lice: _____.
erythematosus	**16-30** Skin changes may be related to specific skin diseases but also may reflect an underlying systemic disorder. Discoid lupus erythematosus (DLE) is a disease primarily of the skin. This chronic disorder is characterized by lesions that are covered with scales. The disorder was so named because of the reddish facial rash that appears in some patients, giving them a wolflike appearance (see Figure 7-14). The combining form *erythemat(o)* means erythema, or redness. Erythema is redness (example, blushing) or inflammation of the skin (example, sunburn) or mucous membranes that is the result of dilation of the superficial capillaries. Write the name of the disorder that is believed to be a problem of autoimmunity: discoid lupus _____.
hardened	**16-31** Sclero/derma (sklēr″o-der′mə) means hardening and thickening of the skin, a finding in various diseases. Literal translation of scleroderma is _____ skin. Systemic scleroderma is an autoimmune disorder of the connective tissue.

■ *Dermatitis and Skin Infections*

skin	**16-32** Dermat/itis (der″mə-ti′tis) is an inflammatory condition of the _____. It may be acute or chronic and is a very general term that applies to any type of inflammation of the skin, including skin infections. A superficial dermatitis, inflammation on the surface of the skin, is called eczema (ek′zə-mə).
light	**16-33** Contact dermatitis is a skin rash resulting from exposure to an irritant or antigen. Figure 16-5 A shows the appearance of the skin of a person who is allergic to a necklace that contains nickel. Sunburn is a type of dermatitis that results from overexposure to the sun. Remembering that phot(o) means light, the literal translation of photodermatitis (fo″to-der″mə-ti′tis) is inflammation of the skin caused by _____. Photodermatitis is an abnormal skin reaction to light and is a common symptom of DLE.

TABLE 16-1 Skin Eruptions Caused by Infectious Organisms

Bacterial	Fungal	Viral
Erysipelas	Candidiasis	Herpes simplex type 1 fever blisters
Furuncles (boils) and carbuncles	Onychomycosis	Herpes zoster (shingles)
Impetigo	Tinea capitis (ringworm of scalp)	Rubella (German measles)
Leprosy	Tinea corporis (generalized)	Rubeola (measles)
Lyme disease	Tinea pedis (athlete's foot)	Varicella (chickenpox)
Meningococcemia		Verrucae (warts)
Paronychia (infection of marginal structures around nail)		
Scarlet fever		
Syphilis		

Complete definitions of the terms can be found in the Index/Glossary.

scabies

16-34 <u>Scabies</u> (**ska′bēz**) is a contagious dermatitis caused by the itch mite and is transmitted by close contact. Write the name of this parasitic disease: _____. The dermatitis results from irritation of the skin by the itch mite and is complicated by scratching caused by the intense itching.

skin

seborrheic

16-35 Seborrheic (**seb″o-re′ik**) dermatitis is an inflammatory condition of the _____ that begins with the scalp but may involve other areas, particularly the eyebrows. <u>Seborrheic dermatitis</u> is commonly called dandruff. The cause is not known, but the sebaceous glands become overactive and the hair and scalp are excessively oily. This skin condition is known as _____ dermatitis.

sebaceous

16-36 <u>Sebo/rrhea</u> (**seb″o-re′ə**) means excessive production of sebum, the oily secretion of the sebaceous glands of the skin. The increased activity of the sebaceous glands at puberty may block the hair follicle and cause blackheads. Bacteria can infect the blocked follicle and result in a pus-filled pimple. Acne, a skin disease common where sebaceous glands are most numerous (face, chest, and upper back), is characterized by blackheads, whiteheads, pimples, nodules, and cysts. (See frame 16-41 for more information about nodules and cysts.) Acne is also called acne vulgaris (**vəl-ga′ris**). Pimples result from bacterial infection of blocked _____ glands.

pyogenesis

16-37 Three words that mean the production of pus are <u>suppuration</u> (**sup″u-ra′shən**), <u>purulence</u> (**pu′roo-ləns**), and <u>pyogenesis</u> (**pi″o-jen′ə-sis**). It is important to remember the meanings of suppuration and purulence, although they do not contain word parts that you necessarily recognize. Like _____, suppuration and purulence mean production of pus.

A <u>furuncle</u> (**fu′rung-kəl**), commonly called a boil, is a localized suppurative (**sup′u-ra″tiv**) infection that begins with infection of a hair follicle or sebaceous gland by pathogenic staphylococci.

verruca

16-38 Skin infections are caused by specific types of bacteria, viruses, and fungi. A <u>verruca</u> (**və-roo′kə**) is a benign warty skin lesion (wart) with a rough surface, caused by a common contagious virus (see Figure 16-5 B). The term for a wart is a _____.

herpes

<u>Herpes simplex virus</u> (HSV) infection is the most common viral infection of adult skin. Type 1 (HSV 1) causes the classic <u>fever blisters</u>. Another type of herpes virus, <u>herpes zoster</u>, causes <u>shingles</u> and occurs with reactivation of the herpes virus in individuals who have previously had chickenpox. The cause of fever blisters is an infection with the type 1 _____ simplex virus. HSV 1 is not to be confused with HSV 2, which causes genital herpes infections that are generally limited to the genital region.

fungus

16-39 A superficial fungal infection is called a <u>dermato/myc/osis</u> (**dər″mə-to-mi-ko′sis**) or <u>myco/dermat/itis</u> (**mi″ko-der″mə-ti′tis**). Either of these terms means a skin infection caused by a _____. Ringworm, or tinea, is a group of dermatomycoses that can affect various parts of the body (see Figure 16-5 C).

Several skin infections caused by infectious microorganism are presented in Table 16-1.

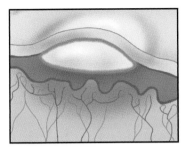

A cyst is a sac filled with fluid or semi-solid material.

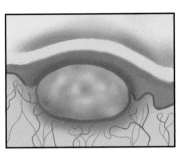

A nodule is a marble-like, solid lesion more than 1 cm wide and deep.

Figure 16-6   Schematic drawing of two types of lesions in cross section. Palpation will usually distinguish between a fluid-filled cyst and a solid nodule.

Exercise 3

Match skin conditions in the left column with their characteristics in the right column.

_____ 1. albinism

_____ 2. dermatitis

_____ 3. ichthyosis

_____ 4. pediculosis

_____ 5. scleroderma

_____ 6. seborrheic dermatitis

_____ 7. xeroderma

A. absence of pigment in the skin, hair, and eyes
B. any inflammatory condition of the skin
C. autoimmune condition that often causes hard and thickened skin
D. dandruff
E. infestation by human lice
F. dry, scaly skin
G. rough, dry skin

■ Skin Lesions

pus

16-40 A skin <u>lesion</u> is any visible, local abnormality of the tissues of the skin, such as a sore, a rash, or a tumor. Most skin lesions are benign, but one type is among the most malignant of all kinds of cancer.

Trauma, such as cuts, punctures, or burns, exposes the underlying tissue to infection. Climate, hygiene, and general health also play a part. An <u>abscess</u> (**ab′ses**) is any pus-containing cavity that is surrounded by inflamed tissue and is usually caused by infection with staphylo/cocci. Healing usually occurs when the abscess drains or is incised. <u>Staphylococci</u>, often abbreviated Staph, are pyo/genic bacteria, which means they produce _____.

nodule (**nod′ūl**)

16-41 Observe the two types of lesions shown in Figure 16-6. Both a <u>cyst</u> and a <u>nodule</u> cause a raised area of the overlying skin, but the cyst is filled with fluid or a semisolid material, whereas the _____ is solid.

macule (**mak′ūl**)

papule

16-42 Examine the appearance of other types of lesions presented in Figure 16-7. The lesions are <u>primary lesions</u> because they are initial reactions to an underlying problem. A freckle is a nonraised, small dark spot on the skin, so it is called a _____.

Both <u>papules</u> (**pap′ūlz**) and <u>plaques</u> (**plaks**) are elevated and circumscribed, but which type is less than 1 cm in diameter? _____. A small mole is a papule. Dandruff represents a type of plaque.

<u>Vesicles</u> (**ves′ĭ-kəlz**), <u>bullae</u> (**bul′e**), and <u>pustules</u> (**pus′tūlz**) are blister-like and contain fluid. Note that the singular form of bullae is bulla (**bul′ə**). The lesions of acne are filled with pus, so they are called _____.

pustules

bullae

Vesicles and bullae are differentiated by size. Which type of lesion is larger? _____.

16-43 <u>Urticaria</u> (**ur″tĭ-kar′e-ə**) is an allergic skin eruption characterized by transient, elevated, irregularly-shaped lesions that are called <u>wheals</u> (**hwēlz, wēlz**). Treatment includes antihistamines and removal of the stimulus or allergen. The name for this allergic skin reaction, also called <u>hives</u>, is

urticaria

_____ (Figure 16-8).

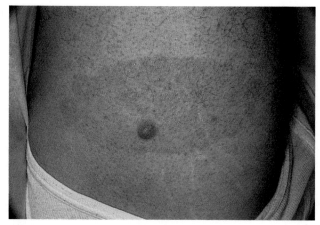

Macules
Nonraised, discolored spots less than 1 cm in diameter

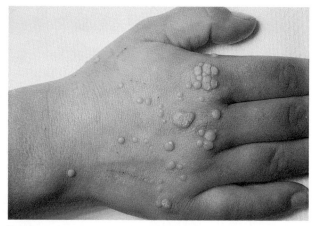

Papules
Elevated lesions less than 1 cm in diameter

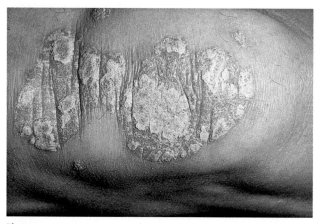

Plaques
Elevated and circumscribed patches more than 1 cm in diameter

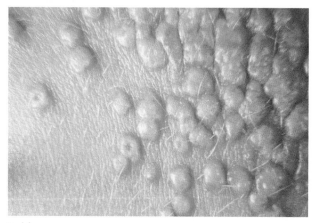

Vesicles
Blisters less than 1 cm and filled with clear fluid

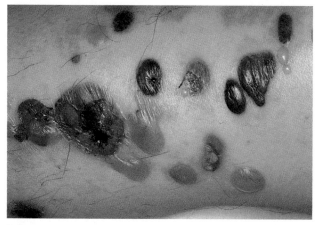

Bullae
Blisters greater than 1 cm and filled with clear fluid.

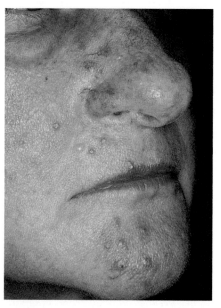

Pustules
Vesicles filled with cloudy fluid or pus

Figure 16-7   Primary lesions of the skin. These are initial reactions to an underlying problem that alters one of the structural components of the skin.

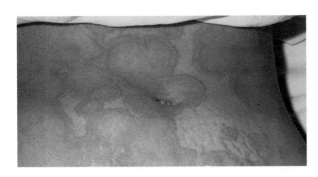

Figure 16-8 Wheals. This elevated, irregularly shaped lesion is seen in urticaria (hives), an allergic skin eruption. Notice the irregular shape, which is caused by edema.

16-44 <u>Secondary lesions</u> are changes in the appearance of the primary lesion and can occur with normal progression of the disease. See Figure 16-9 and use the accompanying information to write words in the blanks in this frame. A/trophy (**at′rə-fe**) of the skin is characterized by thinning with loss of skin markings. Stretch marks are an example of atrophy.

Deep, irregular erosions that extend into the dermis are called

ulcers   _____.

Athlete's foot produces linear cracks in the epidermis that are examples of

fissures (**fish′ərz**)   _____.

16-45 <u>Dried</u> serum, sebum, blood, or pus on the skin surface produces a <u>crust</u>. Crusts frequently result from broken vesicles, bullae, or pustules.

<u>Scales</u> are dried fragments of sloughed epidermis. They appear dry and irregular in size and shape and are usually whitish. They are frequently seen in <u>psoriasis</u> (**sə-ri′ə-sis**), a common chronic skin disease characterized by circumscribed red patches covered by thick, dry, silvery scales (Figure 16-10 A).

<u>Petechiae</u>* (**pə-te′ke-e**) are tiny purple or red spots appearing on the skin as a result of tiny hemorrhages within the dermal or submucosal layers (see Figure 16-10 B). They are flush with the skin and range in size from pinpoint to pinhead size. Write the term for the spots that result from tiny

petechiae   hemorrhages in the skin: _____.

An <u>ecchymosis</u> (**ek″ĭ-mo′sis**) is a hemorrhagic spot, larger than a petechia. It forms a nonelevated blue or purplish patch (see Figure 16-10 C). Write the term for this large hemorrhagic spot:

ecchymosis   _____.

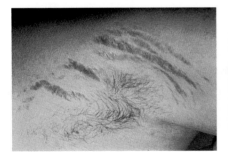

Atrophy
Wasting of the epidermis; skin appears thin and transparent

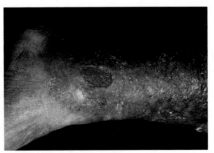

Ulcer
Irregularly shaped erosions that extend into the dermis

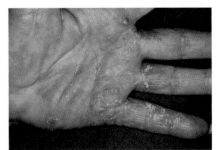

Fissures
Deep linear splits through the epidermis into the dermis

Figure 16-9 Secondary lesions of the skin. The linear lines of atrophy, ulcerations, and fissures result from changes in the initial skin lesion.

*Petechiae (Italian: *petecchie*, flea bite).

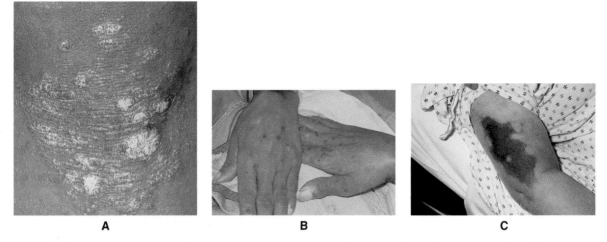

A   **B**   **C**

Figure 16-10   Common benign disorders of the skin. **A,** Psoriasis is characterized by circumscribed red patches covered by thick, dry, silvery scales. **B,** Petechiae appear on the skin as a result of tiny hemorrhages beneath the surface. **C,** An ecchymosis is a hemorrhagic spot.

nevus

tumor

16-46 A new growth of tissue characterized by a disordered growth of cells is a tumor, also called a neoplasm. Several benign tumors have already been mentioned, for example, warts and moles. Another term for a mole is a nevus (ne′vəs); the plural is nevi (ne′vi). Write the term that means a mole: _____.

16-47 The combining form lip(o) means fats. A lip/oma (lip-o′mə) is a common, benign _____ consisting of mature fat cells that usually can be removed easily by excision.

A kerat/oma (ker″ə-to′mə), also called a callus, is a flat, poorly defined mass, often on the sole over a bony prominence, and is caused by pressure. A corn is also caused by pressure or friction but, unlike a callus, is round or conical and usually painful.

16-48 Kerat/osis (ker″ə-to′sis) is a condition of the skin characterized by the formation of horny growths or excessive development of the epithelium. One type of keratosis, sebo/rrhe/ic keratosis (seb″o-re′ik ker″ə-to′sis), is a consequence of aging. The lesion of seborrheic keratosis is a common benign lesion that may occur anywhere on the body of an older person, but it is more commonly found on the face, neck, upper trunk, and arms (Figure 16-11). Lesions such as this, with well-defined edges and definite boundaries, are described as circumscribed lesions because it would be possible to draw a circle around a lesion of this type.

Figure 16-11   Seborrheic keratoses. Numerous seborrheic keratoses are present, some of which are deeply pigmented with melanin. The large lesions show the characteristic stuck-on appearance. Seborrheic keratoses are benign tumors that can be removed by curettage, cryosurgery, and application of caustic agents.

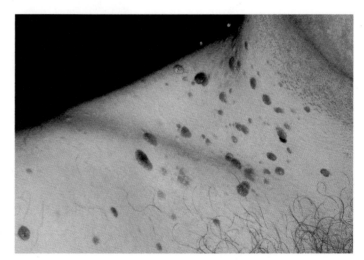

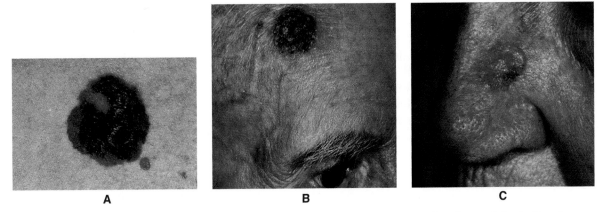

Figure 16-12 Three common types of skin cancer. **A,** Malignant melanoma. **B,** Squamous cell carcinoma. **C,** Basal cell carcinoma.

actinic

Actinic keratosis* (**ak-tin´ik ker″ə-to´sis**) is a premalignant lesion that is common in people with chronically sun-damaged skin. Write the name of the type of keratosis that is considered a premalignant lesion: _____ keratosis. These premalignant lesions may progress to skin cancer if the lesions are not removed. They are usually treated, because this type of keratosis can progress to squamous cell carcinoma.

16-49 Basal and squamous cell cancers are common types of skin cancer that are rarely invasive. In other words, they rarely spread to other organs. One type of skin cancer that is included in cancer statistics is malignant melanoma. Because about half of malignant melanomas (**mel″ə-no´məz**) arise from moles, nevi with irregular edges or variegated colors are usually removed and examined to determine whether they are malignant melanomas. Literal interpretation of melan/oma is a black

tumor

_____.

A malignant melanoma, often shortened to melanoma, is a pigmented neoplasm that originates in the skin and is composed of melano/cytes (**mel´ə-no-sītz, mə-lan´o-sītz**). It is highly metastatic, one of the most malignant of all skin cancers, and causes a high mortality rate in affected individuals. Figure 16-12 shows a melanoma with two other common types of skin cancer. Squamous cell carcinoma, basal cell carcinoma, and malignant melanoma are all types of skin

cancer (or carcinoma)

_____.

16-50 Kaposi's sarcoma (**kah´po-shēz, kap´o-sēz sahr-ko´mə**) is the most common malignancy associated with acquired immunodeficiency syndrome (AIDS). The lesions are small, purplish-brown papules that spread throughout the skin, the lymph nodes, and the internal organs. Other disorders associated with this lesion include diabetes and malignant lymphoma. The name of the

Kaposi's

lesion is _____ sarcoma (see Figure 13-10 B).

Exercise 4

Match skin lesions in the left column with their characteristics in the right column.

_____ 1. bulla

_____ 2. cyst

_____ 3. fissure

_____ 4. macule

_____ 5. papule

_____ 6. pustule

A. blister, larger than 1 cm
B. crack in the skin
C. discolored spot, not elevated
D. fluid-filled sac containing pus
E. sac filled with clear fluid
F. solid elevation, less than 0.5 cm in diameter

*Actinic (Greek: *aktis*, ray).

■ *Injuries to the Skin*

16-51 A <u>wound</u> is a physical injury involving a break in the skin, usually caused by an act or accident other than a disease. Some examples of wounds are puncture wounds, stab wounds, skin scrapes, and burns.

　　A <u>pressure ulcer</u> is a special type of injury to the skin that occurs almost exclusively in people with limited mobility. Also called bedsores or <u>decubitus ulcers</u> (**de-ku′bĭ-təs ul′sərz**), these sores occur as a result of mechanical trauma and lack of adequate blood circulation to the affected area. Once formed, they are slow to heal. Ulcerations that occur almost exclusively in persons with

pressure or decubitus | limited mobility are called _____ ulcers.

16-52 The skin is subject to many injuries because it serves as the external covering and the part of the body that is exposed to the external environment. Trauma to the skin and underlying tissues requires healing to repair the defect, whether the wound was created by a surgical incision or an accident. A surgical incision generally heals faster than other wounds because it is performed aseptically (free of infection) and minimal damage is done to the tissue by the sharp instrument.

　　The combining forms seps(o) and sept(o) mean infection. A/septic means free of pathogenic

infected | organisms or _____ material.

16-53 A <u>laceration</u> (**las″ər-a′shən**) is a torn, jagged wound. A <u>puncture</u> is a wound made by piercing. Skin is scraped or rubbed away by friction in an <u>abrasion</u> (**ə-bra′zhən**). One type of injury, a <u>contusion</u> (**kən-too′zhən**), is caused by a blow to the body that causes subcutaneous bleeding and does not disrupt the integrity of the skin. A contusion is called a bruise and is characterized by swelling, discoloration, and pain.

laceration | 　　A torn, jagged wound is called a _____, whereas a wound that is made by piercing is called a puncture.

abrasion | 　　When skin is scraped away by friction, it is called an _____.

16-54 A mark that is left by healing of a lesion where excess collagen was produced to replace the injured tissue is called a <u>scar</u>. Excessive overgrowth of unsightly scar tissue, called a <u>keloid</u> (**ke′loid**), occurs in some individuals, especially black individuals. Write the word that means overgrowth of

keloid | scar tissue: _____.

16-55 <u>Burns</u> are tissue injuries resulting from excessive exposure to heat, electricity, chemicals, radiation, or gases, in which the extent of the injury is determined by the amount of exposure and the nature of the agent that causes the burn. The magnitude of the injury is based on the depth and extent of the <u>total body surface area</u> (TBSA) that is burned.

　　In the past, burns were classified into first-, second-, third-, and fourth-degree injuries. Currently, the American Burn Association (ABA) advocates categorizing the burn injury according to the depth of tissue destruction as <u>partial-thickness (superficial or deep)</u> and <u>full-thickness (third or fourth degree)</u>. Study Figure 16-13 and read the descriptions of skin layer destruction and appearances of the burns.

　　In comparing superficial partial-thickness burns and full-thickness burns, the

full | _____-thickness burns destroy deeper layers of tissue.

　　The superficial burn does not extend beyond which layer of skin?

epidermis | _____

　　In a deep partial-thickness burn, damage does not extend beyond which layer of skin?

dermis | _____

deep | 　　Muscle and bone are exposed in a _____ full-thickness burn.

partial | 　　Which type of burn is characterized by blisters? deep _____-thickness burn.

16-56 Burned tissue usually represents various levels of damage. In addition to the burn depth, burn severity takes into consideration factors such as the size and location of the burn, mechanism of injury, duration and intensity of the burn, and the age and health of the individual. The very young and older persons are at greatest risk. The magnitude of the burn is determined by how much

surface | of the TBSA is affected. TBSA means total body _____ area.

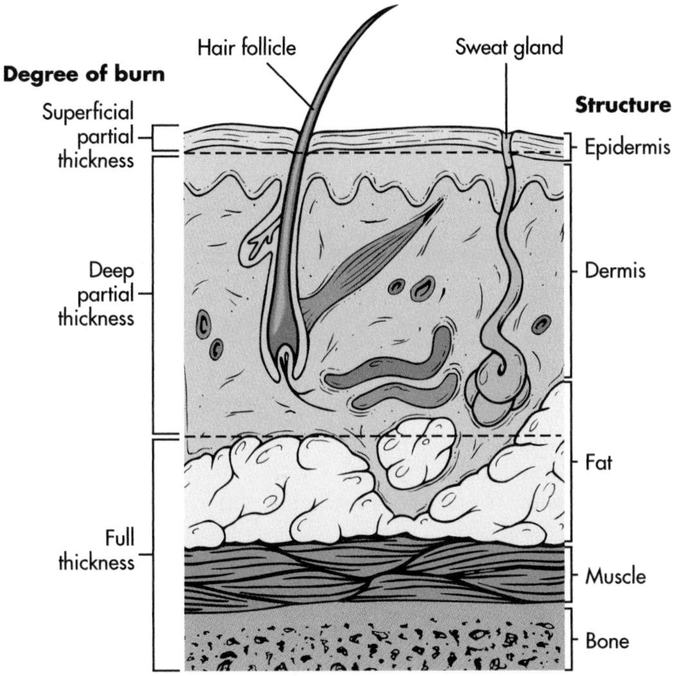

Degree of burn	Structure
Superficial partial thickness	Epidermis
Deep partial thickness	Dermis
Full thickness	Fat
	Muscle
	Bone

Hair follicle   Sweat gland

Type of Burn	Dermal Layers Involved	Appearance of the Skin
Partial-thick: Superficial (1st degree)	Only the epidermis.	Red, no immediate blisters, but may blister after 24 hours.
Deep partial-thickness (2nd degree)	Extends into the dermis.	Red and moist, blistered.
Full-thickness: (3rd degree)	Throughout the dermis and epidermis, sometimes into subcutaneous fat layer.	Hard, dry, and leathery. White, deep red, yellow, brown to black.
Deep: (4th degree)	No skin layers remain. Underlying bone and muscle are damaged.	Wound is blackened and depressed. Muscle and bone are exposed.

Figure 16-13 Cross section of skin indicating the degree of burn and structures involved.

Serious burn injuries can result in systemic disturbances, including fluid and protein losses, and abnormalities in many body systems. In addition, infection is a serious threat when the skin is destroyed and can no longer protect the underlying tissues from microorganisms. Another term for infection is sepsis (**sep′sis**).

16-57 <u>Frostbite</u> is damage to skin, tissues, and blood vessels as a result of prolonged exposure to cold. The extent of injury depends largely on the intensity and the duration of the exposure. Because injury is greater in hypoxic tissue, the individual's health affects the severity of injury. Hyp/oxia (**hi-pok′se-ə**) means a condition in which the amount of oxygen is

below

frostbite

_____ normal.
Damage to tissue as a result of exposure to cold is called _____.

16-58 <u>Necr/osis</u> (**nə-kro′sis**) is localized tissue death that occurs in response to disease or injury, in other words, death of areas of tissue or bone surrounded by healthy parts. When tissue is badly damaged, it becomes necro/tic (**nə-krot′ik**). The combining form *necr(o)* means dead or death. Necro/tic describes a characteristic of tissue that has been broken down. Necrotic tissue is

dead

_____ tissue.

■ *Disorders of Accessory Skin Structures*

16-59 Pathologies also occur with the hair, nails, sebaceous glands, and sweat glands.
Use trich(o) to write a term that means any disease of the hair:

trichopathy
(**trĭ-kop′ə-the**)

_____.

16-60 Infections in intact skin often involve the hair follicles, where bacteria easily accumulate and grow well. <u>Follicul/itis</u> (**fo-lik″u-li′tis**) is a term that refers to superficial bacterial infection involving the hair follicles, and it uses the combining form follicul(o), which means follicle. Write the term that means inflammation of the hair follicles: _____.

folliculitis

Without treatment, folliculitis can progress to <u>cellul/itis</u> (**sel″u-li′tis**), a localized bacterial invasion of subcutaneous tissue. Cellulitis can also occur independently of folliculitis and is characterized by pain, heat, swelling, and redness.

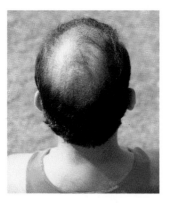

Figure 16-14   Alopecia prematura. This man is in his early 30s and is experiencing premature baldness.

condition

16-61 The literal translation of <u>trich/osis</u> (**tri-ko′sis**) is an abnormal
_____ of the hair. Its extended meaning is abnormal growth or
development of hair in an unusual place.

alopecia

16-62 An equally important problem is loss of hair. Baldness is <u>alopecia</u> (**al″o-pe′she-ə**). Write this
new word for baldness: _____.
   <u>Alopecia prematura</u> is baldness that occurs early in life (Figure 16-14).

onychopathy
  (**on″ĭ-kop′ə-the**)
fungus

16-63 Use onych(o) to write a term that means any disease of the nails:
_____. <u>Onych/osis</u> (**on″ĭ-ko′sis**) is atrophy or other unhealthy condition of the nails, often caused by a fungal infection. <u>Onycho/myc/osis</u> (**on″ĭ-ko-mi-ko′sis**) is a
condition of the nails resulting from a _____.
   <u>Onychomalacia</u> (**on″ĭ-ko-mə-la′shə**) is abnormal softening of the nails.

sweat

16-64 <u>Hidr/aden/itis</u> (**hi″drad-ə-ni′tis**) is inflammation of a
_____ gland. (Hidr[o] loses the "o" when joined with aden[o].)
   A chronic form of hidradenitis is caused by closure of the pores with secondary bacterial infection of apocrine sweat glands, chiefly in the axillary and anogenital areas. It is characterized by
the development of a tender red abscess that enlarges and eventually breaks through the skin or
forms a cyst.

transmission

16-65 <u>Dia/phoresis</u> (**di″ə-fə-re′sis**) means excessive sweating. The suffix *-phoresis* means transmission. Translated literally, dia/phoresis means _____ through, so
you will need to remember that diaphoresis means excessive sweating (or perspiration).
   Perspiration is only one means of ridding the body of excess heat. The level of heat produced
within the body and lost from the body surface is regulated and controlled by the brain.

below

16-66 Prolonged exposure to cold temperatures can lead to <u>hypo/thermia</u> (**hi″po-thər′me-ə**), a
condition in which the body temperature is _____ normal.
Literal translation of hypothermia is a condition of less than normal heat.

16-67 Using hypothermia as a model, write a word that means a greatly increased body
temperature: _____.

hyperthermia
  (**hi″pər-ther′me-ə**)

16-68 In a healthy person, internal body temperature is maintained within a narrow range by the
brain, resulting in a balance between generation and conservation of heat. <u>Pyrexia</u> (**pi-rek′se-ə**),
or fever, is an increased body temperature that is mediated by an increase in the heat regulatory set
point. In contrast, hyperthermia overrides or bypasses normal heat regulation. <u>Heat stroke</u> and
<u>sunstroke</u> are examples of hyperthermia. These conditions are caused by prolonged exposure to
excessive heat or the sun and may be life-threatening. <u>Thermo/plegia</u> (**thər″mo-ple′jə**) is
another name for heatstroke or sunstroke. Translated literally, thermoplegia means heat

paralysis

_____.

Exercise 5

Write a word in each blank to complete these sentences.

1. An _____ is a cavity that contains pus.

2. A _____ is commonly called a boil.

3. Another name for a wart is a _____.

4. A mycodermatitis is a superficial _____ infection of the skin.

5. Tiny purple or red spots that result from tiny hemorrhages within the dermal or submucosal layers are called _____.

6. Another name for a mole is a _____.

7. A condition of the skin characterized by the formation of horny growths or excessive development of the horny growth is called a _____.

8. A common, benign tumor consisting of mature fat cells is called a _____.

9. The most common lesion associated with AIDS is _____ sarcoma.

10. In a deep partial-thickness burn, damage does not extend beyond the layer of skin called the _____.

SURGICAL AND THERAPEUTIC INTERVENTIONS

16-69 Most surgical procedures involving the skin are for the purposes of repairing or treating damaged skin, removing lesions, or penetrating the skin to perform diagnostic or surgical procedures.

Superficial wounds often heal without suturing (**soo′chər-ing**). Deep wounds with gaping edges or wounds located over joints where movement opens the cut edges are generally sutured to stop the bleeding, hold the tissue together, and enhance the healing process. Dermabond is an adhesive spray that is used for closing certain wounds, but deep wounds generally require

suturing   _____.

16-70 A skin graft is transplantation of skin to cover areas where skin has been lost through a burn or other trauma, or to replace diseased skin that has been removed. If the graft is from the patient's own body, it is called an autograft (**aw′to-graft**), for which the literal translation is

self   _____ graft.

An allograft (**al′o-graft**) is a graft of tissue between two genetically different individuals of the same species.

16-71 A skin flap is a special type of skin graft that involves moving a section of skin to a nearby area without cutting off the end of the transplanted tissue. This is done to leave some of the blood circulation intact.

skin   A derma/tome is used to cut thin slices of _____ for grafting.

16-72 Severe burns of the arms or legs can require amputation (**am″pu-ta′shən**), the surgical removal of a limb or part of the body. All depths of burns except superficial partial-thickness burns may involve skin grafting.

Histo/compatibility (**his″to-kəm-pat″ĭ-bil′ĭ-te**) is necessary for a successful transplant of any organ or tissue. Histo/compatibility means that the transplanted _____ is

tissue   capable of surviving without ill effects. If the tissue is not compatible, this is called in/compatibility.

16-73 Remembering that top(o) means place, topical (**top′ĭ-kəl**) medications are placed directly on the skin. Topical antimicrobial (**an″te-, an″ti-mi-kro′be-əl**) agents and dressings are applied to injured or burned tissue to prevent infection, and aseptic procedures are followed. A/septic means

without

_____ infection.

16-74 <u>Escharo/tomy</u> (es″kə-rot′ə-me) is a surgical incision into necrotic tissue resulting from a severe burn; it is done to relieve pressure that results from severe swelling.

<u>Débridement</u> (da-brēd-maw′) is the removal of foreign material and dead or damaged tissue, especially from a wound. To <u>débride</u> (da-brēd′) is to remove by dissection. Write this word that means the removal of foreign material or damaged tissue by excision:

débridement

_____.

16-75 Use onych(o) to write a word that means removal (excision) of the nail:

onychectomy
(on″ĭ-kek′tə-me)

_____.

(Declawing of an animal is also called onychectomy.)

16-76 The treatment of lesions depends on the type of lesion. <u>Anti/septics</u> help to clean a wound and inhibit the growth of microorganisms, <u>antibiotics</u> are used to treat infections, and <u>antipruritics</u> (an″te-, an″ti-proo-rit′ikz) relieve or prevent itching. Write the term that means medications that are used to relieve itching: _____.

antipruritics

Boils or other deep suppurative wounds may require <u>incision and drainage</u> (I & D) to relieve pressure and speed healing.

16-77 Topical medications may be found in many forms: <u>aerosols</u>, <u>ointments</u>, <u>liquids</u>, or <u>creams</u>. An aero/sol (ār′o-sol) medication is a liquid that is vaporized and propelled into the

air

_____ by gas under pressure within the container.

An ointment (ung) is a medicated, fatty, soft substance for external application to the body. In

topical

other words, an ointment is for what type of use? _____

feeling

<u>Topical an/esthetics</u> are applied to produce a lack of _____.

16-78 Wart treatments include <u>salicylic acid</u> and <u>electrodesiccation</u> (e-lek″tro-des″ĭ-ka′shən). In

electricity

electro/desiccation, tissue is destroyed by burning with _____.

Warts may also be destroyed by <u>cryo/therapy</u> (kri″o-ther′ə-pe), a technique of exposing tissues to extreme cold to produce well-defined areas of cell destruction.

16-79 <u>Plastic surgery</u> is the replacement or restoration of parts of the body and is performed to correct a structural or cosmetic defect. Increased expenditures on cosmetics, surgery, and other treatments to improve our appearance attest to how we value our physical appearance.

A reconstructive technique in plastic surgery uses <u>collagen injections</u> to enhance the lips or "plump" sagging facial skin. The collagen injections are replacement of the lost collagen and elastic

dermis

from which layer of the skin? _____. This is sometimes used with injections of <u>Botox</u>, a potent bacterial toxin that relaxes facial wrinkles. (Botox often is used to relax the muscles involved in spasms of the eyelid.)

16-80 A combining form that means wrinkle or wrinkles is _rhytid(o)_. <u>Rhytido/plasty</u> (rit′ĭ-do-plas″te) means face-lift. Literal translation of rhytido/plasty means surgical repair for

wrinkles

_____. Skin of the face is tightened, wrinkles are removed, and the skin is made to appear firm and smooth.

16-81 <u>Derm/abrasion</u> (dər″mə-bra′zhən) is a treatment for removing superficial scars on the skin. This physical "sanding of the skin" to reduce facial scars is called

dermabrasion

_____. This procedure is also used to remove tattoos.

Alternatives to dermabrasion are <u>chemical peels</u> or <u>laser</u> destruction of the outermost epidermal layers. Chemical peels use a strong chemical solution to reduce wrinkles, blemishes, and sun-damaged areas of the skin. The top layers peel away, and new, smoother skin layers replace the old ones.

16-82 It may seem natural to think of excision of a lipoma as <u>lip/ectomy</u> (lĭ-pek′tə-me); however, this is incorrect. Lipectomy originally meant excision of a mass of subcutaneous fat tissue, as from the abdominal wall. The term has been extended to mean removal of fat from the neck, legs, arms,

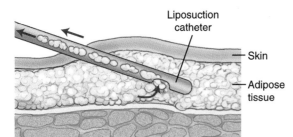

Liposuction
catheter

— Skin

— Adipose
tissue

Figure 16-15 Liposuction. This procedure, also called suction lipectomy, removes adipose tissue with a suction pump device.

belly, and elsewhere by placing a narrow tube under the skin and applying a vacuum. The suction pulls the fat loose. This suction lipectomy is called <u>liposuction</u> (**lip″o-suk′shən**).

fat

Lipo/suction removes adipose tissue with a suction pump device, and it is used primarily as cosmetic surgery to remove or reduce localized areas of _____ (Figure 16-15).

16-83 <u>Electro/lysis</u> (**e″lek-trol′ə-sis**) is sometimes used to destroy the hair follicles when hair is growing in an undesirable place. By its word parts, you know that electro/lysis is

destruction

_____ of a substance by passing electrical current through it. Most electrolysis is done for aesthetic reasons, for example, getting rid of facial hair.

16-84 The most popular aesthetic plastic surgery for male individuals is <u>hair transplantation</u>. Grafts or plugs of skin containing hair follicles are transplanted from some part of the body to the head. An oral medication is effective in restoring hair in certain types of hair loss but must be taken the remainder of one's life to prevent hair loss. You learned earlier of different types of skin grafts. Which type of graft is transplantation of hair from one part of the body to another?

autograft

_____.

16-85 Treatment of acne includes the use of topical and oral antibiotics. Topical antibiotics are

skin

applied directly to the _____. <u>Topical and oral retinoids</u> (**ret′ĭ-noidz**) are also used. Retinoids are compounds that are structurally related to substances that exhibit Vitamin A activity, such as retinal and retinol. Retinoids increase the sloughing of epithelial cells and cause extrusion of blackheads.

16-86 Several physical treatments are available for various skin conditions. <u>UV light therapy</u> is a common physical treatment in psoriasis and other skin conditions. UV radiation, one of the types of energy that is included in sunlight, is more readily accessible and easier to control than exposure to the sun.

treatment

<u>Helio/therapy</u> (**he″le-o-ther′ə-pe**) is _____ of disease by exposing the body to sunlight. The combining form heli(o) means the sun.

16-87 Certain wounds require the use of <u>heat hydro/therapy</u>. By its name, you know that heat

water

hydrotherapy makes use of warm _____.

16-88 The remaining types of physical therapy have to do with treatments for muscle pain, reduction of tissue swelling, or increasing circulation. The skin is involved in many cases, however, because the treatment is delivered through the skin.

<u>Ultrasound</u> is used therapeutically as a penetrating deep-heating agent for soft tissue. Ultrasound

sound

uses high-frequency _____ waves.

Another method of generating heat in soft tissue is <u>diathermy</u> (**di′ə-ther″me**). Both diathermy and ultrasound are used to increase circulation to an inflamed area. Dia/therm/y means passing

heat

high-frequency current through tissue to generate _____ in a particular part of the body.

16-89 Various types of stimulation to the skin and subcutaneous tissue offer pain relief. <u>Trans/cutaneous electrical nerve stimulation</u> (TENS) is one of these methods. Trans/cutaneous means that

skin

the electrical current is delivered across (or through) the _____.

Electrodes are placed over the painful sites, and small amounts of electrical current are delivered to painful areas.

16-90 <u>Transdermal drug delivery</u> is a method of applying a drug to unbroken skin. The drug is absorbed through the skin and then enters the circulatory system. It is used particularly for estrogen, nicotine, and scopolamine (to prevent motion sickness). Not all medications can be administered in this way. Administration of a drug through unbroken skin is called _____ drug delivery.

transdermal

Exercise 6

Match the terms in the surgical list on the left with their descriptions on the right.

_____ 1. allograft

_____ 2. autograft

_____ 3. débridement

_____ 4. escharotomy

_____ 5. liposuction

_____ 6. onychectomy

_____ 7. rhytidoplasty

A. cutting away of dead or damaged tissue in a wound
B. excision of the nail
C. face-lift
D. surgery to remove excess fat
E. surgical incision to relieve pressure after a severe burn
F. tissue graft between two genetically different individuals
G. tissue graft whereby one's tissue is transplanted to another site of one's body

Exercise 7

Match the types of therapy with their characteristics.

_____ 1. diathermy

_____ 2. heat hydrotherapy

_____ 3. heliotherapy

_____ 4. TENS

_____ 5. transdermal drug delivery

A. administers a drug through unbroken skin
B. delivering electric current through the skin to painful areas
C. exposes the body to the sun
D. uses high-frequency current to generate heat for healing
E. uses warm water

SELECTED ABBREVIATIONS

AIDS	acquired immunodeficiency syndrome		**Staph**	*Staphylococcus*
ABA	American Burn Association		**TB**	tuberculosis
bx	biopsy		**TBSA**	total body surface area
DLE	discoid lupus erythematosus		**TENS**	transcutaneous electrical nerve stimulation
HSV	herpes simplex virus		**ung**	ointment
HSV 1	herpes simplex virus type 1		**UV**	ultraviolet
I & D	incision and drainage			

CHAPTER 16 REVIEW

■ Basic Understanding

Listing

I. List five functions of the skin.

1. _____

2. _____

3. _____

4. _____

5. _____

II. List and describe the functions of the accessory skin structures.

1. _____

2. _____

3. _____

4. _____

Matching

III. Match skin lesions in the left column with their characteristics in the right column.

_____ 1. bulla
      A. blister, larger than 1 cm
_____ 2. cyst
      B. blister, smaller than 1 cm
      C. cracklike lesion of the skin
_____ 3. fissure
      D. discolored spot, not elevated
_____ 4. macule
      E. excess collagen production after injury
_____ 5. papule
      F. fluid-filled sac containing pus
_____ 6. pustule
      G. sac filled with clear fluid
      H. solid elevation, less than 0.5 cm in diameter
_____ 7. scar

_____ 8. vesicle

Multiple Choice

IV. Circle the correct answer for each multiple choice question.

1. Which test determines an individual's reaction to a substance by observing the results after injecting the substance or applying it to the skin? (needle aspiration, punch biopsy, skin culture, skin test)

2. Which of the following destroys tissue using very cold temperatures? (cryotherapy, electrodesiccation, heliotherapy, ultrasound)

3. Which of the following means removal of foreign material and dead or contaminated tissue from an infected or traumatic lesion until surrounding healthy tissue is exposed? (débridement, necrosis, pyemia, rhytidectomy)

4. Which term means pertaining to the armpit? (adipose, alopecia, apocrine, axillary)

5. Which of the following is an inflammatory skin disease that begins on the scalp but may involve other areas, particularly the eyebrows? (acne vulgaris, basal cell carcinoma, seborrheic dermatitis, verruca)

6. Which of the following is a test that is used to diagnose cystic fibrosis? (shaved specimen, skin biopsy, sebum analysis, sweat test)

7. Which term means a disease characterized by chronic hardening and thickening of the skin? (ecchymosis, Kaposi's sarcoma, keratosis, scleroderma)

8. Which of the following is a common name for decubitus ulcer? (bedsore, keratoma, mole, wart)

9. In describing a burn by "thickness," which type of burn is characterized by blisters? (deep partial-thickness, deep full-thickness, full-thickness, superficial partial-thickness)

10. Which term means the death of areas of tissue or bone surrounded by healthy parts? (atrophy, erosion, fissure, necrosis)

Fill In the Blanks

V. Complete the sentences by writing a term in each blank space.

1. Cells of the epidermis contain _____, which is a scleroprotein.

2. The corium is another name for the layer of skin called the _____.

3. An oily material secreted by the sebaceous glands is called _____.

4. Sweat glands, also called _____ glands, produce perspiration.

5. Diaphoresis means excessive _____.

Writing Terms

VI. Write words for the following:

1. a boil   _____

2. a contagious dermatitis caused by the itch mite   _____

3. a torn, jagged wound   _____

4. absence of pigment in the skin, hair, and nails   _____

5. another name for a bruise   _____

6. any disease of the nails   _____

7. baldness   _____

8. condition in which the skin is dry and scaly   _____

9. heatstroke or sunstroke   _____

10. superficial infection involving hair follicles   _____

■ Greater Comprehension

Health Care Report

VII. *Find the correct terms in the health report to match the descriptions that follow the report.*

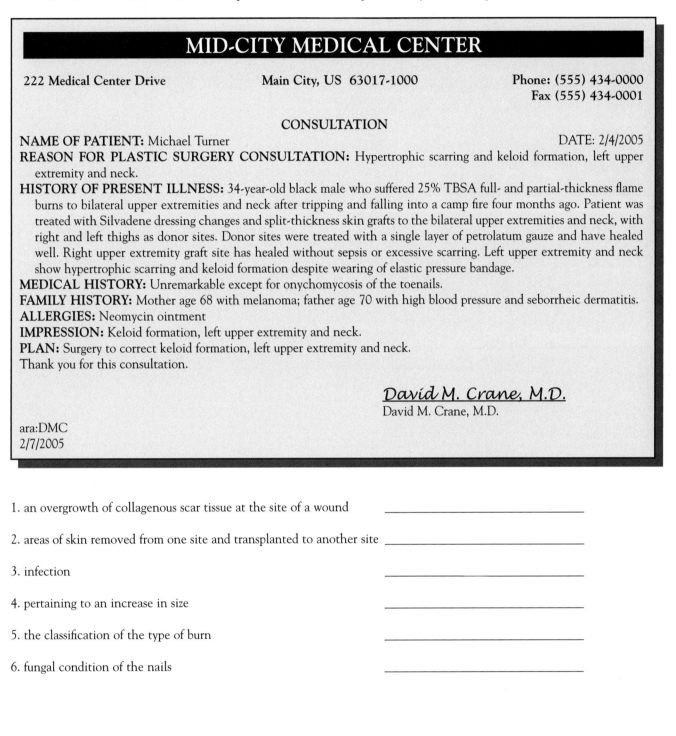

MID-CITY MEDICAL CENTER

222 Medical Center Drive   Main City, US 63017-1000   Phone: (555) 434-0000
                                                                            Fax (555) 434-0001

CONSULTATION

NAME OF PATIENT: Michael Turner   DATE: 2/4/2005

REASON FOR PLASTIC SURGERY CONSULTATION: Hypertrophic scarring and keloid formation, left upper
  extremity and neck.

HISTORY OF PRESENT ILLNESS: 34-year-old black male who suffered 25% TBSA full- and partial-thickness flame
  burns to bilateral upper extremities and neck after tripping and falling into a camp fire four months ago. Patient was
  treated with Silvadene dressing changes and split-thickness skin grafts to the bilateral upper extremities and neck, with
  right and left thighs as donor sites. Donor sites were treated with a single layer of petrolatum gauze and have healed
  well. Right upper extremity graft site has healed without sepsis or excessive scarring. Left upper extremity and neck
  show hypertrophic scarring and keloid formation despite wearing of elastic pressure bandage.

MEDICAL HISTORY: Unremarkable except for onychomycosis of the toenails.

FAMILY HISTORY: Mother age 68 with melanoma; father age 70 with high blood pressure and seborrheic dermatitis.

ALLERGIES: Neomycin ointment

IMPRESSION: Keloid formation, left upper extremity and neck.

PLAN: Surgery to correct keloid formation, left upper extremity and neck.

Thank you for this consultation.

David M. Crane, M.D.
David M. Crane, M.D.

ara:DMC
2/7/2005

---

1. an overgrowth of collagenous scar tissue at the site of a wound   _____

2. areas of skin removed from one site and transplanted to another site   _____

3. infection   _____

4. pertaining to an increase in size   _____

5. the classification of the type of burn   _____

6. fungal condition of the nails   _____

Health Care Report

VIII. Write the meanings of the underlined terms in the following health report.

CASE STUDY

Patient: Rodney Masters (39 years of age)

Symptoms: Warmth, edema, and <u>erythema</u> from right knee to calf with some <u>induration</u>. Temp. 100.8.

History: Scratched an area of probable <u>folliculitis</u> on right lower extremity three days prior to admission. Patient had been water skiing in the river two days prior to that.

Medical history: Insulin-dependent diabetes mellitus for two years and frequent bacterial skin infections.

Family history: Mother—age 60 with <u>discoid lupus erythematosus</u>; father—age 73 with history of <u>eczema</u>.

Physical examination: Right lower extremity red and inflamed. Slight amount of serous drainage from lesion. Edema present.

Laboratory tests: WBC 12.0; wound culture showed light growth of MRSA (methicillin-resistant *Staphylococcus aureus*).

Diagnosis: <u>Cellulitis</u>, right lower extremity.

Plan: Intravenous antibiotic treatment.

Define:

1. erythema   _____

2. induration   _____

3. folliculitis   _____

4. discoid lupus erythematosus _____

5. eczema   _____

6. cellulitis   _____

Spelling

IX. Circle each misspelled term in this list and write the correct spelling.

abrasion   aerosol   ektoderm   hydradenitis   onykectomy

Interpreting Abbreviations

X. Write the meaning of each abbreviation.

1. DLE   _____

2. HSV 1 _____

3. I & D   _____

4. TBSA   _____

5. ung   _____

Pronunciation

XI. Pronunciation is shown for several medical terms. Indicate the primary accent in each term by marking it with an ′.

1. cellulitis (sel u li tis)

2. dermabrasion (dər mə bra shən)

3. ichthyosis (ik the o sis)

4. urticaria (ur tĭ kar e ə)

5. xeroderma (zēr o der mə)

XII. Classify the terms in the left column by selecting A, B, C, D, or E.

_____ 1. diathermy   A. anatomy
                             B. diagnostic test or procedure
_____ 2. eczema   C. pathology
                             D. surgery
_____ 3. escharotomy   E. therapy

_____ 4. liposuction

_____ 5. pediculosis

_____ 6. rhytidectomy

_____ 7. shaved specimen

_____ 8. skin flap

_____ 9. ungual

_____ 10. xerosis

(Check your answers with the solutions in Appendix VI.)

LISTING OF MEDICAL TERMS

Use the practice CD to review the terms that have been presented. Look closely at the spelling of each term as it is pronounced and be sure you know the meaning of each term.

abrasion	alopecia	basal cell carcinoma	cystic fibrosis
abscess	amputation	bulla	débride
acne vulgaris	antimicrobial	cellulitis	débridement
acquired	antipruritic	collagen injection	decubitus ulcer
immunodeficiency	antiseptic	contusion	dermabrasion
syndrome	apocrine gland	corium	dermatitis
actinic keratosis	arrector pili muscle	cryotherapy	dermatologist
adipose	asepsis	curet	dermatology
aerosol	atrophy	curettage	dermatome
albinism	autograft	cutaneous	dermatomycosis
albino	axilla	cyanosis	dermis
allograft	axillary	cyst	diaphoresis

diathermy
discoid lupus
  erythematosus
ecchymosis
ectoderm
eczema
electrodesiccation
electrolysis
endoderm
epidermal
epidermis
erosion
erythema
escharotomy
exfoliation
fissure
folliculitis
frostbite
furuncle
heliotherapy
herpes simplex virus
hidradenitis
histocompatibility
hydrotherapy
hyperthermia
hypothermia
ichthyoid
ichthyosis

incompatibility
induration
integument
integumentary
jaundice
Kaposi's sarcoma
keloid
keratin
keratogenesis
keratoma
keratosis
laceration
lesion
lipectomy
lipoma
liposuction
lunula
macule
melanocyte
melanoma
mesoderm
mycodermatitis
necrosis
necrotic
neoplasm
nevus
nodule
ointment

onychectomy
onychomalacia
onychomycosis
onychopathy
onychophagia
onychophagist
onychosis
papule
pediculicide
pediculosis
perspiration
petechia
photodermatitis
plaque
psoriasis
purulence
pustule
pyogenesis
pyrexia
retinoid
rhytidoplasty
scabies
scleroderma
scleroprotein
sebaceous gland
seborrhea
seborrheic dermatitis
seborrheic keratosis

sebum
squamous cell carcinoma
stimulator
subcutaneous
sudoriferous
suppuration
suppurative
thermoplegia
topical anesthetic
topical antibiotic
topical medication
transcutaneous electrical
  nerve stimulation
transdermal
trichopathy
trichosis
ulcer
ungual
urticaria
verruca
vesicle
wart
wheal
xeroderma
xerosis

español ENHANCING SPANISH COMMUNICATION

ENGLISH	SPANISH (PRONUNCIATION)
allergy	alergia (ah-LEHR-he-ah)
armpit	sobaco (so-BAH-co)
biopsy	biopsia (be-OP-see-ah)
burn	quemadura (kay-mah-DOO-rah)
dermatology	dermatología (der-mah-to-lo-HEE-ah)
eyebrow	ceja (SAY-hah)
eyelash	pestaña (pes-TAH-nyah)
gland	glándula (GLAN-doo-lah)
hair	pelo (PAY-lo)
hives	roncha (RON-chah)
injury	daño (DAH-nyo)
nails	uñas (OO-nyahs)
perspiration	sudor (soo-DOR)
skin	piel (pe-EL)
ulcer	ulcera (OOL-say-rah)
wound	lesión (lay-se-ON)

CHAPTER 17

Endocrine System

FUNCTION FIRST

The endocrine system cooperates with the nervous system to regulate body activities. This is accomplished by endocrine hormones that affect various processes throughout the body, such as growth, metabolism, and secretions from other organs.

ANATOMY AND PHYSIOLOGY

17-1 The endocrine (en′do-krīn, en′do-krin) system and the nervous system work together to maintain homeostasis (ho″me-o-sta′sis). Homeostasis (home[o], sameness or constant, -stasis, stopping or controlling) is a relative constancy in the internal environment of the body.

The nervous system communicates with the endocrine system through nerve impulses. The endocrine system acts through chemical messengers called hormones. Working together, the nervous system and the endocrine system help maintain constancy in the body that is called

homeostasis   _____.

17-2 You have learned that the combining form crin(o) means to _____.
The endocrine (endo- inside, -crine, to secrete) system is composed of the ductless glands and other
secrete   structures that secrete hormones into the bloodstream. The ductless glands are endocrine glands, and they secrete hormones (hor′mōnz), chemical substances, into the blood that are carried to another part of the body, where they exert specific physiologic effects. Write the name of the chemical secretions of
hormones   endocrine glands: _____.

17-3 A gland is an organ that has specialized cells that secrete or excrete substances that are not related to the gland's ordinary metabolism. There are many glands in the body, and they are classified as either exo/crine (ek′so-krin) or endo/crine glands. The prefix *exo-* means outside. Exocrine glands have ducts that enable them to empty secretions onto an external or an internal body surface. A sweat gland is an example of an exocrine gland. Unlike exocrine glands,
ducts   endocrine glands do not have _____, so they secrete their hormones into the bloodstream.

17-4 Dysfunctions in hormone production fall into two categories: either a deficiency or an excess in secretion. A deficiency is called hypo/secretion (hi″po-sə-kre′shən). Excess secretion is called
hypersecretion   _____.
(hi″pər-se-kre′shən)

The organ or structure toward which the effects of a hormone are primarily directed is called the target organ. If a hormone has a specific effect on the thyroid gland, then the thyroid is the target organ. If a hormone has a specific effect on the ovaries, then the ovary is the
target   _____ organ.

17-5 Hormones are either proteins or steroids (ster′oidz). Most hormones in the human body are protein, with the exception of the sex hormones and those from the adrenal cortex. Proteins are quickly inactivated in the digestive tract, so these hormones are administered by injection if there is a deficiency. Sex hormones and other steroids can be taken orally.

17-6 The locations of the major glands of the endocrine system are shown in Figure 17-1. Observe that the pituitary (pĭ-too′ĭ-tar″e) gland is also called the _____ .
hypophysis   This gland is a small, round structure about 1 cm (or 0.5 inch) in diameter that is attached by a
(hi-pof′ə-sis)   stalk at the base of the brain.
An adrenal (ə-dre′nəl) gland lies above each of the two kidneys. Supra/renal (soo″prə-re′nəl)
kidneys   means above the _____, and sometimes the adrenal glands are called the suprarenal glands.
The ovaries and testes are gonads (go′nadz)—glands that provide ova and sperm, respectively.

17-7 Observing the endocrine glands on the right side of Figure 17-1, the pineal* (pin′e-əl) gland, also called the pineal body, is shaped like a pine cone and is attached to the posterior part of the brain.
The thyroid (thi′roid), also called the thyroid gland, is located at the front of the neck. Note that it consists of bilateral lobes that are connected by a narrow strip of thyroid tissue. Parathyroid (par″ə-thi′roid) glands are located near the thyroid (as the name implies). They are actually embedded in its posterior surface.

*Pineal (Latin: *pineus*, pine cone).

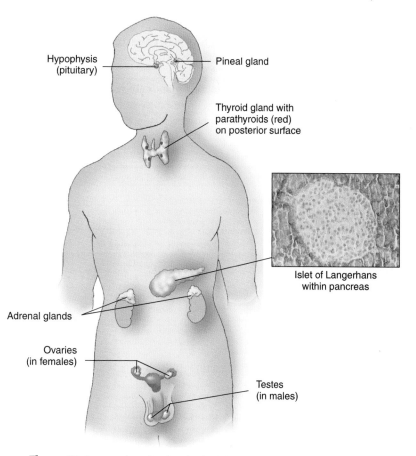

Hypophysis (pituitary)

Pineal gland

Thyroid gland with parathyroids (red) on posterior surface

Islet of Langerhans within pancreas

Adrenal glands

Ovaries (in females)

Testes (in males)

Figure 17-1   Location of major glands of the endocrine system.

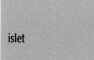

islet

The pancreas is an elongated structure that has digestive functions, as well as endocrine functions. The clusters of cells within the pancreas that perform the endocrine function are shown in Figure 17-1. These clusters of cells are the _____ of Langerhans (**lahng′ər-hahnz**).

Learn the meanings of the following terms.

Word Parts Pertaining to Endocrine Anatomy and Physiology

Combining Forms Associated with Anatomy

COMBINING FORM	MEANING
aden(o)	gland
adren(o), adrenal(o)	adrenal gland
gonad(o)	gonad
mamm(o), mast(o)	breast
pancreat(o)	pancreas
parathyroid(o)	parathyroid glands
pituitar(o)	pituitary gland
thyr(o), thyroid(o)	thyroid gland

Word Parts Associated with Function

COMBINING FORM	MEANING
andr(o)	male or masculine
calc(i)	calcium
gigant(o)	large
gluc(o)	glucose
glyc(o), glycos(o)	sugar
insulin(o)	insulin
iod(o)	iodine
ket(o)	ketone
lact(o)	milk
trop(o)	to stimulate

SUFFIX	MEANING
-crine	secrete
-dipsia	thirst
-physis	growth
-tropic	stimulating
-tropin	that which stimulates

17-8 The pituitary gland supplies numerous hormones that act directly on cells or stimulate other glands that govern many vital processes. The pituitary gland is also called the pituitary, the hypophysis cerebri, or simply the hypophysis. The suffix -*physis* means growth. The hypo/physis was so named because it grows _____ the cerebrum.

under

Some hormones of the endocrine glands are released in response to the nervous system (i.e., the adrenal gland releases adrenaline in response to the sympathetic nervous system in stressful situations). Many endocrine glands, however, respond to hormones produced by the pituitary gland, and it is nicknamed the "master gland" for this reason.

Exercise 1

1. Write the names of six major glands of the endocrine system: _____

_____

Exercise 2

Fill in the blanks in these sentences.

1. The endocrine system and the _____ system cooperate to maintain homeostasis.

2. The name of the master gland is the _____.

3. An organ that has specialized cells that secrete or excrete substances that are not related to its ordinary metabolism is called

   a _____.

4. Chemical substances that are produced in one part or organ and initiate or regulate the activity of an organ in another part

   are called _____.

17-9 Examine the diagram of the pituitary and its target organs in Figure 17-2. The pituitary is divided structurally and functionally into an anterior lobe and a posterior lobe.

nerve

The posterior lobe of the pituitary is called the neurohypophysis (**noor″o-hi-pof′ə-sis**). The combining form neur(o) means _____. This lobe contains ends of neurons, the cell bodies of which are located in the hypothalamus (**hi″po-thal′ə-məs**), a portion of the lower part of the brain. The hormones of the neurohypophysis are stored in the axon endings and are released when a nerve impulse travels down the axon.

neurohypophysis

The portion of the pituitary that releases hormones when stimulated by nervous impulses from the hypothalamus is called the _____.

gland

17-10 The anterior lobe of the pituitary is called the adenohypophysis (**ad″ə-no-hi-pof′ĭ-sis**). The word part *aden(o)* refers to a _____. This lobe is the glandular part of the hypophysis. The release of hormones from the adenohypophysis is controlled by regulating hormones produced by the hypothalamus.

17-11 Look again at Figure 17-2. Abbreviations such as ADH, STH, and MSH stand for pituitary hormones. The two hormones produced by the posterior lobe of the pituitary act directly on specific cells of the kidneys, the breasts, and the uterus.

The anterior lobe of the pituitary produces many hormones, several of which act on other endocrine glands, causing them also to secrete hormones. The green arrows in Figure 17-2 represent anterior pituitary hormones. Which lobe of the pituitary releases the greater number of hormones? _____ lobe.

anterior

■ *Hormones of the Neurohypophysis*

17-12 The hypothalamus plays an important role in hormonal regulation. The hormones of the neurohypophysis, antidiuretic (**an″te-, an″ti-di″u-ret′ik**) hormone and oxytocin (**ok″sĭ-to′sin**), are synthesized in the hypothalamus, and then transported to the neurohypophysis for storage. They are released through nervous stimulation.

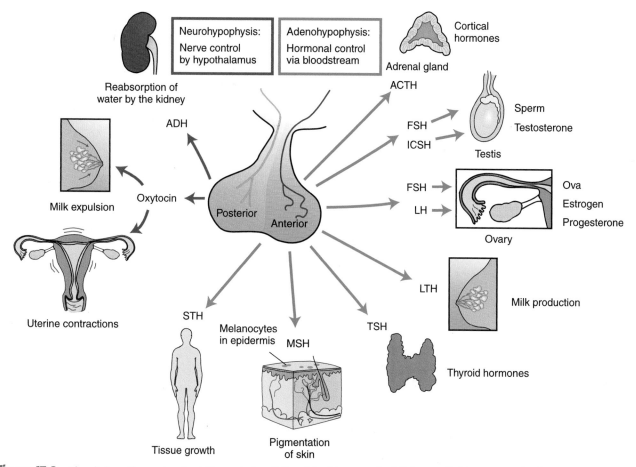

Figure 17-2   The pituitary, the master gland. The posterior pituitary lobe (*shown on the left*) is controlled by nervous stimulation by the hypothalamus and releases two hormones. In contrast, the anterior pituitary lobe is controlled by hypothalamic hormones brought by the bloodstream and secretes many hormones.

against

Antidiuretic hormone (ADH) affects the volume of urine excreted. The prefix *anti-* means _____. Diuretic means increasing urine excretion or the amount of urine. It also means an agent that promotes urine excretion. Anti/diuretic hormone acts against a diuretic. It acts in the kidneys to reabsorb water from the urine, producing concentrated urine. Absence of this hormone produces diuresis (**di″u-re′sis**), passage of large amounts of dilute urine.

17-13 Some common substances such as tea, coffee, and water act as diuretics. Physicians also prescribe diuretic drugs to rid the body of excess fluid in patients with edema. Diuretics (increase or

increase

decrease?) _____ urination. Anti/diuretic hormone causes a decrease in the amount of water lost in urination.

17-14 The second hormone, oxytocin, is released in large quantities just before a female gives birth. It causes uterine contractions, thus inducing childbirth. It also acts on the mammary glands to stimulate the release of milk. Write the name of the pituitary hormone that causes contraction of

oxytocin

the uterus and acts on the mammary glands: _____.

Hormones of the Adenohypophysis

17-15 The hypothalamus regulates the adenohypophysis by producing regulatory and inhibitory hormones, which stimulate or inhibit the secretion of its hormones. When the adenohypophysis secretes its hormones, they travel through the bloodstream and bring about changes in other organs, often another endocrine gland.

The adenohypophysis releases several hormones that regulate a large range of body activities. Look again at the target organs of these hormones (see Figure 17-2). Most of these pituitary secretions stimulate other glands, and many of their names contain *trop(o)*, which means to stimulate or turn. Tropic (**tro′pik**) is an adjective that means to _____.

17-16 Growth hormone (GH) is also called somato/tropic hormone (STH), or somatotropin (**so′mə-to-tro″pin**). The suffix *-tropin* refers to that which stimulates. Somato/tropin is the hormone that _____ body growth.

This hormone increases the rate of growth and maintains size once growth is attained. It is called GH or _____.

17-17 Melanocyte-stimulating hormone (MSH) from the pituitary stimulates melanocytes distributed throughout the epidermis. MSH promotes pigmentation and controls the amount of melanin that melanocytes produce. The name *melanin* (**mel′ə-nin**) implies the color _____. Melanin is a black or dark brown pigment that occurs naturally in the hair, skin, and parts of the eye.

17-18 Remembering the meaning of lact(o), the lactogenic hormone (LTH), also called prolactin (**pro-lak′tin**), is produced by the anterior pituitary and causes _____ production by the mammary glands.

17-19 The combining form *gonad(o)* means gonads (ovaries or testes). Gonado/tropic (**go″nə-do-trop′ik**) hormones stimulate the ovaries of the female and the testes of the male. Follicle-stimulating hormone (FSH) and luteinizing (**loo′te-in-ī″zing**) hormone (LH) are produced by the adenohypophysis. These two hormones have the gonads as target organs.

Write a word that means a hormone that stimulates the gonads: _____. FSH and LH are gonadotropins.

17-20 The adrenal glands are target organs of another pituitary hormone. Because ren(o) means kidney, ad/ren/al (**ə-dre′nəl**) tells us that these glands are located near or toward the _____.

The cortex and medulla of the adrenal gland are stimulated by different means, and they secrete different hormones. The hypothalamus influences both portions, but the medulla receives direct nervous stimulation, and the cortex is stimulated by the adrenocorticotropic (**ə-dre″no-kor″tĭ-ko-trop′ik**) hormone (ACTH) brought by the circulating blood.

17-21 Looking at Figure 17-2, you see that the pituitary secretes TSH, which causes the glandular cells of the _____ to produce thyroid hormones. TSH means thyroid-stimulating hormone, also called thyrotropin (**thi-rot′rə-pin**).

17-22 The next several frames provide additional information about several target organs of the adenohypophysis. The gland located at the front of the neck that is stimulated by TSH is the _____. Eu/thyroid (**u-thi′roid**) means a normally functioning thyroid, because *eu-* means good or normal. The major function of the thyroid is regulation of body metabolism, normal growth and development, and the storage of calcium in bone tissue. It accomplishes these functions by secretion of three hormones: thyroxine (**thi-rok′sin**), triiodothyronine (**tri-i″o-do-thi′ro-nēn**), and thyrocalcitonin (**thi″ro-kal″sĭ-to′nin**).

17-23 The majority of the hormone secreted by the thyroid gland is thyroxine, abbreviated T_4, which is tetra/iodo/thyro/nine, because the molecule contains four atoms of _____ in its chemical structure.

Another hormone produced by the thyroid gland, but in far less quantities, is tri/iodo/thyronine, which is abbreviated T_3. Both of these hormones are synthesized by the thyroid using iodine. If there is a deficiency of _____ in the diet, the thyroid will not be able to produce sufficient T_3 and T_4 for metabolism.

stimulate

stimulates

somatotropin

black

milk

gonadotropin
(**go′nə-do-tro″pin**)

kidney

thyroid

thyroid

iodine

iodine

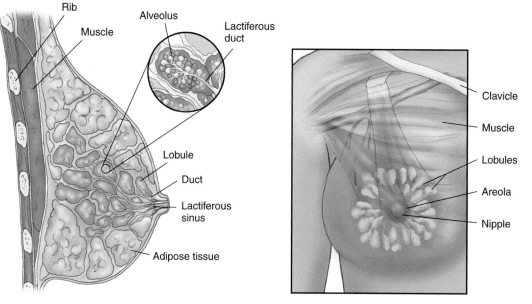

Lateral view   Anterior view

Figure 17-3   Structure of the adult female breast, lateral and anterior views. The breasts are mammary glands and function as part of the endocrine and reproductive systems.

---

thyroid

A third hormone produced by the thyroid gland is thyro/calcitonin (TCT, also called calcitonin). This hormone is involved in the homeostasis of the blood calcium level. TCT is a hormone produced by the _____. The combining form *calc(i)* means calcium.

17-24 The mammary (**mam′ər-e**) glands are the two glands of the female breasts that secrete milk. The female breasts are accessory organs of the reproductive system. The breasts are located anterior to the chest muscles, and each breast contains 15 to 20 lobes of glandular tissue that radiate around the nipple. The milk-producing glands of the female are called the

mammary

_____ glands.

Structural aspects of the breast are shown in Figure 17-3. The circular pigmented area of skin surrounding the nipple is the areola (**ə-re′o-lə**). Lobule (**lob′ūl**) means small lobe. The lobes are separated by connective and adipose (fatty) tissue. The amount of adipose tissue determines the size of the breasts, but not the amount of milk that can be produced.

17-25 Lacto/genic means inducing the secretion of milk (lact[o] means milk). During pregnancy, the mammary glands undergo changes that prepare them for lacto/genesis (**lak′to-jen′ə-sis**), the production of milk. The most important hormone that stimulates milk production is prolactin, also called LTH.

The mammary glands secrete a cloudy fluid called colostrum (**kə-los′trəm**) the first few days after a female gives birth. Because of its high antibody and high protein content, colostrum serves adequately as food for the infant until milk production begins 2 to 3 days after parturition.

17-26 Each breast lobule is drained by its own lactiferous (**lak-tif′ər-əs**) duct, which has a dilated portion called a sinus that serves as a reservoir for milk. The nipple, located near the center of the breast, contains the openings of the milk ducts.

Lactation (**lak-ta′shən**) is the secretion or ejecting of milk. Milk ejection is a normal reflex in a lactating woman and is elicited by tactile stimulation of the nipple (such as nursing by the infant). Impulses from the nipple to the hypothalamus stimulate the release of

oxytocin

_____ by the pituitary gland, which brings about contractions that eject the milk from the breast (Figure 17-4). If a lactating mother stops nursing, milk production usually ceases within a few days.

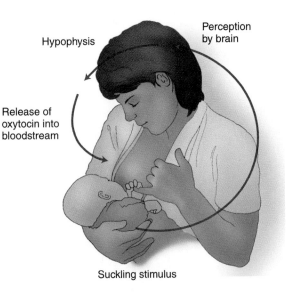

Figure 17-4 Interrelationships of hypothalamus, neurohypophysis, and breast. Suckling by the infant stimulates nerve endings at the nipple. Impulses are carried to the hypothalamus, which causes the neurohypophysis to secrete oxytocin into the bloodstream. The oxytocin is carried to the breast, where it causes milk to be expressed into the ducts. Milk begins to flow within 30 seconds to 1 minute after a baby begins to suckle.

between	**17-27** Several adjectives are used when describing locations near the breasts. Remembering that *inter-* means between, inter/mammary (**in″tər-mam′ə-re**) means situated _____ the breasts. Retro/mammary (**ret″ro-mam′ər-e**) means behind the mammary gland.
gonads	**17-28** Gonad/al (**go-nad′əl**) means pertaining to the _____. Gonadotropic (**go″nə-do-trop′ik**) is an adjective that means stimulating the gonads. The first gonadotropic hormone, FSH, stimulates the ovaries to secrete estrogen and acts on the follicle (as its name implies). FSH stimulates production of sperm in the testes of male individuals. LH stimulates ovulation and production of progesterone in the female ovary. LH often is called interstitial cell–stimulating hormone (ICSH) in male individuals because it promotes the growth of the interstitial cells of the testes and the secretion of testosterone.
testosterone	**17-29** The period of life at which reproduction becomes possible is puberty (**pu′bər-te**). It is recognized by maturation of the genitals and appearance of secondary sex characteristics. The onset of puberty is triggered by the hypothalamus and the anterior pituitary. FSH and LH act on the testes and ovaries (Figure 17-5). Male sex hormones are collectively called androgens (**an′dro-jənz**), with testosterone (**tes-tos′tə-rōn**) being the most abundant. Figure 17-5 reinforces the concept that the main hormones secreted by the ovaries and testes are estrogen and _____, respectively.
cortex glucose	**17-30** The adrenal glands have two parts, the cortex and the medulla, each having its own independent functions. The outer cortex (**kor′teks**) makes up the bulk of the gland, and the inner portion is called the medulla (**mə-dul′ə**). Table 17-1 lists the important hormones produced by the adrenal glands. Mineralocorticoids (**min″ər-əl-o-kor′tĭ-koidz**), glucocorticoids (**gloo″ko-kor′tĭ-koidz**), androgens, and estrogens are secreted by the adrenal _____. Mineralo/corticoids help maintain water balance in the body. As the name implies, gluco/corticoids increase blood _____, but they also inhibit inflammation. Individuals with severe inflammation, as in the joints, may receive injections of cortisone to relieve the pain and inflammation. Cortisone may also be included in topical creams and ointments to relieve skin inflammation. Androgens have masculinizing effects, and estrogens have feminizing effects.
male	**17-31** The combining form *andr(o)* means _____ or masculine. Testosterone is the most potent androgen and is produced in large quantities by the testes, making

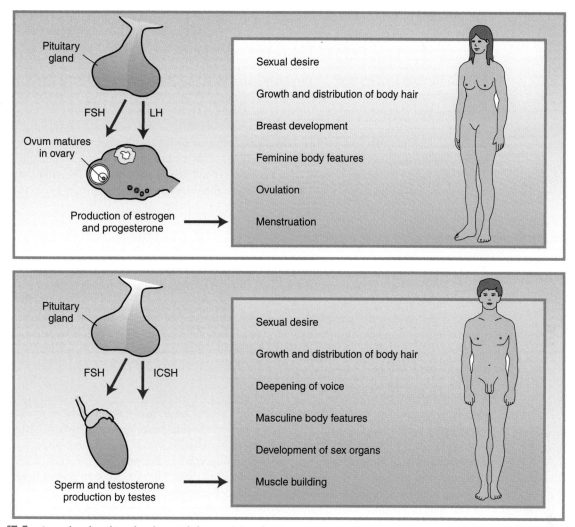

Figure 17-5   Secondary female and male sexual characteristics. The changes that occur at puberty are brought about by the hypothalamus and the anterior pituitary. Changes in the secretions of FSH and LH bring about changes in the ovaries and testes and the hormones they produce.

TABLE 17-1 Hormones Secreted by the Adrenal Gland

Gland	Hormone	Target Tissue	Principal Action
Adrenal cortex	Mineralocorticoids (main one is aldosterone)	Kidney	Increases water retention by changing sodium and potassium reabsorption in the kidney tubules
	Glucocorticoids (main ones are cortisol and cortisone)	Most body tissue	Increases blood glucose levels; inhibits inflammation and the immune response
	Androgens and estrogens	Most body tissue	Secreted in such small amounts that the effect is generally masked by ovarian and testicular hormones
Adrenal medulla	Epinephrine, norepinephrine	Heart and blood vessels, liver, adipose	Increases heart rate and blood pressure, increases blood flow and blood glucose level, helps the body cope with stress

masculine

that produced by the adrenal glands insignificant in most cases. Andro/genic (**an″dro-jen′ik**) means producing _____ characteristics or masculinization. In female individuals, the masculinization effect of androgen secretion may become evident after menopause.

17-32 The hormone secreted by the adenohypophysis that stimulates the adrenal cortex is ACTH. The combining forms *adren(o)* and *adrenal(o)* refer to the adrenal glands. Adreno/cortico/tropin (**ə-dre″no-kor″tĭ-ko-tro′pin**) is another name for ACTH, the hormone that

stimulates

_____ the adrenal glands.

The adrenal medulla secretes two hormones: epinephrine (**ep″ĭ-nef′rin**), also called adrenaline (**ə-dren′ə-lin**), and norepinephrine (noradrenaline). The medulla mostly secretes epinephrine, which stimulates the heart. Norepinephrine causes blood vessels to constrict. Together they prepare the body for strenuous activity and are sometimes called the fight-or-flight hormones.

■ *Other Endocrine Tissues and Homeostasis*

17-33 In addition to the endocrine glands that have been studied in previous sections, the pineal gland, the pancreas, and the parathyroids are considered here with a few other organs that have hormonal activity.

The exact functions of the pineal gland have not been established, but there is evidence that it secretes the hormone melatonin (**mel′ə-to′nin**). The pineal gland usually begins to diminish around the age of 7 years. If degeneration does not occur, the production of melatonin remains high and puberty may be delayed in girls. This indicates that melatonin may inhibit the activities of the ovaries.

pineal

Melatonin is secreted by the _____ gland. In addition to a regulatory function in sexual development, effects of melatonin may influence the sleepiness/wakefulness cycle and mood and may cause a decrease in skin pigmentation.

17-34 Strict regulation of hormonal secretion is important to maintain homeostasis. The body uses three different methods to regulate hormones: direct nervous stimulation, secretion of hormones in response to other hormones, and a negative feedback mechanism.

The adrenal medulla is an example of the first method, direct nervous stimulation. The adrenal medulla secretes epinephrine and norepinephrine in response to stimulation by sympathetic nerves.

Tropic hormones cause secretion of other hormones. For example, thyrotropin (TSH) from the anterior pituitary gland causes the thyroid gland to secrete the

thyroid

_____ hormones.

The interaction between two important pancreatic hormones and the concentration of glucose in the blood is an example of a negative feedback system. In negative feedback, a gland is sensitive to the concentration of a substance that it regulates. Continue reading to see how this works.

17-35 The pancreas has an exocrine portion that secretes digestive enzymes that are carried through a duct to the duodenum and an endocrine portion that secretes hormones into the blood. The endocrine portion consists of many small cell groups called islets of Langerhans. These cells secrete two hormones that have a role in regulating blood glucose levels.

The two hormones secreted by the islets of Langerhans are glucagon (**gloo′kə-gon**) and insulin (**in′sə-lin**). The action of glucagon is to increase blood glucose levels. It is secreted in response to a low concentration of glucose in the blood. This mechanism prevents hypoglycemia (**hi″po-gli-se′me-ə**), a less than normal amount of _____ in the blood, from

sugar

occurring between meals. Glucose, which the body uses for energy, is the type of sugar found in blood; therefore, hypoglycemia means a less than normal amount of blood glucose.

17-36 The action of insulin is opposite or antagonistic to glucagon. Insulin promotes the uptake and utilization of glucose for energy and is secreted in response to a high concentration of glucose in the blood. Because insulin opposes the action of glucagon, the action of insulin brings about a

decrease

_____ in blood glucose levels.

Insufficient insulin activity may be caused by insufficient secretion or by insufficient or defective receptor sites on its target cells.

17-37 The parathyroid gland is an endocrine gland not directly controlled by the pituitary but closely linked with the thyroid gland. Four small parathyroid glands, another type of endocrine gland, secrete parathyroid hormone (PTH) or parathormone (*para-* means near, beside, or abnormal). PTH increases the blood calcium levels and is regulated by a negative feedback mechanism. This means that PTH is secreted in response to low levels of _____ in the blood.

calcium

PTH has the opposite effect, or is antagonistic, to calcitonin secreted by the _____ gland.

thyroid

17-38 In addition to the endocrine glands you have studied, other organs that have some hormonal activity include the stomach, small intestines, thymus, heart, and placenta.

The lining of the stomach produces gastrin (**gas'trin**), which stimulates the production of hydrochloric acid, and the enzyme pepsin (**pep'sin**), each being substances that are used in the digestion of food. The hormone gastrin (*gastr[o]* means stomach) is secreted in response to food in the stomach. Hormones secreted by the lining of the small intestine stimulate the pancreas and the gallbladder to produce substances that aid in digestion.

The thymus (**thi'məs**) is located near the middle of the chest cavity behind the breastbone. It produces thymosin (**thi'mo-sin**), which assists in the development of lymphocytes, blood cells that function in immunity. The thymus, usually largest at puberty, diminishes in size as an individual reaches adulthood. The hormone produced by the thymus is called _____.

thymosin

Special cells in the atria, the upper chambers of the heart, produce a hormone, atriopeptin (**a"tre-o-pep'tin**), which increases the loss of sodium and water in urine.

The placenta of a pregnant female produces human chorionic gonadotropin (HCG), estrogen, and progesterone, which function to maintain the uterine lining during pregnancy.

17-39 The cells of most tissues throughout the body can produce prostaglandins (**pros"tə-glan'dinz**) when stimulated, particularly by injury. Prostaglandins, potent chemical regulators, are hormone-like substances that have a localized, immediate, and short-term effect on or near the cells where they are produced.

Prostaglandins have many effects, and the same substance sometimes has opposite effects on different tissues. Some of the effects include smooth muscle contraction, involvement in blood clotting, and many aspects of fever and pain. They are believed to be implicated in the symptoms of severe menstrual cramps, premenstrual syndrome, and premature labor. Write the name of these hormone-like substances: _____.

prostaglandins

The major endocrine glands and their secretions are summarized in Table 17-2.

TABLE 17-2 Major Endocrine Glands and Their Secretions

Gland	Primary Secretions
Pituitary gland, anterior lobe	ACTH, FSH, GH, ICSH, LH, LTH, MSH, and TSH
Pituitary gland, posterior lobe	ADH and oxytocin
Adrenal glands, cortex	Aldosterone, cortisol, and androgens
Adrenal glands, medulla	Epinephrine and norepinephrine
Gonads, ovaries	Estrogen, progesterone, and HCG
Gonads, testes	Testosterone
Pancreas (islets of Langerhans)	Insulin and glucagon
Parathyroid glands	PTH
Thyroid gland	Thyroxine, triiodothyronine, and calcitonin
Pineal gland	Melatonin and serotonin
Thymus	Thymosin

Exercise 3

Match the hormones on the left with the glands on the right that secrete them.

_____ 1. ACTH

_____ 2. antidiuretic hormone

_____ 3. epinephrine

_____ 4. follicle-stimulating hormone

_____ 5. growth hormone

_____ 6. insulin

_____ 7. luteinizing hormone

_____ 8. melanocyte-stimulating hormone

_____ 9. oxytocin

_____ 10. testosterone

_____ 11. thyrocalcitonin

_____ 12. thyrotropin

A. adrenals
B. gonads
C. pancreas
D. pituitary
E. thyroid

Exercise 4

Name the target organ for each of the following hormones.

1. ACTH   _____

2. antidiuretic hormone   _____

3. follicle-stimulating hormone _____

4. luteinizing hormone   _____

5. prolactin   _____

6. thyrotropin   _____

DIAGNOSTIC TESTS AND PROCEDURES

17-40 Most endocrine glands are not accessible for examination in a routine physical examination; however, the thyroid gland and the male gonads are exceptions. The patient's neck can be observed for any unusual bulging over the thyroid area, and the gland can be palpated (Figure 17-6). Both enlargement and masses are abnormal findings and indicate additional testing is necessary.

Likewise, the testicles are examined visually for a difference in size and palpated for masses. The method of using the hands or fingers to examine an organ is called _____.

palpation

17-41 Hyper/thyroid/ism (hi″pər-thi′roid-iz-əm) is abnormally _____ activity of the thyroid. A classic finding associated with hyper/thyroid/ism is ex/ophthal/mos (ek″sof-thal′mos), that is, protrusion (bulging outward) of the eyeballs. Hyperthyroidism is not always the cause of exophthalmos, and further tests are required. The patient in Figure 17-7 has exophthalmos and a goiter (goi′tər), an enlarged thyroid gland that is usually evident as a pronounced swelling in the neck.

increased

Physical indications of endocrine dysfunctions also include unusually tall or short stature, coarsening of facial features, edema (accumulation of fluid in the interstitial tissues), hair loss, or excessive facial hair in female individuals.

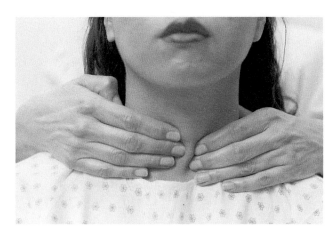

Figure 17-6   Palpation of the thyroid gland.

luteinizing

17-42 Laboratory testing includes blood tests and urine tests, depending on the symptoms. Pituitary studies include <u>blood tests for levels of GH, gonadotropins, and other hormones</u> secreted by the pituitary gland. The gonadotropins are FSH and _____ hormone.

<u>Magnetic resonance imaging</u> (MRI) is useful in identifying tumors involving the pituitary or the hypothalamus.

17-43 There are a number of blood tests and radiologic tests to determine thyroid function. Blood studies include testing for <u>TSH, thyroxine, and T_3</u>.

Because the thyroid gland absorbs iodine from the blood to synthesize T_3 and T_4, radio/iodine can be used to study the gland. Radioiodine, ^{131}I, like all radionuclides (radioisotopes), gives off radiation. The <u>radioactive iodine uptake</u> (RAIU) test measures the ability of the thyroid gland to trap and retain the ^{131}I after oral ingestion. A radiation counter determines the amount of ^{131}I uptake by the thyroid gland. If a less than normal quantity of radioactive iodine is absorbed by the thyroid gland, which condition is expected, hypothyroidism or hyperthyroidism?

hypothyroidism

_____

<u>Thyroid scans</u> consist of administration of a radiopharmaceutical, followed by passing a scanner over the thyroid and making an image of the spatial distribution of the radionuclide.

17-44 Measurement of the levels of <u>PTH, calcium, and phosphate</u> in the blood helps to determine the functioning of the _____ gland.

parathyroid

Several hormones secreted by the adrenal glands can be measured in the blood and urine, as can the <u>level of ACTH</u> in the blood. <u>Computed tomography</u>, sometimes using contrast agents, can be used to detect tumors of the adrenal gland.

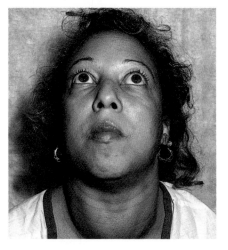

Figure 17-7   Graves' disease. Three important characteristics of Graves' disease are hyperthyroidism, exophthalmos, and goiter. Exophthalmos is the result of fluid accumulation in the fat pads and muscles behind the eyeballs, which causes the eyes to protrude. A goiter is an enlarged thyroid gland, evidenced by the swelling in the neck.

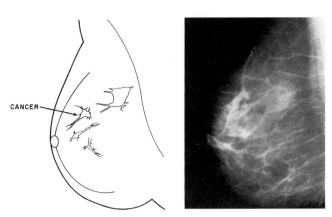

Figure 17-8 Mammogram, including a drawing, of cancer of the breast. The light areas indicate carcinoma.

17-45 Blood tests to study pancreatic function include <u>fasting blood sugar</u> (FBS), glycosylated hemoglobin (Hb AIC), and <u>oral glucose tolerance</u> (GTT). The FBS measures the glucose level in circulating blood. Hyper/glyc/emia is a greater than normal amount of glucose in the blood, and hypo/glyc/emia is a _____ than normal amount of glucose in the blood. <u>Hb AIC</u> is an abbreviation for a type of hemoglobin, Hb A_{IC}, and is also called <u>glycosylated hemoglobin</u>. Hb AIC is more accurate than a fasting blood sugar, because AIC measures the degree of glucose control during the previous three months, rather than a day.

A GTT test is a test of the body's ability to use carbohydrates by giving a standard dose of glucose to the patient and measuring the blood and urine for glucose levels at regular intervals.

17-46 <u>Urine studies</u> to evaluate pancreatic function include <u>testing for glucose and ketones</u> (**ke′tōnz**). Neither glucose nor ketones are detectable in normal urine specimens. Use glycos(o) and *-uria* to write a word that means the presence of sugar, especially glucose, in the urine: _____.

Ketones are products of abnormal use of fat in the body (as in diabetes). Excessive production of ketones leads to their excretion in the urine. Combine ket(o) and *-uria* to write a word that means the presence of ketones in the urine: _____.

Radiologic testing to identify pancreatic tumors or cysts usually includes computed tomography, with or without a contrast medium.

17-47 The breasts are part of several body systems, including the endocrine system. Self-examination of the breasts should be done periodically. A <u>self breast examination</u> includes observing and palpating the breasts for changes that could indicate disease. Early diagnosis of breast cancer greatly improves the chance of survival.

<u>Mammo/graphy</u> (**mə-mog′rə-fe**) is a diagnostic procedure that uses x-rays to study the soft tissues of the breast. It is used as a screening test to detect various benign conditions and malignant tumors of the breast. The radiographic image produced in mammography is called a _____.

Figure 17-8 is a <u>mammogram</u> showing carcinoma of the breast.

less

glycosuria
(gli″ko-su′re-ə)

ketonuria
(ke″to-nu′re-ə)

mammogram
(mam′ə-gram)

Exercise 5

Write terms for these meanings.

1. decreased activity of the thyroid   _____

2. increased activity of the thyroid   _____

3. presence of ketones in the urine   _____

4. presence of sugar in the urine   _____

5. radiographic examination of the breast   _____

PATHOLOGIES

adenopathy
(ad″ə-nop′ə-the)

17-48 Too little or too much of a specific hormone leads to a dysfunction of the endocrine system. Write a term that has a literal translation of any disease of a gland: _____. This term means any disease of a gland, but you need to remember that the term is sometimes used to mean any disease of the lymph nodes.

An <u>aden/oma</u> (ad″ə-no′mə) is a benign tumor in which the cells are clearly derived from glandular tissue. In contrast, <u>adeno/carcinoma</u> (ad″ə-no-kahr″sĭ-no′mə) means any of a large group of malignant tumors of the glands.

antidiuretic

17-49 <u>Pituitary dysfunction</u> can result in <u>hypo/secretion</u> or <u>hyper/secretion</u> of the pituitary hormones. Disorders of the posterior lobe of the pituitary are usually related to a deficiency or excess of ADH, which is the _____ hormone.

<u>Diabetes insipidus</u> (di″ə-be′tēz in-sip′ĭ-dəs) is a disorder associated with a deficiency of ADH or inability of the kidneys to respond to ADH. Do not confuse diabetes insipidus with diabetes mellitus (mel′lĕ-təs, mə-li′tis), the well-known type of diabetes that is associated with insufficient or improper use of insulin. Diabetes insipidus has some of the characteristics of the other type of diabetes, <u>poly/uria</u> (pol″e-u′re-ə) and <u>poly/dipsia</u> (pol″e-dip′se-ə), but it is not associated with insulin deficiency. <u>Poly/uria</u> and <u>poly/dipsia</u> mean excessive urination and excessive _____, respectively.

thirst

Excessive release of ADH leads to an abnormal condition called the <u>syndrome of inappropriate ADH secretion</u> (SIADH) and usually develops in association with other diseases.

17-50 The effects and hormones of anterior pituitary disorders are excessive or deficient growth (somatotropin), metabolism (prolactin, STH, ACTH, and MSH), or sexual development (FSH and LH). Untreated endocrine dysfunctions during childhood generally have longer lasting and greater effects than those that occur after puberty. Because of better knowledge and improved testing, many endocrine dysfunctions in children are treated and long-lasting effects are avoided.

decreased

<u>Hypo/pituitar/ism</u> (hi″po-pĭ-too′ĭ-tə-riz″əm) is _____ activity of the pituitary gland. A person with hypopituitarism is deficient in one or more anterior pituitary hormones, with deficiencies of ACTH and TSH being the most life threatening. This condition is a result of a congenital developmental defect, a tumor that destroys the pituitary or the hypothalamus, or lack of blood circulation to the pituitary.

17-51 Insufficient GH in childhood (Figure 17-9) leads to <u>dwarfism</u> (dworf′iz-əm) and the adult <u>dwarf</u> may be no more than 3 to 4 feet tall. <u>Pituitary dwarfism</u> is caused by a deficiency of which hormone? _____.

somatotropin

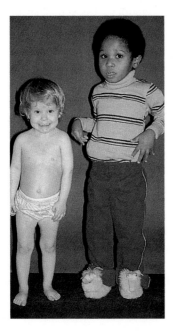

Figure 17-9 Childhood deficiency of growth hormone. Compare the normal 3-year-old boy with the short 3-year-old girl who exhibits the characteristic small stature and "Kewpie doll" appearance, suggesting a deficiency of growth hormone.

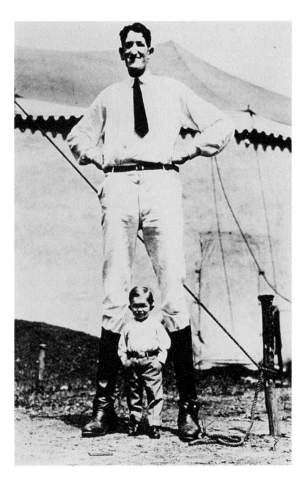

Figure 17-10 Gigantism and dwarfism, resulting from abnormal secretions of growth hormone. Hypersecretion of growth hormone during the early years results in gigantism. The person usually has normal body proportions and normal sexual development. The same hypersecretion in an adult causes acromegaly. Hyposecretion of growth hormone during the early years produces a dwarf unless the child is treated with injections of growth hormone.

pituitary

increased

somatotropin

enlargement

thyropathy
(thi-rop′ə-the)
inflammation

Pituitary insufficiency in childhood has more drastic effects than the same disorder in adults. Atrophy of the pituitary gland in an adult causes a state of ill health, malnutrition, and wasting known as pituitary cachexia **(kə-kek′se-ə)**. Although cachexia may occur in many chronic diseases, pituitary cachexia is caused by hyposecretion of the _____ gland.

17-52 Hyperpituitarism **(hi″pər-pĭ-too′ĭ-tə-riz″əm)** is _____ pituitary activity. A common cause of this overactivity is the presence of a benign tumor, especially a pituitary adenoma. Overproduction of GH during childhood leads to gigantism **(ji-gan′tiz-əm, ji′gan-tiz-əm)**, and the person will become much taller than normal. Two opposite conditions, dwarfism and gigantism, are shown in Figure 17-10.

Pituitary gigantism is caused by hypersecretion of which hormone? _____ .

17-53 Excess of GH in adults does not cause gigantism. Increased secretion of GH in adults causes acromegaly **(ak″ro-meg′ə-le)**. The name acro/megaly denotes a typical feature of the disease, _____ of the extremities. Bones of the feet, hands, cheeks, and jaws thicken in this disease because of oversecretion of GH (Figure 17-11).

Hyperpituitarism almost always involves excessive secretion of GH, but may involve other pituitary hormones as well.

17-54 Using thyr(o), write a word that means any disease of the thyroid gland: _____ . Thyroid disorders include inflammation or enlargement of the thyroid and hypersecretion or hyposecretion of thyroid hormones. Thyroid/itis **(thi″roid-i′tis)** is _____ of the thyroid gland. Acute thyroiditis is generally the result of an infection, but there are also different forms and causes of chronic thyroiditis.

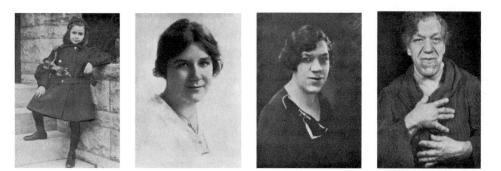

Figure 17-11   Progression of acromegaly. The patient is shown at ages 9, 16, and 33 years with well-established acromegaly, and at age 52 years in the late stages of acromegaly.

excessive

17-55 Hyper/thyroid/ism is a condition caused by _____ secretion of two hormones of the thyroid gland. This increases the metabolic rate, which then causes an increased demand for food to support this metabolic activity.

eyes

The patient with hyperthyroidism becomes excitable and nervous, exhibiting moist skin, rapid pulse, increased metabolic rate, weight loss, and exophthalmos. In ex/ophthalmos, the _____ protrude outward. (One "o" is dropped to prevent double "o.")

17-56 The most common form of hyperthyroidism is Graves' disease, believed to be an autoimmune disease. Three hallmarks of Graves' disease are hyperthyroidism, exophthalmos, and goiter. The patient shown in Figure 17-7 exhibits exophthalmos and goiter.

A goiter is a descriptive term that means an enlarged thyroid gland, usually evident as a pronounced swelling in the neck. It may be associated with hyperthyroidism, hypothyroidism, tumors, or thyroiditis.

17-57 Thyrotoxicosis (thi″ro-tok″sĭ-ko′sis), also called thyroid storm, is a life-threatening event that is usually triggered by a major stressor, such as trauma or infection. Signs and symptoms result from a rapid increase in the metabolic rate and include fever, fast pulse, hypertension, gastrointestinal symptoms, agitation, and anxiety. A term for thyroid storm is

thyrotoxicosis

_____.

decreased

17-58 Hypothyroidism (hi″po-thi′roid-iz-əm) means _____ activity of the thyroid gland.

Hypothyroidism in childhood results in a condition called cretinism (kre′tin-iz-əm) and is caused by insufficient thyroxine. The condition is characterized by arrested physical and mental development (Figure 17-12).

17-59 Myxedema (mik″sə-de′mə) is caused by hyposecretion of thyroxine and T₃ during adulthood. The body retains water, and the resultant edema causes facial puffiness. This condition is caused by decreased secretion of the thyroid gland. Hormone therapy usually alleviates the symptoms.

17-60 Hypo/parathyroid/ism (hi″po-par″ə-thi′roid-iz-əm) is below normal functioning of the parathyroids. Hyper/parathyroid/ism (hi″pər-par″ə-thi′roid-iz-əm) means abnormally

increased

_____ activity of the parathyroids.

Hypoparathyroidism results in hypocalcemia (hi″po-kal-se′me-ə), which is a less than normal

calcium

level of _____ in the blood. Early on, surgeons learned the importance of calcium when they inadvertently removed the parathyroids while removing the thyroid. Hypocalcemia occurred 1 to 2 days after the surgery.

Hyperparathyroidism causes hypercalcemia. Hyper/calc/emia (hi″pər-kal-se′me-ə) is a greater than normal blood calcium level.

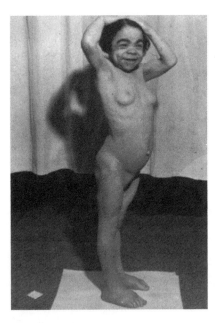

Figure 17-12   Cretinism. This 33-year-old untreated adult cretin exhibits characteristic features. She is only 44 inches tall, has underdeveloped breasts, protruding abdomen, umbilical hernia, widened facial features, and scant axillary and pubic hair.

gonads

adrenopathy
(ad″rən-op′ə-the)
enlargement

adrenals

hair

andropathy
(an-drop′ə-the)

decreased

cortex

17-61 <u>Pituitary hypogonadism</u> (hi″po-go′nad-iz-əm) is caused by a decreased secretion of FSH or LH by the pituitary. <u>Hypo/gonad/ism</u> is decreased functional activity of the
_____ and results in a deficiency in the hormones produced by the affected structures, ovaries or testes.

17-62 Using adren(o), write a word that means any disease of the adrenals:
_____.

   <u>Adreno/megaly</u> (ə-dre″no-meg′ə-le) is _____ of one or both adrenal glands.

17-63 <u>Hyper/adrenal/ism</u> (hi″pər-ə-dre′nəl-iz-əm) is increased secretory activity of the
_____. Hypersecretion of the adrenal cortex causes Cushing's syndrome, which is characterized by increased blood glucose levels, edema resulting from imbalance of water in the body, and masculinization in female individuals.
   Tumors that result in hypersecretion of androgens or estrogens before puberty usually have dramatic effects. This is called the <u>adrenogenital</u> (ə-dre″no-jen′ĭ-təl) <u>syndrome</u>. There is a rapid onset of puberty and sex drive in male individuals. In female individuals, the masculine distribution of body hair develops and the clitoris enlarges to look more like a penis.
   Excessive growth and male distribution of body hair in the female is <u>hirsutism</u>* (hir′soot-iz-əm). Hirsutism, however, means excessive growth of _____. It has several causes, including heredity, hormonal dysfunction, and medication. A decreased estrogen level or other hormonal dysfunction can result from abnormalities of the ovaries or adrenals.

17-64 Write a word that means any disease peculiar to the male gender by joining andr(o) and the suffix for disease: _____.

   Occasionally, an adrenal tumor secretes excess estrogens. When this occurs, the male patient experiences development of gyneco/mast/ia (gi″nə-, jin″ə-ko-mas′te-ə), which translated literally means a female breast condition. <u>Gynecomastia</u> means excessive growth of the male mammary glands.

17-65 <u>Hypo/adrenal/ism</u> (hi″po-ə-dre′nəl-iz-əm) is _____ adrenal activity. The loss of medullary activity does not cause as drastic an effect as the loss of adrenocortical activity. <u>Adreno/cortical</u> pertains to the adrenal _____.

*Hirsutism (Latin: *hirsutus*, shaggy).

Hyposecretion of epinephrine produces no significant effect. Hypersecretion, usually from a tumor, puts the body in a prolonged or continual fight-or-flight mode.

17-66 Hyposecretion of the adrenal cortex in which all three classes of adrenal corticosteroids are reduced leads to <u>Addison's disease</u>. This life-threatening condition is characterized by dehydration, low blood glucose levels, bronzing of the skin, and general ill health. Partial or complete failure of the adrenal glands can result from auto/immune processes, infection, tumors, or hemorrhage within the gland. Addison's disease results from _____ of the adrenal cortex.

17-67 The pancreas is subject to inflammation and cancer, and both conditions can lead to insufficient secretion of insulin. Write a term that means inflammation of the pancreas: _____. This disorder, as well as pancreatic cancer, can result in a deficiency of insulin secretion by the pancreas. <u>Hypo/insulin/ism</u> (**hi″po-in′su-lin-iz″əm**) is a deficient secretion of _____ by the pancreas.

17-68 <u>Diabetes mellitus</u> (DM) is primarily a result of <u>resistance to insulin</u> or a <u>deficiency or complete lack of insulin secretion</u> by the insulin-producing cells of the pancreas. Without insulin, glucose builds up in the blood and hyperglycemia results. <u>Hyper/glycem/ia</u> means a _____ than normal level of glucose in the blood.

Hyperglycemia causes serious fluid and electrolyte imbalances, ultimately resulting in the classic symptoms of diabetes: polyphagia, polyuria, and polydipsia. <u>Polyphagia</u> (**pol″e-fa′jə**) (*poly*, many, and *-phagia*, eating) means excessive hunger and uncontrolled eating. <u>Polyuria</u> (*-uria*, urination) means _____ urination, and <u>polydipsia</u> (*-dipsia*, thirst) means excessive thirst.

17-69 When used alone, the term *diabetes* generally refers to diabetes mellitus, but one should be aware that the term *diabetes* means excessive excretion of urine, and <u>diabetes insipidus</u>, for example, is so named because of its classic symptoms, not because of its relationship to DM.

Broad classifications of DM are type 1, type 2, gestational, and other types. <u>Type 1 diabetes</u> is genetically determined and results in absolute insulin deficiency; however, most people with this gene never develop type 1 diabetes. Individuals with this particular gene are genetically susceptible and may or may not experience development of diabetes _____.
This group was previously called insulin-dependent diabetes mellitus (IDDM).

Chronic complications of DM include vascular diseases and neuro/pathy (**noo-rop′ə-the**). Vascular diseases include diseases of the heart and major vessels, as well as smaller vessels (e.g., <u>diabetic nephro/pathy</u> [**nə-frop′ə-the**], which is damage to the small vessels of the kidneys and is the leading cause of end-stage renal disease in the United States). <u>Diabetic retino/pathy</u>, another complication, is a disorder of the retinal blood vessels of the eye that can eventually lead to blindness. <u>Diabetic neuropathy</u> is nerve damage associated with DM. Foot complications are a common problem for the patient with diabetes, particularly the development of <u>peripheral vascular disease</u> (PVD), which can lead to amputation.

17-70 The specific genetic link and development of <u>type 2 diabetes</u> is unclear. Contributing causes may be genetic and environmental factors, as well as the aging process and obesity. It is characterized by insulin resistance, rather than insufficient _____ secretion. This was formerly called non–insulin-dependent diabetes (NIDDM), but this was misleading, because some individuals with type 2 diabetes require insulin.

17-71 <u>Gestational diabetes mellitus</u> (GDM), first recognized during pregnancy, is carbohydrate intolerance, usually caused by a deficiency of insulin. It disappears after delivery of the infant, but in a significant number of cases, returns years later. This type of diabetes is called _____ diabetes mellitus.

There are some other less common types of DM in addition to type 1, type 2, and gestational. An example is the type of DM associated with hyperthyroidism.

17-72 <u>Hyper/insulin/ism</u> (**hi″pər-in′sə-lin-iz″əm**) is excessive insulin in the blood. Hyperinsulinism results in hypo/glyc/emia, a _____ amount of glucose in the blood.

---

hyposecretion

pancreatitis
  (pan″kre-ə-ti′tis)
insulin

greater

excessive

mellitus

insulin

gestational

decreased

hypoglycemia

Hypo/glycemia is a less than normal amount of glucose in the blood. It is caused by administration of too much insulin, excessive secretion of insulin by the pancreas, or dietary deficiency. An individual with hypoglycemia usually experiences weakness, headache, hunger, visual disturbances, and anxiety. If untreated, hypoglycemia can lead to coma and death. Write the term that means less than normal levels of glucose in the blood: _____.

17-73 The mammary glands are lactiferous glands in the female breasts that are the target organs of oxytocin and LTH. Many problems associated with the breast are not a result of hormones. However, hormones may be related to breast disorders, for example, inappropriate lactation (nipple discharge).

pain

Mamm/algia (mə-mal′jə), masto/dynia (mas″to-din′e-ə), and mast/algia (mas-tal′jə) mean breast _____.

Frequently encountered breast disorders include fibrocystic (fi″bro-sis′tik) disease, breast cancer, and benign tumors.

17-74 Fibro/cystic breast disease is a disorder characterized by single or multiple benign cysts of the breast. The cysts must be considered potentially malignant until diagnostic tests indicate otherwise; thereafter, the breasts should be observed carefully for change. The cysts often occur as a result of cyclic breast changes that accompany the menstrual cycle.

fibrocystic

This disorder characterized by benign cysts of the breast is called _____ breast disease.

17-75 A number of breast tumors are benign and can be differentiated from cancerous tumors by mammography and biopsy. Excluding skin cancer, breast cancer has been the most common malignancy among women in the United States for many years. The cause of breast cancer is still unknown, but early detection and improved treatment have contributed to a decrease in mortality rates. Breast cancer in female individuals is still a major cause of cancer death. Breast cancer in male individuals is rare.

Breast cancer often begins as a small, painless lump, dimpled skin, or nipple retraction. As the cancer progresses, there may be nipple discharge, pain, and ulceration.

cancer

Masto/carcinoma (mas″tə-kahr″sĭ-no′mə) is a term that means breast _____.

breast

17-76 Mast/itis (mas-ti′tis) is an inflammatory condition of the _____ that usually occurs most frequently in lactating women. It is usually caused by bacterial infection. If untreated, abscesses may form.

Exercise 6

Match pathologies in the left column with their characteristics in the right column.

_____ 1. acromegaly

_____ 2. Addison's disease

_____ 3. Cushing's syndrome

_____ 4. cretinism

_____ 5. diabetes mellitus

_____ 6. exophthalmos

_____ 7. gigantism

_____ 8. goiter

_____ 9. hypogonadism

_____ 10. myxedema

A. decreased functional activity of the ovaries or testes
B. enlarged thyroid gland
C. hypersecretion of the adrenal cortex
D. hypersecretion of GH in adults
E. hypersecretion of somatotropin during childhood
F. hyposecretion of the adrenal cortex
G. hyposecretion of thyroxine and T_3 during adulthood
H. hypothyroidism in childhood
I. insufficient secretion or resistance to insulin
J. outward protrusion of the eye

SURGICAL AND THERAPEUTIC INTERVENTIONS

17-77 Because the most common cause of hypopituitarism is a pituitary tumor, treatment consists of <u>surgery</u> or <u>radiation</u> to remove the tumor, followed by <u>administration of the deficient hormones</u>.

Certain types of pituitary tumors can cause overproduction of GH, and the treatment of choice is surgery to remove the tumor. Irradiation of the tumor and drugs may also be indicated. Overproduction of a single tropic hormone (such as TSH) usually causes oversecretion by the target organ (e.g., overproduction of thyroxine and T_3). Drug therapy may be useful to suppress the hormone production.

17-78 The treatment of hyperthyroidism is destruction of large amounts of the thyroid tissue by either surgery or <u>radioactive materials</u> or the use of <u>anti/thyroid drugs</u> to block the production of thyroid hormones. Thyroid/ectomy (**thi″roid-ek′tə-me**) is _____ of the thyroid.

excision

17-79 It may be necessary to surgically remove adrenal tumors that cause the adrenals to produce excess corticoids. Using adrenal(o), write a word that means excision of an adrenal gland: _____ .

adrenalectomy
(ə-dre″nəl-ek′to-me)

17-80 The goal of treatment of DM is to maintain a balance of the body's insulin and glucose. Type 1 diabetes is controlled by <u>administration of insulin</u>, <u>proper diet</u>, and <u>exercise</u>. Insulin is administered by injection on a regular basis, either by <u>sub/cutaneous injection</u> or insulin pump. An insulin pump is a portable battery-operated instrument that delivers a measured amount of insulin through the abdominal wall. It can be programmed to deliver doses of insulin according to the body's needs (Figure 17-13).

The individual with type 1 diabetes requires an outside source of _____ to sustain life.

insulin

Insulin is a <u>glucose-lowering agent</u> (GLA). Type 2 diabetes is controlled by diet, exercise, <u>oral agents</u>, and sometimes insulin. Oral agents are another type of GLA.

Proper nutrition is important in gestational diabetes. Insulin is given if nutritional therapy is insufficient.

17-81 Treatment of hypoglycemia may consist of a glucose paste placed inside the cheek, <u>administration of glucose</u> (dextrose) such as that found in orange juice, or intravenously if the person is unconscious. Strict attention to diet is important for patients with hypoglycemia caused by _____ secretion of insulin.

excessive

17-82 Treatment of breast cancer may require <u>lump/ectomy</u> (removal of the lump or tumor), radiation therapy, <u>chemotherapy</u>, <u>hormone manipulation</u>, or surgical removal of the breast. Use mast(o) to write a term that means surgical removal of a breast: _____ .

mastectomy
(mas-tek′tə-me)

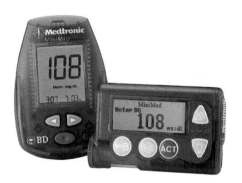

Figure 17-13 External insulin pump. This portable battery-operated instrument delivers a measured amount of insulin through the abdominal wall at preset intervals. The pump can be worn in the patient's pocket.

mastopexy (mas'to-pek-se)	**17-83** Masto/ptosis (mas"to-to'sis) is sagging or prolapsed breasts. Write a word using mast(o) that means surgical fixation of the breasts: _____. 　　Mastopexy is performed to correct a pendulous breast. (This is also called breast-lift.)
reduce	**17-84** Mammo/plasty (mam'o-plas"te) is plastic surgery of the breast. Augmentation mammoplasty is plastic surgery to increase the size of the female breast. Reduction mammoplasty is plastic surgery to _____ the size of the breast.

Exercise 7

Write a term for each of the following:

1. excision of a lump in the breast _____

2. excision of the thyroid _____

3. plastic surgery of the breast _____

4. removal of the adrenal gland _____

5. surgical fixation of the breasts _____

6. surgical removal of a breast _____

SELECTED ABBREVIATIONS

ACTH	adrenocorticotropic hormone		**LH**	luteinizing hormone
ADH	antidiuretic hormone		**LTH**	lactogenic hormone
DM	diabetes mellitus		**MSH**	melanocyte-stimulating hormone
FBS	fasting blood sugar		**PTH**	parathormone (parathyroid hormone)
FSH	follicle-stimulating hormone		**PVD**	peripheral vascular disease
GDM	gestational diabetes mellitus		**RAIU**	radioactive iodine uptake
GH	growth hormone		**STH**	somatotropic hormone
GTT	glucose tolerance test		**TCT**	thyrocalcitonin
Hb AIC	glycosylated hemoglobin		**TSH**	thyroid-stimulating hormone
HCG	human chorionic gonadotropin		T_3	triiodothyronine
^{131}I	radioactive iodine		T_4	thyroxine
ICSH	interstitial cell–stimulating hormone			

Chapter 17 Review

■ Basic Understanding

Listing

I. Write the names of the six major endocrine glands: _____

_____

II. Describe two ways in which the pituitary cooperates with the nervous system to maintain homeostasis.

1. _____

2. _____

Matching

III. Match each hormone with its target gland. (Some selections will be used more than once.)

_____ 1. antidiuretic hormone

_____ 2. follicle-stimulating hormone

_____ 3. luteinizing hormone

_____ 4. oxytocin

_____ 5. thyrotropin

A. breasts
B. gonads
C. kidneys
D. thyroid gland

IV. Match each hormone with the gland(s) that secrete them.

_____ 1. adrenocorticotropin

_____ 2. antidiuretic hormone

_____ 3. epinephrine

_____ 4. follicle-stimulating hormone

_____ 5. growth hormone

_____ 6. insulin

_____ 7. luteinizing hormone

_____ 8. melanocyte-stimulating hormone

_____ 9. oxytocin

_____ 10. testosterone

_____ 11. thyrocalcitonin

_____ 12. thyrotropin

_____ 13. thyroxine

A. adrenals
B. gonads
C. pancreas
D. pituitary
E. thyroid

V. *Match these hormones with their principal action.*

_____ 1. calcitonin

_____ 2. epinephrine

_____ 3. insulin

_____ 4. glucocorticoids

_____ 5. melanocyte-stimulating hormone

_____ 6. mineralocorticoids

_____ 7. parathormone

A. has antidiuretic effect
B. decreases blood calcium level
C. decreases blood glucose level
D. increases blood calcium level
E. increases blood glucose level
F. increases heart rate and blood pressure
G. promotes pigmentation of skin and hair

Multiple Choice
VI. *Circle the correct answer for each of the following questions.*

1. Which of the following is an exocrine gland? (adrenal gland, pituitary, sweat gland, thyroid)

2. Which of the following hormones produce masculine sex characteristics? (androgens, estrogens, prolactins, triiodothyronines)

3. What is the name of the diagnostic procedure that uses x-ray to study the breast? (mammogram, mammography, radioactive iodine uptake test, reduction mammoplasty)

4. Which of the following pathologies is associated with hypersecretion of the glucocorticoids? (Addison's disease, Cushing's syndrome, gigantism, thyrotoxicosis)

5. Which of the following is the expected result of increased secretion of growth hormone in adults? (acromegaly, cretinism, gigantism, gonadopathy)

6. Which of the following disorders is associated with a deficiency of ADH? (cretinism, diabetes insipidus, hyperaldosteronism, pituitary dwarfism)

7. Which of the following disorders is caused by hyposecretion of thyroxine and T_3 during adulthood? (cretinism, Graves' disease, hypogonadism, myxedema)

8. The islets of Langerhans are structures in which of the following organs? (adrenal gland, kidney, pancreas, thyroid)

9. Which of the following tests is more accurate for determining the degree of blood glucose control? (fasting blood sugar, glycosylated hemoglobin, radioactive iodine uptake, urinary ketones)

10. Which of the following terms means an enlarged thyroid gland? (goiter, hyperadenism, hyperthyroidism, hypothyroidism)

Writing Terms
VII. *Write a term for each of the following:*

1. adrenalin   _____

2. decreased thyroid activity   _____

3. excessive growth of hair   _____

4. glands that produce ova or sperm   _____

5. increased level of blood glucose   _____

6. lactogenic hormone   _____

7. master gland   _____

8. producing masculine characteristics   _____

9. stability in the normal body state   _____

10. sugar in the urine   _____

■ Greater Comprehension

Health Care Report
VIII. Write the meaning of underlined terms in the following case study.

CASE STUDY

Patient: W. A. Harter (62-year-old female)
Symptoms: Palpitations, hyperexcitability, weight loss, and <u>exophthalmos</u>.
History: Osteoporosis; currently in hospital with fractured hip after a fall.
Physical examination: <u>Goiter</u> present; pulse 120; blood pressure 170/96 mm Hg; appears anxious.
Diagnosis: <u>Hyperthyroidism</u>.
Plan: Conservative treatment with Tapazole for now. Consider possible <u>thyroidectomy</u>.

---

1. exophthalmos _____

2. goiter _____

3. hyperthyroidism _____

4. thyroidectomy _____

Health Care Report
IX. Write abbreviations or terms from the case study for the descriptions that follow the report.

CASE STUDY

Patient: M.E. Sanders (female, age 50)
Symptoms: Fatigue, polydipsia, polyuria.
History: Obesity, poorly healing skin wounds, frequent urinary tract infections, peripheral vascular disease, carcinoma of right breast with mastectomy, hypercholesteremia. Admitted to hospital for nonhealing leg ulcers.
Family history: Mother—age 75 with history of obesity, hypothyroidism, and fibrocystic breast disease. Father—age 80 with history of hypertension, IDDM with retinopathy and neuropathy, and nephropathy.
Laboratory tests: FBS 150; Hb AIC 9%.
Diagnosis: Diabetes mellitus type 2.
Plan: Weight loss with 1800-calorie diabetic diet; self-monitoring of blood sugar four times a day; oral hypoglycemic medication; repeat Hb AIC every 3 months.

---

1. excessive thirst _____

2. excessive urination _____

3. excision of a breast _____

4. damage to nerves resulting from diabetes _____

5. decreased thyroid activity _____

6. type 1 diabetes _____

7. disease of the retinal blood vessels _____

8. glycosylated hemoglobin _____

9. pertaining to a low blood sugar level _____

10. renal failure resulting from diabetes _____

Spelling

X. *Circle each misspelled term in the following list and write its correct spelling:*

adrenohypophysis   calcitonin   homostasis   neurohypophysis   tyrotropin

Interpreting Abbreviations

XI. *Write the meaning of these abbreviations:*

1. GDM _____

2. GH   _____

3. ICSH _____

4. ^{131}I   _____

5. TSH   _____

Pronunciation

XII. *The pronunciation of several medical terms is shown. Indicate the primary accented syllable by marking it with an ′.*

1. antidiuretic (an te, an tǐ di u ret ik)

2. gynecomastia (gi nə, jin ə ko mas te ə)

3. hypoadrenalism (hi po ə dre nəl iz əm)

4. mammoplasty (mam o plas te)

5. oxytocin (ok sǐ to sin)

Categorizing Terms

XIII. *Classify the terms in the left column by selecting A, B, C, D, or E.*

_____ 1. acromegaly

_____ 2. dwarfism

_____ 3. glucose-lowering agent

_____ 4. hirsutism

_____ 5. hypogonadism

_____ 6. lobule

_____ 7. mammogram

_____ 8. mastectomy

_____ 9. radioactive iodine uptake

_____ 10. thyroiditis

A. anatomy
B. diagnostic test or procedure
C. pathology
D. surgery
E. therapy

(Check your answers with the solutions in Appendix VI.)

LISTING OF MEDICAL TERMS

Use the practice CD to review the terms that have been presented. Look closely at the spelling of each term as it is pronounced and be sure you know the meaning of each term.

acromegaly
Addison's disease
adenocarcinoma
adenohypophyseal
adenohypophysis
adenoma
adenopathy
adrenal
adrenal cortex
adrenal medulla
adrenalectomy
adrenaline
adrenocortical
adrenocorticotropic
adrenocorticotropin
adrenogenital
adrenomegaly
adrenopathy
aldosterone
androgen
androgenic
andropathy
antidiuretic hormone
antithyroid
areola
atriopeptin
cachexia
calcitonin
colostrum
cortex
cortisone
cretinism
Cushing's syndrome
diabetes insipidus
diabetes mellitus
diabetic nephropathy
diabetic neuropathy
diabetic retinopathy
diuresis
diuretic
dwarfism

endocrine
epinephrine
estrogen
euthyroid
exocrine
exophthalmos
fibrocystic
follicle-stimulating
   hormone
gastrin
gestational diabetes
gigantism
gland
glucagon
glucocorticoid
glycosuria
glycosylated hemoglobin
goiter
gonad
gonadal
gonadotropic
gonadotropic hormone
gonadotropin
Graves' disease
gynecomastia
hirsutism
homeostasis
hormonal
hormone
human chorionic
   gonadotropin
hyperadrenalism
hypercalcemia
hyperglycemia
hyperinsulinism
hyperparathyroidism
hyperpituitarism
hypersecretion
hyperthyroidism
hypoadrenalism
hypocalcemia

hypoglycemia
hypogonadism
hypoinsulinism
hypoparathyroidism
hypophysis
hypopituitarism
hyposecretion
hypothalamus
hypothyroidism
insulin
intermammary
islets of Langerhans
ketone
ketonuria
lactation
lactiferous
lactogenesis
lactogenic hormone
lumpectomy
luteinizing hormone
mammalgia
mammary gland
mammogram
mammography
mammoplasty
mastalgia
mastectomy
mastitis
mastocarcinoma
mastodynia
mastopexy
mastoptosis
medulla
melanin
melanocyte-stimulating
   hormone
melatonin
mineralocorticosteroid
myxedema
neurohypophysis
norepinephrine

oxytocin
pancreas
pancreatitis
parathormone
parathyroid
pepsin
peripheral vascular disease
pineal gland
pituitary cachexia
pituitary gland
polydipsia
polyphagia
polyuria
progesterone
prolactin
prostaglandin
puberty
retromammary
somatotropic
somatotropin
steroid
suprarenal
target organ
testosterone
tetraiodothyronine
thymosin
thymus
thyrocalcitonin
thyroid
thyroidectomy
thyroiditis
thyropathy
thyrotoxicosis
thyrotropin
thyroxine
triiodothyronine
tropic

español ENHANCING SPANISH COMMUNICATION

ENGLISH	SPANISH (PRONUNCIATION)
adrenal	suprarenal (soo-prah-ray-NAHL)
adrenaline	adrenalina (ah-dray-nah-LEE-nah)
augmentation	aumento (ah-oo-MEN-to)
beard	barba (BAR-bah)
breasts	senos (SAY-nos)
calcium	calcio (CAHL-se-o)
diabetes	diabetes (de-ah-BAY-tes)
dwarf	enano (ay-NAH-no)
giant	gigante (he-GAHN-tay)
gland	glándula (GLAN-doo-lah)
glucose	glucosa (gloo-CO-sah)
goiter	papera (pah-PAY-rah)
growth	crecimiento (cray-se-me-EN-to)
hormone	hormona (or-MOH-nah)
insulin	insulina (in-soo-LEE-nah)
iodine	yodo (YO-do)
masculine	masculino (mas-coo-LEE-no)
nipple	pezón (pay-SON)
pancreas	páncreas (PAHN-cray-as)
pituitary	pituitario (pe-too-e-TAH-re-o)
same	mismo (MEES-mo)
synthesis	síntesis (SEEN-tay-sis)
thyroid	tiroides (te-RO-e-des)

CHAPTER **18**

Review of Chapters 1 Through 17

LEARNING GOALS

In this chapter, you will learn to do the following:

Basic Understanding
1. Match terms pertaining to anatomy, diagnostic tests or procedures, pathology, surgery, or therapy with their meanings or descriptions.
2. Write terms when presented with their definitions.
3. Categorize terms as anatomy, diagnostic test or procedure, pathology, surgery, or therapy.

Preparing for the Final Examination
This chapter is included to help you test yourself on how well you remember the material. Work all questions in the review if you completed all chapters in the book. Questions are presented within chapter groups. If you did not complete all chapters in the book, do not work the questions relating to chapters that you did not cover.

It is better to do all questions in a set before checking the answers. When you find that you have answered incorrectly, prepare a study sheet of terms that you did not remember. When finished with this chapter, look through the earlier chapters and find the correct answer for all questions that you missed. Analyze the component parts of these items.

The review is a representative sample of chapter material but does not include every term. Before taking the test that your instructor prepares, refer to your study sheet several times and study the list of terms at the end of each chapter, being sure you remember the meaning of each term.

THESE ARE THE MAJOR SECTIONS IN THIS CHAPTER:

CHAPTERS ARE DESIGNATED IN EACH SECTION.
  I. Multiple Choice Questions
  II. Writing Terms
  III. Categorizing Terms

I. Multiple Choice Questions

Circle the correct answer for each of the following questions.

■ *Chapter 2*

1. Cynthia is pregnant. Which type of specialist should she see to care for her during her pregnancy, labor, and delivery? (gerontologist, obstetrician, orthopedist, otologist)
2. Which of the following physicians specializes in the diagnosis and treatment of newborns through the age of 28 days? (geriatrician, gynecologist, neonatologist, urologist)
3. Sally injures her arm while ice skating. The emergency department physician orders an x-ray. Which type of physician is a specialist in interpreting radiographs? (gynecologist, ophthalmologist, plastic surgeon, radiologist)
4. What does the word *neuron* mean? (medical specialty that deals with the nervous system, nerve cell, neurosurgery, specialist in diseases of the nervous system)
5. Which physician specializes in diagnosis of disease using clinical laboratory results? (clinical pathologist, gastroenterologist, internist, surgical pathologist)

■ *Chapter 3*

6. Susie tells the doctor that she has a sore throat. Which term describes the sore throat? (diagnosis, prognosis, sign, symptom)
7. Mr. Jones has plastic surgery on his hand. What is the name of this procedure? (carpectomy, chiroplasty, ophthalmoplasty, otoplasty)
8. An elderly man is told he has an enlarged heart. Which term describes his condition? (cardiomegaly, carditis, coronary artery disease, megalomania)
9. Which term means a record of the electrical impulses of the heart? (electrocardiogram, electrocardiograph, electrocardiography, telecardiography)
10. Which diagnostic procedure produces an image of a detailed cross section of tissue similar to what one would see if the organ were actually cut into sections? (computed tomography, contrast imaging, electrocardiography, nuclear medicine imaging)

■ *Chapter 4*

11. Johnny, a college student, sees the physician and is told that his appendix is inflamed. What is the name of his condition? (appendectomy, appendicitis, appendorrhexis, appendotomy)
12. Karen sustains a severe head injury in which there is herniation of the brain through an opening in the skull. What is the name of this pathology? (cerebritis, cerebrotomy, encephalocele, encephaloplasty).
13. Ken suffers from an abnormal fear of heights. What type of pathology does he have? (dilatation, mania, phobia, ptosis)
14. Which of the following produces insensibility or stupor? (analgesic, anesthetics, narcotic, pharmaceutic)
15. Which of the following is a medication that is used to treat neoplasms? (analgesic, antineoplastic, local anesthesia, regional anesthesia)

■ *Chapter 5*

16. Which term describes a structure that can be seen with the naked eye? (macroscopic, microscopic, ophthalmoscopic, ophthalmoscopy)
17. What does the prefix in antibiotic mean? (against, before, effective, supporting)
18. What is the meaning of the prefix in bilateral? (one, two, three, four)

19. In which type of injection is the needle placed in the subcutaneous tissue? (intradermal, intramuscular, intravenous, subcutaneous)
20. Which term means a set of symptoms that occur together and characterize a particular disease or condition? (dysphoria, symptomatic, syndrome, tachyphasia)

■ Chapter 6

21. Which term means similar cells acting together to perform a function? (body system, organ, organism, tissue)
22. Pete is trying to explain a method of drawing imaginary lines to designate abdominal areas. Which term should he use to describe the areas when the abdomen is divided into four regions? (bilateral areas, nine regions, six regions, quadrants)
23. Dr. Ray explains in a radiology report that a fracture has occurred in the distal portion of the thigh bone. What does distal mean? (farther from the origin, in the middle of the bone, nearer the origin, on the side of the bone)
24. Which plane divides the body into anterior and posterior portions? (frontal, midsagittal, sagittal, transverse)
25. Which of these terms means a muscular partition that separates the thoracic and abdominopelvic cavities? (diaphragm, paracentesis, peritoneum, pyrogen)

■ Chapter 7

26. Which element of the blood is responsible for transportation of oxygen to body cells? (blood platelets, erythrocytes, leukocytes, thrombocytes)
27. Which term means having no tendency to repair itself or to develop into new tissue? (analytic, anisocytosis, aplastic, hemolytic)
28. What is the surgical procedure whereby living organs are transferred from one part of the body to another or from one individual to another? (rejection, transmission, transplant, transreaction)
29. Where is intracellular fluid found? (around, between, inside, outside) cells.
30. What is a decrease in the number of blood platelets called? (hemophilia, leukemia, leukocytosis, thrombopenia)

■ Chapter 8

31. Charlie, a 60-year-old man, has just been diagnosed as having a coronary occlusion. He is most at risk for which of the following? (atrioventricular block, congenital heart disease, myocardial infarction, rheumatic fever)
32. Charlie is told that he has a form of arteriosclerosis in which yellowish plaque has accumulated on the walls of the arteries. What is the name of this form of arteriosclerosis? (aortostenosis, atherosclerosis, cardiomyopathy, coarctation)
33. Jim developed a blood clot in a coronary artery. What is Jim's condition called? (myocardial infarction, coronary artery bypass, coronary thrombosis, fibrillation)
34. Baby Seth is born with cyanosis and a heart murmur. Which congenital heart disease does the neonatologist think is most likely? (atrial septal defect, atrioventricular block, megalocardia, pericarditis)
35. Ten-year-old Zack had a sore throat for several days before painful joints and a fever developed. Which disease does the physician suspect that can cause damage to the heart valves? (aortic valve sclerosis, aortic valve stenosis, mitral valve prolapse, rheumatic fever)

■ Chapter 9

36. Mrs. Smith's doctor tells her that she has pneumonia. What is another name for her diagnosis? (congestive heart disease, pneumonitis, pulmonary edema, pulmonary insufficiency)
37. Which term means coughing up and spitting out sputum? (expectoration, expiration, exhalation, extrapleural)

38. What is the name of the serous membrane that lines the walls of the thoracic cavity? (parietal pleura, rhinorrhea, silicosis, visceral pleura)
39. What is the correct sequence for the first and second leading causes of adult deaths in the United States? (cancer and heart, heart and cancer, heart and colon cancer, lung cancer and colon cancer)
40. Mrs. Sema has difficulty breathing except when sitting in an upright position. What is the term for her condition? (anoxia, hypocapnia, inspiration, orthopnea)

■ *Chapter 10*

41. Cal Stone has radiography of the gallbladder. What is the name of this diagnostic test? (barium enema, barium meal, cholecystography, esophagogastroscopy)
42. Tests show that Cal Stone has a gallstone in the common bile duct. Which of the following is a noninvasive conservative procedure to alleviate Cal's problem? (cholecystostomy, choledochostomy, choledochojejunostomy, extracorporeal shock wave lithotripsy)
43. Linda M., a 16-year-old girl, is diagnosed as having self-induced starvation. Which of the following is the name of the disorder associated with Linda's problem? (anorexia nervosa, aphagia, malaise, polyphagia)
44. Unless there is intervention for Linda's self-induced starvation, which condition will result? (adipsia, atresia, emaciation, volvulus)
45. A 70-year-old man is diagnosed with cancer of the colon. Which term indicates a surgical intervention for this condition? (colectomy, colonoscopy, colonic irrigation, colonic stasis)

■ *Chapter 11*

46. Which of the following terms means making radiographic images of the urinary system after the urine has been rendered opaque by a contrast medium? (cystoscopy, cystoureteroscopy, intravenous pyelography, nephrotomography)
47. Which of the following is indicated if the blood urea nitrogen level is increased? (pyelostomy, pyuria, renal clearance, renal failure)
48. Which term means an inability to control urination? (frequency, hesitancy, incontinence, retention)
49. Which term means excretion of an abnormally large quantity of urine? (anuria, dysuria, oliguria, polyuria)
50. Which of the following is not a type of urinary tract catheterization? (endoscopy tube, nephrostomy tube, suprapubic tube, urethral tube)

■ *Chapter 12*

51. Which term means difficult or painful menstruation? (amenorrhea, dysmenorrhea, metrorrhagia, menorrhea)
52. Which of the following instruments is commonly used in a gynecologic examination? (curet, hysterosalpingograph, hysteroscope, speculum)
53. Which term means surgical fixation of a prolapsed uterus? (cervicectomy, hysterectomy, hysteropexy, leiomyomectomy)
54. Which term means a condition in which tissue that contains typical endometrial elements is present outside the uterus? (endometriosis, endometritis, hysteropathy, salpingopathy).
55. Which term means absence of a testis? (anorchidism, aspermia, oligospermia, orchidectomy)

■ *Chapter 13*

56. Which term means abnormal or difficult labor? (abortion, dystocia, eclampsia, stillbirth)
57. Which of the following is a genetic disorder in which the fetus has an extra chromosome? (Down syndrome, erythroblastosis fetalis, hemolytic anemia, implantation)
58. Which term means the same as pregnancy? (embryonic, gestation, ovulation, parturition)

59. Which of the following is the normal presentation of the fetus during labor? (breech, cephalic, shoulder, transverse)
60. Which of the following is the common name for Condyloma acuminatum? (genital herpes, genital warts, moniliasis, venereal ulcer)

■ Chapter 14

61. Which term means congenital fissure of the breastbone? (costectomy, rachischisis, spondylosyndesis, sternoschisis)
62. Which term means pertaining to two bones of the forearm? (carpopedal, carpophalangeal, humeroulnar, ulnoradial)
63. Which term means any disease of the joints? (arthropathy, bursopathy, chondropathy, osteopathy)
64. Which of the following is the record produced in a procedure that records the response of a muscle to electrical stimulation? (arthrocentesis, electromyogram, myograph, range of motion reading)
65. What is the term for the presence of extra fingers or toes? (carpopedal disease, Paget's disease, phalangitis, polydactylism)

■ Chapter 15

66. Which of the following is the outermost meningeal membrane? (arachnoid, dura mater, epidural, pia mater)
67. Which term means paralysis of the lower portion of the body and both legs? (diplegia, hemiplegia, paraplegia, quadriplegia)
68. Which of the following means hernial protrusion of the meninges through a defect in the vertebral column? (meningitis, meningocele, myelocele, myelomalacia)
69. Which term means incision of the lacrimal sac? (cholecystotomy, cystolithectomy, dacryocystotomy, dacryolithiasis)
70. Which of the following is chronic, progressive mental deterioration that involves irreversible loss of memory, disorientation, and speech and gait disturbances? (Alzheimer's disease, Lou Gehrig's disease, Meniere's syndrome, multiple sclerosis)

■ Chapter 16

71. Which of the following means removal of foreign material and dead or contaminated tissue from an infected or traumatic lesion until surrounding healthy tissue is exposed? (débridement, necrosis, pyemia, rhytidectomy)
72. Which of the following is an inflammatory skin disease that begins on the scalp but may involve other areas, particularly the eyebrows? (acne vulgaris, basal cell carcinoma, seborrheic dermatitis, verruca).
73. Which term means a disease characterized by chronic hardening and thickening of the skin? (ecchymosis, Kaposi's sarcoma, keratosis, scleroderma)
74. In describing a burn by "thickness," which type of burn is characterized by blisters? (deep partial-thickness, deep full-thickness, full-thickness, superficial partial-thickness)
75. Which term means the death of areas of tissue or bone surrounded by healthy parts? (atrophy, erosion, fissure, necrosis)

■ Chapter 17

76. The islets of Langerhans are structures in which of the following organs? (adrenal, kidney, pancreas, thyroid)
77. Which of the following terms means an enlarged thyroid gland? (goiter, hyperadenism, hyperthyroidism, hypothyroidism)
78. What is the name of the diagnostic procedure that uses x-ray to study the breast? (mammogram, mammography, radioactive iodine uptake test, reduction mammoplasty)

79. Which of the following disorders is associated with a deficiency of ADH? (cretinism, diabetes insipidus, hyperaldosteronism, pituitary dwarfism)
80. Which of the following pathologies is associated with hypersecretion of the glucocorticoids? (Addison's disease, Cushing's syndrome, gigantism, thyrotoxicosis)

II. Writing Terms

Write one word for each of the following clues.

■ *Chapter 2*

1. having a severe and relatively short duration   _____
2. method of prioritizing patients according to their need   _____
3. pertaining to the heart   _____
4. study of the characteristics, causes, and effects of disease   _____
5. the secretions of endocrine glands   _____

■ *Chapter 3*

6. excision of the colon   _____
7. incision of the eye   _____
8. instrument used in encephalotomy   _____
9. suture of a vessel   _____
10. swelling of the eyelid   _____

■ *Chapter 4*

11. a substance that causes hemolysis   _____
12. a substance that produces cancer   _____
13. any disease of the eye   _____
14. inflammation of a bone   _____
15. pertaining to the nose   _____

■ *Chapter 5*

16. having no symptoms   _____
17. abnormally slow speech   _____
18. absence of the external ear   _____
19. behind the nose   _____
20. double vision   _____

■ *Chapter 6*

21. affecting only one side

22. lying flat on the back

23. inflammation of the skin

24. pertaining to the abdomen and pelvis

25. a record of electrical impulses of the brain

■ *Chapter 7*

26. any erythrocyte of irregular shape

27. below normal sodium in the blood

28. dissolving of a thrombus

29. neutral-staining granulocyte

30. production of blood

■ *Chapter 8*

31. absence of a heart beat

32. agent that causes dilation of blood vessels

33. increased blood pressure

34. increased pulse

35. inflammation of a lymphatic vessel

■ *Chapter 9*

36. an internal blood clot

37. difficult or weak voice

38. presence of nasal calculi

39. pertaining to the air sacs of the lung

40. radiographic examination of the larynx

■ *Chapter 10*

41. any disease of the stomach

42. enzyme that breaks down starch

43. excessive vomiting

44. excision of the gallbladder

45. inflammation of the stomach

■ *Chapter 11*

46. inflammation of the renal glomeruli _____

47. inflammation of the renal pelvis _____

48. outside the urinary bladder _____

49. radiography of the bladder _____

50. surgical crushing of a stone _____

■ *Chapter 12*

51. incision of the vas deferens _____

52. inflammation of the cervix uteri _____

53. inflammation of the vulva and vagina _____

54. insufficient sperm in the semen _____

55. surgical fixation of a fallopian tube _____

■ *Chapter 13*

56. a woman who has produced many viable offspring _____

57. attachment of a fertilized ovum to the endometrium _____

58. deliberate rupture of the fetal membranes to induce labor _____

59. incision made to enlarge the vaginal opening for delivery _____

60. painless sore of syphilis _____

■ *Chapter 14*

61. degenerative joint disease _____

62. excision of the tailbone _____

63. herniation of a muscle _____

64. inflammation of a bone _____

65. lateral curvature of the spine _____

■ *Chapter 15*

66. radiography of the spinal cord _____

67. recording the electrical activity of the brain _____

68. the presence of lacrimal calculi _____

69. inflammation of the brain and spinal cord _____

70. inflammation of the cornea _____

■ *Chapter 16*

71. another name for a bruise   _____

72. any disease of the nails   _____

73. superficial infection involving hair follicles   _____

74. absence of pigment in the skin, hair, and nails   _____

75. a torn, jagged wound   _____

■ *Chapter 17*

76. master gland   _____

77. producing masculine characteristics   _____

78. decreased thyroid activity   _____

79. glands that produce ova and sperm   _____

80. sugar in the urine   _____

III. Categorizing Terms

Classify each term by writing *A* (anatomy), *D* (diagnostic test or procedure), *P* (pathology), *S* (surgery), or *T* (therapy).

■ *Chapter 2*

1. anesthetic   _____

2. gastric   _____

3. neurosurgery   _____

4. ophthalmic   _____

5. tumor   _____

■ *Chapter 3*

6. adenectomy   _____

7. blepharoplasty   _____

8. colonoscopy   _____

9. colorrhaphy   _____

10. edema   _____

■ *Chapter 4*

11. analgesics _____
12. blepharal _____
13. dermatitis _____
14. jaundice _____
15. electrocardiogram _____

■ *Chapter 5*

16. intramuscular _____
17. microtia _____
18. postnasal _____
19. suprarenal _____
20. tachyphasia _____

■ *Chapter 6*

21. acrocyanosis _____
22. antipyretics _____
23. aplasia _____
24. febrile _____
25. thoracotomy _____

■ *Chapter 7*

26. analgesics _____
27. cyanosis _____
28. leukocyte _____
29. lithotripsy _____
30. staphylococcemia _____

■ *Chapter 8*

31. aneurysm _____
32. angiostomy _____
33. arteriography _____
34. thymus _____
35. ultrasonography _____

■ *Chapter 9*

36. acidosis _____

37. bronchogram _____

38. coryza _____

39. glottis _____

40. thromboembolics _____

■ *Chapter 10*

41. diverticulectomy _____

42. endoscopy _____

43. gingiva _____

44. glossorrhaphy _____

45. pancreatography _____

■ *Chapter 11*

46. dysuria _____

47. hydronephrosis _____

48. lithotrite _____

49. nephrectomy _____

50. renal _____

■ *Chapter 12*

51. candidiasis _____

52. chemotherapeutic _____

53. colporrhaphy _____

54. hydrocele _____

55. scrotal _____

■ *Chapter 13*

56. eclampsia _____

57. extrauterine _____

58. endometrium _____

59. pelvimetry _____

60. stethoscope _____

■ *Chapter 14*

61. arthrocentesis   _____

62. calcaneofibular   _____

63. chondrectomy   _____

64. dystrophy   _____

65. myelosuppressives _____

■ *Chapter 15*

66. cerebellum   _____

67. echoencephalograph _____

68. hydrocephalus   _____

69. neurosclerosis   _____

70. vagotomy   _____

■ *Chapter 16*

71. dermatomycosis _____

72. liposuction   _____

73. rhytidoplasty   _____

74. trichopathy   _____

75. ungual   _____

■ *Chapter 17*

76. adrenalectomy _____

77. exophthalmos _____

78. mastectomy   _____

79. myxedema   _____

80. parathyroids   _____

APPENDIX I Pharmacology

James F. McCalpin, R.Ph.

CHAPTER 2

Pharmacology is the science that deals with the origin, nature, chemistry, effects, and uses of drugs. A drug may modify one or more of the body's functions. Drugs are used in medicine to prevent, diagnose, and treat disease and to relieve pain. Another term for medicines is *pharmaceuticals*. Radioactive pharmaceuticals that are used for medicinal diagnosis or treatment are called radiopharmaceuticals.

Drug abuse is use of any drug in a way that deviates from the manner in which it was prescribed. *Drug addiction* is caused by excessive or continued use of habit-forming drugs.

Giving a drug to a patient is called *drug administration*. The various ways a drug may be administered are called the *routes of administration*. Although most therapeutics are administered orally or by injection, they can sometimes be administered through the skin (transdermal patches) or mucous membranes (e.g., nasal spray). *Parenteral administration* includes all of the ways a drug may be administered except through the digestive tract.

Once administered, a drug may remain at the site of administration or it may enter the blood. The movement of the drug from the administration site into the blood is called *absorption* of the drug. The transportation of the drug to other body tissues is called the *distribution* of the drug. Where and how a drug combines with the tissue is called the *action* of the drug. If the effect is confined to the site of administration, the drug has a *local* effect. If it acts on many sites away from the administration site, the effect is said to be *systemic*. The drug eventually is chemically changed, a process called *biotransformation*.

A measured amount of a drug is called a *dose*. The greater the effect with a single dose, the more potent a drug is.

The *generic name* (e.g., acetaminophen) of a drug may be used by any company, whereas the trade name or *brand name* (e.g., Tylenol) is the property of only one company and cannot be used by other companies. The first letter of the *trade name* is capitalized.

CHAPTER 3

Drugs are generally grouped into several *classes* on the basis of their major effects. The following list indicates the class of various drugs and gives some representative examples. Actions, reactions, and interactions with other drugs often are shared by drugs of the same class. Pharmacists provide information regarding a medication's possible side effects—that is, reactions to or the consequences of taking the particular medication. Adverse drug reactions are harmful, unexpected reactions to a drug.

The drugs are listed by generic name with the trade name in parentheses. The trade name may be the only medication of its type available or the name more commonly used. The drugs listed for this chapter pertain to the whole body rather than to a particular body system. Rather than memorizing the names of the drugs, it is more important to remember the drug classes and their uses. Subsequent chapters also have a pharmacology section.

DRUG CLASS	EFFECTS AND USES
Anesthetics	**Loss of Sensation**
Local anesthetics	*Local loss of sensation*
Benzocaine (Solarcaine)	Topical anesthetic
Cocaine	Topical anesthetic (mucous membrane)
Dibucaine (Nupercaine)	Nerve block, spinal anesthetic
Lidocaine (Xylocaine)	Topical anesthetic, nerve block
Procaine (Novocain)	Nerve block
Tetracaine (Pontocaine)	Spinal anesthetic

General anesthetics	*Loss of all body sensation, loss of consciousness*
Halothane (Fluothane)	Major surgery
Ketamine	Major surgery
Nitrous oxide	Minor surgery
Propofol (Diprivan)	Major surgery
Thiopental (Pentothal)	Minor surgery, induction anesthetic
Neuromuscular Blocking Drugs	**Used in Surgery to Cause Flaccid Paralysis So Surgeon Can Cut Through Muscles Without Reflex Contraction**
Cisatracurium (Nimbex)	
Curare	
Dimethyltubocurarine (Metabine)	
Pancuronium (Pavulon)	Also used to produce respiratory paralysis in some patients who are on intermittent positive pressure respirators, as in the treatment of tetanus
Succinylcholine (Anectine)	Most widely used blocking drug in surgery
Tubocurarine	
Opioid Antagonists	**Used to Reverse Narcotics**
Naloxone (Narcan)	Reverses opioid effects, including respiratory depression
Radiopharmaceuticals	**Used to Assess Many Internal Structures and to Treat Hyperfunction**
Iodine-131 (Iodotope)	Used in thyroid cancer
Strontium-89 (Metastron)	Used for metastatic bone pain

CHAPTER 4

DRUG CLASS	**EFFECTS AND USES**
Antiinfectives/Antimicrobials	**Used Against Microorganisms**
Amebicides	*Kill amebae*
Emetine	For amebic dysentery
Metronidazole (Flagyl)	Used in the treatment of trichomoniasis
Paromomycin (Humatin)	Used to treat acute and chronic intestinal amebiasis
Aminoglycosides	*Generally active against gram-negative bacteria (neurotoxic, ototoxic, and nephrotoxic)*
Amikacin (Amikin)	
Gentamicin (Garamycin)	
Kanamycin (Kantrex)	
Tobramycin (Nebcin)	
Antibacterials	*Used in bacterial infections*
Cephalosporins	
First generation	*Used mainly against gram-negative cocci*
Cefpodoxime (Vantin)	
Cefazolin (Kefzol)	
Cephalexin (Keflex)	
Cephalothin (Keflin)	
Second generation	*Used mainly against gram-positive cocci and H. influenzae*
Cefaclor (Ceclor)	
Cefamandole (Mandol)	

Third generation
Azithromycin (Zithromax)
Cefoperazone (Cefobid)
Ceftazidime (Fortaz)
Chloramphenicol (Chloromycetin)
Clarithromycin (Biaxin)
Erythromycin (E-Mycin)
Nitrofurantoin (Furadantin)
Kanamycin (Kantrex)

Penicillins
Amoxicillin (Amoxil)
Ampicillin (Polycillin)
Penicillin G (K-cillin)
Amoxicillin/Pot. Clavulanate (Augmentin)

Sulfas
Sulfisoxazole (Gantrisin)

Tetracycline (Achromycin)
Vancomycin (Vancocin)

Antifungals
Amphotericin B (Fungizone)
Fluconazole (Diflucan)
Nystatin (Mycostatin)
Terbinafine (Lamisil)

Antihelmintics
Mebendazole (Vermox)
Pyrantel (Antiminth)

Antimalarials
Quinine
Quinacrine (Atabrine)
Mefloquine (Lariam)

Antituberculars
Ethambutol (Myambutol)
Isoniazid (INH)
Rifampin (Rifadin)
Pyrazinamide
Cycloserine (Seromycin)

Antivirals
Acyclovir (Zovirax)
Amantadine (Symmetrel)
Zidovudine (Retrovir)
Stavudine, D4T (Zerit)
Dideoxyinosine, dDi (Videx)
Zalcitabine, ddc (Hivid)
Famciclovir (Famvir)
Foscarnet sodium (Foscavir)

Fluoroquinolones
Ciprofloxacin (Cipro)
Norfloxacin (Noroxin)
Ofloxacin (Floxin)

Expanded spectrum against gram-negative bacteria

Gram-positive and gram-negative (broad spectrum)

Streptococcal infections
Urinary gram-negative microorganisms
Mainly gram-negative, some gram-positive

Most gram-positive and gram-negative aerobes

Mainly gram-positive

Urinary tract infections
Urinary tract—mainly gram-positive

Gram-positive and gram-negative (broad spectrum)
Life-threatening infections

Used in fungal infections
Parenteral drug used in severe fungal infections

Topical candidiasis infections
Treats onychomycosis of toes and fingernails

Destroy worms
Used for pinworms, whipworms
Used to treat *Ascaris*

Used to treat malaria

Used to treat organisms of genus Mycobacterium

Used in some viral infections
Herpes infection
Influenza type A viruses
Human immunodeficiency virus exposure

Use with caution in children younger than 18 years

CHAPTER 5

DRUG CLASS	EFFECTS AND USES
Analgesics	**Relief of Pain**
Non-narcotic analgesics	*No abuse potential; for mild to moderate pain*
Acetaminophen (Tylenol)	
Aspirin (many trade names)	
Ibuprofen (Motrin)	
Tramadol (Ultram)	
Narcotic analgesics	*Potential for abuse*
Codeine	Mild to moderate pain
Meperidine (Demerol)	Moderate pain
Methadone (Dolophine)	Drug detoxification
Morphine	Moderate to severe pain
Propoxyphene (Darvon and Darvocet)	Mild to moderate pain
Oxycodone (Percodan; OxyContin)	Severe pain
Sufentanil (Fentanyl)	Severe pain
Antiinflammatory Drugs	**Reduce Inflammation**
Aspirin	
Cyclooxygenase-2 (COX-2)	New group of nonsteroidal antiinflammatory drugs with fewer side effects
Celecoxib (Celebrex)	
Nonsteroidal antiinflammatory drugs	
Diclofenac (Voltaren)	
Indomethacin (Indocin)	
Ibuprofen (Motrin)	
Naproxen (Naprosyn)	
Prednisone	
Antipyretics	**Drugs Used to Reduce Fever**
Acetaminophen (Tylenol)	
Aspirin	
Ibuprofen (Motrin)	

CHAPTER 6

DRUG CLASS	EFFECTS AND USES
Minerals	
Calcium	Essential for bone and tooth formation, for clotting of blood, and for normal nervous system activity, including heart
Iron, gluconate (Fergon), sulfate (Feosol)	Essential for hemoglobin formation and for function of certain enzymes
Magnesium	Essential for enzymes to function properly
Manganese	Essential for enzymes to function properly
Phosphorus	Essential for bone and tooth formation and for maintaining normal pH of body fluids
Potassium	Essential for normal cardiac and other muscle functions and for nervous system integrity
Sodium	Essential for normal cardiovascular function, maintenance of fluid balance, and nervous system function
Vitamins	
A (β-carotene, retinol)	Prevents night blindness

B-Complex

Folic acid	Used for megaloblastic and macrocytic anemias
Niacin, niacinamide	Used for the treatment of pellagra
Pantothenic acid	Used to stimulate intestinal peristalsis
Pyridoxine, B_6	Prevents gastroenteritis, convulsions, neuritis
Riboflavin, B_2	Used to treat microcytic anemia
Thiamine, B_1	Used to treat beriberi
Cyanocobalamin, B_{12}	Used to treat pernicious anemia

Other Vitamins

C (ascorbic acid)	Used to prevent scurvy
D	Used to treat rickets
E	Used as a vitamin supplement
K, menadione	Used to treat hypoprothrombinemia

CHAPTER 7

DRUG CLASS	EFFECTS AND USES
Anticoagulants	**Prevent Clotting of Blood**
Indirect-acting	*Act in liver to prevent synthesis of clotting factors*
Warfarin (Coumadin)	Can be administered orally or intravenously
Direct-acting	*Act in blood to prevent activation of clotting factors*
Heparin (Panheprin)	
Aspirin (many trade names)	
Pentoxifylline (Trental)	Intermittent claudication
Antihistamines	**Oppose the Action of Histamine**
H_1 *types*	*Inhibit most actions of histamine, particularly block allergic reactions*
Diphenhydramine (Benadryl)	Drowsiness is the main side effect
Fexofenadine (Allegra)	Much less drowsiness
Triprolidine (Actidil)	
Desloratadine (Clarinex)	
Loratadine (Claritin)	Much less drowsiness
H_2 *types*	*Inhibit histamine action on parietal cells, thus reducing gastric acid secretion*
Cimetidine (Tagamet)	Used in the treatment of gastric ulcers
Omeprazole (Prilosec)	Used in the treatment of gastric ulcers
Ranitidine (Zantac)	
Esomeprazole (Nexium)	
Lansoprazole (Prevacid)	A proton pump inactivator used in gastric reflux
Antineoplastic Drugs/ Chemotherapeutics	**Drugs Used to Treat Cancer**
Cisplatin (Platinol)	Used for metastatic carcinoma
Cyclophosphamide (Cytoxan)	Used in myeloma and solid tumors
DTIC-Dome	Used in Hodgkin's disease
Doxorubicin (Adriamycin)	Used in solid tumors
Fluorouracil (5-FU)	Used in carcinoma of the colon
Melphalan (Alkeran)	Used in multiple myelomas
Estramustine (EMCYT)	Prostate carcinoma
Methotrexate	Used to treat trophoblastic neoplasms in women
Tamoxifen (Nolvadex)	Mainly used in mammary cancer

Antiplatelet Drugs (Platelet Aggregation Inhibitors)
Aspirin
Dipyridamole (Persantine)
Ticlopidine (Ticlid)

Reduce Risk of Arterial Thrombin Formation

The most commonly used drug

Hemostatics
Aminocaproic acid
Phytonadione (vitamin K)

Control Bleeding
Used in acute life-threatening situations
Used to control bleeding, an oral preparation

Immunosuppressants
Azathioprine (Imuran)
Mycophenolate (CellCept)
Glatiramer (Copaxone)
Cyclosporine (Neoral)
Tacrolimus (Prograf)

Adjuncts for Prevention of Graft Rejection

Used to prevent kidney transplant rejection
Used to prevent rejection of kidney, liver, and heart allografts

Vaccines
BCG vaccine (bacille Calmette-Guérin vaccine)
Cholera vaccine
Hepatitis A virus vaccine
Hepatitis B virus vaccine

Influenza virus vaccine (Fluzone)
Measles virus vaccine
Mumps vaccine (Mumpsvax)
Plague vaccine

Pneumococcal vaccine
Polio virus (IPOL)
Rabies vaccine

Rubella vaccine (Meruvax)
Typhoid vaccine
Yellow fever vaccine

Used to Prevent or Modulate Diseases
Used to promote active immunity to tuberculosis

Used for prevention of cholera

Used to promote immunity in individuals at high risk for potential exposure to hepatitis B
Used to promote active immunity to influenza
Used to promote active immunity to measles
Used to promote active immunity to mumps
Used to promote active immunity in individuals at high risk for infection after exposure
Used to promote active immunity to pneumonia
Used to promote active immunity to polio
Used to promote active immunity to individuals who have been exposed to rabies
Used to promote active immunity to rubella
Used to promote active immunity to individuals at risk
Used to promote active immunity to yellow fever

CHAPTER 8

DRUG CLASS

EFFECTS AND USES

Antihypertensives
Angiotensin-converting enzyme (ACE) inhibitors
Captopril (Capoten)
Ramipril (Altace)
Fosinopril (Monopril)
Lisinopril (Zestril)
Quinapril (Accupril)
Enalapril (Vasotec)
Trandolapril (Mavik)

Reduce Blood Pressure to Treat Hypertension

Block formation of angiotensin II

Calcium channel blockers   *Inhibit movement of calcium ions across cell membranes*
Nifedipine (Procardia)
Bepridil (Vascor)
Isradipine (DynaCirc)
Amlodipine (Norvasc)
Diltiazem (Cardizem)
Verapamil (Calan)
Nisoldipine (Sular)

Beta-adrenergic blocking agents   *Exert a quinidine-like effect*
Atenolol (Tenormin)
Pindolol (Visken)
Metoprolol (Lopressor)
Nadolol (Corgard)
Propranolol (Inderal)

Diuretics   *Used for edema and hypertension*
Hydrochlorothiazide, HCTZ
   (HydroDIURIL)
Indapamide (Lozol)
Metolazone (Zaroxolyn)
Furosemide (Lasix)   Inhibit reabsorption of water in renal tubules
Bumetanide (Bumex)   Inhibit reabsorption of water in renal tubules
Spironolactone (Aldactone)   A potassium-sparing diuretic
Triamterene (Dyrenium)   A potassium-sparing diuretic
Torsemide (Demadex)

Carbonic anhydrase inhibitors   *Used in glaucoma to decrease intraocular pressure*
Acetazolamide (Diamox)
Methazolamide (Neptazane)

Antianginal Drugs   **Used to Relieve Pain of Acute Angina Pectoris and for Prophylaxis**
Isosorbide mononitrate (ISMO)   Used for angina pectoris
Nitroglycerin (Nitrostat)   Used for the management of angina pectoris
Isosorbide dinitrate (Isordil)   Used for the management of angina pectoris

Antiarrhythmic Drugs   **Regulate Cardiac Arrhythmias**
Moricizine (Ethmozine)
Ibutilide fumarate (Corvert)
Quinidine (Quinora)
Procainamide (Pronestyl)
Disopyramide (Norpace)
Lidocaine (Xylocaine)
Tocainide (Tonocard)
Propafenone (Rythmol)
Adenosine (Adenocard)

Blood Flow Agents   **Peripheral Vasodilators**
Cyclandelate (Cyclospasmol)   Used for intermittent cramping of legs
Isoxsuprine (Vasodilan)   Used for relief of symptoms of cerebral vascular insufficiency
Minoxidil (Loniten)

Cardiac Drugs   **Used in Congestive Heart Failure, Atrial Fibrillation, Atrial Flutter**
Digoxin (Lanoxin)
Amrinone (Inocor)
Flecainide (Tambocor)

Cholesterol-reducing Agents
Antihyperlipidemics   *Reduce lipids (cholesterol) in the blood*
Cholestyramine (Questran)
Colestipol (Colestid)
Lovastatin (Mevacor)
Simvastatin (Zocor)
Pravastatin (Pravachol)
Atorvastatin (Lipitor)
Gemfibrozil (Lopid)

Ophthalmic Vasoconstrictors   **Reduce the Amount of Aqueous Humor in the Eye and Dilate the Pupil**
Tetrahydrozoline (Visine)   Used in the eye (over the counter)
Phenylephrine (Neo-Synephrine)   Used in the eye and nose
Naphazoline (Naphcon)   Used in the eye

Vasoconstrictors   **Used in Shock to Support Blood Circulation**
Isoproterenol (Isuprel)
Dobutamine (Dobutrex)
Epinephrine (Adrenalin)
Metaraminol (Aramine)

CHAPTER 9

DRUG CLASS	EFFECTS AND USES
Antiasthmatic Drugs/Bronchodilators	**Used to Treat Asthma, Relax the Bronchioles to Improve Respiration**
Antiasthmatics	*Used to treat asthma*
Salmeterol (Serevent)	Used by inhalation
Terbutaline (Brethaire)	Used in asthma and bronchospasm
Albuterol (Proventil)	Used in asthma and bronchospasm
Metaproterenol (Alupent)	Used for asthma and bronchospasm
Epinephrine (Primatene Mist)	Used for temporary relief of shortness of breath, wheezing
Theophylline (Elixophyllin)	Used in bronchial asthma
Aminophylline	Used in bronchial asthma
Zileuton (Zyflo)	Used in adults and children 12 years or older
Montelukast (Singulair)	Used in adults and children 6 years or older
Corticosteroids	*Have potent antiinflammatory activity*
Beclomethasone (QVAR)	For patients with asthma in need of a corticosteroid
Triamcinolone (Azmacort)	Prophylactic therapy for patients requiring systemic corticosteroids
Fluticasone (Flovent)	Prophylactic therapy for patients requiring systemic corticosteroids
Flunisolide (AeroBid)	
Anticholinergics	*Dilate the bronchi and bronchioles*
Ipratropium (Atrovent)	Used to treat bronchospasm associated with chronic obstructive pulmonary disease
Miscellaneous	
Cromolyn (Nasalcrom)	Prophylactic treatment of bronchial asthma
Nedocromil (Tilade)	Maintenance therapy for mild to moderate bronchial asthma
Anti–cystic Fibrosis Agents	**Have Pulmonary Mucolytic Activity**
Acetylcysteine (Mucomyst)	Treats pulmonary complications of cystic fibrosis

Antihistamines
Diphenhydramine (Benadryl)
Promethazine (Phenergan)
Hydroxyzine (Atarax)
Loratadine (Claritin)
Fexofenadine (Allegra)

Oppose the Action of Histamine
Used in hypersensitivity reactions
Used in hypersensitivity reactions and for motion sickness
Used for pruritus
Used for allergic rhinitis
Used for allergic rhinitis

Antitussives
Narcotic
Codeine derivatives

Suppress Coughing

The dose is normally less than that to relieve pain

Non-narcotic
Dextromethorphan (Robitussin)

Benzonatate (Tessalon)

Makes nonproductive cough more productive, thus reducing frequency of coughing
Reduces cough reflex

Expectorants
Guaifenesin

Used to remove excess mucus from respiratory tract

Smoking Cessation Adjuncts
Nicotine polacrilex (Nicorette)

Encourage Abstinence from Smoking
Nicotine-containing chewing gum

CHAPTER 10

DRUG CLASS	EFFECTS AND USES

Anorexiants
Benzphetamine (Didrex)
Dextroamphetamine (Dexedrine)
Phentermine (Adipex-P)
Sibutramine (Meridia)
Phenylpropolamine (Dexatrim)
Orlistat (Xenical)

Appetite Suppression
Used for short-term treatment of exogenous obesity
Used for short-term treatment of exogenous obesity
Used for short-term treatment of exogenous obesity
Used for short-term treatment of exogenous obesity
Used for short-term treatment of exogenous obesity
A lipase inhibitor

Anti–Canker Sore Drugs
Carbamide peroxide (Gly-Oxide)
Benzocaine (Tanac)

Relief of Minor Oral Inflammation of Canker Sores
Local oral hygiene preparation
A topical local anesthetic

Antidiabetic Drugs
Sulfonylureas

Used to Treat Diabetes
Adjuncts to diet and exercise for type II diabetes (non–insulin-dependent diabetes mellitus [NIDDM])

Chlorpropamide (Diabinese)
Tolazamide (Tolinase)
Glipizide (Glucotrol)
Glyburide (DiaBeta)
Acarbose (Precose)

Biguanides
Metformin (Glucophage)

Adjuncts to diet and exercise for type II diabetes (NIDDM)

Thiazolidinediones
Troglitazone (Rezulin)
Rosiglitazone (Avandia)

Adjuncts to diet and exercise for type II diabetes (NIDDM)

Insulins	*Used for type I diabetes mellitus (insulin-dependent diabetes mellitus)*
Antidiarrheal Drugs	**Relieve Symptoms of Diarrhea**
Diphenoxylate (Lomotil)	
Loperamide (Imodium)	
Antiemetics	**Prevent or Alleviate Nausea and Vomiting**
Cyclizine (Marezine)	Used to prevent motion sickness
Dimenhydrinate (Dramamine)	Used to prevent motion sickness
Meclizine (Antivert)	Used to prevent motion sickness
Prochlorperazine (Compazine)	Used to control nausea and vomiting
Trimethobenzamide (Tigan)	
Antispasmodics	**Prevent Cramping of Smooth Muscle of Gastrointestinal Tract, Urinary Tract, and Uterus**
Dicyclomine (Bentyl)	Decreases motility of gastrointestinal tract
Antiulcer Drugs	**Prevent or Alleviate Symptoms of Ulcers and Eliminate *H. pylori* Infections**
Antibiotic combinations	
Metronidazole, tetracycline, and bismuth subsalicylate	Used to treat *H. pylori* infections
H₂ antagonists	*Competitive blockers of histamine at H₂ site*
Cimetidine (Tagamet)	
Famotidine (Pepcid)	
Ranitidine (Zantac)	
Sucralfate (Carafate)	
Proton pump inhibitors	*Block final step of gastric acid production*
Omeprazole (Prilosec)	
Lansoprazole (Prevacid)	
Antiflatulents	**Relieve or Prevent Excessive Gas in the Stomach and Intestinal Tract**
Simethicone (Gas-X)	Prevents formation of gas pockets
Miscellaneous	**Action May Be Topical Rather Than Systemic**
Mesalamine (Asacol)	Used in ulcerative colitis
Laxatives	**Promote Bowel Evacuation**
Saline types	*Attract and retain water in intestinal tract*
Milk of magnesia	Increases pressure in the intestinal tract
Epsom salts	Increases pressure in the intestinal tract
Stimulants	*Stimulate intestinal mucosa*
Cascara sagrada	
Sennoside (Ex-Lax)	
Senna (Senokot)	
Castor oil	
Bisacodyl (Dulcolax)	
Bulk-producing	
Psyllium (Metamucil)	Holds water in the stool

Emollient
Mineral oil   Lubricates and softens tissue

Fecal softeners
Docusate (Kasof/Colace)   Facilitates action of fat and water to soften the stool

CHAPTER 11

CLASS	EFFECTS AND USES
Antihypertensives (see Pharmacology section in Chapter 8)	**Reduce Blood Pressure, thus Reducing Blood Pressure in the Kidneys**
Antiinfectives (see also the Antiinfectives section in Chapter 4)	**Used Against Microorganisms**
Trimethoprim (Trimpex)	Used for urinary tract infections (UTIs)
Trimethoprim/sulfamethoxazole	Used for UTIs
Methylene blue	Used for UTIs
Nalidixic acid (NegGram)	Used for UTIs
Nitrofurantoin (Macrobid)	Used for UTIs
Penicillin G	Used for treating gonorrhea
Diuretics	**Increase Urination**
Thiazide diuretics	Prevent formation and recurrence of kidney stones
Chlorothiazide (Diuril) (see Pharmacology section in Chapter 8)	Prevents excess calcium loads in the urine
Uricosuric Drugs	**Treat Gout**
Allopurinol	Manages gout attacks and treats uric acid stones

CHAPTER 12

DRUG CLASS	EFFECTS AND USES
Anti–Benign Prostatic Hyperplasia Drugs	**Used to Treat Benign Prostatic Hyperplasia**
Finasteride (Proscar)	Inhibits androgen
Terazosin (Hytrin)	Treats obstruction of urinary outflow
Doxazosin (Cardura)	Treats obstruction of urinary outflow
Tamsulosin (Flomax)	Treats obstruction of urinary outflow
Estrogen	**Used for Hormonal Replacement in Postmenopausal Women; Used in Combination Birth Control Products and Inoperable Prostatic Cancer**
Conjugated estrogens (Premarin)	Used for hormonal replacement
Estradiol (Estrace)	Used for hormonal replacement
(Climara)	A transdermal product
Estropipate (Ogen)	A cream for intravaginal use
Testosterone	**Used for Testosterone Deficiency in Male Individuals; for Inoperable Breast Cancer in Female Individuals**
Finasteride (Proscar)	Used for benign prostatic hypertrophy and alopecia
Fluoxymesterone (Halotestin)	For androgenetic alopecia and inoperable breast cancer

CHAPTER 13

DRUG CLASS	EFFECTS AND USES
Anti-AIDS Drugs	**Used as Investigational Drugs to Treat AIDS**
Didanosine (Videx)	An antiviral for advanced HIV infection
Zidovudine (Retrovir)	
Ribavirin (Virazole)	An antiviral for asymptomatic HIV-positive patients
Aldesleukin (Proleukin)	A cytokine, involved in immune response
Ganciclovir (Cytovene)	An antiviral
Interferon β-1b (Betaseron)	A cytokine
Oral Contraceptives	**Used to Prevent Pregnancy**
Monophasic types	*Maintain a fixed dose of estrogen:progestin throughout the cycle*
Mestranol/norethindrone (Ortho-Novum)	A fixed dose throughout the cycle
Biphasic types	*Progestin:estrogen varies throughout the cycle*
Norethindrone/estradiol (Ortho-Novum 10/11)	Same ratio for first 21 days, then ratio changes for last 7 days of cycle
Triphasic types	*The estrogen remains the same or varies throughout the cycle; the progestin varies throughout the cycle*
Levonorgestrel/ethinyl estradiol (Tri-Levlen)	Three colors of tablets for phases 1, 2, and 3
Norethindrone/estradiol (Tri-Norinyl)	Three colors of tablets for phases 1, 2, and 3
Progestin only	*Uses the same dose at the same time every day*
Norethindrone (Micronor)	Slightly greater failure rate than progestin:estrogen combinations
Ovulation Stimulants	**Used to Induce Ovulation in Selected Anovulatory Patients Who Desire Pregnancy**
Chorionic gonadotropin (Profasi)	Used to induce ovulation
Clomiphene (Clomid)	Used to treat ovulatory failure
Danazol (Danocrine)	For treating endometriosis
Dinoprostone (Prostin E₂)	Used to remove uterine contents after an intrauterine fetal death
Ergonovine (Ergotrate Maleate)	Used to prevent and treat postpartum and postabortal hemorrhage
Follitropin alfa (Gonal-F)	Used to treat ovulatory failure
Oxytocin (Pitocin)	Used to induce labor
Ritodrine (Yutopar)	Used to manage preterm labor
Progestins	**Used for Progesterone-like Effect to Prepare the Uterus for Implantation in Various Menstrual Disorders, Infertility, and Repeated Spontaneous Abortions**
Medroxyprogesterone (Provera)	Used mainly for treatment of menopause in combination with estrogen
Megestrol (Megace)	Used to relieve symptoms of advanced breast carcinoma

CHAPTER 14

DRUG CLASS	EFFECTS AND USES
Antiarthritics (Nonsteroidal Antiinflammatory Drugs)	**Relieve the Symptoms of Arthritis**
Celecoxib (Celebrex)	Selectively inhibits prostaglandin synthesis
Diclofenac (Voltaren)	Used in chronic arthritis and pain management
Flurbiprofen (Ansaid)	Used in rheumatoid arthritis and osteoarthritis

Ibuprofen (Motrin)	Also used to treat pain
Ketoprofen (Orudis)	Also used to treat pain
Ketorolac (Toradol)	For relief of pain
Nabumetone (Relafen)	Used in treating acute arthritis
Naproxen (Naproxen)	Used in treating acute arthritis
Oxaprozin (Daypro)	Used in treating acute arthritis
Sulindac (Clinoril)	For long-term management of both rheumatoid arthritis and degenerative joint disease

Antigout (Uricosurics)	**Used to Treat Gout**
Allopurinol (Zyloprim)	Increases the urinary excretion of uric acid, thus decreasing uric acid in the serum
Colchicine (Colchicine)	Used to treat acute attacks of gout
Probenecid (Benemid)	Increases the urinary excretion of uric acid
Sulfinpyrazone (Anturane)	Increases the urinary excretion of uric acid

Antiinflammatories (see Pharmacology section in Chapter 5)	**Used to Relieve and Control Inflammation**
Neuromuscular Blocking Drugs (see Pharmacology section in Chapter 3)	
Radiopharmaceuticals	**Used to Diagnose and Treat Metastatic Tumors**
Strontium-89 (Metastron)	Used both in bone scanning and in alleviating metastatic bone pain

CHAPTER 15

DRUG CLASS	EFFECTS AND USES
Antialcoholic Drugs	**For Management of Chronic Alcoholics Who Want or Need Enforced Sobriety**
Disulfiram (Antabuse)	Must be used with the patient's knowledge
Analgesics (see Pharmacology section of Chapter 5)	**For Relief of Pain**
Anesthetics (see Pharmacology section in Chapter 3)	**For Loss of Sensation**
Anti-Alzheimer drugs	**Cholinesterase Inhibitors Relieve the Deficiency of Acetylcholine That Is Thought to Exist in Alzheimer's Disease**
Donepezil (Aricept)	Used to treat mild to moderate dementia
Tacrine (Cognex)	Used to treat mild to moderate dementia
Antianxiety Drugs	**Used to Relieve the Symptoms of Anxiety**
Meprobamate (Equanil)	Used for short-term relief of symptoms
Benzodiazepines	*Used to treat anxiety disorders and are processed by the kidneys*
Alprazolam (Xanax)	Also used for panic disorders
Chlordiazepoxide (Librium)	Also used in alcohol withdrawal
Oxazepam (Serax)	Used for short-term relief
Lorazepam (Ativan)	Used for short-term relief
Diazepam (Valium)	Also used for the relief of tension before surgery
Clorazepate (Tranxene)	Also used for acute alcohol withdrawal

Miscellaneous	*Lack prominent sedative effects*
Buspirone (BuSpar)	Used in anxiety disorders
Doxepin (Sinequan)	Used in depression or anxiety
Hydroxyzine (Atarax)	Also used for pruritus

Anticonvulsants	**Prevent or Reduce the Severity of Epileptic or Other Convulsive Seizures**
Hydantoins	
Mephenytoin (Mesantoin)	Inhibits seizure activity
Phenytoin (Dilantin)	Used to control grand mal seizure
Succinimides	
Ethosuximide (Zarontin)	Used in petit mal seizures
Phensuximide (Milontin)	Used in petit mal seizures
Oxazolidinediones	
Trimethadione (Tridione)	Used in petit mal seizures
Benzodiazepines	
Clonazepam (Klonopin)	Used in petit mal seizures
Clorazepate (Tranxene)	Used to manage partial seizures
Diazepam (Valium)	Used with other drugs to prevent convulsions
Miscellaneous	
Carbamazepine (Tegretol)	Also used to treat trigeminal neuralgia
Gabapentin (Neurontin)	Used in partial seizures
Lamotrigine (Lamictal)	Used in partial onset seizures
Topiramate (Topamax)	Used to treat a broad spectrum of epileptic activity
Valproic acid (Depakote)	Also used in manic episodes of bipolar disorder

Antidepressants	**Used in Depression**
Tricyclic drugs	
Amitriptyline (Elavil)	Used in depression
Amoxapine (Asendin)	Used in depression
Clomipramine (Anafranil)	Used in obsessive–compulsive disorders
Imipramine (Tofranil)	Used for enuresis in children
Nortriptyline (Pamelor)	Used in depression
Tetracyclic drugs	*Used to treat symptoms of depression*
Bupropion (Wellbutrin)	
Maprotiline (Ludiomil)	
Mirtazapine (Remeron)	
Trazodone (Desyrel)	
Venlafaxine (Effexor)	
Selective serotonin reuptake inhibitors	*Used in depression*
Fluoxetine (Prozac)	Used in depression, bulimia nervosa
Fluvoxamine (Luvox)	Used in obsessive–compulsive disorder
Paroxetine (Paxil)	Used in panic disorders also
Sertraline (Zoloft)	Multiple uses
Monoamine oxidase inhibitors (MAOIs)	*Used in depression that is not responsive to other antidepressive therapy*
Phenelzine (Nardil)	Used in atypical depression
Tranylcypromine (Parnate)	Used in depression

Antiemetic Drugs (see Pharmacology section in Chapter 10)	**Used to Relieve or Prevent Vomiting and Lightheadedness**

Antimanic Drug
Lithium   Used in manic episodes of manic depression

Antimigraine Drugs   **Used to Relieve Migraine Headaches**
Rizatriptan (Maxalt)   Not intended for prevention of migraines
Sumatriptan (Imitrex)   Used for treatment of acute migraine or cluster headache
Zolmitriptan (Zomig)   Used for treatment of acute migraine with or without aura

Antiparkinson Drugs   **Used to Relieve the Symptoms of Parkinson's Disease**
Amantadine (Symmetrel)   Thought to release dopamine
Benztropine (Cogentin)   Used as an adjunct treatment for all types of Parkinson's disease
Levodopa (Dopar)   Used in combination with other drugs of this type
Pramipexole (Mirapex)   Used for certain types of Parkinson's disease
Procyclidine (Kemadrin)   Also used as antispasmodic
Selegiline (Eldepryl)   Used in combination with other drugs of this type
Tolcapone (Tasmar)   Used if patient does not respond to other drugs
Trihexyphenidyl (Artane)   Used in all forms of Parkinson's disease

Antipsychotic Drugs   **Used to Relieve the Symptoms of Psychoses**
Phenothiazines
Chlorpromazine (Thorazine)   Also used for manic–depressive disorder
Fluphenazine (Prolixin)   Used to manage psychotic symptoms
Mesoridazine (Serentil)   Used in schizophrenia
Prochlorperazine (Compazine)   Also used for nausea and vomiting
Promazine (Sparine)   Used to manage psychotic symptoms
Thioridazine (Mellaril)   Also used for severe combativeness in children
Trifluoperazine (Stelazine)   Also used for short-term relief of anxiety

Phenylbutylpiperadines
Haloperidol (Haldol)   Also used in Tourette's syndrome

Dibenzapines
Clozapine (Clozaril)   Used for severe schizophrenia
Loxapine (Loxitane)   Manages manifestations of psychoses
Olanzapine (Zyprexa)   Manages manifestations of psychoses
Benzisoxazole
Risperidone (Risperdal)

Emetic
Ipecac   Used for drug overdoses and poisonings

CHAPTER 16

CLASS	EFFECTS AND USES
Anesthetics, Local (see also Pharmacology section in Chapter 3)	**Relieve Superficial Pain**
Benzocaine (Lanacane)	Used to relieve pain and itching from various causes
Lidocaine (Solarcaine)	Often used for sunburn pain
Antiacne Drugs, Topical	**Used to Treat Acne Vulgaris**
Adapalene (Differin)	Retinoid-like action prevents blackheads
Azelaic acid (Azelex)	Has activities similar to other drying antiacne drugs but also is antimicrobial for certain types of bacteria
Benzoyl peroxide (Oxy10 Wash)	Produces a drying effect and is antimicrobial for the most prominent bacteria in sebaceous follicles

Tazarotene (Tazorac)	Also used for the treatment of psoriasis
Tetracyclines, topical (Topicycline)	Has local antiinfective effect
Tretinoin (Retin-A)	Also used to improve photoaged skin, especially wrinkles and liver spots

Antihistamines, Topical
Relieve Itching

Benadryl (see Pharmacology section in Chapter 7)	Produces local anesthetic activity

Antiinfectives, Topical
Inhibit the Growth of or Kill Microorganisms on the Skin

Antibiotics
Inhibit or destroy bacteria on the skin

Mupirocin (Bactroban)	Commonly used in impetigo
Erythromycin (Akne-Mycin)	Used for acne vulgaris and as prophylaxis in wounds and burns
Neomycin (Neomycin sulfate)	Prophylactic treatment of wounds or burns

Antifungals
Inhibit the growth of fungi

Ciclopirox (Loprox)	Used for athlete's foot, jock itch, and ringworm
Clotrimazole (Lotrimin)	Used for athlete's foot, ringworm, and other dermatomycoses

Antivirals
Have inhibitory effect on herpes simplex viruses type 1 and 2

Acyclovir (Zovirax)	Used to manage initial episodes of herpes genitalis and limited viral infections in immunocompromised patients
Penciclovir (Denavir)	Used to treat cold sores on the lips

Anti–Poison Ivy Drugs
Used to Prevent or Relieve the Symptoms Associated with Poison Ivy

Poison ivy treatments

Ivarest	Relieves itching, pain, and discomfort of contact dermatoses
Calamatum	A spray that relieves itching and irritation

Systemic prevention
Recommended for prevention of poison ivy in hypersensitive individuals

Poison ivy extract	Used to counteract dermatitis due to poison ivy

Antipsoriatic Drugs
Used to Treat Psoriasis

Anthralin (Anthra-Derm)	Ointment to treat the lesions of psoriasis
Calcipotriene (Dovonex)	Topical use of synthetic vitamin D to heal the lesions of psoriasis
Methotrexate (Methotrexate)	Systemic drug used for severe psoriasis only; also used as antineoplastic agent and in rheumatoid arthritis

Antiseborrheic Drugs
Reduce the Amount of Sebum Produced by the Sebaceous Glands

Selenium sulfide (Selsun Blue)	Used to treat dandruff and seborrheic dermatitis of the scalp
Tar derivatives (Tegrin Medicated Shampoo)	Decrease epidermal proliferation and are antipruritic and antibacterial

Burn Preparations, Topical
Used to Treat Burned Skin

Nitrofurazone (Furacin)	Antiinfective, also used on skin grafts
Mafenide (Sulfamylon)	Bacteriostatic

Cauterizing Agents
Penetrate and Destroy Tissue

Chloracetic acids	Used to destroy surface lesions that are not malignant

Corticosteroids, Topical
Act Against Inflammation

Amcinonide (Cyclocort)	Relieves inflammation from various causes
Hydrocortisone (Cort-Dome)	Relieves inflammation from various causes

Keratolytics
Salicylic acid (Compound W)

Remove Warts, Calluses, and Corns
Over-the-counter solution for removing warts

Scabicides/Pediculicides
Lindane (Scabene)

Kill Ectoparasites and Eggs
Used for head lice, pubic lice, and body lice

Topical Drugs, Miscellaneous
Fluorouracil (Efudex)

Used to treat multiple actinic or solar keratoses and superficial basal cell carcinomas

Minoxidil (Rogaine)

Stimulates growth of hair in certain types of male baldness

CHAPTER 17

DRUG CLASS	EFFECTS AND USES
Adrenal Cortical Steroids	**Used in Individuals with Inadequate Adrenocorticotropic Hormone Secretion and to Treat Addison's Disease**
Aminoglutethimide (Cytadren)	Used to treat Cushing's syndrome
Cortisone	Used in Addison's disease
Dexamethasone (Decadron)	Used to treat allergic disorders
Fludrocortisone acetate (Florinef)	Used in Addison's disease
Hydrocortisone (Cortef)	Used for allergic states, respiratory disease, osteoarthritis
Methylprednisolone (Medrol)	Used in allergic states
Prednisolone	Used in multiple sclerosis
Prednisone (Deltasone)	Used in multiple sclerosis
Triamcinolone (Aristocort)	Used in respiratory disease, bronchial asthma
Antidiabetic Drugs (see Pharmacology section in Chapter 10)	
Antiosteoporotic Drugs	**Used to Treat and Prevent Osteoporosis Especially in Postmenopausal Women**
Alendronate (Fosamax)	Used to treat osteoporosis and Paget's disease
Calcitonin-salmon (Miacalcin)	Used to treat Paget's disease, postmenopausal osteoporosis
Antithyroid Drugs	**Used to Treat Hyperthyroidism and Goiter**
Methimazole (Tapazole)	
Propylthiouracil (PTU)	
Growth Hormone	**Used to Treat Growth Failure from Various Causes**
Somatrem (Protropin)	Injections for children who have insufficient pituitary hormone
Posterior Pituitary Hormones	**Used for Deficits in Oxytocin or Antidiuretic Hormone**
Oxytocin (Pitocin)	Improves uterine contractions to achieve early vaginal delivery when needed or for expulsion of the placenta
Vasopressin (Pitressin Synthetic)	Exerts an antidiuretic effect on the kidneys
Sex Hormones (see Pharmacology section in Chapter 12)	
Thyroid Drugs	**Used to Treat Hypothyroidism, to Suppress Thyroid-stimulating Hormone, and to Diagnose Thyroid Diseases**
Thyroid	
Levothyroxine (Synthroid)	
Liotrix (Thyrolar)	

^{131}I	radioactive iodine
a.c.	before meals (*ante cibum*)
ABA	American Burn Association
abd	abdomen, abdominal
ABG	arterial blood gas
ABO	blood groups
ACh	acetylcholine
ACS	American Cancer Society
ACTH	adrenocorticotropic hormone
ad lib.	freely as needed, at pleasure (*ad libitum*)
ADD	attention deficit disorder
ADH	antidiuretic hormone
ADHD	attention deficit hyperactivity disorder
ADL	activities of daily living
AFB	acid-fast bacillus (some types cause tuberculosis)
AHF	antihemophilic factor
AI	aortic insufficiency
AIDS	acquired immunodeficiency syndrome
ALL	acute lymphoblastic leukemia
ALP	alkaline phosphatase (liver function test)
ALS	amyotrophic lateral sclerosis
ALT	alanine transferase
AML	acute myelogenous leukemia
ANA	antinuclear antibody
AP	anteroposterior
Aq.	water (*aqua*)
ARDS	acute or adult respiratory distress syndrome
ARF	acute renal failure
ASD	atrial septal defect
ASHD	arteriosclerotic heart disease
AST (formerly SGOT)	aspartate aminotransferase (enzyme increased after myocardial infarction)
AV, A-V	atrioventricular
BBT	basal body temperature
b.i.d.	twice a day (*bis in die*)
b.i.n.	twice a night (*bis in nocte*)
BM	bowel movement
BMI	body mass index
BP	blood pressure
BPH	benign prostatic hyperplasia
BSA	body surface area
BUN	blood urea nitrogen
Bx, bx	biopsy
C	Celsius, centigrade
CA	carcinoma
Ca	calcium
CABG	coronary artery bypass graft
CAD	coronary artery disease
CAL	chronic airflow limitation
CBC, cbc	complete blood cell count
CCU	critical care unit
CDC	Centers for Disease Control and Prevention
CHF	congestive heart failure
CK (CPK)	creatine kinase (formerly called creatine phosphokinase)
C-l, C-2, etc.	cervical vertebrae
CMV	cytomegalovirus
CNS	central nervous system
CO$_2$	carbon dioxide
COLD	chronic obstructive lung disease
COPD	chronic obstructive pulmonary disease
CPAP	continuous positive airway pressure (for sleep apnea)
CPD	cephalopelvic disproportion
CPK	creatine phosphokinase
CPR	cardiopulmonary resuscitation
CRF	chronic renal failure
CS or C-section	cesarean section
CSF	cerebrospinal fluid
CSR	Cheyne-Stokes respiration
CT, CAT	computed tomography, computerized axial tomography, or computed axial tomography
CTS	carpal tunnel syndrome
CVA	cerebrovascular accident, costovertebral angle
Cx	cervix
CXR	chest x-ray
D & C	dilation and curettage
DIC	disseminated intravascular coagulation
diff	differential count (white blood cell counts)
DJD	degenerative joint disease
DLE	discoid lupus erythematosus
DM	diabetes mellitus
DMARDs	disease-modifying antirheumatic drugs
DNA	deoxyribonucleic acid
DOB	date of birth
DSM	Diagnostic and Statistical Manual of Mental Disorders
DTR	deep tendon reflex
Dx	diagnosis
ECG, EKG	electrocardiogram
ECHO	echocardiography
ECMO	extracorporeal membrane oxygenation
ED	emergency department

EDD	expected delivery date	IBS	irritable bowel syndrome
EEG	electroencephalogram	IC	irritable colon
EFM	electronic fetal monitor	ICP	intracranial pressure
EGD	esophagogastroduodenoscopy	ICSH	interstitial cell–stimulating hormone
ELISA	enzyme-linked immunosorbent assay (commonly used in AIDS diagnosis)	ICU	intensive care unit
EMG	electromyography	IgA, IgD, IgG, IgM, IgE	immunoglobulins
ENT	ear, nose, and throat	INR	International Normalized Ratio
ER	emergency room	IUD	intrauterine device
ESR	erythrocyte sedimentation rate	IV	intravenous
ESWL	extracorporeal shock wave lithotripsy	IVF	*in vitro* fertilization
ET	endotracheal	IVP	intravenous pyelogram
F	Fahrenheit	KUB	kidneys, ureters, and bladder
FBS	fasting blood sugar	LA	left atrium
FEMA	Federal Emergency Management Agency	lab	laboratory
FHR	fetal heart rate	lap	laparotomy
FSH	follicle-stimulating hormone	lat.	lateral
fx	fracture	LCA	left coronary artery
G	gravida (pregnant)	LDH	lactate dehydrogenase (enzyme increased after myocardial infarction)
GB	gallbladder		
GC	gonococcus	LE	lupus erythematosus
GDM	gestational diabetes mellitus	LFT	liver function test
GERD	gastroesophageal reflux disease	LH	luteinizing hormone
GFR	glomerular filtration rate	lig	ligament
GH	growth hormone	L-1, L-2, etc.	lumbar vertebrae
GI	gastrointestinal	LLL	left lower lobe
GP	general practitioner	LLQ	left lower quadrant
GTT	glucose tolerance test	LMP	last menstrual period
GU	genitourinary	LPF	low-power field
Gyn	gynecology	LPN	licensed practical nurse
H & P	history and physical	LRT	lower respiratory tract
HAV	hepatitis A virus	LTH	lactogenic hormone
Hb AIC	glycosylated hemoglobin	LUL	left upper lobe
Hb, Hgb	hemoglobin	LUQ	left upper quadrant
HBV	hepatitis B virus	LV	left ventricle
HCG	human chorionic gonadotropin	LVN	licensed vocational nurse
HCT	hematocrit	MCH	mean corpuscular hemoglobin (average amount of hemoglobin in each red blood cell)
HCV	hepatitis C virus		
HDN	hemolytic disease of the newborn		
HDV	hepatitis D virus	MCHC	mean corpuscular hemoglobin concentration (amount of hemoglobin per unit of blood)
HEV	hepatitis E virus		
HIPAA	Health Insurance Portability and Accountability Act		
HIV	human immunodeficiency virus	MCV	mean corpuscular volume (average size of individual red cells)
HLA	human leukocyte antigens		
HPF	high-power field	MI	myocardial infarction
HPV	human papillomavirus	MRI	magnetic resonance imaging
HRT	hormone replacement therapy	MS	multiple sclerosis
HSV	herpes simplex virus	MSH	melanocyte-stimulating hormone
HSV-1	herpes simplex virus type 1	MTP	metatarsophalangeal
HSV-2	herpes simplex virus type 2 (genital herpes)	MVP	mitral valve prolapse
		NG tube	nasogastric tube
hx, Hx	history	Noct.	night (*nocte*)
I & D	incision and drainage	NPO	nothing by mouth (*nil per os*)
I & O	intake and output	NSAID	nonsteroidal antiinflammatory drug
IBD	inflammatory bowel disease	O_2	oxygen
		OB	obstetrics

OCD	obsessive–compulsive disorder
OD	overdose; right eye (*oculus dexter*)
OP	outpatient
OR	operating room
OTC	over the counter (drug that can be obtained without a prescription)
PA	physician assistant or posteroanterior
Pap	Papanicolaou smear, stain, or test
PAT	paroxysmal atrial tachycardia
PCV	packed cell volume
PE	physical examination
PET	positron emission tomography
PFT	pulmonary function test
pH	potential hydrogen or potential of hydrogen
PID	pelvic inflammatory disease
PMN	polymorphonuclear
PMS	premenstrual syndrome
PNS	peripheral nervous system
PO	by mouth (*per os*)
PO_2	oxygen partial pressure
p.r.n.	as the occasion arises, as needed (*pro re nata*)
PSA	prostate-specific antigen
PT	prothrombin time or physical therapy
PTA	percutaneous transluminal angioplasty
PTCA	percutaneous transluminal coronary angioplasty
PTH	parathormone (parathyroid hormone)
PTT	partial thromboplastin time
PVC	premature ventricular contraction
PVD	peripheral vascular disease
q.	every
q.i.d.	four times a day (*quater in die*)
R	respiration
RA	right atrium or rheumatoid arthritis
RAIU	radioactive iodine uptake
RBC	red blood cell, red blood cell count
RCA	right coronary artery
RDA	recommended dietary allowance
RDS	respiratory distress syndrome
RF	rheumatoid factor
Rh	rhesus factor in blood
RLL	right lower lobe
RLQ	right lower quadrant
ROM	range of motion
RPR	rapid plasma reagin or rapid plasma reagin test (for syphilis)
RUL	right upper lobe
RUQ	right upper quadrant
RV	right ventricle
Rx	prescription
SA	sinoatrial
SARS	severe acute respiratory syndrome
SCI	spinal cord injury
SGOT (enzyme test of heart and liver function)	serum glutamic-oxaloacetic transaminase
SGPT (enzyme test of liver function, now called ALT)	serum glutamic-pyruvic transaminase
SIDS	sudden infant death syndrome
SLE	systemic lupus erythematosus
SOB	shortness of breath
SSN	social security number
Staph	Staphylococcus
stat.	immediately (*statim*)
STD	sexually transmitted disease
STH	somatotropic hormone
Sx	symptoms
T & A	tonsillectomy and adenoidectomy
T_3	triiodothyronine
T_4	thyroxine
TB	tuberculosis
TBSA	total body surface area
TCT	thyrocalcitonin
TENS	transcutaneous electrical nerve stimulation
TIA	transient ischemic attack
t.i.d.	three times a day (*ter in die*)
TJR	total joint replacement
T-l, T-2, etc.	thoracic vertebrae
TMJ	temporomandibular joint
TPN	total parenteral nutrition
TSH	thyroid-stimulating hormone
TSS	toxic shock syndrome
TTO	transtracheal oxygen
TUR	transurethral resection
TURP	transurethral resection of the prostate
Tx	treatment
UA, U/A	urinalysis
UGI	upper gastrointestinal series or upper GI
ung	ointment
URI	upper respiratory infection
URT	upper respiratory tract
UTI	urinary tract infection
UV	ultraviolet
VC	vital capacity
VCUG	voiding cystourethrogram
VD	venereal disease
VDRL	Venereal Disease Research Laboratories
VS, v.s.	vital signs
VSD	ventricular septal defect
WBC	white blood cell, white blood cell count
WMD	weapons of mass destruction
WNL	within normal limits
WNV	West Nile virus

ENGLISH	SPANISH (PRONUNCIATION)
abdomen	abdomen (ab-DOH-men), vientre (ve-EN-tray)
acidity	acidez (ah-se-DES)
acute	agudo (ah-GOO-do)
adrenal	suprarenal (soo-prah-ray-NAHL)
adrenaline	adrenalina (ah-dray-nah-LEE-nah)
aged	envejecido (en-vay-hay-SEE-do)
allergy	alergia (ah-LEHR-he-ah)
anatomy	anatomía (ah-nah-to-MEE-ah)
anemia	anemia (ah-NAY-me-ah)
anesthesia	anestesia (ah-nes-TAY-se-ah)
anesthetic	anestésico (ah-nes-TAY-se-co)
ankle	tobillo (to-BEEL-lyo)
antibiotic	antibiótico (an-te-be-O-te-co)
anxiety	ansiedad (an-se-ay-DAHD)
appendix	apéndice (ah-PEN-de-say)
appetite	apetito (ah-pay-TEE-to)
arm	brazo (BRAH-so)
armpit	sobaco (so-BAH-co)
artery	arteria (ar-TAY-re-ah)
asphyxia	asfixia (as-FEEC-se-ah)
aspirate	aspirar (as-pe-RAR)
asthma	asma (AHS-mah)
augmentation	aumento (ah-oo-MEN-to)
bacilli	bacilos (bah-SEE-los)
back	espalda (es-PAHL-dah)
beard	barba (BAR-bah)
belch	eructo (ay-ROOK-to)
belly	barriga (bar-REE-gah)
benign	benigno (bay-NEEG-no)
biopsy	biopsia (be-OP-see-ah)
birth	nacimiento (nah-se-me-EN-to)
black	negro (NAY-gro)
bladder	vejiga (vah-HEE-gah)
blood	sangre (SAHN-gray)
blood pressure	presión sanguínea (pray-se-ON san-GEE-nay-ah)
blood sample	muestra de sangre (moo-AYS-tah de SAHN-gray)
blue	azul (ah-SOOL)
body	cuerpo (coo-ERR-po)
bone	hueso (oo-AY-so)
brain	cerebro (say-RAY-bro)
breast	seno (SAY-no)
breathe	alentar (ah-len-TAR), respirar (res-pe-RAR)
breathing	respiración (res-pe-rah-se-ON)
burn	quemadura (kay-mah-DOO-rah)

ENGLISH	SPANISH (PRONUNCIATION)
calcium	calcio (CAHL-se-o)
calculus	cálculo (CAHL-coo-lo)
cancer	cáncer (CAHN-ser)
capillary	capilar (cah-pe-LAR)
cartilage	cartílago (car-TEE-lah-go)
catheter	catéter (cah-TAY-ter)
cheek	mejilla (may-HEEL-lyah)
chest	pecho (PAY-cho)
chew, to	masticar (mas-te-CAR)
child	niña (NEE-nya), niño (NEE-nyo)
childbirth	parto (PAR-to)
cholesterol	cholesterol (co-les-tay-ROL)
chronic	crónico (CRO-ne-co)
circumcision	circumcisión (ser-coon-se-se-ON)
clot	coágulo (co-AH-goo-lo)
collarbone	clavicula (clah-VEE-coo-lah)
conception	concepción (con-sep-se-ON)
concussion	concusión (con-coo-se-ON)
condom	condón (con-DON)
conscious	consciente (cons-se-EN-tay)
consciousness	conciencia (con-se-EN-se-ah)
constipation	estreñimiento (es-tray-nye-me-EN-to)
contraception	contracepción (con-trah-cep-se-ON)
convulsion	convulsión (con-vool-se-ON)
cough	tos (tos)
cranium	cráneo (CRAH-nay-o)
cream	crema (CRAY-mah)
cry, to	llorar (lyo-RAR)
defecate	evacuar (ay-vah-coo-AR)
dentist	dentista (den-TEES-tah)
dermatology	dermatología (der-mah-to-lo-HEE-ah)
destruction	destrucción (des-trooc-se-ON)
diabetes	diabetes (de-ah-BAY-tes)
diagnosis	diagnóstico (de-ag-NOS-te-co)
diagnostic	diagnóstico (de-ag-NOS-te-co)
dialysis	diálisis (de-AH-le-sis)
diaphragm	diafragma (de-ah-FRAHG-mah)
diarrhea	diarrea (de-ar-RAY-ah)
digestion	digestión (de-hes-te-ON)
disease	enfermedad (en-fer-may-DAHD)
dizziness	vértigo (VERR-te-go)
dwarf	enano (AY-nah-no)
ear	oreja (o-RAY-hah)
edema	hidropesía (e-dro-pay-SEE-ah)
elbow	codo (CO-do)
electricity	electricidad (ay-lec-tre-se-DAHD)

ENGLISH	SPANISH (PRONUNCIATION)
enlargement	aumento (ah-oo-MEN-to)
enzyme	enzima (en-SEE-mah)
epilepsy	epilepsia (ay-pe-LEP-se-ah)
erect, straight	derecho (day-RAY-cho)
erection	erección (ay-rec-se-ON)
esophagus	esófago (ay-SO-fah-go)
excretion	excreción (ex-cray-se-ON)
extremity	extremidad (ex-tray-me-DAHD)
eye	ojo (O-ho)
eyeball	globo del ojo (GLO-bo del O-ho)
eyebrow	ceja (SAY-hah)
eyelash	pestaña (pes-TAH-nyah)
eyelid	párpado (PAR-pah-do)
face	cara (CAH-rah)
fainting	languidez (lan-gee-DES), desmayo (des-MAH-yo)
fatigue	fatiga (fah-TEE-gah)
fear	miedo (me-AY-do)
feces	excremento (ex-cray-MEN-to)
feminine	femenina (fay-may-NEE-na)
fetus	feto (FAY-to)
fever	fiebre (fe-AY-bray)
fiber	fibra (FEE-brah)
finger	dedo (DAY-do)
fingerprint	impresión digital (im-pray-se-ON de-he-TAHL)
fire	fuego (foo-AY-go)
fluid	fluido (floo-EE-do)
foam	espuma (es-POO-mah)
foot (pl., feet)	pie (PE-ay), pies (PE-ays)
forearm	antebrazo (an-tay-BRAH-so)
fracture	fractura (frac-TOO-rah)
gallbladder	vesícula biliar (vay-SEE-coo-la be-le-AR)
gallstone	cálculo biliar (CAHL-coo-lo be-le-AR)
giant	gigante (he-GAHN-tay)
gland	glándula (GLAN-doo-lah)
glucose	glucosa (gloo-CO-sah)
goiter	papera (pah-PAY-rah)
green	verde (VERR-day)
growth	crecimiento (cray-se-me-EN-to)
gum, gingiva	encía (en-SEE-ah)
gynecology	ginecología (he-nay-co-lo-HEE-ah)
hair	pelo (PAY-lo)
hand	mano (MAH-no)
head	cabeza (cah-BAY-sah)
headache	dolor de cabeza (do-LOR day cah-BAY-sa)
heart	corazón (co-rah-SON)
heat	calor (cah-LOR)
heel	talón (tah-LON)
hemorrhage	hemorragia (ay-mor-RAH-he-ah)

ENGLISH	SPANISH (PRONUNCIATION)
hernia	hernia (AYR-ne-ah), quebradura (kay-brah-DOO-rah)
high blood pressure	hipertensión, presión alta (e-per-ten-se-ON, pray-se-ON AHL-tah)
hip	cadera (cah-DAY-rah)
hives	roncha (RON-chah)
hormone	hormona (or-MOH-nah)
hunger	hambre (AHM-bray)
hypodermic	hipodérmico (e-po-DER-me-co)
imperfect	imperfecto (im-per-FEC-to)
impotency	impotencia (im-po-TEN-se-ah)
inflammation	inflamación (in-flah-mah-se-ON)
influenza	gripe (GREE-pay)
injection	inyección (in-yec-se-ON)
injury	daño (DAH-nyo)
instrument	instrumento (ins-troo-MEN-to)
insulin	insulina (in-soo-LEE-nah)
intercourse, sexual	cópula (CO-poo-lah)
intestine	intestino (in-tes-TEE-no)
iodine	yodo (YO-do)
jaw	mandíbula (man-DEE-boo-lah)
joint	articulación (ar-te-coo-lah-se-ON), coyuntura (co-yoon-TOO-rah)
kidney	riñon (ree-NYOHN)
knee	rodilla (ro-DEEL-lyah)
kneecap	rótula (RO-too-lah)
laxative	purgante (poor-GAHN-tay)
leg	pierna (pe-ERR-nah)
leukemia	leucemia (lay-oo-SAY-me-ah)
life	vida (VEE-dah)
ligament	ligamento (le-gah-MEN-to)
light	luz (loos)
lips	labios (LAH-be-os)
liver	hígado (EE-ga-do)
lobe	lóbulo (LO-boo-lo)
lung	pulmón (pool-MON)
lymph	linfa (LEEN-fa)
lymphatic	linfático (lin-FAH-te-co)
malignant	maligno (mah-LEEG-no)
masculine	masculino (mas-coo-LEE-no)
membrane	membrana (mem-BRAH-nah)
menopause	menopausia (may-no-PAH-oo-se-ah)
menstruation	menstruación (mens-troo-ah-se-ON)
microscope	microscopio (me-cros-CO-pe-o)
milk	leche (LAY-chay)
mind	mente (MEN-te)
mouth	boca (BO-cah)
movement	movimiento (mo-ve-me-EN-to)
mucus	moco (MO-co)
murmur	murmullo (moor-MOOL-lyo)
muscle	músculo (MOOS-coo-lo)

ENGLISH	SPANISH (PRONUNCIATION)
nails	uñas (OO-nyahs)
narcotic	narcótico (nar-CO-te-co)
narrow	estrecho (es-TRAY-cho)
navel	ombligo (om-BLEE-go)
neck	cuello (coo-EL-lyo)
nerve	nervio (NERR-ve-o)
nervous	nervioso (ner-ve-O-so)
neurology	neurología (nay-oo-ro-lo-HEE-ah)
newborn	recién nacida (ray-se-EN nah-SEE-dah)
nipple	pezón (pay-SON)
nose	nariz (nah-REES)
nostril	orificio de la nariz (or-e-FEE-se-o day lah nah-REES)
nutrition	nutrición (noo-tre-se-ON)
obstruction	obstrucción (obs-trooc-se-ON)
optic	óptico (OP-te-co)
optician	óptico (OP-te-co)
orange (color)	anaranjado (ah-nah-ran-HAH-do), naranjado (nah-ran-HAH-do)
orthodontist	ortodóntico (or-to-DON-te-co)
ovarian	ovárico (o-VAH-re-co)
ovary	ovario (o-VAH-re-o)
oxygen	oxígeno (ok-SEE-hay-no)
pain	dolor (do-LOR)
painful	doloroso (do-lo-RO-so)
palm	palma (PAHL-mah)
pancreas	páncreas (PAHN-cray-as)
paralysis	parálisis (pah-RAH-le-sis)
parasite	parásito (pah-RAH-se-to)
parturition	parto (PAR-to)
pathology	patología (pah-to-lo-HEE-ah)
penis	pene (PAY-nay)
perspiration	sudor (soo-DOR)
phalanges	falanges (fah-LAHN-hays)
phosphorus	fósforo (FOS-fo-ro)
physical examination	examen físico (ek-SAH-men FEE-se-co)
pink	rosa (RO-sah)
pituitary	pituitario (pe-too-e-TAH-re-o)
pneumonia	neumonía (nay-oo-mo-NEE-ah), pulmonía (pool-mo-NEE-ah)
pregnancy	embarazo (em-bah-RAH-so)
pregnant	embarazada (em-bah-rah-SAH-dah)
prolapse	prolapso (pro-LAHP-so)
prostate	próstata (PROS-ta-tah)
prostatic	prostático (pros-TAH-te-co)
prostatitis	prostatitis (pros-ta-TEE-tis)
protection	protección (pro-tec-se-ON)
psychiatry	psiquiatría (se-ke-ah-TREE-ah)
psychology	psicología (se-co-lo-HEE-ah)
pulse	pulso (POOL-so)
radiation	radiación (rah-de-ah-se-ON)
rectum	recto (REK-to)
red	rojo (ROH-ho)
reduction	reducción (ray-dooc-se-ON)
renal artery	arteria renal (ar-TAY-re-ah ray-NAHL)
renal calculus	cálculo renal (CAHL-coo-lo ray-NAHL)
reproduction	reproducción (ray-pro-dooc-se-ON)
respiration	respiración (res-pe-rah-se-ON)
rhythm	ritmo (REET-mo)
rhythm method	método de ritmo (MAY-to-do day REET-mo)
rib	costilla (cos-TEEL-lyah)
ringing	zumbido (zoom-BEE-do)
rupture	ruptura (roop-TOO-rah)
sacrum	hueso sacro (oo-AY-so SAH-cro)
saliva	saliva (sah-LEE-vah)
same	mismo (MEES-mo)
seizure	ataque (ah-TAH-kay)
sensation	sensación (sen-sah-se-ON)
sexual	sexual (sex-soo-AHL)
shoulder	hombro (OM-bro)
shoulder blade	espaldilla (es-pal-DEEL-lyah)
skeleton	esqueleto (es-kay-LAY-to)
skin	piel (pe-EL)
skull	cráneo (CRAH-nay-o)
sleep	sueño (soo-AY-nyo)
sole	planta (PLAHN-tah)
sound	sonido (so-NEE-do)
spasm	espasmo (es-PAHS-mo)
speech	habla (AH-blah), lenguaje (len-goo-AH-hay)
spinal column	columna vertebral (co-LOOM-nah ver-tay-BRAHL)
spine	espinazo (es-pe-NAH-so)
spiral	espiral (es-pe-RAHL)
spleen	bazo (BAH-so)
sprain, to	torcer (tor-SERR)
starch	almidón (al-me-DON)
sterile	estéril (es-TAY-reel)
sternum	esternón (es-ter-NON)
stiff	tieso (te-AY-so)
stomach	estómago (es-TOH-mah-go)
stone	cálculo (CAHL-coo-lo)
stroke	ataque de apoplejía (ah-TAH-kay de ah-po-play-HEE-ah)
sugar	azúcar (ah-SOO-car)
support	sustento (sus-TEN-to)
surgeon	cirujano(a) (se-roo-HAH-no) (na)
surgery	cirugía (se-roo-HEE-ah)
suture	sutura (soo-TOO-rah)
swallow	tragar (trah-GAR)

ENGLISH	SPANISH (PRONUNCIATION)	ENGLISH	SPANISH (PRONUNCIATION)
sweat	sudor (soo-DOR)	urea	urea (oo-RAY-ah)
swelling	hinchar (in-CHAR)	urinalysis	urinálisis (oo-re-NAH-le-sis)
symptom	síntoma (SEEN-to-mah)	urinary	urinario (oo-re-NAH-re-o)
synthesis	síntesis (SEEN-tay-sis)	urinary system	sistema urinario (sis-TAY-mah oo-re-NAH-re-o)
tears	lágrimas (LAH-gre-mahs)		
temperature	temperatura (tem-pay-rah-TOO-rah)	urinate	orinar (o-re-NAR)
		urination	urinación (oo-re-nah-se-ON)
temple	sien (se-AN)	urine	orina (o-REE-nah)
tendon	tendón (ten-DON)	urology	urología (oo-ro-lo-HEE-ah)
testicle	testículo (tes-TEE-coo-lo)	uterus	útero (OO-tay-ro)
tests	pruebas (proo-AY-bahs)	vagina	vagina (vah-HEE-nah)
therapy	tratamiento (trah-tah-me-EN-to)	varicose veins	venas varicosas (VAY-nahs vah-re-CO-sas)
thigh	muslo (MOOS-lo)		
thirst	sed (sayd)	vein	vena (VAY-nah)
throat	garganta (gar-GAHN-tah)	vertebral column	columna vertebral (co-LOOM-nah ver-tay-BRAHL)
thumb	pulgar (pool-GAR)		
thyroid	tiroides (te-RO-e-des)	vessel	vaso (VAH-so)
toe	dedo del pie (DAY-do del PE-ay)	vision	visión (ve-se-ON)
tongue	lengua (LEN-goo-ah)	voice	voz (vos)
tonsil	tonsila (ton-SEE-lah), amígdala (ah-MEEG-dah-lah)	voiding	urinar (oo-re-NAR)
		vomiting	vómito (VO-me-to)
tooth (pl., teeth)	diente (de-AYN-tay), dientes (de-AYN-tays)	water	agua (AH-goo-ah)
		weakness	debilidad (day-be-le-DAHD)
trachea	tráquea (TRAH-kay-ah)	white	blanco (BLAHN-co)
transfusion	transfusión (trans-foo-se-ON)	wound	lesión (lay-se-ON)
trauma	daño (DAH-nyo), herida (ay-REE-dah)	wrist	muñeca (moo-NYAY-cah)
		x-ray	radiografía (rah-de-o-grah-FEE-ah)
treatment	tratamiento (trah-tah-me-EN-to)	yellow	amarillo (ah-mah-REEL-lyo)
ulcer	ulcera (OOL-say-rah)		

SPANISH	ENGLISH
acidez	acidity
adrenalina	adrenaline
agua	water
agudo	acute
alentar	breathe
alergia	allergy
almidón	starch
amarillo	yellow
amígdala	tonsil
anaranjado	orange-colored
anatomía	anatomy
anemia	anemia
anestesia	anesthesia
anestésico	anesthetic
ansiedad	anxiety
antebrazo	forearm
antibiótico	antibiotic
apéndice	appendix
apetito	appetite
arteria	artery
articulación	joint
asfixia	asphyxia
asma	asthma
aspirar	aspirate
ataque	seizure
ataque de apoplejía	stroke
aumento	augmentation, enlargement
azúcar	sugar
azul	blue
bacilos	bacilli
barba	beard
barriga	belly
bazo	spleen
benigno	benign
biopsia	biopsy
blanco	white
boca	mouth
brazo	arm
cabeza	head
cadera	hip
calcio	calcium
cálculo	calculus, stone
cálculo biliar	gallstone
cálculo renal	renal calculus
calor	heat
cáncer	cancer
capilar	capillary
cara	face
cartílago	cartilage

SPANISH	ENGLISH
catéter	catheter
ceja	eyebrow
cerebro	brain
circuncisión	circumcision
cirugía	surgery
cirujano(a)	surgeon
clavícula	collarbone
coágulo	clot
codo	elbow
colesterol	cholesterol
columna vertebral	spinal column, vertebral column
concepción	conception
conciencia	consciousness
concusión	concussion
condón	condom
consciente	conscious
contracepción	contraception
convulsión	convulsion
cópula	sexual intercourse
corazón	heart
costilla	rib
coyuntura	joint
cráneo	cranium, skull
crecimiento	growth
crema	cream
crónico	chronic
cuello	neck
cuerpo	body
daño	trauma, injury
debilidad	weakness
dedo	finger
dedo del pie	toe
dentista	dentist
derecho	erect, straight
dermatología	dermatology
desmayo	fainting
destrucción	destruction
diafragma	diaphragm
diagnóstico	diagnostic
diálisis	dialysis
diarrea	diarrhea
diente, dientes	tooth (pl., teeth)
dilatación	dilation
dolor	pain
dolor de cabeza	headache
doloroso	painful
electricidad	electricity
embarazada	pregnant
embarazo	pregnancy

SPANISH	ENGLISH
enano	dwarf
encía	gum, gingiva
envejecido	aged
enzima	enzyme
epilepsia	epilepsy
erección	erection
eructo	belch
esófago	esophagus
espalda	back
espaldilla	shoulder blade
espasmo	spasm
espinazo	spine
espiral	spiral
espuma	foam
esqueleto	skeleton
estéril	sterile
esternón	sternum
estómago	stomach
estrecho	narrow
estreñimiento	constipation
evacuar	defecate
examen físico	physical examination
excreción	excretion
excremento	feces
extremidad	extremity
falanges	phalanges
fatiga	fatigue
femenina	feminine
feto	fetus
fibra	fiber
fiebre	fever
fluido	fluid
fósforo	phosphorus
fractura	fracture
fuego	fire
garganta	throat
gigante	giant
ginecología	gynecology
glándula	gland
globo del ojo	eyeball
glucosa	glucose
gripe	influenza
gris	gray
habla	speech
hambre	hunger
hemorragia	hemorrhage
hidropesía	edema
hígado	liver
hinchar	swelling, to swell
hipertensión	high blood pressure
hipodérmico	hypodermic
hombro	shoulder
hormona	hormone
hueso	bone
hueso sacro	sacrum
imperfecto	imperfect

SPANISH	ENGLISH
impotencia	impotency
impresión digital	fingerprint
inflamación	inflammation
instrumento	instrument
insulina	insulin
intestino	intestine
inyección	injection
labios	lips
lágrimas	tears
languidez	fainting
leche	milk
lengua	tongue
lenguaje	speech
lesión	wound
leucemia	leukemia
ligamento	ligament
linfa	lymph
linfático	lymphatic
llorar	to cry
lóbulo	lobe
luz	light
maligno	malignant
mandíbula	jaw
mano	hand
masculino	masculine
masticar	to chew
mejilla	cheek
membrana	membrane
menopausia	menopause
menstruación	menstruation
mente	mind
método de ritmo	rhythm method
microscopio	microscope
miedo	fear
mismo	same
moco	mucus
movimiento	movement
muestra de sangre	blood sample
muñeca	wrist
murmullo	murmur
músculo	muscle
muslo	thigh
nacimiento	birth
naranjado	orange-colored
narcótico	narcotic
nariz	nose
negro	black
nervio	nerve
nervioso	nervous
neumonía	pneumonia
neurología	neurology
niño (a)	child
nutrición	nutrition
obstrucción	obstruction
ojo	eye
ombligo	navel

SPANISH	ENGLISH	SPANISH	ENGLISH
óptico	optician, optic	rosa	pink
oreja	ear	rótula	kneecap
orificio de la nariz	nostril	ruptura	rupture
orina	urine	sangre	blood
orinar	urinate	sanguínea	blood pressure
ortodóntico	orthodontist	sed	thirst
ovárico	ovarian	senos	breasts
ovario	ovary	sensación	sensation
oxígeno	oxygen	sien	temple
palma	palm	síntesis	synthesis
páncreas	pancreas	síntoma	symptom
papera	goiter	sistema urinario	urinary system
parálisis	paralysis	sobaco	armpit
parásito	parasite	sonido	sound
parpado	eyelid	sudor	sweat, perspiration
parto	childbirth, parturition	sueño	sleep
patología	pathology	suprarenal	adrenal
pecho	chest	sustento	support
pelo	hair	sutura	suture
pene	penis	talón	heel
pestaña	eyelash	temperatura	temperature
pezón	nipple	tendón	tendon
pie (pl., pies)	foot (pl., feet)	testículo	testicle
piel	skin	tieso	stiff
pierna	leg	tiroides	thyroid
pituitario	pituitary	tobillo	ankle
planta	sole	tonsila	tonsil
presión alta presión	high blood pressure	torcer	to sprain
prolapso	prolapse	tos	cough
próstata	prostate	tragar	swallow
prostático	prostatic	transfusión	transfusion
prostatitis	prostatitis	tráquea	trachea
protección	protection	tratamiento	treatment, therapy
pruebas	tests	ulcera	ulcer
psicología	psychology	uñas	nails
psiquiatría	psychiatry	urinación	urination
pulgar	thumb	urinálisis	urinalysis
pulmón	lung	urinar	voiding
pulmonía	pneumonia	urinario	urinary
pulso	pulse	urología	urology
purgante	laxative	útero	uterus
quebradura	hernia	varicosas	varicose veins
quemadura	burn	vaso	vessel
radiación	radiation	vejiga	bladder
radiografía	x-ray	vena	vein
recién nacida	newborn	venas varicosas	varicose veins
recto	rectum	verde	green
reducción	reduction	vértigo	dizziness
reproducción	reproduction	vesícula biliar	gallbladder
respiración	breathing, respiration	vida	life
respirar	breathe	vientre	abdomen
riñón	kidney	visión	vision
ritmo	rhythm	vómito	vomiting
rodilla	knee	voz	voice
rojo	red	yodo	iodine
roncha	hives	zumbido	ringing

APPENDIX V Conversion Tables

WEIGHT EQUIVALENTS

1 lb	= 453.6 g = 0.4536 kg = 16 oz
1 oz	= 38.35 g
1 kg	= 1000 g = 2.2046 lb
1 g	= 1000 mg
1 mg	= 1000 μg = 0.001 g
1 μg	= 0.001 mg = 0.000001 g

1 μg/g or 1 mg/kg is the same as parts per million (ppm)

CONVERSION FACTORS

1 milligram	= 1/65 grain	(1/60)*
1 gram	= 15.43 grains	(15)
1 kilogram	= 2.20 pounds	(avoirdupois)
	2.68 pounds	(Troy)
1 milliliter	= 16.23 minims	(16)
1 liter	= 1.06 quarts	(1+)
	33.80 fluid ounces	(34)
1 gram	= 0.065 gm	(60 mg)
1 dram	= 3.9 gm	(4)
1 ounce	= 31.1 gm	(30+)
1 minim	= 0.062 ml	(0.06)
1 fluid dram	= 3.7 ml	(4)
1 fluid ounce	= 29.57 ml	(30)
1 pint	= 473.2 ml	(500)
1 quart	= 946.4 ml	(1000)

*Figures in parentheses are commonly used approximate values.

TEMPERATURE CONVERSION

Degrees Celsius to degrees Fahrenheit: (°C) $^9/_5$ + 32°

Degrees Fahrenheit to degrees Celsius: (°F − 32°) $^5/_9$

WEIGHT—UNIT CONVERSION FACTORS

Units Given	Units Wanted	For Conversion Multiply By
lb	g	453.6
lb	kg	0.4536
oz	g	28.35
kg	lb	2.2046
kg	mg	1,000,000
kg	g	1,000
g	mg	1,000
g	μg	1,000,000
mg	μg	1,000
mg/g	mg/lb	453.6
mg/kg	mg/lb	0.4536
μg/kg	μg/lb	0.4536
Mcal	kcal	1,000
kcal/kg	kcal/lb	0.4536
kcal/lb	kcal/kg	2.2046
ppm	μg/g	1
ppm	mg/kg	1
ppm	mg/lb	0.4536
mg/kg	%	0.0001
ppm	%	0.0001
mg/g	%	0.1
g/kg	%	0.1

VOLUME EQUIVALENTS

Household	Metric
1 drop (gt)	0.06 milliliter (ml)
15 drops (gtt)	1 ml (1 cc)
1 teaspoon (tsp)	= 5 ml
1 tablespoon (tbs)	= 15 ml
2 tablespoons	= 30 ml
1 ounce (oz)	= 30 ml
1 teacup	= 180 ml (6 oz)
1 glass	= 240 ml (8 oz)
1 measuring cup	= 240 ml (0.5 pint)
2 measuring cups	= 500 ml (1 pint)

Modified from Kirk RW, Bistner SI: Appendix IV. In *Handbook of veterinary procedures and emergency treatment*, ed 3, Philadelphia, 1981, WB Saunders, with permission.

CHAPTER 1

Exercise 1
1. frame
2. answer
3. write
4. check

Exercise 2
1. CF
2. CF
3. WR
4. CF
5. WR
6. WR
7. CF
8. WR
9. WR

Exercise 3
1. P
2. S
3. P
4. S
5. CF
6. S
7. P
8. CF
9. S

Exercise 4
1. P
2. S
3. S
4. S
5. P
6. S
7. P

8. P
9. P

Exercise 5
1. CF
2. CF
3. S
4. CF
5. P
6. P
7. S
8. P
9. P
10. CF

Exercise 6
1. acidosis
2. acromegaly
3. antiemesis
4. bronchoscopy
5. dysphagia
6. hypothyroidism
7. leukocytosis
8. malabsorption
9. myometrium
10. thrombophlebitis

Exercise 7
1. six
2. se
3. hi
4. i in hi, e in se, e in me

Exercise 8
1. capsules
2. cataracts

3. calculi
4. cortices
5. diagnoses
6. neuroses
7. protozoa
8. viruses
9. appendix
10. fungus
11. larynx
12. prognosis
13. sarcoma
14. spermatozoon

CHAPTER 1 REVIEW

I.
1. A combining form is a word root with an attached vowel to which prefixes and suffixes can be added.
2. A prefix is placed before a word root to modify its meaning.
3. A suffix is attached to the end of a word or word part to modify its meaning.
4. A word root is the main body of a word.

II.
1. CF
2. CF
3. S
4. CF

5. S
6. P
7. P
8. S
9. S
10. CF

III.
1. hypodermic
2. leukemia
3. melanoid
4. myocardial
5. thrombosis

IV.
1. calculi
2. diagnoses
3. septa
4. vertebrae
5. protozoa

V.
cancer, ophthalmoplasty

VI.
1. ad; pos; ad, i
2. ar; ar, o; sol
3. kor; son; kor, ti
4. lak; tos, lak
5. nef; ro, skop; nef

CHAPTER 2

Exercise 1
1. E
2. E
3. D
4. A
5. E
6. B
7. C
8. F

Exercise 2
1. D
2. I
3. H
4. E
5. G
6. F
7. J
8. C

9. B
10. A

Exercise 3
1. cardiology
2. radiology
3. immunology
4. endocrinology
5. otolaryngology

6. obstetrics
7. gastroenterology
8. urology
9. orthopedics
10. rheumatology

CHAPTER 2 REVIEW

I.
1. cardi/ac: *cardi* is CF: *ac* is S.
2. gyneco/logist: *gyneco* is CF; *logist* is S.
3. ophthalmo/logical: *ophthalmo* is CF; *logical* is S.
4. patho/logy: *patho* is CF; *logy* is S.
5. psych/iatry: *psych* is CF; *iatry* is S.

II.
1. life or living
2. secrete
3. tooth
4. inside
5. vision
6. vision
7. mouth
8. drugs or medicine
9. nose
10. urinary tract or urine

III.
1. B
2. K
3. F
4. J
5. E
6. H
7. L
8. D
9. C
10. A
11. G
12. I

IV.
1. A
2. D
3. B
4. C
5. E

V.
1. cardiologist
2. obstetrician
3. anesthetist
4. neonatologist
5. gastroenterologist
6. radiologist
7. orthopedist
8. nerve cell
9. clinical pathologist
10. radiopaque

VI.
1. internist
2. chronic
3. acute
4. triage
5. radiolucent
6. cardiac
7. pathology
8. neurosurgery
9. malignant
10. hormones

VII.
cardiac, psychiatry

VIII.
1. emergency department
2. ear, nose, and throat
3. intensive care unit
4. obstetrics
5. physician assistant

IX.
1. an es the ze ol'ə je
2. fə ren'zik
3. gas tro en tər ol'ə je
4. or tho pe'diks
5. ra de o loj'ik

CHAPTER 3

Exercise 1
1. G
2. A
3. F
4. H
5. I
6. J
7. B
8. D
9. C
10. E

Exercise 2
1. loosening, freeing, destroying
2. eye
3. suture
4. ear
5. brain
6. surgical repair
7. vessel
8. gland
9. incision
10. eyelid

Exercise 3
1. E
2. B
3. G
4. H
5. F
6. C
7. D
8. A

Exercise 4
1. -penia
2. -rrhea
3. -oid
4. -rrhexis
5. -spasm

Exercise 5
1. contrast
2. tomography
3. radioactive
4. resonance
5. sound

CHAPTER 3 REVIEW

I.
1. E
2. A
3. D
4. F
5. G
6. H
7. B
8. C

II.
1. E
2. A
3. I
4. J
5. H
6. B
7. F
8. C
9. D
10. G

III.
1. surgical puncture of the amnion
2. plastic surgery of the eyelid
3. deficiency of calcium
4. process of imaging deep structures by sending and receiving high-frequency sound waves that are reflected back
5. instrument used in electrocardiography
6. instrument used in fluoroscopy
7. resembling bone
8. record produced in tomography

IV.
1. symptom
2. chiroplasty
3. stasis
4. cardiomegaly
5. electrocardiogram
6. tracheostomy
7. adenectomy
8. ophthalmomalacia
9. otodynia
10. computed tomography

V.
1. hemorrhage
2. colectomy or colonectomy
3. ophthalmotomy
4. encephalotome
5. otoplasty

6. neurolysis
7. colopexy
8. angiorrhaphy
9. blepharedema
10. otoscopy

VI.

neurotripsy, ophthalmo-
plasty, symptom

VII.
1. computed tomography
2. chest x-ray

3. electrocardiogram
4. magnetic resonance
   imaging
5. within normal limits

VIII.
1. ap en dek′ tə me
2. kal sĭ pe′ne ə
3. en sef ə lot′ə me
4. nŏŏ rol′ ĭ sis
5. sə nog′rə fe

CHAPTER 4

Exercise 1
1. condition
2. inflammation
3. fear
4. prolapse
5. -mania
6. -oma
7. -pathy
8. -cele
9. -emia
10. -lith

Exercise 2
1. A
2. C
3. D
4. E
5. B
6. J
7. I
8. G
9. F
10. H

Exercise 3
1. B
2. G
3. D
4. I
5. J
6. E
7. A
8. H
9. C
10. F

Exercise 4
1. C
2. E
3. H
4. A
5. B
6. I
7. G
8. J
9. D
10. F

Exercise 5
1. white
2. green
3. blue
4. red
5. white
6. black
7. yellow

Exercise 6
1. E
2. C
3. B
4. G
5. F
6. A
7. D

Exercise 7
1. analgesic
2. anesthesia
3. neuromuscular
4. therapeutic

5. narcotic
6. radiation

CHAPTER 4 REVIEW

I.
1. F
2. D
3. C
4. B
5. E
6. H
7. A
8. G

II.
1. E
2. C
3. B
4. D
5. A
6. E

III.
1. dermatitis
2. jaundice
3. appendicitis
4. encephalocele
5. phobia
6. biopsy
7. radiation oncology
8. tissue
9. narcotic
10. antineoplastic

IV.
1. erythrocyte
2. hemolysin
3. carcinogen
4. ophthalmopathy
5. pyromania
6. osteitis
7. myalgia
8. nasal
9. pharmacotherapy
10. microscopy

V.

anesthetic, cephalic,
   cerebral

VI.
1. biopsy
2. overdose; right eye
3. over the counter
4. prescription
5. treatment

VII.
1. ad ə nop′ə the
2. sef ə lom′ə tre
3. si to tok′sik
4. he mo lit′ik
5. lak′tōs

CHAPTER 5

Exercise 1
1. B
2. B
3. E
4. F
5. A
6. D
7. C
8. A

Exercise 2
1. double
2. excessive, more than
   normal
3. beneath or below normal
4. none
5. many
6. first
7. half

Exercise 3

1. away from, toward
2. behind
3. inside
4. within
5. above

Exercise 4

1. anesthesia
2. anhydrous
3. aplastic
4. atraumatic

Exercise 5

1. A
2. F
3. A
4. B
5. D
6. B
7. G
8. E

9. E
10. C

CHAPTER 5 REVIEW

I.

1. J
2. C
3. F
4. B
5. G
6. A
7. E
8. D
9. I
10. H

II.

1. first
2. fast
3. difficult

4. beneath
5. macroscopic
6. against
7. half
8. two
9. intradermal
10. syndrome

III.

1. anesthesia
2. anhydrous
3. aplastic
4. asymptomatic
5. atraumatic

IV.

1. bradyphasia
2. anotia
3. retronasal
4. diplopia
5. contralateral

V.

addiction, ipsilateral, postanesthetic

VI.

1. 40 mg every day
2. 1 mg three times daily
3. once every 3 months
4. 120 mg twice a day
5. as the occasion arises or as needed

VII.

1. ab dukt′
2. kon trə sep′tiv
3. hi po dər′mik
4. sin′drōm
5. trans dər′məl

CHAPTER 6

Exercise 1

1. cell
2. tissue
3. organ
4. connective
5. epithelial
6. muscle
7. nervous
8. somatic
9. stem
10. congenital

Exercise 2

1. front, anterior
2. tail or lower part of body, caudal (caudad)
3. head, cephalad
4. distant or far, distal
5. back side, dorsal
6. situated below, inferior
7. side, lateral
8. middle, medial, or median
9. behind (toward the back), posterior
10. near, proximal
11. uppermost, superior
12. belly, ventral

Exercise 3

1. abdomin(o)
2. thorac(o)
3. acr(o)
4. dactyl(o)
5. pelv(i)
6. periton(o)
7. spin(o)
8. crani(o)

Exercise 4

1. pyrexia
2. pyrogen
3. dysplasia
4. aplasia
5. hypoplasia
6. hyperplasia
7. anaplasia
8. umbilicus
9. somatic
10. brain
11. omphalocele
12. somatopsychic

Exercise 5

1. auscultation
2. percussion
3. palpation
4. ambulation

CHAPTER 6 REVIEW

I.

1. cranial
2. spinal
3. thoracic
4. abdominal
5. pelvic

II.

1. RUQ
2. RLQ
3. LUQ
4. LLQ

III.

1. frontal or coronal
2. midsagittal
3. transverse
4. anterior, ventral
5. posterior, dorsal
6. lateral

IV.

1. B
2. H
3. C
4. I
5. F

6. A
7. G
8. D
9. E

V.

1. E
2. D
3. B
4. C
5. H
6. F
7. B
8. G
9. A
10. E

VI.

(no particular order)
1. epithelial
2. connective
3. nervous
4. muscle

VII.

1. 4
2. 1
3. 3
4. 2

VIII.
1. tissue
2. four quadrants
3. mediolateral
4. farther from the origin
5. frontal
6. encephalitis
7. prone
8. dermatosis
9. umbilicus
10. diaphragm

IX.
1. suprathoracic
2. unilateral
3. supine
4. peritoneal
5. plantar
6. dermatitis
7. abdominopelvic
8. chirospasm
9. dysplasia
10. electroencephalogram

X.
abdomen, acrocyanosis

XI.
1. abdomen, abdominal
2. anteroposterior
3. lateral
4. physical examination
5. vital signs

XII.
1. bi lat′ər əl
2. sə fal′ik
3. om fal′ik
4. pos tər o soo pēr′e or
5. vis′ər əl

CHAPTER 7

Exercise 1
1. homeostasis
2. intracellular
3. extracellular
4. interstitial
5. balance
6. hypokalemia
7. hypocalcemia
8. hypernatremia
9. calculus
10. lithotomy

Exercise 2
1. plasma
2. hematopoiesis
3. thrombosis
4. anticoagulant
5. leukocyte (or white)

Exercise 3
1. thrombocyte
2. nuclei
3. clot
4. thrombolysis
5. hemolysis
6. leukemia
7. leukocytes (white blood cells)
8. thrombocytosis
9. anemia
10. fainting

Exercise 4
1. microcyte
2. macrocytosis
3. anisocytosis
4. spherocyte
5. poikilocyte
6. hyperchromia
7. hypochromia
8. hemoglobinopathy

9. aplastic
10. hemoglobin

Exercise 5
1. coagulation
2. agglutination
3. fibrinolysin
4. hemostasis
5. transfusion
6. autologous
7. homologous

Exercise 6
1. C
2. A
3. B

Exercise 7
1. E
2. C
3. A
4. D
5. B
6. F

Exercise 8
1. weapons
2. disease
3. bioterrorism
4. disseminated

Exercise 9
1. antigen
2. susceptible
3. nonspecific
4. specific
5. active
6. immunodeficiency

Exercise 10
1. inpatients
2. outpatients
3. HIPAA

Exercise 11
1. E
2. A
3. B
4. C
5. D

CHAPTER 7 REVIEW

I.
1. A
2. C
3. B
4. C
5. B

II.
1. A
2. C
3. D
4. B

III.
1. B
2. D
3. F
4. C
5. E
6. A

IV.
1. T
2. T
3. F

4. F
5. T

V.
(no particular order)
1. bacteria
2. fungi
3. viruses
4. protozoa

VI.
(any five; no particular order)
1–5. natural barriers (unbroken skin), complement, interferon, phagocytes, inflammation, mucus, cilia, normal flora, urination, chemicals in human tears, and acids of the stomach, vagina, and skin

VII.
(no particular order)
1. cell-mediated immunity
2. antibody-mediated (humoral) immunity

VIII.
1. potassium
2. coagulation
3. interstitial
4. thrombosis
5. anticoagulant
6. wastes
7. homeostasis
8. differential
9. hemolysis
10. leukemia

IX.
1. fibrinogen
2. virulence
3. erythrocytes
4. aplastic
5. transplant
6. inside
7. cell-mediated immunity
8. inflammation
9. intracellular
10. thrombopenia

X.
1. poikilocyte
2. hyponatremia
3. intercellular
4. thrombosis
5. thrombolysis
6. allograft
7. abscess
8. neutrophil
9. hematopoiesis
10. bioterrorism

XI.
1. decrease in the number of neutrophils in the blood
2. decrease in the number of blood platelets
3. a pigmented malignant tumor
4. above the normal dosage needed for treatment
5. internal blood clot
6. deficiency in erythrocytes, hemoglobin, or both
7. twice a day
8. pertaining to hematology
9. pertaining to Staphylococcus, Gram-positive coccal bacteria

XII.
1. pertaining to difficulty in breathing

2. paleness
3. pertaining to both sides
4. swelling caused by excess fluid in interstitial spaces
5. hemoglobin
6. hematocrit
7. decreased blood sodium

XIII.
1. A
2. E
3. B
4. F

XIV.
anaerobic, fibrinolysis, polymorphonuclear, toxicity

XV.
1. acquired immunodeficiency syndrome
2. complete blood cell count

3. human immunodeficiency virus
4. polymorphonuclear
5. red blood cell, red blood count

XVI.
1. ko ag u lop′ə the
2. ə rith ro poi′ə tin
3. al o jen′ik
4. mi kros′kə pe
5. pro fə lak′sis

XVII.
1. B
2. E
3. A
4. C
5. D

CHAPTER 8

Exercise 1
1. B
2. B
3. A
4. D
5. C
6. D
7. D
8. E

Exercise 2
1. aorta
2. atrium
3. endocardium
4. mediastinum
5. myocardium
6. pericardium
7. septum; partition
8. valve
9. valve
10. ventricle

Exercise 3
1. venae cavae
2. atrium
3. right ventricle
4. lungs
5. left atrium
6. bicuspid (or mitral)

7. aorta
8. arterioles
9. capillaries
10. veins

Exercise 4
1. hypertension
2. bradycardia
3. diastole
4. systolic
5. Holter
6. lipids
7. lipoproteins
8. echocardiography

Exercise 5
1. cardiomegaly
2. cyanosis
3. dysrhythmia
4. infarct
5. ischemia
6. cardiovalvulitis
7. pericarditis
8. stenosis
9. endocarditis
10. shock

Exercise 6
1. aneurysm
2. coronary
3. occlusion
4. thrombosis
5. atherosclerosis
6. aortosclerosis
7. thrombophlebitis
8. stenosis

Exercise 7
1. D
2. B
3. F
4. A
5. C
6. E

Exercise 8
1. A
2. D
3. C
4. B

Exercise 9
1. lymphatic
2. lymph
3. veins
4. systemic

5. splenic
6. thymic
7. tonsillar

Exercise 10
1. lymphography
2. lymphadenography
3. biopsy

Exercise 11
1. D
2. B
3. A
4. E
5. C

Exercise 12
1. A
2. C
3. G
4. F

CHAPTER 8 REVIEW

I.
1. lymphangi(o)
2. arter(o), arteri(o)
3. arteriol(o)
4. phlebo, ven(i), ven(o)
5. venul(o)

II.
1. tonsill(o)
2. lymphaden(o)
3. thym(o)
4. lymphangi(o)
5. splen(o)

III.
1. H
2. B
3. D
4. I
5. E
6. F
7. G
8. C
9. J
10. A

IV.
1. E
2. C
3. A
4. B
5. D

V.
(no particular order)
maintains the internal fluid environment by returning proteins and tissue fluids to the blood; aids in the absorption of fats into the bloodstream; helps defend the body against microorganisms and disease

VI.
1. myocardial infarction
2. atherosclerosis
3. coronary artery bypass
4. endocarditis
5. defibrillation
6. coronary thrombosis
7. atrial septal defect
8. rheumatic fever
9. peripheral artery disease
10. aneurysm

VII.
1. thymoma
2. aortsclerosis
3. asystole
4. vasodilator
5. hypertension
6. tachycardia
7. lymphangitis
8. angiostenosis
9. tonsillectomy
10. splenorrhaphy

VIII.
1. cerebrovascular accident: a stroke; an abnormal condition of occlusion or hemorrhage of a vessel in the brain that results in lack of oxygen to brain tissue
2. computed tomography: a radiographic procedure that produces images of cross sections of brain tissue
3. No. Atrial fibrillation is a cardiac arrhythmia characterized by disorganized, rapid electrical activity in the atria.
4. No. Arrhythmia is a disordered pattern of the heart beat.
5. Telemetry is an electronic transmission of data between distant points.
6. Right and left endarterectomies: surgical removal of the lining of the right and left carotid arteries.
7. hypertension: increased blood pressure
congestive heart failure: an abnormal condition that reflects impaired cardiac pumping

myocardial infarction: necrosis of a portion of cardiac muscle
coronary artery disease: a condition of the heart's arteries that causes reduced flow of blood to the myocardium
atherosclerotic heart disease: heart disease caused by decreased blood flow as a result of atherosclerosis of the coronary arteries
hypercholesterolemia: increased levels of cholesterol in the blood

IX.
1. necrosis of a portion of cardiac muscle
2. increased blood pressure
3. increased blood cholesterol levels
4. the act of listening for sounds within the body, either directly with the unaided ear or with the stethoscope
5. electrocardiogram: a record produced in electrocardiography, recording the electrical activity of the heart
6. introduction of a catheter through an incision into a large vein and threaded through the circulatory system to the heart
7. radiographic study of the coronary arteries
8. coronary artery disease: an abnormal condition that may affect the heart's arteries and produce pathologic effects, especially the reduced flow of blood to the heart
9. thoracic pain caused by insufficient oxygen to the heart
10. coronary artery bypass graft: a section of a blood vessel grafted between the aorta and a coronary artery distal to an occluded coronary artery

X.
atherosclerosis, ischemia

XI.
1. arteriosclerotic heart disease
2. atrioventricular
3. carcinoma
4. chronic heart failure
5. creatine kinase
6. cardiopulmonary resuscitation
7. left ventricle
8. myocardial infarction
9. rheumatoid arthritis; right atrium
10. ventricular septal defect

XII.
1. kahr de o mi op' ə the
2. lim fad ə nop'ə the
3. lim fog'rə fe
4. per ĭ kahr'de əl
5. vas o di la'shən

XIII.
1. B
2. C
3. D
4. C
5. C
6. C
7. B
8. D
9. E
10. A

CHAPTER 9

Exercise 1
1. pharynx
2. trachea
3. septum
4. larynx
5. sinuses
6. trachea
7. bronchioles
8. alveoli
9. apex
10. pleura

Exercise 2
1. D
2. B
3. C
4. A
5. E

Exercise 3
1. apnea
2. dyspnea
3. oxygen
4. hyperpnea
5. hyperventilation
6. alkalosis
7. hypercapnia
8. acidemia
9. orthopnea
10. phrenoplegia

Exercise 4
1. B
2. D
3. C
4. A
5. E

Exercise 5
1. D
2. A
3. B
4. C

Exercise 6
1. tracheostenosis
2. broncholithiasis
3. lobar
4. pleural effusion
5. pleuritis
6. embolism
7. pneumoconiosis
8. emphysema

Exercise 7
1. asphyxia or asphyxiation
2. resuscitation
3. ventilator
4. tracheostomy
5. obstructive
6. transtracheal
7. orotracheal
8. lung
9. thoracostomy
10. antitussive
11. heart
12. cancer
13. prostate
14. breast
15. lung

CHAPTER 9 REVIEW

I.
1. G
2. A
3. B
4. F
5. D
6. E
7. C

II.
1. A
2. G
3. D
4. B
5. C
6. E
7. F

III.
1. sin(o)
2. nas(o), rhin(o)
3. pharyng(o)
4. laryng(o)
5. trache(o)
6. bronch(o), bronchi(o)
7. phren(o)
8. alveol(o)
9. bronchiol(o)

IV.
nasal cavity 1; bronchi 5, larynx 3; pharynx 2; trachea 4, alveoli 7; bronchioles 6

V.
(no particular order)
1. provide oxygen and remove carbon dioxide
2. maintain acid-base balance
3. produce speech
4. facilitate smell
5. maintain body's heat and water balance

VI.
1. LRT
2. LRT
3. LRT
4. URT
5. URT
6. URT
7. LRT

VII.
1. pneumonitis
2. expectoration
3. apnea
4. exchanging CO_2 for O_2
5. parietal pleura
6. heart and cancer
7. orthopnea
8. alkalosis
9. spirometry
10. pulmonary edema

VIII.
1. thrombus
2. dysphonia
3. bronchoscopy
4. aspiration
5. pharyngitis
6. rhinolithiasis
7. alveolar
8. laryngography
9. rhinorrhagia
10. intranasal

IX.
1. device for producing a fine spray, often used for intranasal medications
2. an abnormal condition that occurs when the volume of air that enters the alveoli and takes part in gas exchange is inadequate for the body's needs
3. deficiency of oxygen in arterial blood
4. excessive and prolonged contraction of the bronchi and bronchioles
5. widening of the lumen of the bronchi
6. difficulty in breathing
7. chronic obstructive pulmonary disease: a progressive and irreversible condition characterized by diminished respiration

X.
1. malaise
2. pleural effusion
3. wheezes
4. crackle
5. pneumothorax
6. bronchitis
7. dyspnea
8. pulmonary embolism
9. bronchodilator
10. expectorant

XI.
laryngography, pneumonitis

XII.
1. lar ing gop′ə the
2. pə ri′ə təl
3. fə rin′je əl
4. spi rom′ə tər
5. tra ke os′tə me

XIII.
1. arterial blood gas
2. extracorporeal membrane oxygenation
3. herpes simplex virus
4. severe acute respiratory syndrome
5. upper respiratory tract

XIV.
1. C
2. E
3. B
4. C
5. A
6. A
7. B
8. D
9. B
10. C

CHAPTER 10

Exercise 1
1. starch
2. bile
3. sugar
4. milk
5. fats
6. protein
7. thirst
8. appetite
9. digestion
10. contraction

Exercise 2
1. anus
2. gallbladder
3. common bile duct
4. large intestine; colon
5. duodenum
6. small intestine; intestines
7. stomach
8. liver
9. ileum
10. jejunum
11. mouth
12. pancreas
13. rectum
14. salivary gland
15. mouth

Exercise 3
1. oral
2. mandible
3. maxilla
4. palate
5. cheek
6. gingiva
7. tongue
8. tongue
9. pharynx
10. endodontium
11. periodontium
12. orthodontics
13. pedodontics
14. gerodontics
15. salivary
16. esophagus
17. sphincter
18. pyloric

Exercise 4
1. B
2. B
3. B
4. A
5. A
6. A
7. B

Exercise 5
1. choledochal
2. biliary
3. cholecystic
4. hepatic
5. pancreatic

Exercise 6
1. A
2. D
3. B
4. C
5. H
6. F
7. E
8. G

Exercise 7
1. O
2. H
3. C
4. D
5. B
6. I
7. K
8. L
9. P
10. N
11. F
12. E
13. A
14. J
15. M
16. G

Exercise 8
1. gastroenteritis
2. dysentery
3. fistula
4. diverticulosis
5. fissure
6. irritable
7. hemorrhoids
8. impaction
9. intussusception
10. volvulus

Exercise 9
1. A
2. D
3. F
4. E
5. B
6. G
7. C
8. H
9. I

Exercise 10
1. I
2. D
3. E
4. H
5. B
6. G
7. A
8. F
9. J
10. C

CHAPTER 10 REVIEW

I.
1. pharyng(o)
2. sial(o), sialaden(o)
3. hepat(o)
4. cholecyst(o)
5. duoden(o)
6. or(o), stomat(o)
7. esophag(o)
8. gastr(o)
9. pancreat(o)
10. jejun(o)
11. ile(o)
12. col(o)
13. an(o)

II.
1. C
2. B
3. D
4. A

III.
1. D
2. C
3. I
4. A
5. E
6. G
7. J
8. H
9. B
10. F

IV.
1. C
2. B
3. H
4. G
5. F
6. A
7. J
8. D
9. E
10. I

V.
(no particular order)
1. carbohydrates: basic source of cell energy
2. fats: energy reserve, and help cushion and insulate vital organs
3. proteins: building material for development, growth, and maintenance of the body

VI.
(no particular order)
1. liver = hepat(o)
2. gallbladder = cholecyst(o)
3. pancreas = pancreat(o)
4. salivary glands = sial(o) or sialaden(o)

VII.
1. gastroenterology
2. cholecystography
3. extracorporeal shock wave lithotripsy
4. anorexia nervosa
5. emaciation
6. colectomy
7. pyloric stenosis
8. ileocecal valve
9. hiatal hernia
10. lips and mouth
11. enterostasis
12. gastroscope
13. glucose
14. bulimia
15. gastroenterostomy

VIII.
1. adipsia
2. gastropathy
3. amylase
4. hyperemesis
5. cholecystectomy
6. vagotomy
7. gastritis
8. pharyngeal
9. dyspepsia
10. duodenoscopy

IX.
1. large intestine
2. abnormal new growth
3. gallbladder
4. abdominal wall
5. large intestine
6. abdomen
7. T

8. T
9. F
10. T
11. F
12. F

X.
1. large intestine
2. chronic
3. diagnostic procedure
4. pus
5. colonic obstruction
6. cancer of the large intestine (colon and rectum)
7. frequent passage of loose, watery stools
8. inflammation of the stomach and intestines, usually the small intestine

9. enlargement of the liver and spleen
10. that segment of the colon that extends from the ascending colon, across the abdomen, to the beginning of the descending colon

XI.
glossorrhaphy, nasogastric

XII.
1. body mass index
2. gastrointestinal
3. hepatitis B virus
4. herpes simplex virus
5. total parenteral nutrition

XIII.
1. ko lə sis to gas'trik
2. ko led'ə kəl
3. dis'ən ter e
4. fis'tu lə
5. hem ə roid ek'tə me

XIV.
1. C
2. E
3. B
4. A
5. C
6. B
7. D
8. C
9. C
10. C

CHAPTER 11

Exercise 1
1. pelvis
2. ureter
3. urethra
4. nephron
5. bladder
6. glomerulus
7. tubules
8. meatus

Exercise 2
1. urinalysis
2. urea
3. pyuria
4. glycosuria
5. cystometrography
6. electromyography
7. renography
8. nephrotomography

Exercise 3
1. F
2. C
3. A
4. D
5. G
6. B
7. E
8. J
9. I
10. H

Exercise 4
1. bilateral
2. uremia
3. nephromalacia
4. urethrorrhea
5. renovascular
6. cystitis
7. pyelonephritis
8. polycystic
9. glomerulonephritis
10. mellitus
11. hydronephrosis
12. hydroureter
13. cystocele
14. hyperplasia
15. nephrolithiasis
16. insipidus
17. stenosis
18. thrombosis

Exercise 5
1. nephrectomy
2. ureterostomy
3. infection
4. pyelolithotomy
5. anticoagulant therapy
6. transurethral resection

CHAPTER 11 REVIEW

I.
1. ren(o) or nephr(o)
2. ureter(o)
3. cyst(o)
4. urethr(o)

II.
1. E
2. D
3. A
4. C
5. B

III.
(1 through 3, in no particular order)
filtering the blood; maintaining proper balance of water, salts, and acids; excreting waste products

IV.
1. F
2. F
3. T
4. F
5. F
6. F
7. F
8. T

V.
1. glomerulus
2. pyelolithotomy
3. renal enlargement
4. lithotripsy
5. intravenous pyelography
6. renal failure
7. incontinence
8. polyuria
9. endoscopy tube
10. transurethral resection
11. uremia
12. excessive number of white cells
13. hydroureter
14. stenosis
15. pyelonephritis

VI.
1. uropathy
2. interrenal
3. hematuria
4. urethrocele
5. glomerulonephritis
6. pyelitis
7. hemodialysis
8. extracystic
9. cystography
10. lithotripsy

VII.
1. glomerulus

2. proximal convoluted tube
3. Bowman's capsule
4. distal convoluted tubule
5. collecting duct

VIII.
1. difficult or painful
2. inflammation of the bladder and kidney
3. prostate
4. kidney stones
5. stone in the ureter
6. benign prostatic hyperplasia
7. kidney, ureter, and bladder

8. intravenous
9. urinary tract infection

IX.
1. nighttime frequency
2. kidney stones
3. insulin
4. cystoscope
5. urinalysis
6. within normal limits
7. transurethral resection of the prostate

X.
hydronephrosis, gonorrhea

XI.
1. acute renal failure
2. electromyography
3. blood urea nitrogen
4. extracorporeal shock wave lithotripsy
5. voiding cystourethrogram

XII.
1. di u re′sis
2. lith′o trip se
3. nef ro lǐ thi′ə sis

4. pi′ə lo gram
5. u re′tər o plast te

XIII.
1. B
2. E
3. A
4. C
5. E
6. D
7. C
8. B
9. A
10. C

CHAPTER 12

Exercise 1
1. vagina
2. organs of reproduction
3. uterus
4. month
5. measure or uterine tissue
6. ovum
7. ovary
8. ovary
9. uterus
10. vagina
11. perine(o)
12. cervic(o)
13. salping(o)
14. vulv(o)

Exercise 2
1. A
2. D
3. B
4. E
5. C

Exercise 3
1. menstruation
2. climacteric
3. menarche
4. ovulation
5. estrogen

Exercise 4
1. speculum
2. cytology
3. dysplasia
4. gonadotropin
5. colposcopy

6. hysteroscopy
7. hysterosalpingography
8. laparoscopy

Exercise 5
1. B
2. C
3. A
4. D

Exercise 6
1. premenstrual
2. ovulation
3. anovulation
4. ovarian
5. pelvic
6. prolapse
7. retroversion
8. leiomyoma
9. fistula
10. cystocele

Exercise 7
1. hormone
2. vulvectomy
3. colporrhaphy
4. oophoropexy
5. hysterectomy
6. laparohysterectomy
7. salpingectomy
8. ligation
9. salpingostomy
10. curettage
11. cryotherapy or cryosurgery
12. hysteropexy

Exercise 8
1. epididymis
2. testicle
3. rectum
4. urethra
5. vessel, vas deferens

Exercise 9
1. penile
2. prostatic
3. scrotal
4. seminal
5. testicular

Exercise 10
1. spermatogenesis
2. testicle
3. seminiferous
4. testosterone
5. luteinizing

Exercise 11
1. C
2. A
3. B
4. D

Exercise 12
1. urology
2. torsion
3. oligospermia
4. cryptorchidism
5. epididymitis
6. hydrocele
7. varicocele
8. phimosis

9. balanitis
10. hyperplasia

Exercise 13
1. A
2. G
3. D
4. E
5. C
6. F
7. B
8. H

CHAPTER 12 REVIEW

I.
1. oophor(o)
2. salping(o)
3. hyster(o)
4. cervic(o)
5. colp(o)

II.
1. vas(o)
2. urethr(o)
3. pen(o)
4. prostat(o)
5. epididym(o)
6. orchi(o)
7. scrot(o)

III.
1. A
2. B
3. C

IV.
1. A
2. B
3. C
4. A
5. D
6. F
7. E

V.
1. dysmenorrhea
2. speculum
3. laparoscopy
4. oophoritis
5. menarche
6. hysteropexy
7. leukorrhea
8. endometriosis
9. colpoplasty
10. anorchidism
11. sterility
12. prepuce
13. cryptorchidism
14. torsion
15. orchialgia

VI.
1. ovarian
2. ovulation

3. estrogen
4. uterine
5. menstruation (or menses)

VII.
1. hysterectomy
2. menorrhagia
3. salpingocele
4. vasotomy
5. cervicitis
6. vulvovaginitis
7. oligospermia
8. salpingopexy
9. colposcopy
10. prostatectomy

VIII.
1. anteversion
2. retroversion
3. anteflexion
4. retroflexion

IX.
1. ovary
2. uterus
3. inner lining of the uterus
4. dilation and curettage

X.
1. implantation of a fertilized ovum outside the uterine cavity
2. removal of the uterus through the vagina
3. removal of an ovary and its fallopian tube
4. nonmalignant enlargement of the prostate
5. herniation of the urinary bladder through the vaginal wall
6. herniation of the rectum through the vaginal wall
7. loss of support that holds the vagina in place, allowing it to sag
8. surgical repair of the perineum
9. surgical fixation of the vagina

XI.
dysplasia, gynecology, salpingorrhaphy

XII.
1. benign prostatic hyperplasia
2. follicle-stimulating hormone
3. human chorionic gonadotropin
4. Papanicolaou
5. Venereal Disease Research Laboratories

XIII.
1. per ĭ me′tre əm
2. per ĭ ne′əm
3. pro jes′tə rōn
4. tes tik′u lər
5. sper mə to jen′ə sis

XIV.
1. C
2. C
3. B
4. D
5. B
6. C
7. A
8. B
9. D
10. A

CHAPTER 13

Exercise 1
1. gonad
2. gamete
3. zygote
4. ovulation
5. conception
6. implantation
7. fetus
8. chorion
9. spermatoblast
10. progesterone

Exercise 2
1. nat(o)
2. par(o)
3. false
4. pregnancy
5. pregnant female
6. that which stimulates

Exercise 3
1. pregnancy
2. pelvimetry
3. amniocentesis

4. chorionic
5. fetoscope

Exercise 4
1. E
2. A
3. C
4. D
5. B

Exercise 5
1. E
2. B
3. A
4. D
5. C

Exercise 6
1. vasectomy
2. ligation
3. fertilization
4. abortion
5. episiotomy

Exercise 7
1. A
2. B
3. C
4. D
5. E

CHAPTER 13 REVIEW

I.
1. umbilical cord
2. chorion
3. amnion
4. placenta
5. amniotic fluid
6. uterus

II.
1. D
2. C
3. A

4. B
5. E

III.
1. E
2. D
3. A
4. B
5. C

IV.
1. HCG
2. pelvimetry
3. dystocia
4. Down syndrome
5. gestation
6. cephalic
7. spermicide
8. para I
9. genital warts
10. candidiasis

V.
1. neonate
2. multipara
3. spermatoblast
4. implantation
5. amniotomy
6. episiotomy
7. chancre
8. amniochorial or amnio-chorionic
9. fetal
10. ovulation

VI.
1. vaginal swab (collection of fluid from the vagina)
2. cocci in pairs that are located inside and outside a cell
3. gonorrhea
4. Neisseria gonorrhoeae
5. penicillin or another antibiotic if patient is allergic to penicillin

VII.
amniocentesis, contraceptive

VIII.
1. acquired immunodeficiency syndrome
2. cephalopelvic disproportion
3. fetal heart rate
4. gonococcus
5. intrauterine device

IX.
1. am'ne on
2. shang'kər
3. gam'ēt
4. im u no də fish'ən se
5. se kən dip'ə rə

X.
1. D
2. E
3. E
4. A
5. D
6. B
7. C
8. D
9. C
10. C

CHAPTER 14

Exercise 1
1. marrow
2. epiphyses
3. periosteum
4. bone

Exercise 2
1. skeleton
2. skeletal
3. axial
4. appendicular

Exercise 3
1. vertebrae
2. cranium
3. cost(o)
4. spine
5. stern(o)
6. vertebrae
7. cervical
8. coccygeal

Exercise 4
1. tars(o)
2. fibul(o)
3. clavicul(o)
4. phalang(o)
5. calcane(o)
6. patell(o)
7. tibi(o)
8. scapul(o)
9. femor(o)
10. humer(o)
11. carp(o)

Exercise 5
1. (no particular order) ilium, ischium, and pubis
2. (no particular order) ulna and radius

Exercise 6
1. connective
2. articulation
3. synovial
4. joint
5. bursae
6. tendons
7. ligament
8. perichondrium

Exercise 7
1. B
2. A
3. E
4. F
5. H

Exercise 8
1. bone
2. electromyography
3. motion
4. erythrocyte
5. rheumatoid
6. joint
7. arthroscope
8. arthrocentesis

Exercise 9
1. A
2. C
3. D
4. E
5. I
6. F

Exercise 10
1. carpal
2. bursitis
3. arthritis
4. temporomandibular
5. tarsoptosis
6. tumor
7. osteomalacia
8. bifida
9. osteoarthritis
10. myasthenia

Exercise 11
1. C
2. D
3. B
4. A
5. E

Exercise 12
1. arthroclasia
2. costectomy
3. arthrotomy
4. myelosuppression
5. antiinflammatories
6. spondylodesis

7. arthrocentesis
8. chondrectomy
9. cranioplasty
10. myorrhaphy

CHAPTER 14 REVIEW

I.
1. clavicul(o)
2. stern(o)
3. cost(o)
4. ili(o)
5. pub(o)
6. ischi(o)
7. crani(o)
8. scapul(o)
9. humer(o)
10. radi(o)
11. uln(o)
12. carp(o)
13. femor(o)
14. patell(o)
15. tibi(o)
16. fibul(o)
17. tars(o)
18. phalang(o)

II.
1. G
2. B
3. E
4. D
5. A
6. C
7. F

III.
1. J
2. H
3. A
4. D
5. I
6. G
7. C
8. F
9. B
10. E

IV.
1. A
2. B
3. E
4. C
5. D

V.
1. J
2. D
3. H
4. I
5. F
6. E
7. B
8. G
9. C
10. A

VI.
1. 1
2. 5
3. 3
4. 4
5. 2

VII.
1. (no particular order) support for the body, protection of soft body parts, movement, blood cell formation, and storage

VIII.
(no particular order) skeletal: control movement of bones; visceral: contraction of organs and blood vessels; cardiac: contraction of the heart

IX.
1. sternoschisis
2. ulnoradial
3. arthropathy
4. electromyogram
5. decalcification
6. polydactylism
7. bone marrow
8. arthroscopy
9. tarsoptosis
10. osteomalacia

X.
1. reduction
2. intercostal
3. osteoarthritis
4. coccygectomy
5. myocele
6. osteitis
7. scoliosis
8. myofascial

9. articular
10. arthrocentesis

XI.
1. fracture of the right thigh bone resulting in many bone fragments
2. laminectomy: surgical removal of the bony arches of one or more vertebrae; right knee arthroscopy: examination of the interior of the right knee with an arthroscope
3. rupture of the cartilage surrounding an intervertebral disk
4. painful conditions of the joints
5. osteoporosis: abnormal loss of bone density and deterioration of the bone, with increased fracture risk

XII.
1. degenerative joint disease; degenerative changes in the joints
2. chronic, inflammatory, and sometimes deforming disease of the joints that has an autoimmune component

3. osteoarthritis (nonflammatory, degenerative arthritis) of the left knee
4. right knee replacement
5. right leg

XIII.
femoral, iliofemoral

XIV.
1. antinuclear antibody
2. degenerative joint disease
3. electromyography
4. range of motion
5. systemic lupus erythematosus

XV.
1. ahr thro kla′zhə
2. kon dro sahr ko′mə
3. lum′bahr
4. mi əs the′ne ə
5. stər no kos′təl

XVI.
1. E
2. C
3. B
4. A
5. A
6. C
7. A
8. B
9. D
10. A

CHAPTER 15

Exercise 1
1. (no particular order) stimulates movement; senses changes both within and outside the body; provides us with thought, learning, and memory; maintains homeostasis with the help of the hormonal system
2. sensory, integrative, motor
3. (no particular order) central nervous system, peripheral nervous system
4. (no particular order) neurons, neuroglia
5. (no particular order) axons, dendrites

Exercise 2
1. (no particular order) dura mater, arachnoid, pia mater
2. cerebell(o)
3. cerebr(o)
4. mening(o)
5. myel(o)

Exercise 3
1. sensory
2. sense
3. acetylcholine
4. epinephrine
5. chemoreceptors
6. photoreceptors
7. thermoreceptors
8. nociceptors
9. lacrimal
10. audiology

Exercise 4
1. B
2. G
3. C
4. A
5. F
6. E
7. D

Exercise 5
1. A
2. B
3. E
4. C
5. F
6. D

Exercise 6

1. intracerebral
2. subdural
3. cerebrovascular
4. quadriplegia
5. meningocele
6. encephalomyelitis
7. brain
8. skull
9. epilepsy
10. sclerosis
11. myasthenia
12. lacrimal
13. myopia
14. otitis
15. phobia

Exercise 7

1. C
2. B
3. E
4. A
5. D

Exercise 8

1. thrombolytics
2. aneurysmectomy
3. craniectomy
4. neurorrhaphy
5. blepharoplasty

CHAPTER 15 REVIEW

I.

1. A
2. B

3. B
4. B
5. A

II.

1. A
2. D
3. E
4. C
5. B

III.

1. dura mater
2. Alzheimer's disease
3. paraplegia
4. cerebrovascular accident
5. myelogram
6. claustrophobia
7. meningocele
8. contraindication
9. dacryocystotomy
10. sensitivity to pain

IV.

1. meninges
2. cerebrum
3. cerebrospinal
4. neuron
5. neuroglia
6. axon
7. dendrite

V.

1. anotia
2. neurosclerosis
3. encephalomyelitis
4. keratitis

5. myopia
6. semiconscious
7. myelography
8. electroencephalography
9. dacryolithiasis
10. narcolepsy

VI.

1. C
2. A
3. D
4. E
5. B
6. degenerative
7. dementia
8. dysarthria

VII.

1. a slowly progressing degenerative neurologic disorder characterized by resting tremor, a mask-like facial expression, shuffling gait, muscle rigidity, and weakness
2. tumor of the meninges
3. any disorder of the peripheral nervous system
4. sagging of the eyelid
5. slowness of voluntary movement

VIII.

acetylcholine, cerebral

IX.

1. attention deficit hyperactivity disorder
2. amyotrophic lateral sclerosis
3. cerebrospinal fluid
4. deep tendon reflex
5. spinal cord injury

X.

1. ə rak′noid
2. ser ə brot′ə me
3. ef′ər ənt
4. gli o′mə
5. klep to ma′ne ə

XI.

1. A
2. B
3. C
4. C
5. B
6. A
7. B
8. E
9. C
10. D

CHAPTER 16

Exercise 1

1. fat
2. axilla (armpit)
3. skin
4. sweat
5. horny or cornea
6. nail
7. hair
8. sebum
9. hair
10. nail
11. dermis and epidermis
12. ectoderm
13. sebum
14. sudoriferous gland
15. ungual

Exercise 2

1. biopsy
2. needle
3. skin (or allergy)
4. sweat

Exercise 3

1. A
2. B
3. F
4. E
5. C
6. D
7. G

Exercise 4

1. A
2. E
3. B
4. C
5. F
6. D

Exercise 5

1. abscess
2. furuncle
3. verruca
4. fungal
5. petechiae
6. nevus
7. keratosis

8. lipoma
9. Kaposi's
10. dermis

Exercise 6

1. F
2. G
3. A
4. E
5. D
6. B
7. C

Exercise 7

1. D
2. E
3. C
4. B
5. A

CHAPTER 16 REVIEW

I.

(any 5, no particular order)
external body covering; acts as a barrier to microorganisms; helps regulate body temperature; provides information about the environment; helps eliminate wastes; synthesizes vitamin D

II.

(no particular order)
hair protects the scalp, eyes, nostrils, and ears; nails protect the fingers and toes, and fingernails help us pick up small things; sebaceous glands produce sebum to keep hair and skin soft and inhibit bacterial growth; sweat glands eliminate waste and help regulate body temperature

III.

1. A
2. G
3. C
4. D
5. H
6. F
7. E
8. B

IV.

1. skin test
2. cryotherapy
3. débridement
4. axillary
5. seborrheic dermatitis
6. sweat test
7. scleroderma
8. bedsore
9. deep partial thickness
10. necrosis

V.

1. keratin
2. dermis
3. sebum
4. sudoriferous
5. sweating (perspiration)

VI.

1. furuncle
2. scabies
3. laceration
4. albinism
5. contusion

6. onychopathy
7. alopecia
8. ichthyosis
9. thermoplegia
10. folliculitis

VII.

1. keloid
2. grafts
3. sepsis
4. hypertrophic
5. full- and partial-thickness flame burns
6. onychomycosis

VIII.

1. redness of the skin that is the result of dilation and congestion of superficial capillaries
2. hardening of the tissue, usually caused by edema and inflammation
3. inflammation of hair follicles
4. a chronic disease, primarily of the skin, characterized by lesions that are covered with scales
5. a superficial dermatitis
6. a superficial bacterial infection involving the hair follicles

IX.

ectoderm, hidradenitis, onychectomy

X.

1. discoid lupus erythematosus
2. herpes simplex virus type 1
3. incision and drainage
4. total body surface area
5. ointment

XI.

1. sel u li′tis
2. dər mə bra′shən
3. ik the o′sis
4. ur tĭ kar′e ə
5. zēr o der′mə

XII.

1. E
2. C
3. D
4. D
5. C
6. D
7. B
8. D
9. A
10. C

CHAPTER 17

Exercise 1

1. pituitary, adrenals, gonads, thyroid, pancreas, and pineal gland

Exercise 2

1. nervous
2. pituitary
3. gland
4. hormones

Exercise 3

1. D
2. D
3. A
4. D

5. D
6. C
7. D
8. D
9. D
10. B
11. E
12. D

Exercise 4

1. adrenals
2. kidneys
3. ovaries or testes
4. ovaries or testes
5. female breasts
6. thyroid

Exercise 5

1. hypothyroidism
2. hyperthyroidism
3. ketonuria
4. glycosuria
5. mammography

Exercise 6

1. D
2. F
3. C
4. H
5. I
6. J
7. E
8. B

9. A
10. G

Exercise 7

1. lumpectomy
2. thyroidectomy
3. mammoplasty
4. adrenalectomy
5. mastopexy
6. mastectomy

CHAPTER 17 REVIEW

I.
(no particular order)
pituitary, adrenals, gonads, pineal gland, thyroid, pancreas

II.
(no particular order) nervous system stimulates endocrine glands by nerve impulses; endocrine glands release hormones

III.
1. C
2. B
3. B
4. A
5. D

IV.
1. D
2. D
3. A
4. D
5. D
6. C
7. D
8. D

9. D
10. B
11. E
12. D
13. E

V.
1. B
2. F
3. C
4. E
5. G
6. A
7. D

VI.
1. sweat gland
2. androgens
3. mammography
4. Cushing's syndrome
5. acromegaly
6. diabetes insipidus
7. myxedema
8. pancreas
9. glycosylated hemoglobin
10. goiter

VII.
1. epinephrine
2. hypothyroidism
3. hirsutism
4. gonads

5. hyperglycemia
6. prolactin
7. pituitary
8. androgenic (or masculinizing)
9. homeostasis
10. glycosuria

VIII.
1. bulging outward of the eyes
2. enlarged thyroid
3. increased activity of the thyroid
4. excision of the thyroid

IX.
1. polydipsia
2. polyuria
3. mastectomy
4. neuropathy
5. hypothyroidism
6. IDDM
7. retinopathy
8. Hb AIC
9. hypoglycemic
10. nephropathy

X.
adenohypophysis, homeostasis, thyrotropin

XI.
1. gestational diabetes mellitus
2. growth hormone
3. interstitial cell hormone
4. radioactive iodine
5. thyroid-stimulating hormone

XII.
1. (an tǐ di u ret′ik)
2. (jin ə ko mas′te ə)
3. (hi po ə dre′nəl iz əm)
4. (mam′o plas te)
5. (ok sǐ to′sin)

XIII.
1. C
2. C
3. E
4. C
5. C
6. A
7. B
8. D
9. B
10. C

CHAPTER 18

I.
1. obstetrician
2. neonatologist
3. radiologist
4. nerve cell
5. clinical pathologist
6. symptom
7. chiroplasty
8. cardiomegaly
9. electrocardiogram
10. computed tomography
11. appendicitis
12. encephalocele
13. phobia
14. narcotic
15. antineoplastic
16. macroscopic
17. against
18. two
19. intradermal
20. syndrome
21. tissue
22. quadrants
23. farther from the origin
24. frontal
25. diaphragm
26. erythrocytes
27. aplastic
28. transplant
29. inside
30. thrombopenia
31. myocardial infarction
32. atherosclerosis
33. coronary thrombosis
34. atrial septal defect
35. rheumatic fever
36. pneumonitis
37. expectoration
38. parietal pleura
39. heart and cancer
40. orthopnea
41. cholecystography
42. extracorporeal shock wave lithotripsy
43. anorexia nervosa
44. emaciation
45. colectomy
46. intravenous pyelography
47. renal failure
48. incontinence
49. polyuria
50. endoscopy tube
51. dysmenorrhea
52. speculum
53. hysteropexy
54. endometriosis
55. anorchidism
56. dystocia
57. Down syndrome
58. gestation
59. cephalic
60. genital warts
61. sternoschisis
62. ulnoradial
63. arthropathy
64. electromyogram
65. polydactylism
66. dura mater
67. paraplegia
68. meningocele
69. dacryocystotomy
70. Alzheimer's disease
71. débridement
72. seborrheic dermatitis
73. scleroderma
74. deep partial thickness
75. necrosis
76. pancreas
77. goiter
78. mammography
79. diabetes insipidus
80. Cushing's syndrome

II.

1. acute
2. triage
3. cardiac (sometimes, coronary)
4. pathology
5. hormones
6. colectomy or colonectomy
7. ophthalmotomy
8. encephalotome
9. angiorrhaphy
10. blepharedema
11. hemolysin
12. carcinogen
13. ophthalmopathy
14. osteitis
15. nasal
16. asymptomatic
17. bradyphasia
18. anotia
19. retronasal
20. diplopia
21. unilateral
22. supine
23. dermatitis
24. abdominopelvic
25. electroencephalogram
26. poikilocyte
27. hyponatremia
28. thrombolysis
29. neutrophil
30. hematopoiesis
31. asystole
32. vasodilator
33. hypertension
34. tachycardia
35. lymphangitis
36. thrombus
37. dysphonia
38. rhinolithiasis
39. alveolar
40. laryngography
41. gastropathy
42. amylase
43. hyperemesis
44. cholecystectomy
45. gastritis
46. glomerulonephritis
47. pyelitis
48. extracystic
49. cystography
50. lithotripsy
51. vasotomy
52. cervicitis
53. vulvovaginitis
54. oligospermia
55. salpingopexy
56. multipara
57. implantation
58. amniotomy
59. episiotomy
60. chancre
61. osteoarthritis
62. coccygectomy
63. myocele
64. osteitis
65. scoliosis
66. myelography
67. electroencephalography
68. dacryolithiasis
69. encephalomyelitis
70. keratitis
71. contusion
72. onychopathy
73. folliculitis
74. albinism
75. laceration
76. pituitary
77. androgenic (or masculinizing)
78. hypothyroidism
79. gonads
80. glycosuria

III.

1. T
2. A
3. S
4. A
5. P
6. S
7. S
8. D
9. S
10. P
11. T
12. A
13. P
14. P
15. D
16. A
17. P
18. A
19. A
20. P
21. P
22. T
23. P
24. P
25. S
26. T
27. P
28. A
29. S
30. P
31. P
32. S
33. D
34. A
35. D
36. P
37. D
38. P
39. A
40. T
41. S
42. D
43. A
44. S
45. D
46. P
47. P
48. S
49. S
50. A
51. P
52. T
53. S
54. P
55. A
56. P
57. A
58. A
59. D
60. D
61. S
62. A
63. S
64. P
65. T
66. A
67. D
68. P
69. P
70. S
71. P
72. S
73. S
74. P
75. A
76. S
77. P
78. S
79. P
80. A

APPENDIX VII Word Parts

Alphabetized Word Parts and Meanings

WORD PART	MEANING
a-	no, not, without
ab-	away from
abdomin(o)	abdomen
-able, -ible	capable of, able to
-ac	pertaining to
acid(o)	acid
acr(o)	extremities (arms and legs)
ad-, -ad	toward
aden(o)	gland
adenoid(o)	adenoids
adip(o)	fat
adren(o), adrenal(o)	adrenal gland
aer(o)	air or gas
-al	pertaining to
alb(o), albin(o)	white
albumin(o)	albumin
algesi(o)	sensitivity to pain
-algia	pain
alkal(o)	alkaline, basic
alveol(o)	alveoli
amni(o)	amnion
amyl(o)	starch
an-	no, not, without
an, -ary	pertaining to
an(o)	anus
andr(o)	male or masculine
aneurysm(o)	aneurysm
angi(o)	vessel
ankyl(o)	stiff
-ant	that which causes
ante-	before in time or in place
anter(o)	anterior
anthrac(o)	coal
anti-	against
aort(o)	aorta
append(o), appendic(o)	appendix
arachn(o)	spider or arachnoid membrane
arter(o), arteri(o)	artery
arteriol(o)	arteriole
arthr(o), articul(o)	joint; articulation
-ary	pertaining to
-ase	enzyme
-asthenia	weakness
-ate	to cause an action or the result of an action
atel(o)	imperfect or incomplete

WORD PART	MEANING
ather(o)	yellowish, fatty plaque
-ation	process
atri(o)	atrium
audi(o)	hearing
aut(o)	self
axill(o)	axilla (armpit)
bacter(i), bacteri(o)	bacteria
balan(o)	glans penis
bi-	two
bi(o)	life or living
bil(i), chol(e)	bile or gall
blast(o), -blast	immature, embryonic form
blephar(o)	eyelid
brady-	slow
bronch(o), bronchi(o)	bronchi
bronchiol(o)	bronchioles
bucc(o)	cheek
burs(o)	bursa
calc(i)	calcium
calcane(o)	calcaneus
cancer(o)	cancer
-capnia	carbon dioxide
carcin(o)	cancer
cardi(o)	heart
carp(o)	carpus (wrist)
caud(o)	tail or toward the tail
cec(o)	cecum
-cele	hernia
cellul(o)	little cell or compartment
-centesis	surgical puncture to aspirate or remove fluid
centi-	one hundred or one-hundredth
cephal(o)	head
cerebell(o)	cerebellum
cerebr(o)	brain, cerebrum
cervic(o)	neck; cervix uteri
cheil(o)	lip
chem(o)	chemical
chir(o)	hand
chlor(o)	green
chol(e)	bile
cholecyst(o)	gallbladder
choledoch(o)	common bile duct
chondr(o)	cartilage
chori(o)	chorion
chrom(o)	color

WORD PART	MEANING	WORD PART	MEANING
-cidal	killing	encephal(o)	brain
circum-	around	endocardi(o)	endocardium
-clasia	break	enter(o)	small intestine; intestines
clavicul(o)	clavicle (collarbone)	epi-	above, on
coagul(o)	coagulation	epididym(o)	epididymis
coccyg(o)	coccyx (tail bone)	epiglott(o)	epiglottis
col(o), colon(o)	colon or large intestine	-er	one who
colp(o)	vagina	erythemat(o)	erythema or redness
coni(o)	dust	erythr(o)	red
contra-	against	esophag(o)	esophagus
coron(o)	crown	esthesi(o)	feeling or sensation
cost(o)	costae (ribs)	-esthesia	sensitivity to pain
crani(o)	cranium (skull)	eu-	good, normal
crin(o)	to secrete	-eum	membrane
-crine	secrete	ex-, exo-	out, without, away from
cry(o)	cold	extra-	out, without, away from
crypt(o)	hidden	fasci(o)	fascia
cutane(o)	skin	femor(o)	femur
cyan(o)	blue	fet(o)	fetus
-cyesis	pregnancy	fibr(o)	fiber or fibrous
cyst(o)	bladder, cyst, fluid-filled sac	fibrin(o)	fibrin
cyt(o), -cyte	cell	fibul(o)	fibula
dacry(o), lacrim(o)	tear	fluor(o)	emitting or reflecting light
dactyl(o)	finger or toe	follicul(o)	follicle
de-	down, from or reversing	fung(i)	fungus
dendr(o)	tree	gastr(o)	stomach
dent(i), dent(o)	tooth	gen(o)	beginning, origin
-derm	skin or germ layer	-genesis	producing or forming
derm(a), dermo, dermat(o)	skin	-genic	produced by or in
		genit(o)	organs of reproduction
-desis	binding, fusion	ger(a), ger(o), geront(o)	elderly
di-	two	gigant(o)	large
dia-	through	gingiv(o)	gums
diplo-	double	gli(o)	neuroglia or a sticky substance
-dipsia	thirst	glomerul(o)	glomerulus
dist(o)	distant, far	gloss(o)	tongue
diverticul(o)	diverticula	gluc(o)	glucose
dors(o)	dorsal, back	glyc(o), glycos(o)	sugar
duoden(o)	duodenum	gon(o)	genitals or reproduction
-dynia	pain	gonad(o)	gonad
dys-	bad, difficult	-gram	a record
-eal	pertaining to	gram(o)	to record
ech(o)	sound	-graph	instrument for recording
-ectasia, ectasis	dilatation (dilation, enlargement) or stretching of a structure or part	-graphy	process of recording
		-gravida	pregnant female
		gynec(o)	female
ecto-	out, without, away from	heli(o)	sun
-ectomy	excision (surgical removal or cutting out)	hem(a), hem(o), hemat(o)	blood
-edema	swelling	hemi-	half, partly
electr(o)	electricity	hemoglobin(o)	hemoglobin
embol(o)	embolus	hepat(o)	liver
-emesis	vomiting	herni(o)	hernia
-emia	condition of the blood	hidr(o)	perspiration, sweat
en-, end-, endo-	inside	hist(o)	tissue

WORD PART	MEANING	WORD PART	MEANING
home(o)	sameness, constant	log(o)	knowledge, words
humer(o)	humerus (upper arm bone)	-logic, -logical	pertaining to
hydr(o)	water	-logist	one who studies; specialist
hyper-	excessive, more than normal	-logy	study or science of
hypo-	beneath or below normal	lumb(o)	lower back
hyster(o), uter(o)	uterus	lymph(o)	lymph, lymphatics
-ia-, -iasis	condition	lymphaden(o)	lymph node
-iac	one who suffers	lymphangi(o)	lymph vessel
iatr(o)	physician or treatment	lymphat(o)	lymphatics
-iatrician	practitioner	lys(o)	destruction, dissolving
-iatrics, -iatry	medical profession or treatment	-lysin	that which destroys
-ic, -ive	pertaining to	-lysis	process of loosening, freeing, or destroying
ichthy(o)	fish		
idi(o)	individual	-lytic	capable of destroying
ile(o)	ileum	macro-	large or great
ili(o)	ilium	mal-	bad
immun(o)	immune	malac(o)	soft, softening
in-	not or inside (in)	-malacia	soft; abnormal softening
infer(o)	lowermost or below	mamm(o)	breast
infra-	beneath, under	mandibul(o)	mandible
insulin(o)	insulin	-mania	excessive preoccupation
inter-	between	-maniac	one who shows excessive preoccupation
intestin(o)	intestines		
intra-	within	mast(o)	breast
iod(o)	iodine	maxill(o)	maxilla
ipsi-	same	mechan(o)	mechanical
ir(o), irid(o)	iris	medi(o), medio-	middle
is(o)	equal	mediastin(o)	mediastinum
ischi(o)	ischium	mega-, megalo-	large, enlarged, or great
-ism	condition or theory	-megaly	enlargement
-ist	one who	melan(o)	black
-itis	inflammation	men(o)	month
-itrics, -iatry	medical profession or treatment	mening(i), mening(o)	meninges
-ium	membrane	ment(o)	mind
-ive	pertaining to	meso-	middle
jejun(o)	jejunum	meta-	change; next, as in a series
kal(i)	potassium	-meter	instrument used to measure
kary(o)	nucleus	metr(o)	measure, uterine tissue
kerat(o)	cornea; hard, horny	-metry	process of measuring
ket(o), keton(o)	ketone bodies	micro-	small
kinesi(o)	movement	mid-	middle
-kinesia, -kinesis	movement, motion	milli-	one-thousandth
lacrim(o)	tear	mono-	one
lact(o)	milk	morph(o)	shape; form
lapar(o)	abdominal wall	muc(o)	mucus
laryng(o)	larynx	multi-	many
later(o)	side	muscul(o), my(o)	muscle
leps(o)	seizure	myc(o)	fungus
-lepsy	seizure	myel(o)	bone marrow or spinal cord
leuk(o); occasionally leuc(o)	white	myocardi(o)	myocardium
lingu(o)	tongue	narc(o)	stupor
lip(o)	fat, lipid	nas(o)	nose
lith(o), -lith	stone; calculus	nat(o)	birth
lob(o)	lobe	natr(o)	sodium
		ne(o)	new

WORD PART	MEANING
necr(o)	death
nephr(o)	kidney
neur(o)	nerve
noc(i)	cause harm, injury, or pain
noct(i)	night
norm(o)	normal
nos(o)	disease
nucle(o)	nucleus
nulli-	none
nyct(o)	night
o(o)	ovum
obstetr(o)	midwife
ocul(o)	eye
odont(o)	tooth
-oid	resembling
-ole	small
olig(o)	few, scanty
-oma	tumor
omphal(o)	umbilicus (navel)
onc(o)	tumor
onych(o)	nail
oophor(o)	ovary
ophthalm(o)	eye
-opia	vision
opt(o), optic(o)	vision
or(o)	mouth
orchi(o), orchid(o)	testis
-orexia	appetite
orth(o)	straight
-ose	sugar
-osis	condition (often an abnormal condition; sometimes, an increase)
oste(o)	bone
ot(o)	ear
-ous	pertaining to or characterized by
ovari(o)	ovary
ox(i)	oxygen
palat(o)	palate
pan-	all
pancreat(o)	pancreas
par(o)	bearing offspring
para-	near, beside, or abnormal
-para	woman who has given birth
patell(o)	patella
path(o)	disease
-pathy	disease
ped(o)	child (sometimes, foot)
pelv(i)	pelvis
pen(o)	penis
-penia	deficiency
-pepsia	digestion
per-	through or by
peri-	around

WORD PART	MEANING
pericardi(o)	pericardium
perine(o)	perineum
periton(o)	peritoneum
pex(o), -pexy	surgical fixation
phag(o)	eat, ingest
-phagia, -phagic-, -phagy	eating, swallowing
phalang(o)	phalanx (bones of fingers or toes)
pharmac(o), pharmaceut(i)	drugs or medicine
pharyng(o)	pharynx
phas(o), -phasia	speech
phil(o)	attraction
phleb(o)	vein
-phobia	abnormal fear
phon(o)	voice
-phoresis	transmission
phot(o)	light
phren(o)	mind or diaphragm
-phylaxis	protection
-physis	growth
pil(o), trich(o)	hair
pituitar(o)	pituitary gland
plas(o), -plasia	formation, development
plast(o)	repair
-plasty	surgical repair
pleg(o), -plegia	paralysis
pleur(o)	pleura
-pnea	breathing
pneum(o)	lungs or air
pneumon(o)	lungs
pod(o)	foot
-poiesis	production
-poietin	that which causes production
poikil(o)	irregular
poly-	many
post-	after, behind
poster(o)	back
pre-	before in time or in place
primi-	first
pro-	favoring, supporting
proct(o)	anus, rectum
prostat(o)	prostate
prote(o), protein(o)	protein
proxim(o)	near
pseudo-	false
psych(o)	mind
-ptosis	prolapse (sagging)
-ptysis	spitting
pub(o)	pubis
pulm(o), pulmon(o)	lung
py(o)	pus
pyel(o)	renal pelvis
pylor(o)	pylorus
pyr(o)	fire

WORD PART	MEANING
quad-, quadri-	four
rach(i), rachi(o)	vertebral or spinal column, spine (backbone)
radi(o)	radiant energy (sometimes, radius)
rect(o)	rectum
ren(o)	kidney
retro-	behind, backward
rheumat(o)	rheumatism
rhin(o)	nose
rhythm(o), rrhythm(o)	rhythm
rhytid(o)	wrinkle
-rrhage, -rrhagia	excessive bleeding or hemorrhage
-rrhaphy	suture (uniting a wound by stitches)
-rrhea	flow or discharge
-rrhexis	rupture
sacr(o)	sacrum
salping(o)	fallopian tube
-sarcoma	malignant tumor from connective tissue
scapul(o)	scapula (shoulder blade)
schis(o), schiz(o), schist(o), -schisis	split, cleft
scler(o)	hard
-sclerosis	hardening
scop(o)	to examine, to view
-scope	instrument used for viewing
-scopy	visual examination with a lighted instrument
scrot(o)	scrotum
seb(o)	sebum
semi-	half, partly
semin(o)	semen
seps(o)	infection
sept(i), sept(o)	infection; septum
sial(o)	saliva; salivary glands
sialaden(o)	salivary glands
sigmoid(o)	sigmoid colon
sin(o)	sinus
som(a), somat(o)	body
son(o)	sound
-spasm	twitching, cramp
sperm(o), spermat(o)	spermatozoa
spher(o)	round
spin(o)	spine
spir(o)	to breathe
splen(o)	spleen
spondyl(o)	vertebrae
-stalsis	contraction
staphyl(o)	grapelike cluster; uvula
-stasis	stopping, controlling
-stenosis	narrowing; stricture
stern(o)	sternum

WORD PART	MEANING
steth(o)	chest
stomat(o)	mouth
-stomy	formation of an opening
strept(o)	twisted
sub-	beneath, under
super-	above, beyond, excessive
super(o), supra-	above, beyond
sym-, syn-	joined, together
synov(o), synovi(o)	synovial membrane
tachy-	fast
tars(o)	ankle (sometimes, edge of eyelid)
tel(e)	distant
ten(o), tend(o), tendin(o)	tendon
test(o), testicul(o)	testicle
tetra-	four
therapeut(o), -therapy	treatment
therm(o)	heat
thorac(o)	thorax (chest)
thromb(o)	thrombus; clot
thym(o)	thymus
thyr(o), thyroid(o)	thyroid gland
tibi(o)	tibia
-tic	pertaining to
tom(o)	to cut
-tome	an instrument used for cutting
-tomy	incision (cutting into tissue)
tonsill(o)	tonsil
top(o)	place or position
tox(o), toxic(o)	poison
trache(o)	trachea
trans-	across
tri-	three
trich(o)	hair
-tripsy	surgical crushing
trop(o)	to stimulate
troph(o), -trophic, -trophy	nutrition
-tropic	stimulating
-tropin	that which stimulates
uln(o)	ulna (a bone of the forearm)
ultra-	excessive
umbilic(o)	umbilicus
ungu(o)	nail
uni-	one
ur(o)	urinary tract, urine
ureter(o)	ureter
urethr(o)	urethra
-uria	urine or urination
urin(o)	urine
uter(o)	uterus
vag(o)	vagus nerve
vagin(o)	vagina
valv(o), valvul(o)	valve
varic(o)	twisted and swollen

WORD PART	MEANING	WORD PART	MEANING
vas(o)	vessel; ductus deferens	vesic(o)	bladder or blister
vascul(o)	vessel	vir(o), virus(o)	virus
ven(i), ven(o)	vein	viscer(o)	viscera
ventr(o)	belly	vulv(o)	vulva
ventricul(o)	ventricle	xanth(o)	yellow
venul(o)	venule	xer(o)	dry
vertebr(o)	vertebra	-y	state or condition

English Words and Corresponding Word Parts

MEANING	WORD PART	MEANING	WORD PART
abdomen	abdomin(o)	beginning	gen(o), -gen, -genic, -genesis, -genous
abdominal wall	lapar(o)	behind	poster(o), post-, retr(o)
able to	-able, -ible	belly side	ventr(o)
abnormal	par-, para-	below or beneath	hypo-, sub-
above	epi-	below normal	hypo-
acid	acid(o)	beside	par-, para-
across	trans-	between	inter-
adenoids	adenoid(o)	beyond	supra-
adrenaline	adrenalin(o)	bile	bil(i), chol(e)
adrenals	adren(o), adrenal(o)	binding	-desis
after	post-	birth	nat(o)
again	ana-	birth (give birth)	par(o)
against	anti-, contra-	woman who has given birth	-para
air	aer(o), pneum(o)		
air sac	alveol(o)	black	melan(o)
albumin	albumin(o)	bladder	cyst(o), vesic(o)
alkaline	alkal(o)	blister	vesic(o)
all	pan-	blood	hem(a), hem(o), hemat(o), -emia
alveolus	alveol(o)		
amnion	amni(o)	blue	cyan(o)
aneurysm	aneurysm(o)	body	som(a), somat(o)
ankle bone	tars(o)	bone	oste(o)
anus	an(o)	bone marrow	myel(o)
anus and rectum	proct(o)	brain	cerebr(o), encephal(o)
aorta	aort(o)	break	-clasia
appendix	append(o), appendic(o)	breast	mamm(o), mast(o)
appetite	-orexia	breast bone	stern(o)
arachnoid	arachn(o)	breathe, breathing	-pnea, spir(o)
armpit	axill(o)	bronchi	bronch(o), bronchi(o)
arms and legs	acr(o)	bronchiole	bronchiol(o)
around	circum-, peri-	bursa	burs(o)
arteriole	arteriol(o)	calcaneus	calcane(o)
artery	arter(o), arteri(o)	calcium	calc(i)
atrium	atri(o)	calculus	lith(o), -lith
attraction	phil(o)	capable of	-able, -ible
auditory tube	salping(o)	cancer	cancer(o), carcin(o)
away from	ab-, ex-	carbon dioxide	-capnia
back	dors(o)	carpus	carp(o)
backward	retr(o)	cartilage	chondr(o)
bacteria	bacter(i), bacteri(o)	cause harm or injury	noc(i)
bad	dys-, mal-	cecum	cec(o)
before	ante-, pre-, pro-		

MEANING	WORD PART	MEANING	WORD PART
cell	cyt(o), -cyte	duct	vas(o)
cerebellum	cerebell(o)	ductus deferens	vas(o)
cerebrum	cerebr(o)	(vas deferens)	
cervix uteri	cervic(o)	duodenum	duoden(o)
change	meta-	dust	coni(o)
cheek	bucc(o)	ear	ot(o)
chemical	chem(o)	eat	phag(o)
chest	steth(o), thorac(o)	edge of eyelid	tars(o)
child	ped(o)	egg (ovum)	o(o)
chorion	chori(o)	electricity	electr(o)
clavicle	clavicul(o)	embolus	embol(o)
clot (thrombus)	thromb(o)	embryonic form	-blast, blast(o)
cluster	staphyl(o)	emitting or reflecting light	fluor(o)
coagulation	coagul(o)	endocardium	endocardi(o)
coal	anthrac(o)	enzyme	-ase
coccyx	coccyg(o)	epididymis	epididym(o)
cold	cry(o)	epiglottis	epiglott(o)
collarbone	clavicul(o)	equal	is(o)
colon	col(o)	erythema	erythemat(o)
color	chrom(o)	esophagus	esophag(o)
common bile duct	choledoch(o)	examine	scop(o)
compartment	cellul(o)	instrument used	-scope
condition	-ia, -iasis, -ism, -osis, -y	process of examining	-scopy
constant	home(o)	excessive	hyper-, super-, ultra-
controlling	-stasis	excision	-ectomy
cornea	kerat(o)	extremities	acr(o)
cramp	-spasm	eye	ocul(o), ophthalm(o)
cranium	crani(o)	eyelid	blephar(o)
crown	coron(o)	false	pseudo-
cut (to cut)	tom(o)	far	dist(o)
incision or cutting	-tomy	fascia	fasci(o)
instrument used to cut	-tome	fast	tachy-
cyst	cyst(o)	fat	adip(o), lip(o)
death	necr(o)	fear (abnormal)	-phobia
decreased or deficient	-penia	feeling	esthesi(o), -esthesia
destruction	lys(o)	female	gynec(o)
that which destroys	-lysin	femur	femor(o)
process of destroying	-lysis	fetus	fet(o)
capable of destroying	-lytic	few	olig(o)
development	plas(o), -plasia	fiber, fibrous	fibr(o)
diaphragm	-phren(o)	fibula	fibul(o)
difficult	dys-	fingers or toes	dactyl(o)
digestion	-pepsia	fire	pyr(o)
digit	dactyl(o)	first	primi-
dilation	-ectasia, -ectasis	fish	ichthy(o)
discharge	-rrhea	flow	-rrhea
disease	nos(o), path(o), -osis, -pathy	follicle	follicul(o)
dissolving	lys(o)	foot	ped(o), pod(o), pes-, -pod
distant	dist(o), tel(e)	for	pro-
diverticula	diverticul(o)	form	morph(o)
double	dipl(o)	formation	plas(o), -plasia
down	de-	formation of an opening	-stomy
drooping	-ptosis	four	quad-, quadri-, tetra-
drugs	pharmac(o), pharmaceut(i)	from	de-
dry	xer(o)	front	anter(o)

MEANING	WORD PART
fungus	fung(i), myc(o)
fusion	-desis
gall	chol(e)
gallbladder	cholecyst(o)
gland	aden(o)
glans penis	balan(o)
glomerulus	glomerul(o)
glucose	gluc(o)
gonads (ovaries and testes)	gonad(o)
good	eu-
green	chlor(o)
growth	-physis
gums	gingiv(o)
hair	pil(o), trich(o)
half	hemi-, semi-
hand	chir(o)
hard	kerat(o), scler(o)
hardening	scler(o), -sclerosis
head	cephal(o)
hearing	audi(o)
heart	cardi(o)
heat	therm(o)
heel bone	calcane(o)
hemoglobin	hemoglobin(o)
hemorrhage	-rrhagia
hernia	-cele, herni(o)
hidden	crypt(o)
horny	kerat(o)
humerus	humer(o)
ileum	ile(o)
ilium	ili(o)
immune	immun(o)
imperfect	atel(o)
incision	tom(o), -tomy
instrument used	-tome
incomplete	atel(o)
increase	-osis
individual	idio-
infection	seps(o), sept(o)
inferior	infer(o)
inflammation	-itis
ingest	phag(o)
inside	in-, en-, end-, endo-
insulin	insulin(o)
intestine	enter(o), intestin(o)
iodine	iod(o)
iris	ir(o), irid(o)
irregular	poikil(o)
irrigation	-clysis
ischium	ischi(o)
jejunum	jejun(o)
joined together	syn-, sym-
joint	arthr(o), articul(o)

MEANING	WORD PART
ketone bodies	ket(o), keton(o)
kidney	nephr(o), ren(o)
killing	-cidal
kneecap	patell(o)
large	gigant(o), macr(o), megal(o), mega-, -megaly
large intestine	col(o)
larynx	laryng(o)
life	bi(o)
light	phot(o)
lip	cheil(o)
liver	hepat(o)
living	bi(o)
lobe	lob(o)
location	top(o)
lower back	lumb(o)
lung	pneum(o), pneumon(o), pulm(o), pulmon(o)
lymph	lymph(o)
lymph node	lymphaden(o)
lymph vessel	lymphangi(o)
lymphatics	lymph(o), lymphat(o)
male	andr(o)
mandible	mandibul(o)
many	multi-, poly-
masculine	andr(o)
maxilla	maxill(o)
measure	metr(o)
instrument used	-meter
process	-metry
mechanical	mechan(o)
mediastinum	mediastin(o)
medicine	-iatrics, pharmac(o)
membrane	-eum, -ium
meninges	mening(o)
middle	mid-, medi(o), meso-
midwife	obstetr(o)
milk	lact(o)
mind	ment(o), phren(o), psych(o)
month	men(o)
more than normal	hyper-
mouth	or(o), stomat(o)
movement	kinesi(o), -kinesia
mucus	muc(o)
muscle	muscul(o), my(o)
myocardium	myocardi(o)
nail	onych(o), ungu(o)
narrowing	-stenosis
nature	physi(o)
near	par-, para-, proxim(o)
neck	cervic(o)
nerve	neur(o), nerv(o)
neuroglia	gli(o)
new	neo-

MEANING	WORD PART	MEANING	WORD PART
new opening	-stomy	pregnant female	-gravida
next (as in a series)	meta-	preoccupation (excessive)	-mania
night	noct(i), nyct(o)	process	-ation
no	a-, an-	production	-poiesis
none	nulli-	production, causes	-poietin
normal	norm(o), eu-	prolapse	-ptosis
nose	nas(o), rhin(o)	prostate gland	prostat(o)
not	a-, an-, in-	protection	-phylaxis
nucleus	kary(o), nucle(o)	protein	prote(o), protein(o)
nutrition	troph(o), -trophy	pubis	pub(o)
obsessive preoccupation	-mania	pus	py(o)
old, elderly	ger(a), ger(o), geront(o)	pylorus	pylor(o)
one	uni-, mon(o)	radiant energy	radi(o)
one hundred, one-hundredth	centi-	radius	radi(o)
one-thousandth	milli-	record (the record)	-gram
one who	-er, -ist	to record	gram(o)
one who studies	-logist	recording instrument	-graph
one who suffers	-iac	the recording process	-graphy
one with excessive preoccupation	-maniac	rectum	rect(o)
		red, redness	erythr(o), erythemat(o)
organs of reproduction	genit(o), gon(o)	removal	-ectomy
origin	gen(o), -gen, -genic, -genesis, -genous	renal pelvis	pyel(o)
		reproduction	gon(o)
out	ex-	resembling	-oid
outside	ecto-, exo-, extra-	reversing	de-
outward	exo-	rheumatism	rheumat(o)
ovary	oophor(o)	rhythm	rhythm(o), rrhythm(o)
oxygen	ox(i)	ribs	cost(o)
pain	-algia, -dynia	round	spher(o)
painful	dys-	rupture	-rrhexis
palate	palat(o)	sac	cyst(o)
pancreas	pancreat(o)	sacrum	sacr(o)
paralysis	pleg(o), -plegia	sag	-ptosis
parathyroid gland	parathyroid(o)	saliva	sial(o)
patella (kneecap)	patell(o)	salivary gland	sialaden(o)
pelvis	pelv(i)	same	ipsi-
penis	pen(o)	sameness	home(o)
pericardium	pericardi(o)	scapula (shoulder blade)	scapul(o)
perineum	perine(o)	scrotum	scrot(o)
peritoneum	periton(o)	sebum	seb(o)
perspiration	hidr(o)	secrete	crin(o), -crine
pertaining to	-ac, -al, -ary, -eal, -ic, -ive, -logic, -logical, -ous, -tic	seizure	-lepsy, leps(o)
		self	aut(o)
phalanges	phalang(o)	semen	semin(o)
pharynx	pharyng(o)	sensation	esthesi(o)
physician or treatment	iatr(o)	sensitivity to pain	algesi(o)
pituitary gland	pituitar(o)	septum	sept(o)
place (position)	top(o)	shape	morph(o)
pleura	pleur(o)	shoulder blade	scapul(o)
poison	tox(o), toxic(o)	side	later(o)
potassium	kal(i)	sigmoid colon	sigmoid(o)
practitioner	-iatrician	single	mon(o)
pregnancy	-cyesis	sinus	sin(o)
		situated above	super(o), super-, supra-

MEANING	WORD PART	MEANING	WORD PART
situated below	infer(o), infra-	theory	-ism
skin	cutane(o), derm(a), dermat(o)	thirst	dips(o), -dipsia
skull	crani(o)	thorny	spin(o)
slow	brady-	three	tri-
small	micr(o), -ole	throat	pharyng(o)
small intestine	enter(o)	thrombus	thromb(o)
sodium	natr(o)	through	dia-, trans-
soft, softening	malac(o), -malacia	thymus	thym(o)
sound	ech(o), son(o)	thyroid gland	thyr(o), thryoid(o)
specialist	-ist	tibia	tibi(o)
speech	phas(o), -phasia	tissue	hist(o)
sperm, spermatozoa	spermat(o), sperm(o)	together	sym-, syn-
spider	arachn(o)	tongue	gloss(o), lingu(o)
spinal cord	myel(o)	tonsil	tonsill(o)
spine	rach(i), rachi(o), spondyl(o), spin(o)	toward	ad-, -ad
		trachea	trache(o)
spiral	spir(o)	transmission	-phoresis
spitting	-ptysis	treatment	therapeut(o), -therapy
spleen	splen(o)	tree	dendr(o)
split	schis(o), schist(o), schiz(o), -schisis	tumor	onc(o), -oma
		turn	trop(o)
starch	amyl(o)	twice	di-
sternum (breastbone)	stern(o)	twisted	strept(o)
sticky substance	gli(o)	twitching	-spasm
stiff	ankyl(o)	two	bi-, di-
stimulate	trop(o), -tropic	ulna	uln(o)
that which stimulates	-tropin	umbilicus	omphal(o), umbilic(o)
stomach	gastr(o)	under	sub-
stone	lith(o), -lith	up	ana-
stopping	-stasis	upon	epi-
straight	orth(o)	uppermost	super(o)
stretching	-ectasia, -ectasis	ureter	ureter(o)
stricture	-stenosis	urethra	urethr(o)
structure	-id	urinary tract	ur(o)
study or science of	-logy	urination	urin(o), -uria
stupor	narc(o)	urine	ur(o), -uria, urin(o)
sugar	glyc(o), glycos(o), -ose	uterine tissue	metr(o)
sun	heli(o)	uterine tube	salping(o)
surgical crushing	-tripsy	uterus	hyster(o), uter(o)
surgical fixation	pex(o), -pexy	uvula	staphyl(o)
surgical puncture	-centesis	vagina	colp(o), vagin(o)
surgical repair	-plasty	vagus nerve	vag(o)
suture	-rrhaphy	valve	valv(o), valvul(o)
sweat	hidr(o)	varicose vein	varic(o)
swelling	-edema	vein	phleb(o), ven(o), ven(i)
symptom	sympt(o)	ventral	ventr(o)
synovial membrane	synov(o), synovi(o)	ventricle	ventricul(o)
tail	caud(o)	venule	venul(o)
tail bone	coccyg(o)	vertebra	spondyl(o), vertebr(o)
tarsals (ankle bones)	tars(o)	vessel	angi(o), vas(o), vascul(o)
tear (crying)	dacry(o), lacrim(o)	virus	vir(o), virus(o)
teeth	dent(i), dent(o), odont(o)	viscera	viscer(o)
tendon	ten(o), tend(o), tendin(o)	vision	opt(o), optic(o)
testis, testicle	orchi(o), orchid(o), test(o)	voice	phon(o)

MEANING	WORD PART
vomiting	-emesis
vulva	vulv(o)
washing out	-clysis
water	hydr(o)
weakness	-asthenia
white	alb(o), albin(o), leuk(o)
windpipe	trache(o)

MEANING	WORD PART
within	intra-
without	a-, an-, ex-
wrinkle	rhytid(o)
wrist bone	carp(o)
yellow	xanth(o)
yellow, fatty plaque	ather(o)

BIBLIOGRAPHY

American Cancer Society: *Ca—A cancer journal for clinicians*, vol 54, no 1, Atlanta, 2004.

American Cancer Society: *Ca—A cancer journal for clinicians*, vol 55, no 1, Atlanta, 2004.

Applegate EJ: *The anatomy and physiology learning system: textbook*, Philadelphia, 2000, WB Saunders.

Bedolla M: *Essential Spanish for health care*, New York, 1997, Living Language, A Random House Company.

BJC Health Care: Weapons of mass destruction awareness training, St. Louis, 2002, BJC Health Care.

Bonewit K: *Clinical procedures for medical assistants*, ed 6, Philadelphia, 2004, WB Saunders.

Centers for Disease Control and Prevention, Atlanta, 1999, www.cdc.gov.

Destafano C, Federman FM: *Essentials of medical transcription, a modular approach*, Philadelphia, 2001, WB Saunders.

Dorland's illustrated medical dictionary, ed 30, Philadelphia, 2003, WB Saunders.

Dunmore CW, Fleischer RM: *Medical terminology, exercises in etymology*, ed 2, Philadelphia, 1985, FA Davis.

Frederick PM, Kinn ME: *Medical office assistant*, ed 5, Philadelphia, 1981, WB Saunders.

Fuller JR: *Surgical technology principles and practices*, ed 2, Philadelphia, 1986, WB Saunders.

Ignatavicius DD, Workman ML, Mishler MA: *Medical-surgical nursing: critical thinking for collaborative care*, ed 4, Philadelphia, 2003, WB Saunders.

Joyce EV, Villanueva ME: *Say it in Spanish: a guide for health care professionals*, Philadelphia, 1996, WB Saunders.

Lewis SM, Heitkemper MM, Dirksen SR: *Medical-surgical nursing, assessment and management of clinical problems*, ed 6, St. Louis, 2004, Mosby.

Mosby's medical, nursing, and allied health dictionary, ed 6, St. Louis, 2002, Mosby.

Polaski AL, Tatro SE: *Luckmann's core principles and practice of medical-surgical nursing*, Philadelphia, 1996, WB Saunders.

Seidel HM, Ball JW, Dains JE, Benedict GW: *Mosby's guide to physical examination*, ed 5, St. Louis, 2003, Mosby.

Taber's cyclopedic medical dictionary, ed 18, Philadelphia, 1997, FA Davis.

Velasquez M: *Velasquez Spanish and English dictionary*, Clinton, NJ, 1985, New Win Publishing.

INDEX/GLOSSARY

Note: Page numbers followed by the letter *f* refer to figures; those followed by the letter *t* refer to tables.

anterolateral (an″tər-o-lat′ər-əl) situated anteriorly and to one side. 87

anteromedial (an″tər-o-me′de-əl) situated anteriorly and to the medial side. 86

anteroposterior (an″tər-o-pos-tēr′e-ər) from front to back of the body, such as the direction of a radiographic projection. 86

anterosuperior (an″tər-o-soo-pēr′e-ər) situated anteriorly and superiorly. 87

anteversion (an″te-vər′zhən) the forward tipping or tilting of an organ; displacement in which the uterus is tipped forward but is not bent at an angle. 325

anthracosis (an-thrə-ko′sis) a usually asymptomatic form of pneumoconiosis caused by deposition of coal dust in the lungs. 209

anthrax (an′thraks) an infectious bacterial disease usually transmitted to humans by contact with infected animals or their discharges or with contaminated animal products. 132

antianxiety (an″te-ang-zi′ə-te) reducing anxiety. 455

antiarrhythmic (an″te-a-rith′mik) preventing or alleviating cardiac arrhythmia; an agent that prevents or alleviates arrhythmia. 172

antiarthritic (an″te-ahr-thrit′ik) an agent that alleviates arthritis; alleviating arthritis. 412

antiasthmatic (an″te-az-mat′ik) alleviating asthma; a drug that alleviates asthma. 538

antibiotic (an″te-, an″ti-bi-ot′ik) destructive of life; a chemical substance produced by a microorganism that inhibits the growth of or kills other microorganisms. 96, 482

antibody (an″ti-bod″e) an immunoglobulin that interacts only with the antigen that induced its synthesis or with an antigen closely related to it. 134

anticancer (an″ti-kan′sər) against cancer; a drug used to treat cancer. 216

anticoagulant (an″te-, an″ti-ko-ag′u-lənt) preventing blood clotting; any substance that prevents blood clotting. 114

anticonvulsant (an″te-, an″ti-kən-vul′sənt) preventing or relieving convulsions; an agent that prevents or relieves convulsions. 454

antidepressant (an″te-, an″ti-de-pres′ənt) preventing or relieving depression; an agent that is used to treat the symptoms of depression. 455

antidiarrheal (an″te-, an″ti-di″ə-re′əl) counteracting diarrhea; an agent that is effective in combating diarrhea. 264

antidiuretic (an″te-, an″ti-di″u-ret′ik) suppressing the rate of urine formation; an agent that suppresses urine formation. 494, 495
   a. hormone, a hormone produced by the hypothalamus that decreases the amount of water lost in urination. 494, 495

antiemetic (an″te-ə-met′ik) preventing or alleviating nausea and vomiting; an agent that prevents or alleviates nausea and vomiting. 264

antifebrile (an″te-, an″ti-feb′ril) relieving or reducing fever; an agent that relieves or reduces fever. 95

antigen (an′ti-jən) any substance that is capable, under appropriate conditions, of inducing a specific immune response and of reacting with the products of that response. 133

antihemophilic (an″te-, an″ti-he″mo′fil′ik) counteracting hemophilia; an agent that acts to counteract hemophilia. 118
   a. factor, blood factor VIII. 118

antihistamine (an″te-, an″ti-his′tə-mēn) a drug that counteracts the action of histamine. 135, 217

antihypertensive (an″te-, an″ti-hi″pər-ten′siv) counteracting high blood pressure; an agent that reduces high blood pressure. 172

antiimpotence (an″ti-im′pə-təns) acting against the failure to initiate an erection or to maintain an erection in male individuals. 339

antiinfective (an″te-in-fek′tiv) capable of killing or preventing the multiplication of infectious agents; an agent that so acts. 95

antiinflammatory (an″te-in-flam′ə-to″re) counteracting or suppressing inflammation; an agent that counteracts or suppresses the inflammatory process. 96, 412
   nonsteroidal a., any of a group of drugs acting against fever, pain, and inflammation by inhibiting prostaglandin synthesis. 412

antilipidemic (an″ti-lip″ĭ-de′mik) promoting a reduction of lipid levels in the blood; an agent that reduces lipids in the blood. 172

antimicrobial (an″te-, an″ti-mi-kro′be-əl) killing microorganisms or suppressing their multiplication or growth; an agent that kills microorganisms or suppresses their multiplication or growth. 95

antineoplastic (an″te-, an″ti-ne″o-plas′tik) inhibiting or preventing the development of neoplasms; checking the maturation and proliferation of malignant cells; an agent having such properties. 61, 136, 217

antinuclear antibody test (an″te-, an″ti-noo′kle-ər) a blood test used primarily to help diagnose systemic lupus erythematosus, although a positive result may also indicate other autoimmune diseases. 395

antiperspirant (an″te-, an″ti-pər′spər-ant) inhibiting or preventing perspiration; an agent that inhibits or prevents perspiration. 74

antipruritic (an″te-, an″ti-proo-rit′ik) relieving or preventing itching; an agent that relieves or prevents itching. 482

antipsychotic (an″te-, an″ti-si-kot′ik) drugs that are effective in the treatment of psychosis. 455

antipyretic (an″te-, an″ti-pi-ret′ik) relieving or reducing fever; an agent that relieves or reduces fever. 95, 454

antiseptic (an″tĭ-sep′tik) pertaining to asepsis; a substance that inhibits the growth and development of microorganisms without necessarily killing them. 129, 482

antispasmodic (an″te-, an″ti-spaz-mod′ik) relieving spasm, usually of smooth muscle; an agent that relieves muscle spasms. 301

antithyroid (an″te-thi′roid) counteracting the functioning of the thyroid. 547

antitussive (an″te-, an″ti-tus′iv) relieving or preventing cough; an agent that relieves or prevents cough. 217

anuria (an-u′re-ə) complete suppression of urinary secretion by the kidneys. 291

anuric (an-u′rik) pertaining to or characterized by lack of secretion of urine. 291

anus (a′nəs) the distal or terminal opening of the alimentary canal. 231, 239

aorta (a-or′tə) the main trunk from which the systemic arterial system proceeds. 154

abdominal a., continuation of the thoracic aorta. 157

arch of a., the continuation of the ascending aorta that gives rise to the descending aorta. 157

ascending a., the proximal portion of the aorta arising from the left ventricle, giving origin to the right and left coronary arteries before continuing as the arch of the aorta. 157

coarctation of the a., a localized malformation of the aorta, which causes narrowing of the lumen of the vessel. 163

descending a., the continuation of the aorta from the arch of the aorta, in the thorax, to the point of its division into the common iliac arteries. 157

thoracic a., the proximal portion of the descending aorta. 154

aortic (a-or′tik) of or pertaining to the aorta. 157
   a. insufficiency, aortic regurgitation. 167
   a. regurgitation, blood flow from the aorta back into the left ventricle during diastole. 167
   a. stenosis, a narrowing or stricture of the aortic valve. 167

aortitis (a″or-ti′tis) inflammation of the aorta. 7, 167

aortogram (a-or′to-gram) the radiographic record resulting from aortography. 161

aortography (a″or-tog′rə-fe) radiography of the aorta after the injection of an opaque medium. 161, 167

aortosclerosis (a-or″to-sklə-ro′sis) abnormal hardening of the aorta. 167

apex (a′peks) anatomical nomenclature for the superior aspect of a body, organ, or part, or the pointed extremity of a conical structure. 194

aphagia (ə-fa′jə) refusal or loss of the ability to swallow. 247

aphasia (ə-fa′zhə) defect or loss of the power of expression by speech, writing, or signs, or of comprehending spoken or written language, because of injury or disease of the brain. 204, 439

aphasic (ə-fa′zik) pertaining to or affected with aphasia; a person affected with aphasia. 204

aphonia (a-fo′ne-ə) loss of voice. 204

apical (ap′ĭ-kəl) pertaining or located at the apex. 194

aplasia (ə-pla′zhə) lack of development of an organ or tissue. 96, 206

aplastic (a-plas′tik) pertaining to or characterized by aplasia. 123

apnea (ap′ne-ə) cessation of breathing. 199, 437
   sleep a., transient periods of cessation of breathing during sleep. 199, 437

appendectomy (ap″en-dek′tə-me) surgical removal of the vermiform appendix. 35, 38, 263

appendicitis (ə-pen″dĭ-si′tis) inflammation of the vermiform appendix. 52, 252

appendicular (ap″en-dik′u-lər) pertaining to the vermiform appendix; pertaining to an appendage. 239, 377

appendix (ə-pen′diks) a general term used to designate a supplementary, accessory, or dependent part attached to a main structure; also called appendage. It is frequently used alone to refer to the appendix vermiformis. 239
   vermiform a., a wormlike appendage of the cecum. 239

approximate (ə-prok′sĭ-māt″) to bring close together. 260

approximation (ə-prok″sĭ-ma′shən) the act or process of bringing closer. 260

arachnoid (ə-rak′noid) resembling a spider's web; the middle of the three meninges. 428

areola (ə-re′o-lə) a circular area of a different color, surrounding a central point. 497

arrhythmia (ə-rith′me-ə) any variation from the normal rhythm of the heartbeat. 163

arterial (ahr-tēr′e-əl) pertaining to an artery or to the arteries. 150

arteriogram (ahr-tēr′e-o-gram) a radiograph of an artery after injection of a radiopaque medium. 161

arteriograph (ahr-tēr′e-o-graf) a film produced by arteriography. 161

arteriography (ahr″tēr-e-og′rə-fe) radiography of arteries after injection of radiopaque material into the bloodstream. 161
   coronary a., radiography of the coronary arteries. 161

arteriole (ahr-tēr′e-ōl) a minute arterial branch, especially one just proximal to a capillary. 150

arteriopathy (ahr-tēr″e-op′ə-the) any arterial disease. 167

arteriosclerosis (ahr-tēr″e-o-sklə-ro′sis) a group of diseases characterized by thickening and loss of elasticity of arterial walls. 160, 166

arteriosclerotic (ahr-tēr″e-o-sklə-rot′ik) pertaining to or affected with arteriosclerosis. 166
   a. cardiovascular disease, arteriosclerotic heart disease. 166

arteritis (ahr″tə-ri′tis) inflammation of an artery. 167

artery (ahr′tə-re) a vessel through which the blood passes away from the heart to the various parts of the body. 150
   renal a., one of two arteries that carries blood to the kidneys. 277f, 278
   renal a. stenosis, narrowing of a renal artery. 289f, 297

arthralgia (ahr-thral′jə) pain in a joint. 406

arthrectomy (ahr-threk′tə-me) the excision of a joint. 412

arthritis (ahr-thri′tis) inflammation of joints. 406
   rheumatoid a., a chronic systemic disease primarily of the joints, marked by inflammatory changes in the synovial membranes and articular structures and by muscle atrophy and rarefaction of the bones. In late stages, deformity and ankylosis develop. 406

arthrocentesis (ahr″thro-sen-te′sis) puncture and aspiration of a joint. 394, 412

arthrochondritis (ahr″thro-kon-dri′tis) inflammation of the cartilage of a joint. 399

arthroclasia (ahr″thro-kla′zhə) the surgical breaking down of an ankylosed joint. 412

arthrodesis (ahr″thro-de′sis) the surgical fixation of a joint. 412

arthrodynia (ahr″thro-din′e-ə) pain in a joint. 406

arthrogram (ahr′thro-gram) a radiographic record after introduction of opaque contrast material into a joint. 394

arthrography (ahr-throg′rə-fe) radiography of a joint after injection of opaque contrast material. 394

blood (blud) the fluid that circulates through the heart and blood vessels, carrying nutrients and oxygen to the body cells. 113
  b. cells, red and white corpuscles. 114, 116f
  b. pressure, the pressure existing in the large arteries at the height of the pulse wave. 158
  b. vessels, the arteries, veins, and capillaries. 158
  b. urea nitrogen, the amount of urea in the blood. 285
body system (bod′e sis′təm) several organs of the body that work together to accomplish a set of functions. 81
bolus (bo′ləs) a rounded mass of food or a pharmaceutical preparation ready to swallow, or such a mass passing through the gastrointestinal tract. 230
bone (bōn) the rigid connective tissue constituting most of the skeleton of vertebrates. 373
  b. densitometry, determining blood mass by measuring radiation absorption by the skeleton. 393
  b. density, the amount of bone mass in a given volume. 393
  b. grafting, transplanting a piece of bone from one part of the body to another. 410
  b. marrow, the soft material filling the cavities of bones. 373
botulism (boch′ə-liz-əm) a type of food poisoning caused by a neurotoxin produced by the growth of *Clostridium botulinum* in improperly canned or preserved foods. 129, 444
Bowman's capsule (bo′mənz kap′səl) part of the kidney that functions as a filter in the formation of urine. 279
bradycardia (brad″e-kahr′de-ə) slow heartbeat, as evidenced by slowing of the pulse rate to less than 60 beats per minute. 159
bradyphasia (brad″ĭ-fa′zhə) slow speech. 74
bradypnea (brad″e-ne′ə, brad-ip′ne-ə) abnormal slowness of breathing. 202
brain (brān) that part of the central nervous system contained within the cranium, consisting of the cerebrum, cerebellum, pons, medulla oblongata, and midbrain. 427, 428f
  b. stem, the stemlike portion of the brain connecting the cerebral hemispheres with the spinal cord and constituting the pons, medulla oblongata, and mesencephalon. 429
breast (brest) the anterior aspect of the chest; mammary gland. 497
  b. augmentation, insertion of an implant behind the breast to increase its size. 512
  b. reduction, surgical removal of excess breast and skin tissue. 512
Bright's disease (brīts dĭ-zēz′) a vague term for kidney disease, usually referring to degenerative kidney disease. 294
bronchiectasis (brong″ke-ek′tə-sis) chronic dilatation of the bronchi. 207
bronchiole (brong′ke-ōl) one of the fine divisions of the bronchial tree. 193
bronchiolectasis (brong″ke-o-lek′tə-sis) dilation of the bronchioles. 207
bronchiolitis (brong″ke-o-li′tis) inflammation of the bronchioles; bronchopneumonia. 207
bronchitis (brong-ki′tis) inflammation of the bronchi. 207
bronchoalveolar (brong″ko-al-ve′ə-lər) pertaining to a bronchus and alveoli. 193
bronchoconstriction (bron″ko-kən-strik′shən) the act or process of decreasing the caliber of a bronchus; bronchostenosis. 207
bronchodilator (brong″ko-di′la-tor) stretching or expanding the air passages; an agent that causes dilation of the bronchi. 217
bronchogenic (brong-ko-jen′ik) originating in a bronchus. 207
bronchogram (brong′ko-gram) the record obtained by bronchography. 196
bronchography (brong-kog′rə-fe) radiography of the bronchial tree after injection of an opaque solution. 196
broncholithiasis (brong″ko-lĭ-thi′ə-sis) a condition in which calculi are present within the lumen of the tracheobronchial tree. 207
bronchopathy (brong-kop′ə-the) any disease of the bronchi. 207
bronchoplasty (brong′ko-plas″te) plastic surgery of the bronchus. 207
bronchopneumonia (brong″ko-nōō-mo′ne-ə) a name given to an inflammation of the lungs that usually begins in the terminal bronchioles. These become clogged with a mucopurulent exudate forming consolidated patches in adjacent lobules. 207
bronchopulmonary (brong″ko-pool′mə-nar″e) pertaining to the lungs and their air passages; both bronchial and pulmonary. 207
bronchoscope (brong′ko-skōp) instrument for viewing the bronchi. 196
bronchoscopic (brong″ko-skop′ik) pertaining to either bronchoscopy or the bronchoscope. 196
bronchoscopy (brong-kos′kə-pe) examination of the bronchi through a bronchoscope. 196, 196f
bronchospasm (brong′ko-spaz″əm) spasmodic contraction of the smooth muscle of the bronchi, as occurs in asthma. 207
bronchus (brong′kəs) either of the two main branches of the trachea. 193
buccal (buk′əl) pertaining to or directed toward the cheek. 233
  b. cavity, the vestibule of the mouth, specifically the area lying between the teeth and cheeks. 233
  b. mucosa, the mucous membrane lining the inside of the mouth. 248
bulbourethral glands (bul″bo-u-re′thrəl glandz) Cowper's glands; two small glands, one on each side of the prostate gland. They secrete a viscid fluid that forms part of the seminal fluid. 331
bulimia (bōō-le′me-ə) an emotional disorder characterized by episodic binge eating, usually followed by purging behaviors. 246
bulla (bul′ə) a large vesicle, greater than 1 cm in circumference, containing fluid. 473
bunionectomy (bun″yən-ek′tə-me) excision of an abnormal prominence on the first metatarsal head. 412
burn (bərn) injury to tissues caused by contact with dry heat (fire), moist heat (steam or hot liquid), chemicals (e.g., corrosive substances), electricity (current or lightning), friction, or radiant and electromagnetic energy. 478
  deep partial-thickness b., one in which damage extends through the epidermis into the dermis; second-degree burn. 478
  full-thickness b., one in which the epidermis and dermis are destroyed and damage extends into the underlying tissue; third-degree burn. Burn is classified as fourth-degree burn if underlying bone and muscle are damaged. 478
  superficial b., a burn in which damage is limited to the epidermis; first-degree burn. 478

bursa (bər′sə) a sac or saclike cavity filled with a viscid fluid and situated at places in the tissues at which friction would otherwise develop. 387
bursectomy (bər-sek′tə-me) excision of a bursa. 411
bursitis (bər-si′tis) inflammation of a bursa. 399
bypass (bi′pas) an auxiliary flow; a shunt. 170
  coronary artery b., a section of saphenous vein or other material grafted between the aorta and a coronary artery distal to an obstructive lesion. 170
  coronary artery b. graft, use of a vessel from elsewhere in the patient's body to provide an alternate route for the blood to circumvent an obstructed coronary artery. 170
  gastric b., a surgical procedure that reduces the size of the stomach. 259
cachexia (kə-kek′se-ə) general ill health and malnutrition. 506
  pituitary c., generalized insufficiency of pituitary hormones. 506
calcaneal (kal-ka′ne-əl) pertaining to the calcaneum, or heel bone. 385
calcaneitis (kal-ka″ne-i′tis) inflammation of the heel bone. 399
calcaneodynia (kal-ka″ne-o-din′e-ə) pain in the heel. 399
calcaneofibular (kal-ka″ne-o-fib′u-lər) pertaining to the heel bone and the fibula. 385
calcaneoplantar (kal-ka″ne-o-plan′tər) pertaining to the heel bone and the sole. 385
calcaneotibial (kal-ka″ne-o-tib′e-əl) pertaining to the heel bone and the tibia. 385
calcaneum, calcaneus (kal-ka′ne-əm, kal-ka′ne-əs) the irregular quadrangular bone at the back of the tarsus. It is also called the heel bone or os calcis. 385
calcification (kal″sĭ-fĭ-ka′shən) process whereby tissue becomes hardened by a deposit of calcium salts. 375
calcipenia (kal″sĭ-pe′ne-ə) deficiency of calcium. 402
calcitonin (kal″sĭ-to′nin) a hormone elaborated by the thyroid gland in response to hypercalcemia. 507
calciuria (kal″se-u′re-ə) calcium in the urine. 396
calculus (kal′ku-ləs) an abnormal concretion, occurring within the animal body, chiefly in hollow organs or their passages. 54
  renal c., a stone occurring in the kidney. 300
callus (kal′əs) localized hyperplasia of the horny layer of the epidermis caused by pressure or friction. 476
calorie (kal′ə-re) a unit of heat defined as the amount of heat required to increase the temperature of kilogram of water 1 degree Celsius at a specified temperature. 229
cancer (kan′sər) a neoplastic disease the natural course of which is fatal. Cancer cells, unlike benign tumor cells, exhibit the properties of invasion and metastasis and are highly anaplastic. Cancer includes the two broad categories of carcinoma and sarcoma, but in normal usage it is often used synonymously with carcinoma. 21
Candida albicans (kan′dĭ-də al′bĭ-kanz) a species of yeastlike fungi that is part of the normal flora of human skin and mucous membranes and is the most frequent cause of candidiasis. 247
candidiasis (kan″dĭ-di′ə-sis) infection with a fungus of the genus *Candida,* especially *C. albicans.* It is usually a superficial infection of the moist cutaneous areas of the body. 323, 367
canker (kang′kər) ulceration, chiefly of the mouth and lips; canker sores. 247, 364
cannula (kan′u-lə) a tube for insertion into a duct or cavity. 213
  nasal c., a device for delivering oxygen by way of two small tubes inserted into the nares. 213
capillary (kap′ĭ-lar″e) one of the minute vessels connecting the arterioles and venules. Walls of capillaries act as a semipermeable membrane for exchange of various substances between the blood and tissue fluid. In a less common meaning, capillary also means pertaining to or resembling a hair (Latin: *capillaris,* hairlike). 150
carbohydrate (kahr′bo-hi′drāt) any of a group of organic compounds, the most important of which are the saccharides, starch, cellulose, and glycogen. 228
carcinogen (kahr-sin′ə-jen) any substance that produces cancer. 56
carcinogenesis (kahr″sĭ-no-jen′ə-sis) the origin of cancer. 56
carcinoma (kahr″sĭ-no′mə) a malignant tumor; cancerous tumor. 52
  basal cell c., an epidermoid carcinoma common on the face in the elderly and having a low degree of malignancy. 477
  renal c., cancer of a kidney. 298
  squamous cell c., carcinoma developed from squamous epithelium. 477
cardiac (kahr′de-ak), pertaining to the heart. 19
  c. arrest, ceasing of heart activity. 19
  c. arrhythmia, irregular heart action or irregular pulse. 163
  c. catheterization, passage of a small plastic tube into the heart through a blood vessel for the purpose of diagnosis of heart disorders. 161
  c. muscle, special striated muscle of the myocardium. 152
  c. pacemaker, an electrical device that can substitute for a defective sinoatrial node and control the beating of the heart by a series of electrical discharges. 163
  c. region, the portion of the stomach that is immediately adjacent to and surrounding the esophageal orifice. 260
  c. sphincter, a plain muscle about the esophagus at the cardiac opening into the stomach. 235
cardiologist (kahr″de-ol′ə-jist) a physician who is specially trained in the prevention, diagnosis, and treatment of heart disease. 19
cardiology (kahr″de-ol′ə-je) the study of the heart and its functions. 19
cardiomegaly (kahr″de-o-meg′ə-le) enlargement of the heart. 40, 164
cardiomyopathy (kahr″de-o-mi-op′ə-the) a general diagnostic term designating primary disease of the heart muscle itself. 165
cardioplegia (kahr″de-o-ple′jə) arrest of myocardial contraction, as may be induced in performance of surgery on the heart. 170
cardioplegic (kahr″de-o-plej′ik) pertaining to arrest of myocardial contraction. 170
  c. solutions, drugs that are used to stop myocardial contractions so that surgery can be performed on the heart. 170
cardiopulmonary (kahr″de-o-pool′mə-nar-e) pertaining to the heart and lungs. 169
  c. resuscitation, the re-establishing of heart and lung action as indicated for cardiac arrest or apparent sudden death. 169

chondropathy (kon-drop′ə-the) any disease of the cartilage. 399

chondroplasty (kon′dro-plas″te) surgical repair of the cartilage. 412

chondrosarcoma (kon″dro-sahr-ko′mə) a malignant tumor derived from cartilage cells or their precursors. 402

chorion (kor′e-on) the outermost fetal membrane, which forms the fetal part of the placenta. 350

chorionic (kor″e-on′ik) pertaining to the chorion. 320

  c. gonadotropin, a gonad-stimulating hormone produced by the chorionic villi of the placenta. 320, 356, 496

  c. villi, the tiny vascular fibrils on the surface of the chorion that infiltrate the maternal endometrium and help form the placenta. 357

  c. villi sampling, the sampling of placental tissues for prenatal diagnosis of potential genetic defects. 357

chromosome (kro′mo-sōm) a structure in the nucleus of animal cells that contains DNA, which transmits genetic information. 81

chronic (kron′ik) showing little change or slow progression over a long period. 24

  c. obstructive pulmonary disease (COPD), any disorder marked by persistent obstruction of bronchial air flow; same as chronic obstructive lung disease (COLD). 209

chyme (kīm) the semifluid, homogeneous material produced by gastric digestion of food. 230

circumcision (sər″kəm-sizh′ən) surgical removal of all or part of the foreskin. 339

circumduction (sər″kəm-duk′shən) the active or passive circular movement of a limb or the eye. 393

cirrhosis (sĭ-ro′sis) a chronic liver disease characterized by marked degeneration of liver cells with eventual increased resistance to flow of blood through the liver. 257

cisterna chyli (sis-tər′nə ki′li) a dilated portion of the thoracic duct that receives lymph from several lymph-collecting vessels. 173

claustrophobia (klaws″tro-fo′be-ə) morbid fear of closed places. 451

clavicle (klav′ĭ-kəl) the collarbone; an elongated curved bone, connecting the breastbone to a scapula. 381

cleft lip (kleft) a congenital anomaly consisting of one or more fissures in the upper lip. 249

cleft palate (kleft pal′ət) a congenital defect characterized by a fissure in the palate. 249

climacteric (kli-mak′tər-ik) the syndrome of endocrine, somatic, and psychic changes that occur at the termination of the reproductive period in the female sex; menopause. 316

clitoris (klit″o-ris, kli′tə-ris, klĭ-tor′is) a small erectile body in the female homologous to the male penis. 313

Clostridium (klos-trid′e-əm) a genus of bacteria, containing obligate anerobic, gram-positive, rod-shaped bacilli. 129, 444

coagulant (ko-ag′u-lənt) promoting, accelerating, or making possible the coagulation of blood; an agent that promotes or accelerates the coagulation of blood. 114

coagulate (ko-ag′u-lāt) to become clotted or to cause clotting. 114

coagulation (ko-ag″u-la′shən) formation of a clot. 113

coagulopathy (ko-ag″u-lop′ə-the) any disorder of blood coagulation. 114

cocci (kok′si) spherical bacteria; plural of coccus. 127

coccygeal (kok-sij′e-əl) pertaining to or located in the region of the coccyx. 379

coccygectomy (kok″sĭ-jek′tə-me) excision of the coccyx. 411

coccyx (kok′siks) the tailbone, the small bone that forms the caudal extremity of the vertebral column. 379

cochlea (kok′le-ə) anything of a spiral form; a spirally wound tube, resembling a snail shell, which forms part of the inner ear. 448

coitus (ko′ĭ-tus) sexual connection per vagina between male and female. 332

  c. interruptus, withdrawal of the penis from the vagina before ejaculation. 362t

colectomy (ko-lek′tə-me) removal of part of the large intestine. 37, 262

colic (kol′ik) painful spasm of a hollow or tubular soft organ; pertaining to the large intestine. 231

colitis (ko-li′tis) inflammation of the large intestine. 252

collagen injection (kol′ə-jen) a reconstructive technique in cosmetic surgery to enhance the lips or plump sunken facial skin. 482

colon (ko′lən) the part of the large intestine extending from the cecum to the rectum. 238

  ascending c., the portion of the colon that rises on the right side of the abdomen from the cecum to the transverse colon. 239, 239f

  descending c., the portion of the colon on the left side of the abdomen that extends from the transverse colon to the sigmoid colon. 239, 239f

  sigmoid c., the S-shaped part of the colon. 239, 239f

  spastic c., irritable bowel syndrome. 254

  transverse c., the part of the colon that runs transversely across the upper part of the abdomen. 239

colonic (ko-lon′ik) pertaining to the colon. 231

  c. irrigation, a procedure for washing the inner wall of the colon. 260

  c. polyp, a growth of epithelium tissue protruding from the wall of the colon. 254

  c. stasis (sta′sis), failure of food to be moved along the intestinal tract. 254

colonoscope (ko-lon′o-skōp) a flexible endoscope that permits visual examination of the colon; colonoscope. 37, 244

colonoscopy (ko″lən-os′kə-pe) examination by means of the colonoscope. 37, 244

colopexy (ko′lo-pek″se) surgical fixation or suspension of the colon. 37

colorectal (ko″lo-rek′təl) pertaining to or affecting the colon and rectum. 239

colorrhaphy (ko-lor′ə-fe) suture of the colon. 37, 260

coloscope (kol′o-skōp) colonoscope. 37

coloscopy (ko-los′ko-pe) examination of the colon by means of an elongated flexible endoscope; same as colonoscopy. 37, 244

colostomy (kə-los′tə-me) surgical formation of a new opening from the large intestine to the surface of the body. 262

colostrum (kə-los′trəm) the thin, milky fluid secreted by the mammary gland the first few days before or after birth. 497

colpectomy (kol-pek′tə-me) excision of the vagina. 328

colpitis (kol-pi′tis) inflammation of the vagina; vaginitis. 322

colpocervical (kol″po-sər′vĭ-kəl) pertaining to the vagina and cervix. 314

colpocystitis (kol″po-sis-ti′tis) inflammation of the vagina and of the bladder. 313

colpodynia (kol″po-din′e-ə) vaginal pain. 326

colpohysterectomy (kol″po-his″tər-ek′tə-me) surgical removal of the uterus by way of the vagina. 329

colpoplasty (kol′po-plas″te) plastic surgery of the vagina. 328

colporrhagia (kol″po-ra′jə) vaginal hemorrhage. 326

colporrhaphy (kol-por′ə-fe) suture of the vagina. 328

colposcope (kol′po-skōp) an instrument for examining the vagina and cervix. 320

colposcopy (kol-pos′kə-pe) examination of the vagina and cervix using a colposcope. 320

coma (ko′mə) a profound unconsciousness from which the patient cannot be aroused. 439

comminuted (kom′ĭ-nōōt′əd) broken or crushed into small pieces. 397

  c. fracture, a broken bone in which the bone is splintered or crushed. 397

complement (kom′plə-mənt) proteins in the blood that play a vital role in the body's immune defenses. 133, 133f

compound fracture (kom′pound frak′chər) a break in a bone in which there is an external wound leading to the break; an open fracture. 397

computed tomography (kom-pūt′əd to-mog′rə-fe) a special noninvasive roentgenographic technique that involves reconstruction of the body in cross section from x-ray transmission measurements through the patient. Also called computerized axial tomography, CT, CAT. 394, 436

  c. axial t., same as computed tomography. 394, 436

conception (kən-sep′shən) the onset of pregnancy, marked by implantation of the blastocyst in the endometrium. 361

concussion (kən-kush′ən) an injury resulting from impact with an object; loss of function associated with a blow or fall. 439

  cerebral c., loss of consciousness caused by a blow to the head. 439

condom (kon′dəm) a cover for the penis, worn during coitus to prevent impregnation or infection. 362t

condyloma acuminatum (kon″də-lo′mə ə-ku′mĭ-nat′um) a papilloma usually occurring on the mucous membrane or skin of the external genitals or in the perianal region, caused by an infectious virus; venereal wart. 366

congenital (kən-jen′ĭ-təl) present at or existing from the time of birth. 58, 82

  c. heart disease, any structural or functional abnormality or defect of the heart or great vessels present at birth. 163

congestive (kən-jes′tiv) pertaining to or associated with abnormal accumulation of blood or fluid in a part. 164

  c. heart failure, a condition characterized by weakness, breathlessness, and edema in lower portions of the body resulting from venous stasis and reduced outflow of blood. 164

conjunctiva (kən-jənk′ti-və) the thin membrane lining the eyelids and covering the exposed whites of the eyes. 432

conjunctivitis (kən-junk″tĭ-vi′tis) inflammation of the conjunctiva, the membrane that lines the eyelids and covers the exposed surface of the sclera. 446

constipation (kon″stĭ-pa′shən) infrequent or difficult evacuation of the feces. 254

continence (kon′tĭ-nəns) self-restraint, used especially in reference to the ability to control urination and defecation, or to refraining from sexual indulgence. 292

contraception (kon″trə-sep′shən) prevention of conception or impregnation. 361

contraceptive (kon″trə-sep′tiv) anything used to diminish likelihood of or to prevent impregnation. 74, 328

  oral c., a hormonal compound taken orally that blocks ovulation. 361

contraindication (kon″trə-in″dĭ-ka′shən) any condition that renders some particular line of treatment improper or undesirable. 454

contralateral (kon″trə-lat′ər-əl) associated with a particular part on an opposite side. 72

contusion (kən-too′zhən) a bruise; an injury of a part without a break in the skin. 439, 478

convulsion (kən-vul′shən) a violent involuntary contraction or series of contractions of the involuntary muscles; seizure. 445

copulation (kop″u-la′shən) sexual union between male and female; coitus. 332

corium (kor′e-əm) alternative for dermis. 466

cornea (kor′ne-ə) the transparent structure forming the anterior part of the fibrous tunic of the eye. 454

corneal (kor′ne-əl) pertaining to the cornea. 454

coronal (kor′ə-nəl) pertaining to the crown of the head or to any corona. 84

  c. plane, the frontal plane that divides the body into front and back portions. 84

coronary (kor′ə-nar″e) encircling in the manner of a crown. This term is applied to vessels and ligaments, but especially to the heart's arteries. 152

  c. arteriography, radiographic examination of the coronary arteries. 161

  c. artery bypass, open heart surgery in which a prosthesis or a section of a blood vessel is grafted onto one of the coronary arteries. 170

  c. artery bypass graft, a section of vein or other conduit grafted between the aorta and a coronary artery distal to an obstruction. 170, 171f

  c. artery disease (CAD), myocardial damage caused by insufficient blood supply; also called coronary heart disease (CHD). 166

  c. occlusion, complete obstruction of an artery of the heart, usually from progressive atherosclerosis. 167

  c. stent, a rodlike device used to maintain patency of a coronary artery. 171

  c. thrombosis, development of an obstructive thrombus in a coronary artery. 167

coronavirus (kə-ro′nə-vi″rəs) any virus belonging to the family Coronaviridae, which causes respiratory disease and possibly gastroenteritis in humans. 205

corpus luteum (kor′pəs loo-te′um) a yellow mass in the ovary formed by an ovarian follicle that has matured and discharged its ovum. 316

corpuscle (kor′pəs-əl) any small mass or body. 114

cortex (kor'teks) the outer layer of an organ. 498

    adrenal c., the outer portion of the adrenal, which makes up the bulk of the gland. 492, 498, 499t

    cerebral c., the convoluted layer of gray matter covering each cerebral hemisphere. 498

cortisone (kor'tĭ-sōn) a natural glucocorticoid secreted by the adrenal cortex. 498

coryza (ko-ri'zə) an acute condition of the nasal mucous membrane, with a profuse discharge from the nostrils. 203

costa (kos'tə) rib. 380

costal (kos'təl) pertaining to the ribs. 380

costectomy (kos-tek'tə-me) removal of a rib. 411

costoclavicular (kos″to-klə-vik'u-lər) pertaining to the ribs and collarbone. 382

costovertebral (kos″to-vər'tə-brəl) pertaining to the ribs and vertebrae. 380

Coumadin (koo'mə-din) trademark for preparations of warfarin sodium. 535

COX-2 inhibitors (koks) a group of nonsteroidal antiinflammatory drugs (NSAIDs) that have fewer gastrointestinal side effects than other NSAIDs. 412

crackle (krak'əl) an abnormal nonmusical sound heard on auscultation, primarily during inhalation. 198

cranial (kra'ne-əl) pertaining to the cranium or skull. 377

    c. cavity, the space within the skull that contains the brain. 92

craniectomy (kra″ne-ek'tə-me) excision of a segment of the skull. 411, 453

craniocele (kra'ne-o-sēl″) protrusion of the brain through a defect in the skull. 404

craniocerebral (kra″ne-o-ser'ə-brəl) pertaining to the cranium and the cerebrum. 428

cranioplasty (kra'ne-o-plas″te) plastic surgery of the skull. 410, 453

craniotome (kra'ne-o-tōm″) an instrument used in craniotomy. 411

craniotomy (kra″ne-ot'ə-me) cutting into the skull. 411, 453

cranium (kra'ne-əm) the skull; the skeleton of the head. 427

creatine kinase test (kre'ə-tin ki'nās) a blood test used to detect damage to the cardiac muscle. Also called creatine phosphokinase. 160

creatinine (kre-at'ĭ-nin) a substance formed from the metabolism of creatine. 283

    c. clearance, the rate at which creatinine is cleared from the blood by the kidneys. 285

cretinism (kre'tin-iz-əm) a condition caused by congenital lack of thyroid secretion, marked by arrested physical and mental development. 507

Crohn's disease (krōnz dĭ-zēz') a chronic inflammatory disease involving any part of the gastrointestinal tract from mouth to anus, but commonly involving the terminal ileum with scarring and thickening of the bowel wall. 252

croup (kroōp) a condition resulting from acute obstruction of the upper airway caused by allergy, foreign body, infection, or new growth, occurring chiefly in infants and children, and characterized by resonant barking cough and hoarseness. 204

cryosurgery (kri″o-sər'jər-e) destruction of tissue by application of extreme cold. 329

cryotherapy (kri″o-ther'ə-pe) treatment of tissue using cold temperatures. 329, 482

cryptorchidism (krip-tor'kĭ-diz″əm) a developmental defect in which the testes remain in the abdominal cavity; undescended testes. 336

curet (ku-ret') a spoon-shaped instrument for removing material from a surface. 469

curettage (ku″rə-tahzh') scraping of a cavity for removal of a growth or other material; curettement. 469

    dilation and c., surgical scraping of the uterus with a curette to remove contents of uterus after incomplete abortion, to obtain specimens for diagnosis, or to remove polyps. 329

Cushing's syndrome (koosh'ingz sin'drōm) a group of signs and symptoms associated with hypersecretion of the glucocorticoids by the adrenal cortex. 508

cuspid (kus'pid) having one point; a canine tooth. 234

    c. valve, a flap of tissue that controls the blood flow between an atrium and ventricle of the heart. 154

cutaneous (ku-ta'ne-əs) pertaining to the skin. 466

cyanosis (si″ə-no'sis) blueness of the skin and mucous membranes. 58, 163, 470

cyst (sist) any sac that contains a fluid, either normal or abnormal, and is lined by epithelium. 473

cystectomy (sis-tek'tə-me) excision of a cyst; excision or resection of the urinary bladder. 298

cystic (sis'tik) pertaining to a cyst; pertaining to the urinary bladder or to the gallbladder. 278

cystic fibrosis (sis'tik fi-bro'sis) an inherited disease of exocrine glands that affects the pancreas, the respiratory system, and the sweat glands. 210, 469

cystitis (sis-ti'tis) inflammation of the bladder. 293

cystocele (sis'to-sēl) herniation of the urinary bladder into the vagina. 296, 326

cystogram (sis'to-gram) the record produced after the bladder has been rendered opaque in cystography. 288

cystography (sis-tog'rə-fe) roentgenography of the bladder after injection of the organ with an opaque solution. 288

cystolith (sis'to-lith) a calculus within the bladder. 296

cystolithectomy, cystolithotomy (sis″to-lĭ-thek'tə-me, sis″to-lĭ-thot'ə-me) the removal of a calculus by incision of the bladder. 300

cystometrography (sis″to-mə-trog'rə-fe) the graphic recording of the pressure exerted at varying degrees of filling of the urinary bladder. 286

cystoplasty (sis'to-plas″te) plastic surgery of the bladder. 300

cystoscope (sis'to-skōp″) an instrument used for visual examination of the bladder. 289

cystoscopy (sis-tos'kə-pe) visual examination of the urinary tract with an instrument inserted through the urethra. 289

cystostomy (sis-tos'tə-me) formation of an opening into the urinary bladder. 301

cystotomy (sis-tot'ə-me) incision of the bladder. 301

cystoureteroscopy (sis″to-u-re″tər-os'kə-pe) visual examination of the urinary bladder and ureters using a cystoscope. 289

cystourethritis (sis″to-u″re-thri'tis) inflammation of the bladder and urethra. 293

cystourethrogram (sis″to-u-re'thro-gram) a radiograph of the urinary bladder and urethra. 288

cystourethrography (sis″to-u″rə-throg'rə-fe) x-ray examination of the urinary bladder and the urethra. 288

cystourethroscopy (sis″to-u″re-thros'kə-pe) examination of the urethra and bladder with a cystourethroscope. 289

cytology (si-tol'ə-je) study of cells. 318

cytotoxic (si″to-tok″sik) pertaining to or exhibiting a deleterious effect on cells. 136

cytotoxicity (si″to-tok-sis'ĭ-te) having a deleterious effect on cells. 136

cytotoxin (si″to-tok″sin) a toxin or antibody that has specific toxic action on cells of special organs. 136

dacryocyst (dak're-o-sist″) the lacrimal sac; tear sac. 433

dacryocystitis (dak″re-o-sis-ti'tis) inflammation of the lacrimal sac. 448

dacryocystography (dak″re-o-sis-tog'rə-fe) x-ray examination of the tear sac. 436

dacryocystorhinostomy (dak″re-o-sis″to-ri-nos'tə-me) surgical creation of a communication between the nasal cavity and the lacrimal sac. 454

dacryocystotomy (dak″re-o-sis-tot'ə-me) incision of the lacrimal sac. 454

dacryolith (dak're-o-lith″) a stone in the lacrimal sac or duct. 448

dacryolithiasis (dak″re-o-lĭ-thi'ə-sis) formation of tear stones. 448

dacryosinusitis (dak″re-o-si″nəs-i'tis) inflammation of the lacrimal duct and the ethmoidal sinus. 448

dactylitis (dak″tə-li'tis) inflammation of a finger or toe. 94

dactylogram (dak-til'o-gram) a fingerprint taken for purposes of identification. 94

dactylography (dak″tə-log'rə-fe) the study of fingerprints. 94

dactylospasm (dak'tə-lo-spaz-əm) cramping or twitching of the fingers or toes. 94

débride (da-brēd') to remove foreign material and contaminated or devitalized tissue by sharp dissection. 482

débridement (da-brēd-maw') the removal of foreign material and necrotized or contaminated tissue from or adjacent to an infected or traumatic lesion until surrounding healthy tissue is exposed. 482

decalcification (de-kal″sĭ-fĭ-ka'shən) the loss of calcium from bone. 402

decongestant (de″kən-jes'tənt) tending to reduce congestion or swelling; an agent that reduces congestion or swelling. 217

defecation (def″ə-ka'shən) the evacuation of fecal material from the rectum. 239

defibrillation (de-fib″rĭ-la'shən) termination of fibrillation, usually by electroshock. 164

defibrillator (de-fib″rĭ-la'tər) an apparatus used to stop fibrillation by application of brief electroshock to the heart, directly or through electrodes placed on the chest wall. 164

degenerative joint disease (de-jen'ər-ə-tiv joint dĭ-zēz') a chronic disease involving the joints, especially those bearing weight, characterized by destruction of articular cartilage, overgrowth of bone with lipping and spur formation, and impaired function; osteoarthritis. 406

dehydration (de″hi-dra'shən) removal of water from a substance; the condition that results from excessive loss of body water. 252

dementia (də-men'shə) loss of intellectual function caused by organic brain disease. 445, 446

dendrite (den'drīt) one of the threadlike extensions of a neuron's cytoplasm. 425

dental (den'təl) pertaining to the teeth. 233

    d. caries, tooth decay. 242

dentalgia (den-tal'jə) toothache. 248

dentilingual (den″tĭ-ling'wəl) pertaining to the teeth and tongue. 233

dentist (den'tist) a person who has received a degree in dentistry and is authorized to practice dentistry. 27, 234

dentistry (den'tis-tre) the branch of the healing arts concerned with the teeth, oral cavity, and associated structures, including prevention, diagnosis, and treatment of disease and restoration of defective or missing tissue; the creation of restorations, crowns, and bridges; surgical procedures performed in and about the oral cavity; the practice of the dental profession collectively. 27, 234

denture (den'chər) a complement of teeth, either natural or artificial; ordinarily used to designate artificial replacement for the natural teeth. 233

depression (de-presh'ən) a hollow or depressed area; downward or inward displacement; a lowering or decrease of functional activity; a mental state of depressed mood characterized by feelings of sadness, despair, and discouragement. 438

dermabrasion (dər″mə-bra'zhən) a surgical procedure that uses an abrasive disk or other mechanical method to plane the skin. 482

dermal (dər'məl) pertaining to the skin. 18

dermatitis (der″mə-ti'tis) inflammation of the skin. 53, 94, 471

    contact d., acute or chronic dermatitis caused by materials or substances coming in contact with the skin. 471

dermatologic, dermatological (dər″mə-to-loj'ik, dər″mə-to-loj'ĭ-kəl) pertaining to dermatology; of or affecting the skin. 18

dermatologist (dər″mə-tol'o-jist) a specialist in skin diseases. 18, 466

dermatology (dər″mə-tol'o-je) the study of the skin and skin diseases. 18, 466

dermatome (dər-mə-tōm″) an instrument for cutting thin skin slices for skin grafts; the area of skin supplied with afferent nerve fibers by a single posterior spinal root. 481

dermatomycosis (dər″mə-to-mi-ko'sis) a superficial infection of the skin or its appendages by fungi. 472

dermatoplasty (dər″mə-to-plas″te) plastic surgery of the skin; operative replacement of destroyed or lost skin. 94

dermatosis (dər″mə-to'sis) any skin condition not characterized by inflammation. 94

dermis (dər'mis) the layer of skin that lies under the epidermis. 72, 465

diabetes insipidus (di″ə-be'tēz in-sip'ĭ-dəs) a metabolic disease characterized by polyuria and polydipsia. It is caused by inadequate secretion or release of antidiuretic hormone (ADH), or inability of the kidney tubules to respond to ADH. 291, 505

echoencephalograph (ek″o-en-sef″ə-lo-graf″) the instrument used in echoencephalography. 435

echoencephalography (ek″o-en-sef″ə-log′rə-fe) a diagnostic technique in which ultrasonic waves are beamed through the head from both sides, and echoes are recorded as graphic tracings. 436

echography (ə-kog′rə-fe) a diagnostic aid in which ultrasonic waves are directed at the tissues. A record is made of the sound waves reflected back through the tissues to differentiate structures. 160

    Doppler e., a technique in which ultrasonography is used to evaluate the direction and pattern of blood flow within the heart. 160

eclampsia (ə-klamp′se-ə) convulsions occurring in a pregnant woman with hypertension, proteinuria, and/or edema. 358

ectoderm (ek′to-dərm) in embryology, the outermost layer of cells in the blastoderm. 466

ectopic (ek-top′ik) out of the usual place. 324, 357

    e. pregnancy, the implantation of a fertilized egg in any place other than the uterus. 324, 357

eczema (ek′zə-mə) a dermatitis occurring as a reaction to many endogenous and exogenous agents, characterized in the acute stage by erythema, edema associated with a serous exudate oozing and vesiculation, and crusting and scaling. 471

edema (ə-de′mə) an abnormal accumulation of fluid in intercellular spaces in the tissues. 40, 111, 164

    pulmonary e., abnormal diffuse, extravascular accumulation of fluid in the pulmonary tissues. 197, 208

effacement (ə-fās′mənt) the taking up or obliteration of the cervix in labor when it is so changed that only the thin external os remains. 354

efferent (ef′ər-ənt) conveying away from a center. 424

effusion (ə-fu′zhən) the escape of fluid into a part or tissue; an effused material. 165

    pleural e., presence of liquid in the pleural space. 207, 208f

ejaculation (e-jak″u-la′shən) a sudden act of expulsion, as of the semen. 331

ejaculatory (e-jak′u-lə-to″re) pertaining to ejaculation. 331

electrocardiogram (e-lek″tro-kahr′de-o-gram″) a tracing produced by the electrical impulses of the heart. 41, 60, 160

electrocardiograph (e-lek″tro-kahr′de-o-graf″) an instrument used to record the electrical current produced by the heart contractions. 41, 160

electrocardiography (e-lek″tro-kahr″de-og′rə-fe) recording the electrical currents of the heart muscle. 41, 41f, 160

electrodesiccation (e-lek″tro-des″ĭ-ka′shən) dehydration of tissue by the use of a high-frequency electric current. 482

electroencephalogram (e-lek″tro-en-sef′ə-lo-gram″) a record produced by the electrical impulses of the brain. 97, 435

electroencephalograph (e-lek″tro-ən-sef′ə-lo-graf″) a machine used to record the electrical impulses of the brain. 97, 435

electroencephalography (e-lek″tro-ən-sef″ə-log′rə-fe) the recording of the electrical currents of the brain by means of electrodes applied to the scalp, to the surface of the brain, or placed within the substance of the brain. 97, 435

electrolysis (e″lek-trol′ə-sis) destruction by passage of a galvanic electrical current, as in removal of excessive hair from the body. 483

electrolyte (e-lek′tro-līt) a substance that dissociates into ions when fused or in solution, and thus becomes capable of conducting electricity. 112

electromyogram (e-lek″tro-mi′o-gram) the record obtained by electromyography. 393

electromyography (e-lek″tro-mi-og′rə-fe) the recording and study of the intrinsic electrical properties of skeletal muscle. 287, 393

electrophoresis (e-lek″tro-fə-re′sis) the separation of ionic solutes in a liquid under the influence of an applied electric field. 123

electrophysiologic studies (e-lek″tro-fis″ĭ-o-loj′ik stud′ēz) evaluations of the mechanisms of production of electrical phenomena and the use of electrode catheters to study the effects of electricity on tissue, such as study of the heart rhythm. 161

elephantiasis (el″ə-fən-ti′ə-sis) a disease caused by a parasitic infestation and characterized by inflammation and obstruction of the lymphatics and increased size of nearby tissue. 40, 40f, 176

elimination (e-lim″ĭ-na′shən) the act of expulsion or of extrusion, especially of expulsion from the body; omission or exclusion, as in an elimination diet. 227

emaciation (e-ma″she-a′shən) excessive leanness; a wasted condition of the body. 246

embolectomy (em″bə-lek′tə-me) surgical removal of an embolus from a blood vessel where it has lodged. 172

embolism (em′bə-liz-əm) the sudden blocking of a vessel by a clot or foreign material brought to its site of lodgment by the bloodstream. 167, 209

embolus (em′bo-ləs) a clot or other plug brought by the bloodstream and forced into a smaller vessel where it lodges, thus obstructing circulation. 167, 209

embryo (em′bre-o) derivatives of the fertilized ovum that eventually become the offspring. 351, 351f

emesis (em′ə-sis) vomiting; an act of vomiting. 40, 246

emphysema (em″fə-se′mə) an accumulation of air in tissues or organs; pulmonary disease characterized by destruction of many of the alveolar walls. 210

empyema (em″pi-e′mə) accumulation of pus in a cavity of the body. If used without a descriptive qualifier, it refers to thoracic empyema. 207

enamel (ə-nam′əl) the hard substance covering the dentin of the crown of a tooth. 234

encephalitis (en-sef″ə-li′tis) inflammation of the brain. 97, 443

encephalocele (en-sef′ə-lo-sēl″) hernia of part of the brain and meninges through a skull defect. 53, 404

encephalography (en-sef″ə-log′rə-fe) radiography of the brain. 436

encephalomeningitis (en-sef″ə-lo-men″in-ji′tis) inflammation of the brain and its membranes. 443

encephalomyelopathy (en-sef″ə-lo-mi″əl-op′ə-the) a disease involving the brain and spinal cord. 440

encephalopathy (en-sef″ə-lop′ə-the) any disease of the brain. 97

encephalotome (en-sef′ə-lə-tōm) an instrument for incision of the brain. 38

encephalotomy (en-sef″ə-lot′ə-me) incision of the brain. 38

endarterectomy (end-ahr″tər-ek′tə-me) excision of the atheromatous tunica intima of an artery. 170

    carotid e., surgical excision of atheromatous segments of the inner walls of a carotid artery. 171

endocardial (en″do-kahr′de-əl) pertaining to the endocardium; situated or occurring within the heart. 153

endocarditis (en″do-kahr-di′tis) inflammation of the inner lining of the heart. 165

endocardium (en″do-kahr′de-um) the membrane lining the inner surface of the heart. 153

endocrine (en′do-krīn, en′do-krin) secreting internally; applied to organs that secrete hormones into the bloodstream. 19, 492

endocrinologist (en″do-krĭ-nol′ə-jist) a physician who treats diseases arising from disordered internal secretions. 19

endocrinology (en″do-krĭ-nol′ə-je) the science that studies the endocrine glands and the hormones they produce. 19

endoderm (en′do-dərm) the innermost of the three primary germ layers of the embryo. 466

endodontics (en″do-don′tiks) the branch of dentistry concerned with the cause, prevention, diagnosis, and treatment of conditions that affect the tooth pulp, root, and periapical tissues. 235

endodontist (en″do-don′tist) a dentist who specializes in prevention and treatment of conditions that affect the tooth pulp, root, and periapical tissues. 235

endodontitis (en″do-don-ti′tis) inflammation of the dental pulp. 248

endodontium (en″do-don′she-əm) dental pulp. 234

endogastric (en″do-gas′trik) pertaining to the interior of the stomach. 237

endogenous (en-doj′ə-nəs) produced within or caused by factors within an organism. 246

endometrial (en″do-me′tre-əl) pertaining to the endometrium. 314

    e. biopsy, a microscopic examination of a sample of endometrial tissue. 320

endometriosis (en″do-me″tre-o′sis) ectopic endometrium located in various places, usually in the pelvic cavity. 326

endometritis (en″do-me-tri′tis) inflammation of the lining of the uterus. 326

endometrium (en″do-me′tre-əm) the membrane that lines the cavity of the uterus. 314

endonasal (en″do-na′zəl) within the nose. 192

endorphin (en-dor′fin, en′dor-fin) any of three amino acid residues that bind to opioid receptors in the brain and have potent analgesic activity. 426

endoscope (en′do-skōp) an instrument for the examination of the interior of a hollow viscus. 243

endoscopic sphincterotomy (en″do-skop′ik sfingk″tər-ot′ə-me) incision of a constricting sphincter through an endoscope. 265

endoscopy (en-dos′kə-pe) visual inspection of any cavity of the body by means of an endoscope. 243, 282

endothelium (en″do-the′le-əm) the layer of epithelial cells that lines the cavities of the heart, blood and lymph vessels, and the serous cavities of the body. 156

endotracheal (en″do-tra′ke-əl) within the trachea. 193

    e. intubation, a procedure in which a tube is placed through the nose or mouth into the trachea to establish an airway. 213

enema (en′ə-mə) a liquid that is injected or is to be injected into the rectum. 260

enteral, enteric (en′tər-əl, en-ter′ik) pertaining to the small intestine. 231

enteral feeding (en′tər-əl) the introduction of nutrients directly into the gastrointestinal tract by feeding tube; enteral tube feeding. 259

enteritis (en″tər-i′tis) inflammation of the intestine, especially the small intestine. 231

enterostasis (en″tər-o-sta′sis) the stopping of food in its passage through the intestine. 254

enuresis (en″u-re′sis) involuntary discharge of urine after the age at which urinary control should have been achieved; often used with specific reference to involuntary discharge of urine occurring during sleep at night (bed-wetting). 292

enzyme (en′zīm) a protein molecule that catalyzes chemical reactions of other substances without itself being destroyed or altered. 109

eosinophil (e″o-sin′o-fil) a granular leukocyte with a nucleus that usually has two lobes and cytoplasm containing coarse, round granules that are readily stained by eosin. 116f

epicardium (ep″ĭ-kahr′de-um) the layer of serous pericardium on the surface of the heart. 153

epidemic (ep″ĭ-dem′ik) occurring suddenly in numbers clearly in excess of normal expectancy. 24

epidemiologist (ep″ĭ-de″me-ol′o-jist) a specialist in epidemiology. 24

epidemiology (ep″ĭ-de″me-ol′o-je) the study of the relationships of factors determining the frequency and distribution of diseases in the human community; the field of medicine dealing with the determination of causes of localized outbreaks of infection or other disease of recognized cause. 24

epidermal (ep″ĭ-dər′məl) pertaining to or resembling epidermis. 468

epidermis (ep″ĭ-dər′mis) the outermost, nonvascular layer in the skin. 465

epididymis (ep″ĭ-did′ə-mis) the elongated cordlike structure along the posterior border of the testis that provides for storage, transit, and maturation of spermatozoa and is continuous with the ductus deferens. 331

epididymitis (ep″ĭ-did″ə-mi′tis) inflammation of the epididymis. 337

epidural (ep″ĭ-doo′rəl) situated on or outside of the dura mater. 440

epigastric (ep″ĭ-gas′trik) pertaining to the epigastrium, or upper middle region of the abdomen. 91

epiglottiditis, epiglottitis (ep″ĭ-glot″ĭ-di′tis, ep″ĭ-glŏ-ti′tis) inflammation of the epiglottis. 193, 204

sweat g., a gland in the skin that is responsible for production of sweat. 467, 467f

thyroid g., a two-lobed gland in the front of the neck that produces hormones necessary for normal growth and metabolism. 492

glans penis (glanz pe′nis) the cap-shaped expansion at the end of the penis. 332

glaucoma (glaw-, glou-ko′mə) a group of eye diseases characterized by an increase in intraocular pressure, which causes pathologic changes in the optic disk and typical defects in the field of vision. 447

glia cell (gli′ə) one of the cells that makes up the supporting nerve of nervous tissue. 424

glioma (gli-o′mə) a tumor composed of tissue that represents neuroglia. The term is sometimes extended to include all the primary intrinsic neoplasms of the brain and spinal cord. 444

glomerular filtration rate (glo-mer′u-lər) a kidney function test that can be determined from the amount of filtrate formed by the glomeruli of the kidney. 281

glomeruli (glo-mer′u-li) plural of glomerulus. 279

glomerulonephritis (glo-mer″u-lo-nə-fri′tis) a type of nephritis in which there is inflammation of the glomeruli. 294

glomerulopathy (glo-mer″u-lop′ə-the) any disease of the renal glomeruli. 294

glomerulus (glo-mer′u-ləs) a small cluster, as of blood vessels or nerve fibers; often used alone to designate one of the renal glomeruli, which act as filters. 279

glossal (glos′əl) pertaining to the tongue. 233

glossectomy (glos-ek′tə-me) surgical removal of the tongue. 261

glossitis (glos-i′tis) inflammation of the tongue. 248

glossopathy (glos-op′ə-the) any disease of the tongue. 248

glossopharyngeal (glos″o-fə-rin′je-əl) pertaining to the tongue and the pharynx. 233

glossoplasty (glos′o-plas″te) plastic surgery of the tongue. 261

glossoplegia (glos′o-ple′je-ə) paralysis of the tongue. 248

glossopyrosis (glos″o-pi-ro′sis) pain, burning, itching, and stinging of the mucous membranes of the tongue without apparent lesions of the affected areas. 248

glossorrhaphy (glos-or′ə-fe) suture of the tongue. 260

glottis (glot′is) the vocal apparatus of the larynx. 193

glucagon (gloo′kə-gon) hormone secreted by the alpha cells of the islets of Langerhans in response to hypoglycemia, acetylcholine, some amino acids, and growth hormone. 241, 500

glucocorticoid (gloo″ko-kor′tĭ-koid) any or group of steroids produced by the adrenal cortex. 498

glucose (gloo′kōs) a sugar found in certain foodstuffs, especially fruit, and normal blood; dextrose. 228

g. lowering agent, a drug that lowers the blood glucose. 511

glycosuria (gli″ko-su′re-ə) the presence of sugar in the urine. 283, 504

goiter (goi′tər) enlargement of the thyroid gland, causing a swelling in the front part of the neck. 502

gonad (go′nad) an organ that produces eggs or sperm; ovary or testis. 311, 349, 492, 496

gonadal (go-nad′al) pertaining to the ovaries or the testes. 498

gonadotropic (go″nə-do-trop′ik) capable of stimulating the ovaries or the testes. 496, 498

g. hormone, a general term that means a hormone that stimulates the gonads and includes follicle-stimulating hormone and luteinizing hormone. 496

gonadotropin (go′nə-do-tro″pin) a substance that stimulates the gonads, especially the hormone secreted by the pituitary gland that stimulates the ovaries or testes. 320, 356, 496

human chorionic g., a hormone present in the urine and many body fluids of pregnant female individuals that forms the basis of testing for pregnancy. 320, 356, 496

gonococcus (gon″o-kok′əs) an organism of the species *Neisseria gonorrhoeae,* the cause of gonorrhea. 363

gonorrhea (gon″o-re′ə) infection caused by *Neisseria gonorrhoeae* transmitted sexually in most cases, but also by contact with infected exudates in neonatal children at birth, or by infants in households with infected inhabitants. It is characterized by discharge and painful urination in male individuals and often is asymptomatic in female individuals. 297, 363

gout (gout) hereditary metabolic disease that is a form of acute arthritis and is marked by inflammation of the joints. Gout is characterized by hyperuricemia and deposits of urates in and around joints. Any joint may be affected, but gout usually begins in the knee or foot. 396, 407

graafian follicle (grah′fe-ən fol′ĭ-kəl) development of the primary oocyte in the ovary to the stage where the ovum is fully developed. 316

graft (graft) any tissue or organ for implantation or transplantation; to implant or transplant such tissues. 481

skin g., a part of skin implanted to cover areas where skin has been lost. 481

grafting (graft′ing) the implanting or transplanting of any organ or tissue. 481

Gram stain (gram stān) a special staining procedure in which microorganisms can be classified as gram-positive, gram-negative, or gram variable. 127, 319

granulocyte (gran′u-lo-sīt″) a leukocyte containing neutrophil, basophil, or eosinophil granules in its cytoplasm. 115

gravid (grav′id) pregnant. 351

gravida (grav′ĭ-də) a pregnant woman. 351

g. I, primigravida; during the first pregnancy. 352

guaiac test (gwi′ək) a test for detection of occult blood. 244

gynecologic (gi″nə-, jin″ə-kə-loj′ik) pertaining to female individuals, particularly to the female genitourinary system. 311

gynecologist (gi″nə-, jin″ə-kol′ə-jist) a physician who treats diseases of the female sex. 20

gynecology (gi″nə-, jin″ə-kol′ə-je) the branch of medicine that treats female diseases, especially those of the genital and urinary systems. 20, 311

gynecomastia (gi″nə-, jin″ə-ko-mas′te-ə) excessive development of the male mammary glands, sometimes even to the functional state. 508

halitosis (hal″ĭ-to′sis) offensive breath. 248

hallux valgus (hal′əks val′gəs) angulation of the great toe away from the midline of the body, or toward the other toes. 400

hammertoe (ham′ər to) a toe with dorsal flexion of the first phalanx and plantar flexion of the second and third phalanges. 400

haversian canals (ha-var′zhən kə-nalz′) the channels of compact bone that contain blood vessels, lymph vessels, and nerves. 373, 374f

headache (hed′āk) pain in the head. 438

cluster h., a headache similar to migraine, recurring as often as two or three times a day over a period of weeks; then there may be absence of symptoms for weeks or months. 439

migraine h., paroxysmal attacks of headache frequently unilateral, usually accompanied by disordered vision and gastrointestinal disturbances. 439

heart block (hahrt blok) impairment in conduction of an impulse in heart excitation. 164

Heimlich maneuver (hīm′lik) an emerging procedure for dislodging a bolus of food or other obstruction from the trachea to prevent asphyxiation. 212, 213f

heliotherapy (he″le-o-ther′ə-pe) treatment of disease by exposing the body to sunlight. 483

hemangioma (he-man″je-o′mə) an extremely common benign tumor, occurring most commonly in infancy and childhood, made up of newly formed blood vessels, and resulting from malformation of angioblastic tissue of fetal life. 167

hematemesis (he″mə-tem′ə-sis) vomiting of blood. 246

hematocrit (he-mat′ĭ-krit) a tube with graduated markings used to determine the volume of packed red cells in a blood specimen by centrifugation; by extension, the measurement obtained using this procedure or the corresponding measurements produced by automated blood cell counters. 115

hematologic (he″mə-to-loj′ik) pertaining to the blood and the blood-forming tissues. 113, 394

hematologist (he″mə-tol′ə-jist) a specialist in hematology. 113

hematology (he″mə-tol′ə-je) the study of blood and blood-forming tissues and their physiology and pathology. 113

hematoma (he″mə-to′mə) any localized collection of blood, usually clotted, in an organ, tissue, or space. 109, 440

epidural h., accumulation of blood in the epidural space. 440

intracerebral h., accumulation of blood in the brain tissue. 441

subdural h., accumulation of blood in the subdural space. 441

hematopoiesis (he″mə-to-, hem″ə-to-poi-e′sis) the formation and development of blood cells. 113

hematopoietic (he″mə-to-, hem″ə-to-poi-et′ik) pertaining to or affecting hematopoiesis. 117

hematuria (he″mə-, hem″ə-tu′re-ə) the presence of blood in the urine. 283

hemiplegia (hem″e-ple′jə) paralysis of one side of the body. 442

hemodialysis (he″mo-di-al′ə-sis) the process of diffusing blood through a semipermeable membrane for the purpose of removing toxic materials and maintaining acid–base balance in cases of impaired kidney function. 298

hemoglobin (he″mo-glo′bin) the oxygen-carrying red pigment of red blood cells. 56

glycosylated h., a hemoglobin A molecule in which the concentration represents the average blood glucose level over the previous several weeks. 504

h. A, normal adult hemoglobin, composed of two alpha and two beta chains. 123

hemoglobinopathy (he″mo-glo″bin-op′ə-the) a hematologic disorder caused by genetically determined abnormal hemoglobin. 121

hemolysin (he-mol′ə-sin) a substance that causes destruction of red blood cells. 56, 117

hemolysis (he-mol′ə-sis) destruction of red blood cells that results in the liberation of hemoglobin. 56, 117

hemolytic (he″mo-lit′ik) pertaining to, characterized by, or producing hemolysis. 56, 359

hemolyze (he′mo-līz) to subject to or to undergo hemolysis. 56

hemopericardium (he″mo-per″ĭ-kahr′de-əm) an effusion of blood within the pericardium. 165

hemophilia (he″mo-fil′e-ə) a hereditary hemorrhagic disorder caused by deficiency of antihemophilic factor VIII or IX. 118

hemoptysis (he-mop′tĭ-sis) the spitting of blood or blood-stained sputum. 211

hemorrhage (hem′ə-rəj) bleeding; the escape of blood from the vessels. 40

hemorrhoid (hem′ə-roid) a varicose dilation of a vein of the anal canal inside or just outside the rectum that causes pain, itching, and bleeding. 254

hemorrhoidectomy (hem″ə-roid-ek′tə-me) excision of hemorrhoids. 264

hemostasis (he″mo-sta′sis, he-mos′tə-sis) the checking of the flow of blood either by coagulation or surgical means; interruption of blood flow through any vessel or to any part of the body. 124

hemothorax (he″mo-thor′aks) a collection of blood in the chest cavity. 208, 209f

heparin (hep′ə-rin) a naturally occurring substance that acts in the body as an antithrombin factor to prevent intravascular clotting. Heparin sodium is used therapeutically as an anticoagulant. 124

hepatectomy (hep″ə-tek′tə-me) excision of part of the liver. 264

hepatic (hə-pat′ik) pertaining to the liver. 240

h. lobectomy, excision of a lobe of the liver. 264

hepatitis (hep″ə-ti′tis) inflammation of the liver. 256, 366

viral h., hepatitis caused by a viral infection, such as HAV, HBV, or HCV. 256, 257

hepatolytic (hep″ə-to-lit′ik) destructive to the liver; hepatotoxic. 240

hepatoma (hep″ə-to′mə) a tumor of the liver, especially hepatocellular carcinoma. 257

hepatomegaly (hep″ə-to-meg′ə-le) enlargement of the liver. 256

hepatopathy (hep″ə-top′ə-the) any disease of the liver. 257

hepatorenal syndrome (hep″ə-to-re′nəl sin′drōm) functional renal failure, without pathologic renal changes, associated with cirrhosis and ascites or with obstructive jaundice. 256

hepatosplenomegaly (hep″ə-to-sple″no-meg′ə-le) enlargement of the liver and spleen. 257

laryngotracheal (lə-ring″go-tra′ke-əl) pertaining to the larynx and the trachea. 207

laryngotracheitis (lə-ring″go-tra″ke-i′tis) inflammation of the larynx and the trachea. 207

laryngotracheobronchitis (lə-ring″go-tra″ke-o-brong-ki′tis) inflammation of the larynx, trachea, and bronchi. 206

larynx (lar′inks) the organ of voice; the air passage between the lower pharynx and the trachea. 191

lateral (lat′ər-əl) pertaining to a side; denoting a position farther from the median plane or midline of the body or of a structure. 87

lavage (lah-vahzh′) the irrigation or washing out of an organ; to wash out or irrigate. 260

laxative (lak′sə-tiv) mildly cathartic; an agent that acts to promote evacuation of the bowel; a cathartic or purgative. 264

leiomyoma (li″o-mi-o′mə) a benign tumor derived from smooth muscle, most commonly of the uterus; called also fibroid and fibroid tumor. 325

lesion (le′zhən) any pathologic or traumatic discontinuity of tissue or loss of function of a part. 97, 473

lethargic (lə-thar′jik) pertaining to lethargy. 205

lethargy (leth′ər-je) a lowered level of consciousness marked by listlessness, drowsiness, and apathy; a condition of indifference. 205

leukemia (loo-ke′me-ə) a disease of the blood-forming organs characterized by a marked increase in the number of leukocytes, including young forms of leukocytes not usually seen in circulating blood. 117, 402

leukocyte (loo′ko-sīt) a white blood cell. 115

l. count, enumeration of the number of white blood cells in a blood sample. 115

leukocytopenia (loo″ko-si″to-pe′ne-ə) a deficiency in the number of white blood cells. 117

leukocytosis (loo″ko-si-to′sis) a transient increase in the number of leukocytes in the blood. 119

leukopenia (loo″ko-pe′ne-ə) a deficiency in the number of leukocytes in the blood. 117

leukoplakia (loo″ko-pla′ke-ə) a white patch on a mucous membrane. 248

leukorrhea (loo″ko-re′ə) a white, viscid discharge from the vagina or uterine cavity. 326

ligament (lig′ə-mənt) a band of fibrous tissue that connects bones or cartilages and supports and strengthens joints. 387

ligation (li-ga′shən) application of a ligature, a material for tying or constricting a structure. 264

lingual (ling′gwəl) pertaining to or near the tongue. 233

lipase (lip′ās, li′pās) an enzyme that breaks down fats. 229

lipectomy (li-pek′tə-me) excision of a mass of subcutaneous adipose tissue. 259, 482

suction-assisted l., removal of fat by placing a narrow tube under the skin and applying a vacuum. 483, 483f

lipid (lip′id) a fat. 160

lipoid (lip′oid) resembling fat. 229

lipoma (lip-o′mə) a tumor composed of fatty tissue. 476

lipopenia (lip″o-pe′ne-ə) a deficiency of fats in the body. 256

lipoprotein (lip″o-, li″po-pro′tēn) any of the lipid-protein complexes in which lipids are transported in the blood. 160

high-density l., a plasma protein that contains ~50% lipoprotein along with cholesterol, triglycerides, and phospholipid and is associated with decreased cardiac risk profiles. 160

low-density l., a plasma protein containing relatively more cholesterol and triglycerides than protein. 160

liposuction (lip″o-suk′shən) surgical removal of localized fat deposits using high-pressure vacuum, applied by means of a subdermal cannula. 259, 483

lithiasis (li-thi′ə-sis) a condition marked by formation of stones. 203, 296

litholysis (li-thol′i-sis) the dissolving of a stone. 299

lithotomy (li-thot′ə-me) incision of a duct or organ for removal of a calculus. 112

lithotripsy (lith′o-trip′se) the crushing of a calculus within the urinary system or gallbladder, followed at once by the washing out of the fragments. 112, 265, 299, 300f

extracorporeal shock wave l., a procedure for treating gallstones and upper urinary tract stones. The patient is immersed in a large tub of water or placed in contact with a water cushion. A high-energy shock wave is focused on the stone, which disintegrates into particles small enough to be expelled. 264, 299

lithotriptor (lith′o-trip″tər) an instrument for crushing calculi. 264

lithotrite (lith′o-trīt) an instrument for crushing a urinary calculus. 299

lobectomy (lo-bek′tə-me) excision of a lobe, as removal of a lobe of the lung, brain, or liver. 216

hepatic l., excision of a lobe of the liver. 264

loop of Henle (lūp əv hen′le) a long, *U*-shaped part of the renal tubule, extending through the medulla from the end of the proximal convoluted tubule to the beginning of the distal convoluted tubule. 279, 280f

lordosis (lor-do′sis) the anterior concavity in the curvature of the lumbar and cervical spine as viewed from the side. The term is used to refer to abnormally increased curvature (swayback) and to the normal curvature (normal lordosis). 404

lumbar (lum′bahr) pertaining to the lower back. 379

l. puncture, the introduction of a hollow needle into the subarachnoid space of the lumbar part of the spinal canal. 394, 435

lumpectomy (ləm-pek′tə-me) surgical excision of only the palpable lesion in carcinoma of the breast; surgical removal of a mass. 511

lunula (loo′nu-lə) a small crescent- or moon-shaped area. 468

lupus erythematosis (LE) (loo′pəs er″ə-them″ə-to′sis) a group of connective tissue disorders primarily affecting women, comprising a spectrum of clinical forms in which cutaneous disease may occur with or without systemic involvement. 134, 407

cutaneous l. e., a form of lupus erythematosus in which the skin may be the only organ involved, or it may precede the involvement of other systems. 407

discoid l. e. (DLE), a chronic form of cutaneous lupus erythematosus in which the skin lesions mimic those of the systemic form but systemic signs are rare, although multisystem manifestations may develop after many years. 471

systemic l. e., a chronic inflammatory, collagen disease affecting many systems of the body. 407

luteinizing hormone (loo′te-in-ī″zing hor′mōn) a hormone secreted by the anterior lobe of the hypophysis that stimulates development of the corpus luteum. 316, 496

Lyme disease (līm di-zēz′) a recurrent multisystemic disorder, beginning with a rash and followed by arthritis of the large joints, myalgia, malaise, and neurologic and cardiac manifestations. It is caused by the bacteria *Borrelia burgdorferi,* carried by the deer tick *Ixodes dammini.* 408

lymph (limf) a transparent fluid found in lymphatic vessels consisting of a liquid portion and cells that are mostly lymphocytes. 108, 173

l. node, any of the small knots of lymphatic tissue found at intervals along the course of the lymphatic vessels. 173

lymphadenectomy (lim-fad″ə-nek′tə-me) surgical excision of a lymph node or nodes. 178

lymphadenitis (lim-fad″ə-ni′tis) inflammation of a lymph node. 176, 177f

lymphadenopathy (lim-fad″ə-nop′ə-the) any disease of the lymph nodes. 176

lymphangiography (lim-fan″je-og′rə-fe) roentgenography of the lymphatic vessels after the injection of contrast medium. 175

lymphangioma (lim-fan″je-o′mə) a tumor composed of newly formed lymph channels. 167

lymphangitis (lim″fan-ji′tis) inflammation of a lymphatic vessel. 177

lymphatics (lim-fat′iks) a system of vessels that collects tissue fluids from all parts of the body and returns the fluids to the blood circulation. 173, 174f

lymphedema (lim″fə-de′mə) chronic edema of an extremity because of obstruction within the lymph vessels or the lymph nodes, resulting in accumulation of interstitial fluid. 176

lymphocyte (lim′fo-sīt) any of the mononuclear leukocytes found in the blood, lymph, and lymphoid tissues that are responsible for humoral and cellular immunity. 173

B cell l., a type of lymphocyte that synthesizes antibodies; B cells. 173

T cell l., a type of lymphocyte that is involved in cell-mediated immunity; T cells. 173

lymphogenous (lim-foj′ə-nəs) producing lymph; produced from lymph or in the lymphatics. 173

lymphogram (lim′fo-gram) a roentgenogram of the lymphatic vessels and lymph nodes. 175

lymphography (lim-fog′rə-fe) roentgenography of the lymphatic vessels and nodes after injection of radiopaque material. 175

lymphoma (lim-fo′mə) a lymphatic tumor; any neoplastic disorder of lymphoid tissue. 177

non-Hodgkin's l., any of a group of malignant tumors involving lymphoid tissue, differing from Hodgkin's disease. 177

lymphostasis (lim-fos′tə-sis) stoppage of lymph flow. 176

macrocyte (mak′ro-sīt) a very large cell, usually referring to a very large red blood cell. 120

macrocytosis (mak″ro-si-to′sis) an increase in the number of large red blood cells. 120

macrophage (mak′ro-fāj) any of the mononuclear phagocytes found in the walls of blood vessels and in loose connective tissue. 133

macroscopic (mak″ro-skop′ik) visible with the unaided eye or without the microscope. 74, 121

macroscopy (mə-kros′kə-pe) examination with the naked eye; macroscopic examination. 121

macule (mak′ūl) a discolored spot on the skin that is not elevated above the surface. 473

magnetic resonance imaging or scan (MRI) (mag-net′ik rez′o-nəns im′ə-jing) a noninvasive method of creating images of body parts based on the magnetic properties of chemical elements within the body. 44, 394, 436

malabsorption (mal″əb-sorp′shən) faulty nutritive absorption. 246

m. syndrome, a complex of symptoms resulting from disorders in the intestinal absorption of nutrients, characterized by anorexia, weight loss, abdominal bloating, muscle cramps, bone pain, and an abnormal amount of fat in the feces. 256

malacia (mə-la′shə) a morbid softness or softening of a tissue or part. 40

malaise (mah-lāz′) a general feeling of ill health. 205, 245

malaria (mə-lar′e-ə) an infectious disease mainly found in parts of Africa, Asia; Turkey, the West Indies, Central and South America, and Oceania, caused by intracellular protozoa of the genus *Plasmodium* and usually transmitted by the bites of infected mosquitoes. 131

malignant (mə-lig′nənt) tending to grow worse and threatening to result in death. 21

malnutrition (mal″noo-trish′ən) poor nutrition. 246

malocclusion (mal″o-kloo′zhən) improper position of the teeth resulting in the faulty meeting of the teeth or jaws. 248

mammalgia (mə-mal′jə) painful breast. 510

mammary (mam′ər-e) pertaining to the breast. 54, 497

mammogram (mam′ə-gram) a roentgenogram of the breast. 504

mammography (mə-mog′rə-fe) the use of x-ray examination to diagnose diseases of the breast. 504

mammoplasty (mam′o-plas″te) surgical repair of the breast. 38, 512

augmentation m., plastic surgery to increase the size of the female breast. 38, 512

reduction m., plastic surgery to reduce the size of the female breast. 512

mandible (man′di-bəl) the bone of the lower jaw. 233

mandibular (man-dib′u-lər) pertaining to the lower jaw bone, or mandible. 233

mania (ma′ne-ə) a phase of bipolar disorder characterized by expansiveness, elation, agitation, hyperexcitability, hyperactivity, and increased speed of thought and speech (flight of ideas); also called manic syndrome; as a combining form, it signifies obsessive preoccupation. 451

marrow (mar′o) the soft material that fills the cavities of bones. 373

mastalgia (mas-tal′jə) pain in the breast. 510

mastectomy (mas-tek′tə-me) surgical removal of a breast. 38, 511

mastitis (mas-ti′tis) inflammation of the breast. 52, 510

mastocarcinoma (mas″tə-kahr″si-no′mə) cancerous tumor of the breast. 510

mastodynia (mas″to-din′e-ə) painful breast. 510

mastoiditis (mas″toid-i′tis) inflammation of the mastoid antrum and cells. 448

mastopexy (mas′to-pek-se) plastic surgery to correct a pendulous breast. 512

mastoptosis (mas″to-to′sis) sagging breasts. 512

maxilla (mak-sil′ə) the irregularly shaped bone that helps form the upper jaw. 233

maxillary (mak′sĭ-lar″e) pertaining to the maxilla. 233

measles (me′zəlz) a highly contagious viral disease common in children, but also seen in nonimmune individuals of any age. 136

mechanoreceptor (mek′ə-no-re-sep′tor) a receptor that is excited by mechanical pressures or distortions, as those responding to sound, touch, and muscular contractions. 431

medial, median (me′de-əl, me′de-ən) pertaining to the middle or midline of a body or structure; pertaining to the middle layer of structures. 86

mediastinoscope (me″de-ə-sti′no-skōp) an endoscope used to examine the mediastinum. 196

mediastinoscopy (me″de-as″tĭ-nos″kə-pe) examination of the mediastinum using an endoscope inserted through an anterior midline incision just above the thoracic inlet. 196

mediastinum (me″de-əs-ti′nəm) a median partition; an area in the middle of the chest that contains the heart and its large vessels, trachea, esophagus, thymus, and lymph nodes. 152

medical (med′ĭ-kəl) pertaining to medicine. 19

   m. pathologist, a physician who specializes in the study of disease in general. 19

   m. technician, one who has received formal training in laboratory techniques in a 2-year associate degree program. 19

   m. technologist, one who is skilled in the performance of clinical laboratory procedures used in the diagnosis of disease and evaluation of patient progress. In general, the technologist has completed 4 years of specialized education in medical technology. 19

medicine (med′ĭ-sin) a drug or remedy; the science of diagnosis and treatment of disease and the maintenance of health; the nonsurgical treatment of disease. 17

   forensic m., a branch of medicine that deals with the application of medical knowledge to the purposes of law. 25

   internal m., a branch of medicine that deals specifically with diagnosis and medical treatment of diseases and disorders of internal structures of the body. 18

   preventive m., the branch of medicine that aims at prevention of disease and promotion of health. 24

   rehabilitation m., the branch of medicine that deals with restoring a person's ability to live and work as normally as possible after a disabling injury or illness. 27

mediolateral (me″de-o-lat′ər-əl) pertaining to the middle and to one side. 87

medulla (mə-dul′ə) the innermost part of an organ or structure. 429, 498

   adrenal m., the inner portion of the adrenal gland, which secretes epinephrine. 496

medullary cavity (med′ə-lar″e, med′u-lar″e kav′ĭ-te) the space in the diaphysis of a long bone; marrow cavity. 374

megalocyte (meg′ə-lo-sīt″) an extremely large red blood cell. 121

megalomania (meg″ə-lo-ma′ne-ə) a disordered mental state characterized by delusions of grandeur. 451

melanin (mel′ə-nin) the dark pigment of the skin, hair, eye, and certain tumors. 58, 496

melanocyte (mel′ə-no-sīt, mə-lan′o-sīt) a black cell; a cell that produces melanin. 477

melanoma (mel″ə-no′mə) a tumor arising from the melanocytic system of the skin and other organs. When used alone, the term refers to malignant melanoma. 477

   malignant m., a malignant neoplasm of melanocytes that occurs most often in the skin but may occur elsewhere. 477

melatonin (mel″ə-to′nin) a hormone synthesized by the pineal gland, the secretion of which increases during exposure to light; in mammals it influences hormone production, and in many species it regulates seasonal changes such as reproductive pattern and fur color. In humans it is implicated in the regulation of sleep, mood, puberty, and ovarian cycles. 500

membrane (mem′brān) A thin layer of tissue that covers a surface, lines a cavity, or divides a space or organ. 55

   mucous m., any one of four major kinds of tissue that cover or line cavities or canals of the body that open to the outside. 58

   serous m., the membrane lining the exterior of the walls of various body cavities. 93

menarche (mə-nahr′ke) the beginning of the menstrual function. 316

Ménière's disease (mĕ-nyārz′ dĭ-zēz′) hearing loss, tinnitus, and vertigo resulting from noninfectious disease of the ear. 448

meningeal (mə-nin′je-əl) of or pertaining to the meninges. 428

meninges (mə-nin′jēz) the three membranes covering the brain and the spinal cord: dura mater, arachnoid, and pia mater. 427

meningioma (mə-nin″je-o′mə) a benign, slow-growing tumor of the meninges. 444

meningitis (men″in-ji′tis) inflammation of the meninges, the membranes that cover the brain and the spinal cord. Meningitis is caused by a variety of infectious microorganisms. 443

meningocele (mə-ning′go-sēl″) a hernial protrusion of meninges through a defect in the skull or vertebral column. 442

meningomyelocele (mə-ning″go-mi′ə-lo-sēl″) hernial protrusion of the spinal cord and the meninges, through a defect in the spine. 442

menopause (men′o-pawz) that period in a female individual's life when menstruation ceases. 316

menorrhagia (men″o-ra′jə) abnormally profuse menstruation. 322

menorrhea (men″o-re′ə) menstruation; too profuse menstruation. 322

menses (men′sēz) menstruation, the monthly flow of blood from the female genital tract. 317, 322

menstrual (men′stroo-əl) pertaining to the menses. 317

menstruation (men″stroo-a′shən) the cyclic, physiologic discharge through the vagina of blood and mucosal tissues from the nonpregnant uterus. 316

mental (men′təl) pertaining to the mind. 450

   m. retardation, abnormally low intellectual functioning. 450

mesenteric (mez″ən-ter′ik) pertaining to the mesentery, a fold of the peritoneum. 256

   m. occlusion, a binding or closing off of a segment of the intestine by the mesentery. 255f, 256

mesoderm (mez′o-dərm) in embryology, the middle layer of cells in the blastoderm. 466

mesothelioma (mez″o-the″le-o′mə) a tumor derived from mesothelial tissue. 209

mesothelium (mez″o-the′le-əm) the layer of flat cells forming the squamous epithelium that covers all true serous membranes in adults. 209

metabolism (mə-tab′o-liz″əm) the sum of all the physical and chemical processes by which living organized substance is produced and maintained (anabolism), and also the transformation by which energy is made available for the uses of the organism (catabolism). 228

metacarpal (met″ə-kahr′pəl) pertaining to the metacarpus, the part of the hand between the wrist and fingers; one of the bones of the metacarpus. 381, 382

metastasis (mə-tas′tə-sis) a growth of pathogenic microorganisms or of abnormal cells distant from the site primarily involved by the morbid process. 174

metastatic (met″ə-stat′ik) pertaining to or of the nature of metastasis. 174

metatarsal (met″ə-tahr′səl) pertaining to the metatarsus; a bone of the metatarsus. 385

metatarsophalangeal (met″ə-tahr″so-fə-lan′je-əl) pertaining to the metatarsus and the phalanges of the toes. 400

metritis (mə-tri′tis) inflammation of uterine tissue. 314

metrorrhagia (me″tro-ra′je-ə) uterine bleeding, usually of normal amount, occurring at completely irregular intervals, the period of flow sometimes being prolonged. 322

microbe (mi′krōb) a minute living organism, such as bacteria, protozoa, or fungi. 95

microbiologist (mi″kro-bi-ol′ə-jist) one specializing in microbiology. 127

microbiology (mi″kro-bi-ol′ə-je) the science that deals with the study of microorganisms. 127

microcardia (mi″kro-kahr′de-ə) smallness of the heart. 164

microcyte (mi′kro-sīt) an abnormally small erythrocyte, microns or less in diameter. 120

microcytosis (mi″kro-si-to′sis) an increase in the number of undersized red blood cells. 120

microorganism (mi″kro-or′gən-iz-əm) a minute living organism, usually microscopic, including bacteria, rickettsiae, viruses, molds, yeasts, and protozoa. 127

microscope (mi′kro-skōp) an instrument for viewing small objects that must be magnified to be seen. 56

microscopic (mi″kro-skop′ik) of extremely small size and visible only by the aid of a microscope. 74

microscopy (mi-kros′kə-pe) viewing things with a microscope. 56, 121

microtia (mi-kro′shə) severe hypoplasia or aplasia of the pinna of the ear, with a blind or absent external auditory meatus. 74, 75f

micturition (mik″tu-rĭ-′shən) urination. 281

midbrain (mid′brān″) the part of the brain that connects the pons and the cerebellum with the hemispheres of the cerebrum; mesencephalon. 429f

midphalangeal (mid″fə-lan′je-əl) pertaining to a middle phalanx, a bone of a finger or toe. 400

midsagittal (mid-saj′ĭ-təl) the plane vertically dividing the body through the midline into right and left halves. 84

migraine (mi′grān) an often familial symptom complex of periodic attacks of vascular headache, usually temporal and unilateral in onset, commonly associated with irritability, nausea, vomiting, constipation or diarrhea, and often photophobia. 439, 439f

mineralocorticoid (min″ər-əl-o-kor′tĭ-koid) any of the group of corticosteroids, principally aldosterone, predominantly involved in the regulation of electrolyte and water balance in the body. 498

mitral (mi′trəl) pertaining to the mitral or bicuspid valve; shaped like a miter. 154

   m. valve, a bicuspid valve situated between the left atrium and the left ventricle; bicuspid valve. 154

   m. valve prolapse, protrusion of one or both cusps of the mitral valve back into the left atrium during ventricular contraction. 165

mittelschmerz (mit′əl-shmertz) pain associated with ovulation, usually occurring in the middle of the menstrual cycle. 322

molar (mo′lər) a posterior tooth that is used for grinding food and acts as a major jaw support in the dental arch. 234

Monilia (mo-nil′e-ə) a genus of fungi. 367

moniliasis (mon-ĭ-li′ə-sis) candidiasis; any infection caused by a species of *Candida,* especially *Candida albicans.* 367

monocyte (mon′o-sīt) a mononuclear phagocytic leukocyte that is 13 to 25 microns in diameter and has an ovoid or kidney-shaped nucleus and abundant gray-blue cytoplasm. 115, 116f

mononucleosis (mon″o-noo″kle-o′sis) an excessive number of monocytes in the blood; the term also refers to infectious mononucleosis. 117, 176

monoplegia (mon″o-ple′jə) paralysis of a limb. 442

mons (monz) a general term for an elevation, or eminence. 313

   m. pubis, the rounded fleshy prominence over the symphysis pubis. 313

mucoid (mu′koid) resembling mucus. 232

mucolytic (mu″ko-lit′ik) dissolving mucus; an agent that dissolves or destroys mucus. 217

mucosa (mu-ko′sə) mucous membrane. 232

mucous (mu′kəs) pertaining or relating to, or resembling mucus; mucoid; covered with mucus; secreting, producing, or containing mucus. 109, 232

   m. colitis, irritable bowel syndrome. 254

mucus (mu′kəs) the free slime of the mucous membranes, composed of secretion of the glands, various salts, desquamated cells, and leukocytes. 109, 231

multigravida (mul″tĭ-grav′ĭ-də) a female who has been pregnant more than once. 352

multipara (mul″tip′ə-rə) a female who has produced more than one viable offspring. 354

multiple myeloma (mul″tĭ-pəl mi′ə-lo′mə) a disseminated type of plasma cell dyscrasia characterized by multiple bone marrow tumors. 402

multiple sclerosis (mul′tĭ-pəl sklə-ro′sis) a chronic disease of the central nervous system in which there is development of disseminated demyelinated glial patches called plaques. 446

mumps (mumps) an acute infectious disease caused by a virus, usually seen in children younger than 15 years, although adults may also be affected. 249

murmur (mur′mər) an auscultatory sound, particularly a periodic sound of short duration of cardiac or vascular origin. 159

  heart m., an abnormal sound heard in auscultation of the heart, caused by altered blood flow into a chamber or through a valve. 159, 163

muscle (mus′əl) an organ that produces movement of an animal by contraction. 389

  arrector pili m., minute smooth muscle attached to the connective tissue sheath of the hair follicle, capable of causing the hair to stand erect. 467

  cardiac m., the muscle of the heart. 152

  m. relaxant, an agent that causes the muscles to relax. 411

  skeletal m., striated muscles that are attached to bones and bring about voluntary movement. 389f

  visceral m., muscle that is associated chiefly with the hollow viscera. 389, 389f

muscular (mus′ku-lər) pertaining to or composing muscle; having a well-developed musculature. 60, 389

  m. dystrophy, a genetically determined myopathy characterized by atrophy and wasting away of muscles. 404

musculoskeletal (mus″ku-lo-skel′ə-təl) pertaining to or comprising the skeleton and the muscles, as musculoskeletal system. 373

myalgia (mi-al′jə) pain in a muscle or muscles. 60, 397

myasthenia (mi″əs-the′ne-ə) muscle weakness. 408

  m. gravis, a disease characterized by muscle weakness, caused by a functional abnormality. 408, 445, 446

mycodermatitis (mi″ko-der″mə-ti′tis) inflammation of the skin caused by a fungus. 472

myelin sheath (mi′ə-lin shēth) the sheath surrounding the axon of some (the myelinated) nerve cells. 425f, 426

myelinated (mi′ə-lĭ-nāt″əd) having a myelin sheath. 426

myelitis (mi″ə-li′tis) inflammation of the bone marrow; inflammation of the spinal cord. 401

myeloblast (mi′ə-lo-blast) embryonic form of blood cell found in the bone marrow. 375

myelocyte (mi′ə-lo-sīt) a cell found in the bone marrow. 375

myelogram (mi′ə-lo-gram) X-ray film of the spinal cord. 436

myelography (mi″ə-log′rə-fe) roentgenography of the spinal cord after injection of a contrast medium into the subarachnoid space. 436

myelosuppression (mi″ə-lo-sə-presh′ən) inhibition of bone marrow activity. 413

myelosuppressive (mi″ə-lo-sə-pres′iv) inhibiting bone marrow activity; an agent that inhibits bone marrow activity. 413

myoblast (mi′o-blast) embryonic cell that becomes a cell of the muscle fiber. 389

myocardial (mi″o-kahr′de-əl) pertaining to the muscular tissue of the heart. 153

  m. infarction, development of an infarct in the myocardium, usually the result of ischemia after occlusion of a coronary artery. 164

myocarditis (mi″o-kahr-di′tis) inflammation of the heart muscle. 165

myocardium (mi″o-kahr′de-əm) the middle and thickest layer of the heart wall, made up of cardiac muscle. 153, 389

myocele (mi′o-sēl) hernia of the muscle. 408

myocellulitis (mi″o-sel″u-li′tis) inflammation of cellular tissue and muscle. 401

myodynia (mi″o-din′e-ə) pain in a muscle. 397

myofascial (mi″o-fash′e-əl) pertaining to or involving the fascia surrounding and associated with muscle tissue. 408

myofibroma (mi″o-fi-bro′mə) a tumor composed of muscular and fibrous elements. 401

myofibrosis (mi″o-fi-bro′sis) replacement of muscle tissue by fibrous tissue. 408

myolysis (mi-ol′ĭ-sis) destruction of muscle tissue. 408

myomalacia (mi″o-mə-la′shə) morbid softening of muscle. 408

myometritis (mi″o-mə-tri′tis) inflammation of the myometrium, the muscular substance of the uterus. 326

myometrium (mi-o-me′tre-əm) the smooth muscle of the uterus. 314

myopathy (mi-op′ə-the) any disease of muscle. 408

myopia (mi-o′pe-ə) the error of refraction in which rays of light entering the eye are brought to a focus in front of the retina; also called nearsightedness. 448

myoplasty (mi′o-plas″te) surgical repair of a muscle. 411

myorrhaphy (mi-or′ə-fe) suture of divided muscle. 411

myxedema (mik″sə-de′mə) a condition resulting from hypothyroidism characterized by dry, waxy swelling of the skin. 507

narcolepsy (nahr′ko-lep″se) recurrent, uncontrollable brief episodes of sleep. 445

narcotic (nahr-kot′ik) pertaining to or producing narcosis, nonspecific and reversible depression of function of the central nervous system marked by stupor or insensibility produced by drugs; an agent that produces insensibility or stupor, applied especially to the opioids. 63, 455

nares (na′rēz) the nostrils, the external opening of the nose. 191

nasal (na′zəl) pertaining to the nose. 60, 192

nasogastric (na″zo-gas′trik) pertaining to the nose and stomach. 249

  n. tube, any tube passed into the stomach through the nose. 249, 259f

nasolacrimal (na″zo-lak′rĭ-məl) pertaining to the nose and lacrimal apparatus. 433

  n. duct, a tubular passage that carries tears from the eye to the nose. 433

nasopharyngeal (na″zo-fə-rin′je-əl) pertaining to the nasopharynx. 192

nasopharyngitis (na″zo-far″in-ji′tis) inflammation of the nasopharynx. 203

nasopharynx (na″zo-far′inks) the upper part of the pharynx, continuous with the nasal passages. 192

nasoscope (na′zo-skōp) instrument for examining inside the nose. 195

nasotracheal (na″zo-tra′ke-əl) pertaining to the nose and trachea. 214

natal (na′təl) pertaining to birth. 351

nebulizer (neb′u-li″zər) a device for creating and throwing an aerosol spray. 217

necrosis (nə-kro′sis) death of tissue. 109, 479

necrotic (nə-krot′ik) pertaining to or characterized by necrosis. 479

neonatal (ne″o-na′təl) pertaining to a newborn child, usually designating the first weeks after birth. 355

neonate (ne′o-nāt) a newborn child. 355

neonatologist (ne″o-na-tol′ə-jist) a physician who specializes in care of the newborn. 20, 355

neonatology (ne″o-na-tol′ə-je) the branch of medicine dealing with treatment of the newborn infant. 20, 355

neoplasm (ne′o-plaz-əm) tumor; any new and abnormal growth. Neoplasms may be benign or malignant. 61, 249, 476

neoplastic (ne″o-plas′tik) tending to produce neoplasms. 249

nephrectomy (nə-frek′tə-me) surgical excision of a kidney. 298

nephritis (nə-fri′tis) inflammation of the kidney. 294

nephrolith (nef′ro-lith) a kidney stone. 296

nephrolithiasis (nef″ro-lĭ-thi′ə-sis) a condition marked by the presence of kidney stones. 112, 296

nephrolithotomy (nef″ro-lĭ-thot′ə-me) removal of renal calculi by cutting into the kidney. 300

nephrolysis (nə-frol′ə-sis) destruction of kidney tissue; freeing of a kidney from adhesions. 292

nephromalacia (nef″ro-mə-la′shə) softening of the kidney. 292

nephromegaly (nef″ro-meg′ə-le) enlargement of the kidney. 292

  bilateral n., enlargement of both kidneys. 292

nephron (nef′ron) the structural and functional unit of the kidney. 279, 280f

nephropathy (nə-frop′ə-the) any disease of the kidneys. 509

  obstructive n., a kidney disease caused by obstruction of the urinary tract. 294

nephropexy (nef′ro-pek″se) surgical fixation of a floating kidney. 301

nephroptosis (nef″rop-to′sis) downward displacement of the kidney; floating kidney. 301

nephrosclerosis (nef″ro-sklə-ro′sis) hardening of the kidney caused by renovascular disease. 297

nephroscope (nef′ro-skōp) an instrument inserted into an incision in the renal pelvis for viewing the interior of the kidney. 290, 290f

nephroscopy (nə-fros′kə-pe) visualization of the kidney using a nephroscope. 290

nephrosonography (nef″ro-so-nog′rə-fe) ultrasonic scanning of the kidney. 289

nephrostomy (nə-fros′tə-me) the creation of a fistula leading directly into the renal pelvis. 299f

  percutaneous n., placement of a catheter into the kidney through the skin, providing for diversion of the renal output, certain surgical procedures, including biopsies, and infusion of substances to dissolve calculi. 286, 287f, 299

  n. tube, a tube inserted into the renal pelvis for direct drainage of the urine through a percutaneous opening. 286

nephrotic syndrome (nə-frot′ik sin′drōm) a clinical classification that includes all diseases of the kidney characterized by chronic loss of protein in the urine and subsequent depletion of body protein. 294

nephrotomogram (nef″ro-to′mo-gram) a sectional radiograph of the kidney obtained by nephrotomography. 289

nephrotomography (nef″ro-to-mog′rə-fe) radiologic visualization of the kidney by tomography after intravenous introduction of contrast medium. 289

nephrotoxic (nef′ro-tok″sik) destructive to kidney cells. 292

nephroureterectomy (nef″ro-u-re″tər-ek′tə-me) excision of a kidney and all or part of the ureter. 298

neural (noor′əl) pertaining to a nerve or the nerves. 54, 424

neuralgia (noo-ral′jə) pain of a nerve. 438

neurasthenia (noor″əs-the′ne-ə) a nervous condition characterized by chronic weakness, easy fatigability, and sometimes exhaustion. 451

neurectomy (noo-rek′to-me) excision of a part of a nerve. 35, 453

neuritis (noo-ri′tis) inflammation of a nerve. 52

neuroglia (noo-rog′le-ə) the supporting structure of nervous tissue. 424

neurohypophysis (noor″o-hi-pof′ə-sis) the posterior lobe of the pituitary gland. 494

neurologic (noor″o-loj′ik) pertaining to neurology or the nervous system. 22

neurologist (noo-rol′ə-jist) a specialist in the treatment of nervous diseases. 22

neurology (noo-rol′ə-je) the branch of medicine that deals with the study of the nervous system. 22

neurolysis (noo-rol′ĭ-sis) release of a nerve sheath by cutting it longitudinally; operative breaking up of perineural adhesions; relief of tension on a nerve; exhaustion of nervous energy; destruction of nerve tissue. 36, 453

neuroma (noo-ro′mə) a tumor made up of nerve cells and nerve fibers. 445

  Morton's n., a neuroma resulting from compression of a branch of the plantar nerve by the metatarsal heads. 400

neuromuscular (noor″o-mus′ku-lər) pertaining to the nerves and muscles. 426

  n. blocking agent, a drug used to stop muscle contraction. 62

neuron (noor′on) any of the conducting cells of the nervous system. 22, 424, 425, 425f

  motor n., one of various efferent nerve cells that transmit impulses from either the brain or spinal cord. 426

  sensory n., an afferent nerve cell conveying sensory impulses. 426

neuropathy (noo-rop′ə-the) a functional disturbance or pathologic change in the peripheral nervous system. 442, 509

neuroplasty (noor′o-plas″te) plastic repair of a nerve. 453

neurorrhaphy (noo-ror′ə-fe) suturing of a cut nerve. 453

neurosclerosis (noor″o-sklə-ro′sis) hardening of nerve tissue. 438

neurosis (noo-ro′sis) former name for a category of mental disorders characterized by anxiety and avoidance behavior. In general, the term refers to disorders in which the symptoms are distressing to the person, behavior does not violate gross social norms, and there is no apparent organic cause. 53

neurosurgeon (noor″o-sur′jən) a surgeon who specializes in work on the nervous system. 22

neurosurgery (noor′o-sər″jər-e) surgery of the nervous system. 22

neurosyphilis (noor″o-sif′ĭ-lis) the central nervous system manifestations of syphilis. 364

neurotoxin (noor′o-tok″sin) a toxin that is poisonous to or destroys nerve tissue. 129

neurotransmitter (noor″o-trans′mit-ər) any of a group of substances that are released on excitation from the axon terminal of a neuron and travel across the synaptic cleft either to excite or inhibit the target cell. 426

neurotripsy (noor″o-trip′se) surgical crushing of a nerve. 36, 453

neutrophil (noo′tro-fil) a granular leukocyte having a nucleus with three to five lobes and cytoplasm containing fine inconspicuous granules. 116, 116f

nevus (ne′vəs) any congenital lesion of the skin; a birthmark. 476

nitroglycerin (ni″tro-glis′ə-rin) a drug used chiefly in the prophylaxis and treatment of angina pectoris, administered sublingually. 172

nociceptor (no″sĭ-sep′tər) a receptor for pain caused by injury to body tissues. 431

nocturia (nok-tu′re-ə) excessive urination at night. 292

node (nōd) a small mass of tissue as a swelling, knot, or protuberance, either normal or abnormal.

   cervical lymph n., a group of lymph nodes on each side of the neck. 176, 177f

   inguinal n., any of a group of lymph glands in the upper femoral triangle of the thigh. 174

   n. of Ranvier, one of several constrictions in the medullary substance of a nerve fiber. 426

nodule (nod′ūl) a small node that is solid and can be detected by touch. 473

nonarticular (non″ahr-tik′u-lər) not associated with a joint. 408

noninflammatory (non″in-flam′ə-tor″e) not characterized by inflammation. 252, 254

norepinephrine (nor″ep-ĭ-nef′rin) one of the naturally occurring catecholamines; a neurohormone and a major neurotransmitter. It is also secreted by the adrenal medulla and is released predominantly in response to hypotension and stress. 500

normochromic (nor″mo-kro′mik) having a normal color; having normal hemoglobin content. 122

normocyte (nor′mo-sīt) a normal-sized red blood cell. 121

normocytic (nor″mo-sit′ik) relating to an erythrocyte that is normal in size, shape, and color. 121

nosocomial (nos″o-ko′me-əl) pertaining to or originating in a hospital. 126

   n. infection (in-fek′shən), an infection acquired while one is hospitalized. 126

nucleoid (noo′kle-oid) resembling a nucleus. 117

nucleoprotein (noo″kle-o-pro′tēn) a protein found in the nuclei of cells. 117

nullipara (nə-lip′ə-rə) a female individual who has never borne a child. 354

nurse (ners) one who makes a profession of caring for the sick or disabled or of aiding in the maintenance of health; to care for the sick; to nourish at the breast. 26

   licensed practical n., one who is a graduate of a school of practical nursing and who performs certain services to the sick under the supervision of a registered nurse. 26

   licensed vocational n., a graduate of a school of practical nursing who has been legally authorized to practice. 26

   n. anesthetist, a registered nurse with advanced education and training in administering anesthetics. 26

   n. midwife, an individual educated in the two disciplines of nursing and midwifery. 26

   n. practitioner, a registered nurse who has well-developed competencies in using a broad range of cues. These cues are used for prescribing and implementing both direct and indirect nursing care and for articulating nursing therapies with other planned therapies. 26

   registered n., a graduate nurse who is registered and licensed to practice by a state board of nurse examiners or other state authority. 26

nutrition (noo-trĭ′shən) the sum of the processes involved in taking in nutrients and assimilating and using them; nutriment. 227

   total parenteral n., the intravenous administration of the total nutrient requirements of a patient with gastrointestinal dysfunction. 259

nycturia (nik-tu′re-ə) frequent urination during the night, especially the passage of more urine at night than during the day. 292

obesity (o-bēs′ĭ-te) an increase in body weight beyond the limitation of skeletal and physical requirement, as the result of an excessive accumulation of fat in the body. 246

obstetric, obstetrical (ob-stet′rik, ob-stet′rĭ-kəl) pertaining to obstetrics. 20

obstetrician (ob″stə-trĭ′shən) a physician who is specialized in the treatment of pregnancy, labor, and delivery. 20, 351

obstetrics (ob-stet′riks) a branch of surgery that deals with the management of pregnancy and delivery. 20, 351

occipital (ok-sip′ĭ-təl) pertaining to the occiput, the posterior part of the head; located near the occipital bone, as the occipital lobe of the brain. 429

   o. lobe, one of the five lobes of each cerebral hemisphere. 429

occlusion (o-kloo′zhən) the act of closing or state of being closed; the relation of the teeth of both jaws during mandibular activity; an obstruction. 166

occult blood (ŏ-kult′) blood that is not obvious on examination from a nonspecific source. 244

ocular (ok′u-lər) of, pertaining to, or affecting the eye. 432

ointment (oint′mənt) a medication that contains fat and is of such consistency that it melts when applied to the skin. 482

olfaction (ol-fak′shən) the sense of smell; the act of smelling. 192, 434

olfactory (ol-fak′tə-re) pertaining to the sense of smell. 192, 434

oligospermia (ol″ĭ-go-sper′me-ə) deficiency in the number of spermatozoa in the semen. 336

oliguria (ol″ĭ-gu′re-ə) excretion of a diminished amount of urine in relation to the fluid intake, usually defined as less than 400 ml per 24 hours. 291

omphalic (om-fal′ik) pertaining to the navel. 97

omphalitis (om″fə-li′tis) inflammation of the navel. 98

omphalocele (om′fə-lo-sēl″) hernia of the navel. 97

omphaloma (om″fə-lo′mə) tumor of the navel. 98

omphalorrhagia (om″fə-lo-ra′jə) hemorrhage from the umbilicus. 98

omphalorrhexis (om″fə-lo-rek′sis) rupture of the umbilicus. 98

omphalus (om′fə-ləs) the navel. 97

oncologist (ong-kol′ə-jist) a specialist in the study and treatment of tumors. 20

oncology (ong-kol′ə-je) study of tumors. 20

onychectomy (on″ĭ-kek′tə-me) excision of a nail or nail bed; removal of the claws of an animal. 482

onychomalacia (on″ĭ-ko-mə-la′shə) softening of the nails. 480

onychomycosis (on″ĭ-ko-mi-ko′sis) a disease of the nails caused by a fungus. 480

onychopathy (on″ĭ-kop′ə-the) any disease of the nails. 480

onychophagia (on″ĭ-ko-fa′jə) habit of biting the nails. 468

onychophagist (on″ĭ-kof′ə-jist) one who has the habit of nail biting. 468

onychosis (on″ĭ-ko′sis) a condition of atrophy or dystrophy of the nails. 480

ooblast (o′o-blast) an embryonic egg. 350

oogenesis (o″o-jen′ə-sis) the origin and formation of eggs in the female sex. 317

oophoralgia (o″of-ər-al′jə) ovarian pain. 323

oophorectomy (o″of-ə-rek′tə-me) the removal of an ovary or ovaries. 329

oophoritis (o″of-ə-ri′tis) inflammation of an ovary. 323

oophorohysterectomy (o-of″ə-ro-his″tər-ek′tə-me) surgical removal of the uterus and ovaries. 329

oophoropathy (o-of″ə-rop′ə-the) any disease of the ovaries. 323

oophoropexy (o-of″ə-ro-pek″se) surgical fixation of the ovary. 328

oophorosalpingectomy (o-of″ə-ro-sal″pin-jek′tə-me) surgical removal of an ovary and uterine tube. 329

oophorosalpingitis (o-of″ə-ro-sal″pin-ji′tis) inflammation of an ovary and uterine tube. 323

oophorosalpingohysterectomy (o-of″ə-ro-sal-ping″go-his″tər-ek′tə-me) surgical removal of the ovaries, uterine tubes, and uterus. 329

ophthalmalgia (of″thəl-mal′jə) pain in the eye. 447

ophthalmic (of-thal′mik) pertaining to the eye. 19, 432

ophthalmitis (of″thəl-mi′tis) inflammation of the eye. 52

ophthalmodynia (of-thal″mo-din′e-ə) pain in the eye. 39

ophthalmologist (of″thəl-mol′ə-jist) a physician who specializes in the diagnosis and treatment of eye disease. 19

ophthalmology (of″thəl-mol′ə-je) the study of the eye and its diseases. 19

ophthalmomalacia (of-thal″mo-mə-la′shə) abnormal softness of the eye. 39, 40, 447

ophthalmometer (of″thəl-mom′ə-tər) an instrument for measuring the eye. 436

ophthalmopathy (of″thəl-mop′ə-the) any disease of the eye. 54, 56

ophthalmoplasty (of-thal″mo-plas″te) plastic surgery of the eye or its appendages. 36

ophthalmoplegia (of-thal″mo-ple′jə) paralysis of the eye muscles. 447

ophthalmorrhagia (of-thal″mo-ra′je-ə) hemorrhage from the eye. 447

ophthalmoscope (of-thal′mə-skōp) an instrument used to examine the interior of the eye. 436

ophthalmoscopy (of″thəl-mos′kə-pe) examination of the eye using an ophthalmoscope. 41, 436

ophthalmotomy (of″thəl-mot′ə-me) incision of the eyeball. 36

opioid (o′pe-oid) any synthetic narcotic that has opiate-like activities but is not derived from opium; any of a group of naturally occurring peptides that bind at or otherwise influence opiate receptors of cell membranes. 453, 532

   o. analgesics, a class of compounds that block the perception of pain or affect the emotional response to pain. 453

optical (op′tĭ-kəl) pertaining to vision. 27

optician (op-tish′ən) a specialist in the translation, filling, and adapting of ophthalmic prescriptions, products, and accessories. 27

optometrist (op-tom′ə-trist) a specialist in optometry. 27

optometry (op-tom′ə-tre) the professional practice of primary eye and vision care for the diagnosis, treatment, and prevention of associated disorders and for the improvement of vision by the prescription of spectacles and by use of other functional, optical, and pharmaceutical means regulated by state law. 27

oral (or′əl) pertaining to the oral cavity or mouth. 27, 192, 231

   o. cavity, the mouth. 27

   o. surgeon, a physician specialized in oral surgery. 27

   o. thermometer, an instrument designed for measuring temperature by mouth. 60

orchialgia (or″ke-al′jə) pain in a testis. 336

orchidalgia (or″kĭ-dal′jə) pain in a testis. 336

orchiditis (or″kĭ-di′tis) inflammation of a testicle. 337

orchidopexy (or′kĭ-do-pek″se) orchiopexy. 339

orchiectomy (or″ke-ek′tə-me) excision of one or both testes. 339

orchiepididymitis (or″ke-ep″ĭ-did″ĭ-mi′tis) inflammation of a testicle and an epididymis. 337

orchiopathy (or″ke-op′ə-the) any disease of the testes. 337

Parkinson's disease (pahr″kin-sənz dĭ-zēz′) a chronic nervous disease characterized by a fine, slowly spreading tremor; muscular weakness and rigidity; and a peculiar gait. 445

parotid (pə-rot′id) situated or occurring near the ear. 249

parotitis (par″o-ti′tis) inflammation of the parotid gland. 249
epidemic p., mumps. 249

parous (par′əs) having borne one or more offspring. 352

paroxysmal (par″ok-siz′məl) occurring in sudden, periodic attacks or recurrence of symptoms of a disease. 164

parturition (pahr″tu-rĭ′shən) childbirth. 351

patella (pə-tel′ə) the kneecap, a lens-shaped bone situated in front of the knee. 384

patellar response (pə-tel′ər) a deep tendon reflex elicited by a sharp tap on the tendon just distal to the patella. 426

patellofemoral (pə-tel″o-fem′ə-rəl) pertaining to the kneecap and the femur. 384

patent (pa′tənt) open, unobstructed, or not closed. 213
p. ductus arteriosus, an abnormal opening between the pulmonary artery and the aorta. 163

pathogen (path′o-jən) any disease-producing agent or microorganism. 56, 132

pathogenic (path-o-jen′ik) disease causing. 56

pathologic, pathological (path″o-loj′ik, path″o-loj′ĭ-kəl) indicating or caused by some morbid process. 19

pathologist (pə-thol′ə-jist) a physician who is specialized in the study of the essential nature of disease. 19
clinical p., a physician specialized in the branch of pathology that is applied to the solution of clinical problems, especially the use of laboratory methods in clinical diagnosis. 19
surgical p., a physician specialized in the study of disease processes that are surgically accessible for diagnosis or treatment. 19

pathology (pə-thol′ə-je) the study of the changes caused by disease in the structure or functions of the body. 19
cellular p., the study of cellular changes in disease. 19
clinical p., the study of disease by the use of laboratory tests and methods. 19

pediatric (pe″de-at′rik) pertaining to pediatrics. 20

pediatrician (pe″de-ə-trĭ-′shən) a physician who specializes in the treatment of children's diseases. 20

pediatrics (pe″de-at′riks) the branch of medicine that is devoted to the study of children's diseases. 20

pediculicide (pə-dik′u-lĭ-sīd) destroying lice; an agent that destroys lice. 547

pediculosis (pə-dik″u-lo′sis) infestation with lice of the family Pediculidae. 471

pedodontics (pe-do-don′tiks) the branch of dentistry that deals with the teeth and mouth conditions of children. 235

pedodontist (pe-do-don′tist) a dentist who specializes in the teeth and mouth conditions of children. 235

pelvic (pel′vik) pertaining to the pelvis. 92
p. cavity, the space within the walls of the pelvis, forming the inferior and lesser part of the abdominopelvic cavity. 92
p. girdle, a bony ring formed by the hip bones, the sacrum, and the coccyx. 381
p. inflammatory disease, an ascending pelvic infection involving the genital tract beyond the cervix uteri. 324

pelvimetry (pel-vim′ə-tre) the measurement of the dimensions and capacity of the pelvis. 356

pelvis (pel′vis) the lower portion of the trunk. The word also means any basin-like structure. 92
renal p. (re′nəl), in the kidney, the funnel-shaped structure at the upper end of the ureter. 281

penile (pe′nīl) pertaining to or affecting the penis. 332

penis (pe′nis) the male organ of urination and copulation. 332

pepsin (pep′sin) any of several enzymes of gastric juice that break down proteins. 501

peptic (pep′tik) pertaining to pepsin or digestion; related to action of gastric juices. 250

percussion (pər-kŭ′shən) the act of striking a part with short, sharp blows as an aid in diagnosing the condition of the underlying parts by the sound obtained. 99
abdominal p., assessing the organs of the abdomen by percussion. 242

percutaneous (per″ku-ta′ne-əs) performed through the skin. 171

pericardial (per″ĭ-kahr′de-əl) around the heart. 153
p. cavity, the space between the two pericardial layers. 153

pericarditis (per″ĭ-kahr-di′tis) inflammation of the pericardium. 165

pericardium (per″ĭ-kahr′de-əm) the sac enclosing the heart and the roots of the great vessels. 153
parietal p., the outer layer of the double membrane that surrounds the heart. 153
visceral p., the innermost of the double membrane that surrounds the heart. 153

perichondrial (per″ĭ-kon′dre-əl) pertaining to or composed of perichondrium. 388

perichondrium (per″ĭ-kon′dre-əm) the layer of fibrous connective tissue that invests all cartilage except the articular cartilage of synovial joints. 388

pericolic (per″ĭ-ko′lik) around the colon. 239

perimetrium (per″ĭ-me′tre-əm) the serous coat of the uterus. 314

perineal (per″ĭ-ne′əl) pertaining to the perineum. 287, 314
p. muscles, the muscles that form the perineum. 314

perineum (per″ĭ-ne′əm) the pelvic floor and the associated structures occupying the pelvic outlet; it is bounded anteriorly by the pubic symphysis, laterally by the ischial tuberosities, and posteriorly by the coccyx, the region between the thighs, bounded in the male sex by the scrotum and anus and in the female sex by the vulva and anus. 314

periodontal (per″e-o-don′təl) around a tooth; pertaining to the periodontium. 234

periodontics (per″e-o-don′tiks) the branch of dentistry that deals with the study and treatment of the periodontium. 234

periodontist (per″e-o-don′tist) a dentist who specializes in periodontics. 234

periodontitis (per″e-o-don-ti′tis) inflammation of the periodontium, caused by residual food, bacteria, and tartar that collect in the spaces between the gum and the lower part of the tooth crown. 248

periodontium (per″e-o-don′she-əm) the tissues investing and supporting the teeth. 234

periosteum (per″e-os′te-əm) a tough fibrous membrane that surrounds a bone. 373

peripheral (pə-rif′ər-əl) pertaining to the outside, surface, or surrounding areas of a structure or field of vision. 424, 430
p. nervous system, the various nerve processes that connect the brain and the spinal cord with receptors, muscles, and glands. 424
p. vascular disease, any abnormal condition that affects the blood vessels and lymphatic vessels, except those that supply the heart. 167

peristalsis (per″ĭ-stawl′sis) movement by which the alimentary canal propels its contents. It consists of a wave of contraction passing along the tube for variable distances. 227

peritoneal (per″ĭ-to-ne′əl) pertaining to the peritoneum. 93
p. cavity, the potential space between the parietal and visceral layers of the peritoneum. 93

peritoneum (per″ĭ-to-ne′əm) the serous membrane that lines the walls of the abdominal and pelvic cavities and invests the internal organs in those cavities. 55, 92, 93f
parietal p., the peritoneum that lines the abdominal and pelvic walls and the undersurface of the diaphragm. 93
visceral p., a continuation of the parietal peritoneum reflected at various places over the viscera. 93

peritonitis (per″ĭ-to-ni′tis) inflammation of the peritoneum. 252

perspiration (per″spĭ-ra′shən) sweating; sweat. 108

pertussis (pər-tus′is) an acute, highly contagious infection of the respiratory tract, most frequently affecting young children, usually caused by *Bordetella pertussis*. 205

petechia (pə-te′ke-ə) a pinpoint, nonraised, perfectly round, purplish red spot caused by intradermal or submucous hemorrhage. 475

phagocyte (fag′o-sīt) any cell that ingests something else. The term usually refers to polymorphonuclear leukocytes, macrophages, and monocytes. 56, 133

phagocytosis (fag″o-si-to′sis) the engulfing of microorganisms, other cells, and foreign particles by phagocytes. 133

phalangectomy (fal″ən-jek′tə-me) excision of a finger or toe. 411

phalanges (fə-lan′jēz) bones of the fingers or toes. 93, 381, 382

pharmaceuticals (fahr″mə-soo′tĭ-kəlz) pertaining to pharmacy or to drugs; medicinal drugs. 44

pharmacist (fahr′mə-sist) one who is licensed to prepare, sell, or dispense drugs and compounds and to make up prescriptions. 26

pharmacology (fahr″mə-kol′ə-je) the study of drugs and their origin, properties, and effects on living systems. 26

pharmacotherapy (fahr″mə-ko-ther′ə-pe) treatment of disease with medicines. 62

pharmacy (fahr′mə-se) the science of preparing, compounding, and dispensing medicines; a place where drugs and medicinal supplies are prepared, compounded, and dispensed. 26

pharyngalgia (far″in-gal′jə) pain in the pharynx. 203

pharyngeal (fə-rin′je-əl) pertaining to the throat. 193, 231

pharyngitis (far″in-ji′tis) inflammation of the throat. 203

pharyngodynia (fə-ring″go-din′e-ə) pain in the throat; sore throat. 203

pharyngomycosis (fə-ring″go-mi-ko′sis) any fungal infection of the pharynx. 203

pharyngopathy (far″ing-gop′ə-the) any disease of the pharynx. 203

pharyngoscope (fə-ring′go-skōp) an instrument for examining the throat. 195

pharynx (far′inks) the throat; the cavity behind the nasal cavities, mouth, and larynx, communicating with them and with the esophagus. 191

phimosis (fi-mo′sis) constriction of the preputial orifice so that the prepuce cannot be retracted back over the glans. 337

phlebectomy (flə-bek′to-me) removal of a vein or a segment of a vein. 171

phlebitis (flə-bi′tis) inflammation of a vein. 168

phleboplasty (fleb′o-plas″te) plastic repair of a vein. 171

phlebostasis (flə-bos′tə-sis) controlling the flow of blood in a vein. 169

phlebotomist (flə-bot′ə-mist) one who practices phlebotomy. 150

phlebotomy (flə-bot′ə-me) incision of a vein, as for the letting of blood; needle puncture of a vein for the drawing of blood; venipuncture. 150

phlegm (flem) abnormally thick mucus secreted by the mucosa of the respiratory passages during certain infectious processes. 199

phobia (fo′be-ə) a persistent, irrational, intense abnormal fear or dread. 53, 451

photodermatitis (fo″to-der″mə-ti′tis) an abnormal skin reaction produced by light. 471

photophobia (fo″to-fo′be-ə) abnormal intolerance of light. 439

photoreceptor (fo″to-re-sep′tor) a nerve ending that detects light, found in the human eye. 431

phrenic (fren′ik) pertaining to the diaphragm; pertaining to the mind. 194

phrenitis (frə-ni′tis) inflammation of the diaphragm. 202

phrenodynia (fren″o-din′e-ə) pain in the diaphragm. 202

phrenoplegia (fren″o-ple′jə) paralysis of the diaphragm. 202

phrenoptosis (fren″op-to′sis) downward displacement of the diaphragm. 202

physician (fĭ-zish′ən) an authorized practitioner of medicine, as one graduated from a college of medicine or osteopathy and licensed by the appropriate board; one who practices medicine as distinct from surgery. 17
p. assistant, one who has been trained in an accredited program and certified by an appropriate board to perform certain physician's duties, including history taking, physical examination, diagnostic tests, treatment, certain minor surgical procedures, all under the responsible supervision of a licensed physician. 25

pia mater (pi′ə ma′tər, pe′ə mah′tər) the innermost of the three meninges covering the brain and the spinal cord. 428

pituitary, pituitary gland (pĭ-too′ĭ-tar″e) the hypophysis, a small oval two-lobed body at the base of the brain. It regulates other glands by secretions of hormones. 492
  p. cachexia, a profound and marked state of constitutional disorder with general ill health caused by hypopituitarism. 506

placenta (plə-sen′tə) an organ characteristic of true mammals during pregnancy, joining mother and offspring. 355
  p. previa, a placenta that develops in the lower uterine segment, in the zone of dilatation, so that it covers or adjoins the internal os. 358

plague (plāg) a severe bacterial infection caused by *Yersinia pestis*, which occurs both endemically and epidemically worldwide. 132

plane (plān) a flat surface determined by the position of three points in space; a specified level; to rub away or abrade; a superficial incision in the wall of a cavity or between layers of tissue. 84
  body p., an imaginary flat surface used to identify the position of the body. 84
  coronal p., the frontal plane that divides the body into front and back portions. 84
  frontal p., the body plane that divides the body into front and back portions. 84
  sagittal p., the body plane that divides the body into left and right sides. 84
  transverse p., the body plane that divides the body into upper and lower portions. 84

plantar (plan′tər) pertaining to the sole of the foot. 84

plaque (plak) any patch or flat area; a superficial, solid, elevated skin lesion equal to or greater than 1.0 cm (0.5 cm according to some authorities) in diameter; a patch of atherosclerosis. 473

plasma (plaz′mə) the fluid portion of the blood. 110, 114f
  p. cell, a cell found in the bone marrow, connective tissue, and sometimes the blood. 175

plastic surgery (plas′tik sur′jər-e) the branch of surgery that deals with the repair or reconstruction of tissue or organs. 24, 482

pleura (ploor′ə) serous membrane investing the lungs and lining the walls of the thoracic cavity. 194
  parietal p., pleura that lines the walls of the thoracic cavity. 194
  visceral p., pleura that surrounds the lungs. 194

pleural (ploor′əl) pertaining to the pleura. 194
  p. adhesion, a sticking together of the parietal and visceral pleura, causing pain on inspiration. 208
  p. cavity, the space between the parietal and visceral pleurae. 208
  p. effusion, the presence of liquid in the pleural space. 207, 208f

pleurisy (ploor′ĭ-se) inflammation of the pleura. 208

pleuritis (ploo-ri′tis) inflammation of the pleura, or pleurisy. 208

pleurocentesis (ploor″o-sen-te′sis) thoracentesis; puncture of the chest wall for aspiration of fluid. 215

pleurodynia (ploor″o-din′e-ə) pain of the pleura; pleurisy. 208

pleuropneumonia (ploor″o-noo-mo′ne-ə) pain of the pleura complicated by pneumonia. 208

pneumectomy (noo-mek′tə-me) removal of lung tissue. 215

pneumocentesis (noo″mo-sən-te′sis) surgical puncture of a lung. 214

pneumococci (noo″mo-kok′si) plural of pneumococcus; an individual organism of the species *Streptococcus pneumoniae*. 207

pneumoconiosis (noo″mo-ko″ne-o′sis) any lung condition caused by permanent deposition of substantial amounts of dust particles in the lungs. 209

pneumohemothorax (noo″mo-he″mo-thor′aks) gas or air and blood in the pleural cavity. 208

pneumonectomy (noo″mo-nek′tə-me) surgical removal of all or part of a lung. 215

pneumonia (noo-mo′ne-ə) inflammation of the lung with consolidation; pneumonitis. 207
  lobar p., a severe infection of one or more of the five major lobes of the lung. 207

pneumonitis (noo″mo-ni′tis) inflammation of the lung; pneumonia. 207

pneumothorax (noo″mo-thor′aks) air or gas in the pleural space, which may occur spontaneously (*spontaneous p.*) or as a result of trauma or disease process or which may be introduced deliberately (*artificial p.*). 208, 209f

podiatrist (po-di′ə-trist) one who specializes in the care of the human foot. 95

podiatry (po-di′ə-tre) the specialized field dealing with the study and care of the foot, including its anatomy, pathology, and medical and surgical treatment. 95

podogram (pod′o-gram) a print of the foot. 95

poikilocyte (poi′kĭ-lo-sīt″) an abnormally shaped red blood cell. 121

poikilocytosis (poi″kĭ-lo-si-to′sis) the presence of abnormally shaped red blood cells. 121

poliomyelitis (po″le-o-mi″ə-li′tis) an acute viral disease characterized clinically by fever, sore throat, headache, and vomiting, often with stiffness of the neck and back. In its more severe form, the central nervous system is involved and paralysis can result; polio. 444

polyarthritis (pol″e-ahr-thri′tis) inflammation of several joints. 407

polycystic (pol″e-sis′tik) containing many cysts. 294
  p. kidney, a condition in which multiple cysts occur in both kidneys. 294, 294f
  p. ovary syndrome, a clinical symptom complex associated with polycystic ovaries. 323

polycythemia (pol″e-si-the′me-ə) an increase in the total red cell mass of the blood. 119
  p. vera, a proliferative disorder of the hematopoietic bone marrow and an absolute increase in red cell mass and total blood volume. 119

polydactylism (pol″e-dak′təl-iz-əm) the presence of supernumerary digits on the hands or feet. 404

polydipsia (pol″e-dip′se-ə) excessive thirst. 246, 505

polymorph (pol′e-morf) a term for polymorphonuclear leukocyte. 116

polymorphonuclear (pol″e-mor″fo-noo′kle-ər) having a nucleus that is so divided that it appears to be multiple; a polymorphonuclear leukocyte. 116

polymyalgia (pol″e-mi-al′jə) pain affecting more than one muscle. 408
  p. rheumatica, a syndrome in the elderly characterized by proximal joint and muscle pain and a self-limiting course. 408

polymyositis (pol″e-mi″o-si′tis) a chronic, progressive inflammatory disease of skeletal muscle, characterized by symmetrical weakness of the limb girdles, neck, and pharynx, usually associated with pain and tenderness. 408

polyneuralgia (pol″e-noo-ral′jə) pain of several nerves. 438

polyneuritis (pol″e-noo-ri′tis) inflammation of many nerves simultaneously. 438

polyneuropathy (pol″e-noo-rop′ə-the) a disease involving several nerves. 438

polyp (pol′ip) any growth or mass protruding from a mucous membrane. 195, 204, 292
  nasal p., a rounded, elongated piece of mucosa that projects into the nasal cavity. 195
  bladder p., growths, usually benign, protruding from the lining of the bladder. 292

polypectomy (pol″ĭ-pek′tə-me) surgical removal of a polyp. 254

polyphagia (pol″e-fa′jə) excessive eating; craving for all kinds of food. 246, 509

polyuria (pol″e-u′re-ə) excessive urination. 291, 301, 505

pons (ponz) the part of the central nervous system that lies between the medulla oblongata and the mesencephalon and ventral to the cerebellum; also called pons varolii. 429

postanesthetic (pōst″an″əs-thet′ik) after anesthesia is administered. 74

posterior (pos-tēr′e-or) situated behind. 86

posteroanterior (pos″tər-o-an-tēr′e-or) from back to front. 86

posteroexternal (pos″tər-o-ek-ster′nəl) situated on the outside of a posterior part. 86

posterointernal (pos″tər-o-in-tər′nəl) situated within and to the rear. 86

posterolateral (pos″tər-o-lat′ər-əl) situated on the side and toward the posterior aspect. 87

posteromedial (pos″tər-o-me′de-əl) situated in the middle of the back side. 87

posterosuperior (pos″tər-o-soo-pēr′e-or) situated behind and above. 87

postesophageal (pōst-ə-sof″ə-je′əl) behind the esophagus. 235

postmortem (pōst-mor′təm) occurring or performed after death. 60

postnasal (pōst-na′zəl) behind the nose. 71, 355

postnatal (pōst-na′təl) occurring after birth. 355

postpartum (pōst-pahr′təm) after childbirth. 355

precancerous (pre-kan′sər-əs) used to describe an abnormal growth that is likely to become cancerous. 74

pre-eclampsia (pre″e-klamp′se-ə) a complication of pregnancy characterized by hypertension, edema, and/or proteinuria; when convulsions and coma are associated, it is called eclampsia. 358

premalignant (pre″mə-lig′nənt) precancerous. 248

premenstrual (pre-men′stroo-əl) occurring before menstruation. 322
  p. syndrome, a condition that occurs several days before the onset of menstruation, characterized by one or more of the following: irritability, emotional tension, anxiety, depression, headache, breast tenderness, and water retention. 322

prenatal (pre-na′təl) referring to the time period before birth. 351

prepuce (pre′pūs) a foreskin; a fold over the glans penis. 313, 331

presbyopia (pres″be-o′pe-ə) farsightedness and impairment of vision because of advancing years or to old age. 448

presentation (pre″zən-ta′shən) in obstetrics, that portion of the fetus that is touched by the examining finger through the cervix, or during labor, is bounded by the girdle of resistance. 359
  breech p., presentation of the buttocks or feet of the fetus in labor. 359
  cephalic p., presentation of any part of the fetal head in labor, including occiput, brow, or face. 359
  transverse p., the situation of the fetus when the long axis of its body crosses the long axis of the maternal body. 359

primary health care provider a physician who usually is the first physician to examine a patient and who recommends secondary care physicians with expertise in the patient's specific health problem, if further treatment is needed. 17

primigravida (pri″mĭ-grav′ĭ-də) a woman who is pregnant for the first time. 352

primipara (pri-mip′ə-rə) a female individual who is bearing or has borne her first child. 353

proctologist (prok-tol′ə-jist) a physician who specializes in diseases of the rectum. 239

proctoplasty (prok′to-plas″te) plastic surgery of the rectum. 263

proctosigmoidoscopy (prok″to-sig″moi-dos′kə-pe) examination of the rectum and sigmoid with the sigmoidoscope. 244

progesterone (pro-jes′tə-rōn) the hormone produced by corpus luteum in the ovaries, adrenal cortex, and placenta. It prepares and maintains the uterus during pregnancy. 315, 350

prognosis (prog-no′sis) prediction of the probable outcome of a disease. 39

prolactin (pro-lak′tin) one of the hormones of the anterior pituitary gland that stimulates lactation in postpartum mammals. 496

prolapse (pro-laps′) dropping or sagging of a body part. 296

pronation (pro-na′shən) assuming the prone position, or being prone (lying face downward). Applied to the hand, the act of turning the palm backward or downward. 88, 393

prone (prōn) lying face downward. 88, 89f

prophylaxis (pro″fə-lak′sis) protection against disease. 136

prostaglandin (pros″tə-glan′din) any of a group of components derived from unsaturated 20-carbon fatty acids. They are extremely potent mediators of a diverse group of physiologic processes. 278, 501

prostate (pros′tāt) a gland that surrounds the neck of the bladder and the urethra in the male sex. 332
  p. specific antigen, a protein produced by the prostate that may be elevated in prostatic cancer or other diseases of the prostate. 335

prostatectomy (pros″tə-tek′tə-me) surgical removal of the prostate or part of it. 340
  transurethral p., resection of the prostate by means of a cystoscope passed through the urethra. 340

reduction (re-duk′shən) pulling the broken ends of a fractured bone into alignment. 409
closed r., restoring a fractured bone to its normal position by manipulation without surgery. 409
open r., exposing a fractured bone by surgery to realign it. 409
reflex arc (ark) a simple neurologic unit of a sensory neuron that carries a stimulus impulse to the spinal cord, where it connects with a motor neuron that carries the reflex impulse back to an appropriate muscle or gland. 426
reflex hammer a percussion mallet with a rubber head used to tap tendons. 393
regurgitation (re-gur″jĭ-ta′shən) flow in the opposite direction from normal; vomiting. 250
rejection (re-jek′shən) an immune reaction against transplanted tissue. 136
remission (re-mish′ən) a diminution or abatement of the symptoms of a disease; also the period during which such diminution occurs. 21
renal (re′nəl) pertaining to the kidney. 278
r. clearance, removal of certain substances from the blood by the kidneys. 285
r. dialysis, diffusion of blood across a semipermeable membrane to remove materials that would normally by removed by the kidneys if they were present or were functioning properly. 292
r. failure, inadequate functioning of the kidneys, which leads to uremia. 292
r. pelvis, a funnel-shaped cavity in the kidney that collects urine from many nephrons. 278
r. threshold, that concentration of any of certain substances in the blood plasma above which the substance is excreted by the kidneys and below which it is not excreted. 283
r. transplant, replacement of a diseased kidney with a healthy one from a donor. 298
r. tubule, the part of a nephron in which urine forms. 283
r. vein, the large vein by which blood leaves the kidney. 277f
r. vein thrombosis, a blood clot in a renal vein. 297
renin (re′nin) an enzyme produced by the kidneys that affects blood pressure. 278
renography (re-nog′rə-fe) radiography of the kidney. 289
renovascular (re″no-vas′ku-lər) pertaining to or affecting the blood vessels of the kidney. 297
resection (re-sek′shən) removal of a portion of an organ or other structure. 301
resistance (re-zis′təns) the natural ability of an organism to resist microorganisms or toxins produced in diseases. 133
respiration (res″pĭ-ra′shən) the exchange of oxygen and carbon dioxide between the atmosphere and the cells of the body; the metabolic processes in living cells by which molecular oxygen is taken in, organic substances are oxidized, free energy is released, and carbon dioxide, water, and other oxidized products are given off by the cell. 190
Cheyne-Stokes r., an abnormal pattern of respiration, characterized by alternating periods of apnea and deep, rapid breathing. 199
respiratory (res′pĭ-rə-tor″e) pertaining to respiration. 190
r. distress syndrome, a condition of newborns formerly known as hyaline membrane disease, marked by dyspnea and cyanosis. 206
severe acute r. syndrome, an acute respiratory disease caused by a coronavirus; SARS. 205
resuscitation (re-sus″ĭ-ta′shən) restoration of life to one who is apparently dead or whose respiration has ceased. 169
cardiopulmonary r., an emergency first aid procedure to reestablish heart and lung action, consisting of external heart massage and artificial respiration. 169
retention (re-ten′shən) the process of keeping in position, as the persistent keeping within the body of matters normally excreted or the maintaining of a dental prosthesis in proper position in the mouth. 291
retina (ret′ĭ-nə) the nervous tissue membrane of the eyeball, continuous with the optic nerve, that receives images of external objects. 447
retinal detachment a separation of the retina in the back of the eye. 447, 447f
retinoid (ret′ĭ-noid) resembling the retina; retinol, retinal, or any structurally similar natural derivative or synthetic compound. 483
retinopathy (ret″ĭ-nop′ə-the) any disease of the retina. 447
retrocecal (ret″ro-se′kəl) behind the cecum. 239
retrocolic (ret″ro-kol′ik) behind the large intestine. 239
retroflexion (ret″ro-flek′shən) the bending of an organ so that its top is turned backward; the bending of the body of the uterus toward the cervix. 325
retromammary (ret″ro-mam′ər-e) behind the breast. 498
retronasal (ret″ro-na′zəl) behind the nose. 192
retrosternal (ret″ro-ster′nəl) situated or occurring behind the breastbone. 379
retroversion (ret″ro-ver′zhən) the tipping of an entire organ backward. 325
rheumatic (roo-mat′ik) heart disease damage to heart muscle and heart valves caused by episodes of rheumatic fever. 165
rheumatic fever (roo-mat′ik fe′vər) a systemic inflammatory disease that may develop as a reaction to an inadequately treated infection by group A beta-hemolytic streptococci of the upper respiratory tract. 165
rheumatism (roo′mə-tiz-əm) any of a variety of disorders marked by inflammation, degeneration, or metabolic derangement of the connective tissue structures of the body, especially the joints and related structures. 21
rheumatoid arthritis (roo′mə-toid ahr-thri′tis) a chronic systemic disease characterized by inflamed joints and related structures that often results in crippling deformities. 406
rheumatoid factor (roo′mə-toid fak′tor) antibodies found in the serum of most patients with a clinical diagnosis of rheumatoid arthritis, but may be present in other conditions. 395, 396t
rheumatologist (roo″mə-tol′ə-jist) a specialist in rheumatic conditions. 21
rheumatology (roo″mə-tol′ə-je) the branch of medicine dealing with rheumatic disorders. 21

rhinitis (ri-ni′tis) inflammation of the mucous membranes of the nose. 203
rhinodacryolith (ri′no-dak′re-o-lith″) a tear stone in the nasal duct. 448
rhinolith (ri′no-lith) a calculus or stone in the nose. 203
rhinolithiasis (ri″no-lĭ-thi′ə-sis) a condition marked by the presence of nasal calculi or stones. 203
rhinologist (ri-nol′ə-jist) a specialist in rhinology. 21
rhinology (ri-nol′ə-je) the medical specialty that deals with the nose and its diseases. 21
rhinoplasty (ri′no-plas″te) plastic surgery of the nose. 216
rhinorrhagia (ri″no-ra′je-ə) nosebleed. 203
rhinorrhea (ri″no-re′ə) a discharge from the nose; a runny nose. 203
rhonchus (rong′kəs) a continuous sound consisting of a dry, low-pitched, noise produced in the throat or bronchial tube caused by a partial obstruction. 198
rhytidoplasty (rit′ĭ-do-plas″te) plastic surgery to eliminate wrinkles from the facial skin by excising loose or redundant tissue. 482
rib (rib) any one of the paired bones, 12 on either side, forming the major part of the thoracic skeleton. 379, 380f
false r., one of the five ribs on each side of the body that is not attached to the sternum. 380f
floating r., one of the last two pairs of false ribs, so called because it is attached only on the posterior side. 380f
true r., the upper seven ribs on each side, which directly join the sternum. 380, 380f
rickets (rik′əts) a condition caused by a deficiency of vitamin D, especially in infancy and childhood, with disturbance of normal ossification. 404
roentgenology (rent″gən-ol′ə-je) the branch of radiology that deals with x-rays. 21
rotation (ro-ta′shən) the process of turning around an axis. 392f, 393
rotator cuff a musculotendinous structure about the capsule of the shoulder joint. 399
rugae (roo′je) ridges, wrinkles, or folds, as of mucous membranes. 236
sacral (sa′krəl) pertaining to the sacrum, the triangular bone below the lumbar vertebrae. 379
sacrodynia (sa″kro-din′e-ə) pain in the sacrum, the triangular bone below the lumbar vertebrae. 399
sacrum (sa′krəm) the triangular bone at the base of the spine. 379
sagittal (saj′ĭ-təl) shaped like an arrow; denotes a plane that is parallel to the midsagittal line vertically dividing the body into right and left portions. 84
s. plane, the anteroposterior plane. 84
saliva (sə-li′və) the clear, alkaline, somewhat viscid secretion from the salivary glands of the mouth. 108
salivary (sal′ĭ-var-e) pertaining to saliva. 109, 235
s. gland, any of several glands of the oral cavity that produce saliva. 109, 235
Salmonella (sal″mo-nel′ə) a genus of gram-negative bacteria, made up of nonspore-forming rods and usually motile. 253
salmonellosis (sal″mo-nal-o′sis) any disease caused by infection with a species of *Salmonella.* 253
salpingectomy (sal″pin-jek′tə-me) excision of a uterine tube. 329
salpingitis (sal″pin-ji′tis) inflammation of a fallopian tube. 324
salpingocele (sal-ping′go-sēl) hernial protrusion of a uterine tube. 324
salpingopexy (sal-ping′go-pek″se) surgical fixation of a uterine tube. 330
salpingorrhaphy (sal″ping-gor′ə-fe) suture of the uterine tube. 330
salpingostomy (sal″ping-gos′tə-me) formation of an opening into a uterine tube for the purpose of drainage; surgical restoration of the patency of a uterine tube. 329
sanguinous (sang′gwi-nəs) pertaining to blood. 109
sarcoma (sahr-ko′mə) any of a group of tumors usually arising from connective tissue, although the term includes some of epithelial origin; most are malignant. 366
scabies (ska′bēz) a contagious dermatitis of humans and various wild and domestic animals caused by the itch mite. 472
scan (skan) shortened form of *scintiscan,* as in brain scan, thyroid scan, etc; a visual display of ultrasonographic echoes. 394, 436, 503
scapula (skap′u-lə) the shoulder blade, the flat triangular bone in the back of the shoulder. 381
scapular (skap′u-lər) of or pertaining to the scapula. 382
scapuloclavicular (skap″u-lo-klə-vik′u-lər) pertaining to the scapula and the clavicle. 382
schizophrenia (skiz″o-fre′ne-ə, skit″so-fre′ne-ə) a mental disorder or group of disorders comprising most major psychotic disorders and characterized by disturbances in form and content of thought, mood, and sense of self and relationship to the external world and behavior. 452
sciatic nerve (si-at′ik nərv) the largest nerve in the body, arising in the pelvis and passing down the back of the leg. 429
sciatica (si-at′ĭ-kə) a syndrome characterized by pain radiating from the back into the buttock and into the lower extremity along its posterior or lateral aspect; pain anywhere along the course of the sciatic nerve. 438
sclera (sklēr′ə) the tough, white, outer coat of the eyeball. 58
scleroderma (sklēr″o-der′mə) chronic hardening and thickening of the skin. 407, 471
scleroprotein (sklēr″o-pro′tēn) a protein that is characterized by its insolubility and fibrous structure. 465
sclerosis (sklə-ro′sis) hardening, chiefly applied to hardening of the nervous system or to hardening of the blood vessels. 167
multiple s., a chronic disease of the central nervous system in which disseminated glial patches called plaques develop. 446
systemic s., a systemic disorder of the connective tissue characterized by induration and thickening of the skin, abnormalities involving both the microvasculature (telangiectasia) and larger vessels (Raynaud's phenomenon), and by fibrotic degenerative changes in various body organs, including the heart, lungs, kidneys, and gastrointestinal tract. 407

scoliosis (sko″le-o′sis) lateral curvature of the vertebral column. 404

scrotal (skro′təl) pertaining to the scrotum. 332

scrotum (skro′təm) the pouch that contains the testes and their accessory organs. 331

sebaceous (sə-ba′shəs) pertaining to sebum or secreting sebum. 466
> *s. gland,* oil-secreting gland of the skin. 466

seborrhea (seb″o-re′ə) excessive secretion of sebum; seborrheic dermatitis. 472

seborrheic (seb″o-re′ik) affected with seborrhea. 472
> *s. dermatitis,* an inflammatory skin condition caused by overactive sebaceous glands. 472

sebum (se′bəm) the oily material secreted by a sebaceous gland. 467

secrete (se′krēt) to separate or elaborate cell products. 108

secretion (se-kre′shən) the process of elaborating a specific product as a result of the activity of a gland; material that is secreted. 108

secundipara (se″kən-dip′ə-rə) a woman who has had two pregnancies that resulted in viable offspring. 354

semen (se′mən) fluid consisting of gland secretions and sperm, discharged at ejaculation. 332

semicircular canals (sem″e-sər′kə-lər kə-nalz′) the bony fluid-filled loops in the internal ear that are associated with balance. 433f, 434

semiconscious (sem″e-kon′shəs) only partially aware of one's surroundings. 439

semilunar (sem″e-loo′nər) resembling a half-moon. 154
> *s. valve,* a valve with half-moon–shaped cusps, such as the aortic valve and the pulmonary valve. 153f, 154

seminal (sem′ĭ-nəl) pertaining to semen. 332
> *s. fluid,* semen; the fluid discharged from the penis at the height of sexual excitement. 334
> *s. vesicles,* paired saclike glandular structures in the male sex that produce a fluid that is added to the secretion of the testes and other glands to form the semen. 334

seminiferous tubules (sem″ĭ-nif′ər-əs too′būlz) channels in the testis in which the spermatozoa develop. 333

sensitivity test (sen″sĭ-tiv′ĭ-te) a laboratory method for testing the effectiveness of antibiotics. 129

sensory (sen′sə-re) pertaining to sensation. 424
> *s. nerve cells,* cells of the afferent nervous system that pick up stimuli. 426, 427f

sepsis (sep′sis) the presence in the blood or other tissues of pathogenic microorganisms or their toxins. 479

septal (sep′təl) pertaining to a septum. 153
> *s. deviation,* a deviation in a normally straight septum, such as the nasal septum. 195

septic (sep′tik) produced by or caused by decomposition by microorganisms. 126t, 129, 293

septicemia (sep″tĭ-se′me-ə) a morbid condition caused by the presence of bacteria or their toxins in the blood. 129, 293, 324

septoplasty (sep′to-plas″te) surgical reconstruction of the nasal septum. 216

septorhinoplasty (sep″to-ri′no-plas″te) plastic surgery of the nasal septum and the external nose. 216

septum (sep′təm) a dividing wall or partition. 153
> *cardiac s.,* the membranous partition that divides the heart's left and right sides. 153
> *nasal s.,* the partition between the two nasal cavities. 192

serosa (sēr-o′sə, sēr-o′zə) any serous membrane; the chorion. 236, 238

serotonin (ser″o-to′nin) a vasoconstrictor, found in various animals, in bacteria, and in many plants. It has many physiologic properties. 426

sexually transmitted disease (sek″shoo-əl-le trans-mit′əd dĭ-zēz) a contagious disease usually acquired by sexual intercourse or genital contact. 363

shock (shok) a sudden disturbance of mental equilibrium; a condition of profound hemodynamic and metabolic disturbance characterized by failure of the circulatory system to maintain adequate perfusion of vital organs. 165

shoulder girdle (shōl′dər gər′dəl) a partial arch at the top of the trunk formed by the scapula and clavicle. 381

shunt (shunt) to turn to one side, divert, or bypass; a passage or anastomosis between two natural channels, especially between blood vessels. 112, 454

sialadenitis (si″əl-ad″ə-ni′tis) inflammation of a salivary gland. 248, 258

sialography (si″ə-log′rə-fe) radiographic demonstration of the salivary glands after injection of radiopaque substances. 243

sialolith (si-al′o-lith) a chalky concretion or calculus in the salivary ducts or glands. 243

sialolithiasis (si″ə-lo-lĭ-thi′ə-sis) a condition characterized by the presence of stones in the salivary ducts or glands. 248, 258

sickle cell (sik′əl sel) abnormal red blood cell that has a crescent shape. 121

sigmoid (sig′moid) having the shape of the letter *S* or *C;* the sigmoid colon. 239

sigmoidoscope (sig-moi′do-skōp) a rigid or flexible endoscope with appropriate illumination for examining the sigmoid colon. 244

sigmoidoscopy (sig″moi-dos′kə-pe) inspection of the sigmoid colon through a sigmoidoscope. 244

sign (sīn) an indication of the existence of something as opposed to the subjective sensations (symptoms) of the patient. 39

silicosis (sil″ĭ-ko′sis) pneumoconiosis caused by inhalation of the dust of stone, sand, or flint containing silicon dioxide, with formation of generalized nodular fibrotic changes in both lungs. 209

sinoatrial (si″no-a′tre-əl) pertaining to the sinus venosus and the atrium of the heart. 155
> *s. node,* a node in the wall of the right atrium that is the source of impulses that initiate the heartbeat. 155, 169

sinus (si′nəs) a recess, cavity, or channel. 155
> *paranasal s.,* one of several cavities that communicate with the nasal cavity and are lined with a mucous membrane. 192, 192f
> *s. rhythm,* a cardiac rhythm stimulated by the sinus node. 160

sinusitis (si″nə-si′tis) inflammation of a sinus. 203

Sjögren's syndrome (shər′grenz sin′drōm) a symptom complex of unknown cause, usually occurring in middle-aged or older women, marked by keratoconjunctivitis, xerostomia, and the presence of a connective tissue disease, usually rheumatoid arthritis but sometimes systemic lupus erythematosus, scleroderma, or polymyositis. 407

skin cancer (skin kan′sər) cancer that arises on the surface of the body and manifests as a small ulcer, pimple, or mole. 477, 477f

smallpox (smawl′poks) an acute, highly contagious, often fatal infectious disease characterized by a fever and distinctive, progressive skin eruptions. 132

somatic (so-mat′ik) pertaining to the body. 82, 431
> *s. cell,* all of the body cells that have the diploid number of chromosomes. 82
> *s. death,* absence of electrical activity of the brain for a specified period of time under rigidly defined circumstances. 96

somatogenic (so″mə-to-jen′ik) originating in the cells of the body. 97

somatopsychic (so″mə-to-si′kik) pertaining to both body and mind, denoting a physical disorder that produces mental symptoms. 97

somatotropic (so″mə-to-trop′ik) having an affinity for or stimulating the body or the body cells; having a stimulating effect on body nutrition and growth; having the properties of somatotropin. 496

somatotropin (so′mə-to-tro′pin) growth hormone. 496

somesthetic (so″mes-thet′ik) pertaining to body feeling or sensation. 97

sonography (sə-nog′rə-fe) the process of using sound waves bouncing off body tissue to form a picture of an internal organ; ultrasonography. 44, 356

spasm (spaz′əm) a sudden, violent, involuntary contraction of a muscle or a group of muscles, attended by pain and interference with function, producing involuntary movement and distortion; a sudden but transitory constriction of a passage, canal, or orifice. 40

specific gravity (spə-sif′ik grav′ĭ-te) the ratio of the density of a substance to the density of another substance accepted as a standard, water often being the standard for liquids or solids. 283

speculum (spek′u-ləm) an instrument used to examine a body orifice or cavity. 318
> *vaginal s.,* an instrument used to hold open the vaginal opening for inspection of the vaginal cavity. 318

spermatic (spər-mat′ik) pertaining to spermatozoa. 332

spermatoblast (sper′mə-to-blast″) embryonic form of a sperm. 350

spermatocele (sper′mə-to-sēl) a swelling of the epididymis or of the rete testis containing spermatozoa. 337

spermatocyte (sper′mə-to-sīt) an early male germ cell that eventually gives rise to spermatozoa. 333

spermatogenesis (sper″mə-to-jen′ə-sis) the process of formation of sperm. 333

spermatozoon (sper″mə-to-zo′on) a mature male sperm cell, which serves to fertilize the ovum; the plural is spermatozoa. 333, 333f, 350

spermicide (sper′mĭ-sīd) an agent that destroys spermatozoa. 361

spherocyte (sfēr′o-sīt) an abnormally round red blood cell. 121

spherocytosis (sfēr″o-si-to′sis) the presence of spherocytes in the blood. 121

sphincter (sfingk′tər) a ringlike band of muscle fibers that constricts a passage or closes a natural opening. 235

sphygmomanometer (sfig″mo-mə-nom′ə-tər) an instrument that is used to measure blood pressure in the arteries. 158

spina bifida (spi′nə bif′ĭ-də, bi′fə-də) a developmental abnormality marked by defective closure of the bony encasement of the spinal cord. 404

spinal (spi′nəl) pertaining to the vertebral column. 378
> *s. cavity,* a bone cavity formed by the vertebrae of the backbone and containing the spinal cord and the beginnings of spinal nerves. 92
> *s. fluid,* the fluid that flows through and protects the brain and spinal cord; cerebrospinal fluid. 108
> *s. fusion,* the fixation of an unstable segment of the spine. 411
> *s. puncture,* insertion of a needle into the lumbar region of the spine for the purpose of removing spinal fluid or introducing substances; lumbar puncture. 435

spine (spīn) the backbone or vertebral column, which encases the spinal cord. 378

spirilla (spi-ril′ə) plural of spirillum; any organism of the genus *Spirillum,* a genus of spiral and curved bacteria of the family Spirillaceae, consisting of short, rigid, helical cells with bipolar flagella. 127

spirochete (spi′ro-kēt) a spiral bacterium. 130

spirometer (spi-rom′ə-tər) the instrument used in spirometry. 197, 197f
> *incentive s.,* an instrument used to encourage voluntary deep breathing by providing visual feedback about inspiratory volume. 217, 217f

spirometry (spi-rom′ə-tre) a measurement of the breathing capacity of the lungs. 197

spleen (splēn) a large, glandlike organ situated in the upper left part of the abdominal cavity, which destroys erythrocytes at the end of their usefulness and serves as a blood reservoir. 175

splenectomy (sple-nek′tə-me) removal of the spleen. 178

splenic (splen′ik) pertaining to the spleen. 175

splenolymphatic (sple″no-lim-fat′ik) pertaining to the spleen and the lymph nodes. 175

splenomegaly (sple″no-meg′ə-le) enlargement of the spleen. 177

splenopathy (sple-nop′ə-the) any disease of the spleen. 177

splenopexy (sple′no-pek″se) surgical fixation of the spleen. 178

splenoptosis (sple″no-to′sis) downward displacement of the spleen. 178

splenorrhagia (sple″no-ra′jə) hemorrhage from the spleen. 177

splenorrhaphy (sple-nor′ə-fe) suture of the spleen. 178

spondylalgia (spon″dĭ-lal′jə) a painful vertebra. 399

spondylarthritis (spon″dəl-ahr-thri′tis) inflammation of joints between the vertebrae. 406

spondyloarthropathy (spon″də-lo-ahr-throp′ə-the) any disease of the joints and spine. 407

topical (top′ĭ-kəl) pertaining to a particular surface area, as a topical antiinfective applied to a certain area of the skin and affecting only the area to which it is applied. 263, 481

t. anesthetic, a medication that produces superficial analgesia. 263, 482

t. antibiotic, a chemical substance produced by a microorganism that is applied to the skin to inhibit the growth of or to kill microorganisms. 482

t. medication, any drug that is applied to the skin or a mucous membrane. 482

tourniquet (toor′nĭ-kət) a device applied around an extremity to control the circulation and prevent the flow of blood to or from the distal area. 169

toxemia (tok-se′me-ə) the condition resulting from the spread of bacterial products (toxins) by the bloodstream. 129

toxic (tok′sik) poisonous; pertaining to poisoning. 63

t. shock syndrome, a severe infection with *Staphylococcus aureus* characterized by high fever of sudden onset, vomiting, diarrhea, and myalgia, followed by hypotension and, in severe cases, shock. The syndrome affects almost exclusively menstruating women using tampons, although a few women who do not use tampons and a few male individuals have been affected. 324

toxicity (tok-sis′ĭ-te) the quality of being poisonous, especially the degree of virulence of a toxic microbe or of a poison. 136

toxicologist (tok″sĭ-kol′ə-jist) one who specializes in the study of poisons. 63

toxicology (tok″sĭ-kol′ə-je) the science that deals with poisons. 63

toxin (tok′sin) a substance produced by certain animals, some higher plants, and pathogenic bacteria that is highly poisonous for other living organisms. 63

toxoid (tok′soid) a toxin treated in a way that destroys its deleterious properties without destroying its ability to stimulate antibody production. 136

trabeculae (trah-bek′u-le) plural of trabecula, a supporting or anchoring strand of connective tissue, such as one extending from a capsule into the substance of the enclosed organ. 374

trachea (tra′ke-ə) the windpipe. 191

tracheal (tra′ke-əl) pertaining to the trachea. 193

trachealgia (tra″ke-al′jə) pain in the trachea. 207

tracheomalacia (tra″ke-o-mə-la′shə) softening of the windpipe. 207

tracheoplasty (tra′ke-o-plas″te) plastic surgery of the windpipe. 216

tracheoscopic (tra″ke-o-skop′ik) pertaining to or of the character of tracheoscopy. 196

tracheoscopy (tra″ke-os′kə-pe) examination of the interior of the windpipe. 196

tracheostenosis (tra″ke-o-stə-no′sis) narrowing or contraction of the trachea. 207

tracheostomy (tra″ke-os′tə-me) surgical formation of a new opening into the windpipe from the neck. 37, 213

tracheotomy (tra″ke-ot′ə-me) surgically cutting into the windpipe. 37, 213

traction (trak′shən) the act of drawing or exerting a pulling force. 408

transabdominal (trans″ab-dom′ĭ-nəl) through the abdominal wall. 356

transcutaneous electrical nerve stimulation (TENS) (trans″ku-ta′ne-əs e-lek′trə-kəl nərv stim″u-la′shən) a method for relief of pain by placement of electrodes over the painful site and delivery of small amounts of electrical current. 453, 483

transdermal (trans-dər′məl) entering through or passing through the skin. 484

transfusion (trans-fu′zhən) the introduction of blood directly into the bloodstream of a person. 124

t. reaction, an adverse reaction to blood received in a transfusion. 124

transient (tran′shent, tran′se-ənt) pertaining to a condition that is temporary. 200

t. ischemic attack, a brief attack (from a few minutes to an hour) of cerebral dysfunction of vascular origin, with no persistent neurologic deficit. 441

transmission (trans-mish′ən) the transfer, as of disease, from one person to another. 126

transplant (trans′plant) an organ or tissue used for grafting; the process of removing and grafting such an organ or tissue; (trans-plant′) to transfer tissue from one part to another. 135

renal t., surgical implantation of a donor kidney to replace one removed from a patient. 298

transthoracic (trans″thə-ras′ik) through the chest cavity or across the chest wall. 84

transtracheal (trans-tra′ke-əl) through the wall of the trachea. 213

transureteroureterostomy (trans″u-re″ter-o-u-re″tər-os′tə-me) surgical connection of one ureter to another. 299

transurethral (trans″u-re′thrəl) performed through the urethra. 301

t. resection, resection of the prostate by means of an instrument passed through the urethra. 301

t. resection of the prostate, resection of the prostate by means of a cystoscope passed through the urethra. 301, 339

transverse (trans-vərs′) extending from side to side; at right angles to the long axis. 84

t. plane, an imaginary line that divides the body into upper and lower portions. 84

trauma (traw′mə, trou′mə) an injury or wound, whether physical or psychic. 73

traumatic (trə-mat′ik) pertaining to, occurring as the result of, or causing injury. 73

triage (tre-ahzh′, tre′ahzh) the sorting and prioritizing of patients for treatment. 24

Trichomonas (trik″o-mo′nəs) a genus of parasitic flagellated protozoa. 131, 131f, 319

trichomoniasis (trik″o-mo-ni′ə-sis) infection with *Trichomonas*, a genus of parasitic protozoa found in the intestinal and genitourinary tracts. 131, 367

trichopathy (trĭ-kop′ə-the) any disease of the hair. 479

trichosis (tri-ko′sis) any disease or abnormal growth of the hair; growth of hair in an unusual place. 480

tricuspid (tri-kus′pid) having three points of cusps; pertaining to the tricuspid valve of the heart. 154

tricuspid v., a valve with three main cusps situated between the right atrium and the right ventricle of the heart. 154

triglyceride (tri-glis′ər-īd) a neutral fat synthesized from carbohydrates for storage in animal adipose cells. 160

tri-iodothyronine (tri-i″o-do-thi′ro-nēn) one of the thyroid hormones. Its symbol is T₃. 496

trimester (tri-mes′tər) a period of three months. 351

tripara (trip′ə-rə) a female who has borne three children. 354

trophic (trof′ik) of or pertaining to nutrition. 446

tropic (tro′pik) to stimulate. 496

tubal ligation (too′bəl lĭ-ga′shən) cauterization or tying off of the uterine tubes to prevent passage of eggs and thus prevent pregnancy. 329, 361

tubal pregnancy (tu′bəl preg′nən-se) an ectopic pregnancy in which the product of conception implants in the uterine tube. 357

tubercle (too′bər-kəl) any of the small, rounded, granulomatous lesions produced by infection with *Mycobacterium tuberculosis*; it is the characteristic lesion of tuberculosis. A nodule, or small eminence, such as a rough, rounded eminence on a bone. 210

tuberculosis (too-ber″ku-lo′sis) an infectious bacterial disease caused by species of *Mycobacterium* that is chronic in nature and commonly affects the lungs. 210, 469

tubule (too′būl) a small tube. 279

distal t., the portion of the nephron lying between the descending loop of Henle and the collecting duct in the kidney. 279

proximal t., the portion of the nephron between the glomerulus and the loop of Henle. 279

renal t., the terminal channels of the nephrons in which urine is formed. 283

seminiferous t., one of several small channels of the testes in which spermatozoa develop. 333

tularemia (too″lə-re′me-ə) an infectious, plaguelike disease caused by infection with a bacillus found primarily in rodents, but also affects humans and other animals. 132

tumor (too′mər) a new growth of tissue in which the multiplication of cells is uncontrolled and progressive; neoplasm. 61, 249, 476

tunica (too′nĭ-kə) a general term for a membrane or other structure covering or lining a body part or organ. 156f

t. adventitia, the outer coat of many tubular body structures. 156f

t. intima, the innermost coat of blood vessels. 156f

t. media, the middle coat of blood vessels. 156f

tympanic (tim-pan′ik) of or pertaining to the tympanic cavity or the tympanic membrane; bell-like; resonant. 434

t. membrane, the thin membranous partition between the external acoustic meatus and the tympanic cavity. 434

typhoid (ti′foid) typhuslike; a bacterial infection usually caused by *Salmonella typhi*, transmitted by contaminated milk, water, or food. 136

ulcer (ul′sər) a local defect or excavation of the surface of an organ or tissue, produced by sloughing of necrotic inflammatory tissue. 247

decubitus u., a sore in the skin over a bony prominence that results from ischemic hypoxia of the tissues caused by prolonged pressure; pressure ulcer. 478

peptic u., a loss of tissue lining the lower esophagus, the stomach, or the duodenum. 250

pressure u., a skin defect caused by prolonged pressure from lying too still in bed for too long a time; bed sore. 478

ulceration (ul″sər-a′shən) the formation or development of an ulcer. 246

ulcerative colitis (ul′sə-ra″tiv, ul′sər-ə-tiv ko-li′tis) chronic, recurrent ulceration in the colon, chiefly of the mucosa and submucosa, of unknown cause. 252

ulna (ul′nə) the inner and larger bone of the forearm. 381

ulnoradial (ul″no-ra′de-əl) pertaining to the ulna and radius, the bones of the lower arm. 382

ultrasonography (ul″trə-sə-nog′rə-fe) the visualization of deep structures of the body by recording the reflections of pulses of ultrasonic waves directed into the tissues. 44

ultrasound (ul′trə-sound) mechanical radiant energy with a frequency greater than 20,000 cycles per second; ultrasonography. 44, 410, 483

umbilical (əm-bil′ĭ-kəl) pertaining to the umbilicus. 91

umbilicus (əm-bil′ĭ-kəs) the navel. 97

ungual (ung′gwəl) pertaining to the nails. 468

unilateral (u″nĭ-lat′ər-əl) pertaining to only one side. 87

unmyelinated (ən-mi′ə-lĭ-nāt″ed) not possessing a myelin sheath. 426

urea (u-re′ə) the chief nitrogenous constituent of urine and the major nitrogenous end product of protein metabolism. 283

uremia (u-re′me-ə) an accumulation of toxic products in the blood, owing to inadequate functioning of the kidneys. 292

ureter (u-re′tər) the tubular organ through which urine passes from the kidney to the bladder. 277

ureteral (u-re′tər-əl) pertaining to or used on the ureter. 278

ureterectomy (u-re″tər-ek′tə-me) surgical removal of all or a part of a ureter. 300

ureteritis (u-re″tər-i′tis) inflammation of a ureter. 293

ureterocele (u-re″tər-o-sēl″) hernia of the ureter. 296

ureterocystoneostomy (u-re″tər-o-sis″to-ne-os′tə-me) surgical transplantation of the ureter to a different site of attachment to the bladder. 300

ureterocystostomy (u-re″tər-o-sis-tos′tə-me) surgical transplantation of a ureter to a different site in the bladder. 300

ureterolith (u-re′tər-o-lith) a stone that is lodged or has formed in the ureter. 296

ureterolithiasis (u-re″tər-o-lĭ-thi′ə-sis) formation of stones in a ureter. 296

ureterolithotomy (u-re″tər-o-lĭ-thot′ə-me) the removal of a calculus from the ureter by incision. 300

ureteroneocystostomy (u-re″tər-o-ne″o-sis-tos′tə-me) surgical transplantation of a ureter to a different site in the bladder. 300

ureteropathy (u-re″tər-op′ə-the) any disease of the ureter. 293

ureteroplasty (u-re″tər-o-plas″te) surgical repair of the ureter. 300

ureteropyelitis (u-re″tər-o-pi-ə-li′tis) inflammation of a ureter and the renal pelvis. 293

ureteropyelonephritis (u-re″tər-o-pi-ə-lo-nə-fri′tis) inflammation of the ureter, renal pelvis, and the kidney. 293

ILLUSTRATION CREDITS

Chapter 1

Figures 1-1 and 1-4 From Polaski AL, Tatro SE: *Luckmann's core principles and practice of medical-surgical nursing,* Philadelphia, 1996, Saunders.

Chapter 2

Figure 2-2 From Seidel HM, Ball JW, Dains JE, Benedict GW: *Mosby's guide to physical examination,* ed 4, St. Louis, 1999, Mosby.

Figure 2-3 Ballinger PW, Frank ED: *Merrill's atlas of radiographic positions and radiologic procedures,* vol 1, ed 9, St. Louis, 1999, Mosby.

Figure 2-5 From Ignatavicius DD, Workman M: *Medical-surgical nursing: critical thinking for collaborative care,* ed 4, Philadelphia, 2002, Saunders.

Figure 2-6 From Seidel HM, Ball JW, Dains JE, Benedict GW: *Mosby's guide to physical examination,* ed 5, St. Louis, 2003, Mosby.

Figure 2-7 From Polaski AL, Tatro SE: *Luckmann's core principles and practice of medical-surgical nursing,* Philadelphia, 1996, Saunders.

Figure 2-8 From Gerdin J: *Health careers today,* ed 3, St. Louis, 2003, Mosby.

Chapter 3

Figure 3-2 From Goldstein BJ, Goldstein AO: *Practical dermatology,* ed 2, St. Louis, 1997, Mosby.

Figure 3-3A From Bonewit-West K: *Clinical procedures for medical assistants,* ed 6, Philadelphia, 2004, Saunders.

Figure 3-4 From Zitelli BJ, Davis HW: *Pediatric physical diagnosis,* ed 4, St. Louis, 2002, Mosby.

Figures 3-5 and 3-7 From Ballinger PW, Frank ED: *Merrill's atlas of radiographic positions and radiologic procedures,* vol 2, ed 10, St. Louis, 2003, Mosby.

Figure 3-6A From Perkin GD et al: *Atlas of clinical neurology,* London, 1986, Gower Medical Publishing. B From Seeley RS, Stephens TD, Tate P: *Anatomy and physiology,* ed 3, St. Louis, 1995, Mosby.

Figure 3-8A from Mourad LA: *Orthopedic disorders,* St. Louis, 1991, Mosby. B Courtesy of Professor A. Jackson, Department of Diagnostic Radiology, University of Manchester.

Figure 3-9 From Curry RA, Tempkin BB: *Sonography: introduction to normal structure and function,* St. Louis, 2004, Saunders.

Chapter 4

Figure 4-1 From Zacarian SA: *Cryosurgery,* St. Louis, 1985, Mosby.

Figure 4-2 From Weston WL, Lane AT, Morelli JG: *Color textbook of pediatric dermatology,* ed 3, St. Louis, 2002, Mosby.

Figure 4-3 From Palay DA, Krachmer JH, editors: *Ophthalmology for the primary care physician,* St. Louis, 1998, Mosby.

Figure 4-4 From Zitelli BJ, Davis HW: *Pediatric physical diagnosis,* ed 4, St. Louis, 2002, Mosby.

Figures 4-5 and 4-6 From Kamal A, Brockelhurst JC: *Color atlas of geriatric medicine,* ed 2, St. Louis, 1991, Mosby.

Chapter 5

Figure 5-2 From Moore KL, Persaud TVN: *The developing human: clinically oriented embryology,* ed 7, Philadelphia, 2003, Saunders.

Chapter 6

Figure 6-2A and D From Herlihy B, Maebius NK: *The human body in health and illness,* ed 2, Philadelphia, 2003, Saunders. B and C From Gartner LP, Hiatt JL: *Color textbook of histology,* ed 2, Philadelphia, 2001, Saunders.

Figure 6-4BCD From Kelley LL, Petersen CM: *Sectional anatomy for imaging professionals,* St. Louis, 1997, Mosby-Year Book.

Figure 6-5 From Ballinger PW, Frank ED: *Merrill's atlas of radiographic positions and radiologic procedures,* vol 1, ed 10, St. Louis, 2003, Mosby.

Figure 6-7A, From Thompson JM, Wilson SF: *Health assessment for nursing practice,* St. Louis, 1996, Mosby. B from Jacob S: *Atlas of human anatomy,* Philadelphia, 2002, Churchill Livingstone.

Figure 6-11 From Ignatavicius MS, Workman ML, Mishler MA: *Medical-surgical nursing across the health care continuum,* ed 3, Philadelphia, 1999, Saunders.

Figure 6-13 From Seidel HM, Ball JW, Dains JE, Benedict GW: *Mosby's guide to physical examination,* ed 5, St. Louis, 2003, Mosby.

Chapter 7

Figures 7-1, 7-2, 7-5, 7-13, and 7-15 From Applegate EJ, Thomas P: *The anatomy and physiology learning system: textbook,* Philadelphia, 1995, Saunders.

Figure 7-3 From Hart CA, Broadhad RL: *Color atlas of pediatric infectious diseases,* London, 1992, Mosby-Wolfe.

Figure 7-4 From Dennis Kunkel Microscopy, Inc., 1994.

Figure 7-6 From Rodak BF: *Hematology, clinical principles and applications,* ed 2, Philadelphia, 2002, Saunders.

Figure 7-7 From Hayhoe FGJ, Flemans RJ: *Color atlas of hematological cytology,* ed 3, London, 1992, Mosby-Wolfe.

Figure 7-8A From Murray PR, Rosenthal KS, Kobayashi GS, Pfaller MA: *Medical microbiology,* ed 3, St. Louis, 1994, Mosby. B From Forbes BA, Sahm DF, Weissfeld AS: *Bailey & Scott's diagnostic microbiology,* ed 11, St. Louis, 2002, Mosby.

Figure 7-9C and D, From Forbes BA, Sahm DF, Weissfeld AS: *Bailey & Scott's diagnostic microbiology,* ed 11, St. Louis, 2002, Mosby. F, From Murray PR, Rosenthal KS, Kobayashi GS, Pfaller MA: *Medical microbiology,* ed 3, St. Louis, 1994, Mosby.

Figure 7-10 From Atlas RM: *Principles of microbiology,* St. Louis, 1995, Mosby.

Figure 7-11 From Zitelli BJ, Davis HW: *Atlas of pediatric physical diagnosis,* ed 4, St. Louis, 2002, Mosby.

Figure 7-12 From Cotran RS, Kumar V, Collins T: *Robbin's pathologic basis of disease,* ed 7, Philadelphia, 2004, Saunders.

Figure 7-14 From Behrman R, Kliegman R, Jenson HB: *Nelson's textbook of pediatrics,* ed 17, Philadelphia, 2004, Saunders.

Chapter 8

Figure 8-10 From Applegate EJ: *The anatomy and physiology learning system: textbook,* Philadelphia, 1995, Saunders.

Figure 8-12 From Ballinger PW, Frank ED: *Merrill's atlas of radiographic positions and radiologic procedures,* vol 3, ed 10, St. Louis, 2003, Mosby.

Figure 8-20 From Seidel HM, Ball JW, Dains JE, Benedict GW: *Mosby's guide to physical examination,* ed 5, St. Louis, 2003, Mosby.

Figure 8-21 From Behrman R, Kliegman R, Jenson HB: *Nelson's textbook of pediatrics,* ed 17, Philadelphia, 2004, Saunders.

Figure 8-22 From Stone DR, Gorbach SL: *Atlas of infectious diseases,* Philadelphia, 2000, Saunders.

Chapter 9

Figures 9-2 and 9-12 From Ignatavicius MS, Workman ML, Mishler MA: *Medical-surgical nursing across the health care continuum,* ed 4, Philadelphia, 2002, Saunders.

Figure 9-4 From Monahan FD, Neighbors M: *Medical-surgical nursing: foundations for clinical practice,* ed 2, Philadelphia, 1998, Saunders.

Figure 9-6 From Talbot LA, Myers-Marquardt M: *Pocket guide to critical care assessment,* ed 3, St. Louis, 1997, Mosby.

Figure 9-7 From Wilson SF, Thompson JM: *Respiratory disorders,* St. Louis, 1990, Mosby.

Figure 9-8 Courtesy of Ohmeda, Boulder, CO.

Figure 9-9 and 9-14B From Seidel HM, Ball JW, Dains JE, Benedict GW: *Mosby's guide to physical examination,* ed 5, St. Louis, 2003, Mosby.

Figure 9-13 From Earis JE, Pearson MG: *Respiratory medicine,* London, 1995, Times Mirror International Publishers.

Figure 9-14A, From Lemmi FO, Lemmi CAE: *Physical assessment findings CD-ROM,* Philadelphia, 2000, Saunders.

Figure 9-15 From Wilson SF, Giddens JF: *Health assessment for nursing practice,* ed 2, St. Louis, 2001, Mosby.

Figure 9-18 From Lewis SM, Heitkemper MM, Dirksen SR: *Medical-surgical nursing: assessment and management of clinical problems,* ed 6, St. Louis, 2004, Mosby.

Figure 9-23 From Potter PA, Perry AG: *Fundamentals of nursing,* ed 5, St. Louis, 2001, Mosby.

Chapter 10

Figure 10-9 From Carlson K, Eisenstat S: *Primary care of women,* St. Louis, 1995, Mosby.

Figure 10-12 Lemmi FO, Lemmi CAE: *Physical assessment findings CD-ROM,* Philadelphia, 2000, Saunders.

Figure 10-13 Callen JP, Greer KE, Hood et al: *Color atlas of dermatology,* Philadelphia, 1992, Saunders.

Figure 10-16 From Damjanov I, Linder J: *Anderson's pathology,* ed 10, St. Louis, 1996, Mosby.

Figures 10-20 and 10-22 From Lewis SM, Heitkemper MM, Dirksen SR: *Medical-surgical nursing,* ed 6, St. Louis, 2004, Mosby.

Chapter 11

Figure 11-6 From Brunzel NA: *Fundamentals of urine & body fluid analysis,* ed 2, St. Louis, 2004, Saunders.

Figures 11-9 From Lewis SM, Heitkemper MM, Dirksen SR: *Medical-surgical nursing, assessment and management of clinical problems,* ed 6, St. Louis, 2004, Mosby.

Figure 11-10 From Price S, Wilson L: *Pathophysiology: clinical concepts of disease processes,* ed 6, St. Louis, 2003, Mosby.

Figure 11-13 From Brundage DJ: *Renal disorders,* St. Louis, 1992, Mosby.

Chapter 12

Figure 12-9 From Walter JB: *An introduction to the principles of disease,* ed 2, Philadelphia, 1982, Saunders.

Figure 12-10 From Polaski AL, Tatro SE: *Luckmann's core principles and practice of medical-surgical nursing,* Philadelphia, 1996, Saunders.

Figure 12-18B Courtesy of Fisher Scientific Company.

Chapter 13

Figure 13-2 From Moore KL: *The developing human,* ed 7, Philadelphia, 2003, Saunders.

Figure 13-4A From Curry RA, Tempkin BB: *Sonography: introduction to normal structure and function,* St. Louis, 2004, Saunders.

Figure 13-7 From Zitelli BJ, Davis HW: *Atlas of pediatric physical diagnosis,* ed 4, St. Louis, 2002, Mosby.

Figure 13-9 From Forbes BA, Sahm DF, Weissfeld AS: *Bailey & Scott's diagnostic microbiology,* ed 10, St. Louis, 1998, Mosby.

Figure 13-10 From Noble J, editor: *Textbook of primary care medicine,* ed 3, St. Louis, 2001, Mosby.

Chapter 14

Figures 14-2, 14-7, 14-8, 14-21, and 14-28 From Ballinger PW, Frank ED: *Merrill's atlas of radiographic positions and radiologic procedures,* vol 1, ed 10, St. Louis, 2003, Mosby.

Figure 14-11 From Thibodeau GA, Patton KT: *Anatomy and physiology,* ed 3, St. Louis, 1996, Mosby.

Figure 14-15 From Herlihy B, Maebius NK: *The human body in health and illness,* ed 2, Philadelphia, 2003, Saunders.

Figure 14-20 From Canale ST: *Operative orthopaedics,* ed 9, St. Louis, 1998, Mosby.

Figure 14-22 From Kamal A, Brockelhurst JC: *Color atlas of geriatric medicine,* ed 2, St. Louis, 1991, Mosby.

Figure 14-23 From Walter JB: *An introduction to the principles of disease,* ed 2, Philadelphia, 1982, Saunders.

Figures 14-25B and 14-27 From Zitelli BJ, Davis HW: *Atlas of pediatric physical diagnosis,* St. Louis, 1997, Mosby.

Figures 14-25AC and 14-26B From Zitelli BJ, Davis HW: *Atlas of pediatric physical diagnosis,* ed 4, St. Louis, 2002, Mosby.

Figure 14-26A Courtesy Dr. Christine L. Williams, New York Medical College.

Figure 14-29 From Monahan FD, Neighbors M. *Medical-surgical nursing: foundations for clinical practice,* ed 2, Philadelphia, 1998, Saunders.

Chapter 15

Figure 15-9B From Thibodeau GA, Patton KT: *Anatomy & physiology,* ed 5, St. Louis, 2003, Mosby.

Figures 15-10 and 15-19 From Palay DA, Krachmer JH, editors: *Ophthalmology for the primary care physician,* St. Louis, 1998, Mosby.

Figure 15-11 From Chipps EM, Clanin NJ, Campbell VG: *Neurologic disorders,* St. Louis, 1992, Mosby.

Figure 15-12 From Polaski AL, Tatro SE: *Luckmann's core principles and practice of medical-surgical nursing,* Philadelphia, 1996, Saunders.

Figure 15-17 From Zitelli BJ, Davis HW: *Atlas of pediatric physical diagnosis,* ed 3, St. Louis, 1997, Mosby.

Figure 15-18 From Osborn AG: *Diagnostic neuroradiology,* St. Louis, 1994, Mosby.

Figure 15-22 From Ignatavicius DD, Workman ML: *Medical-surgical nursing: critical thinking for collaborative care,* ed 4, Philadelphia, 2002, Saunders.

Chapter 16

Figure 16-4 From Wilson SF, Giddens JF: *Health assessment for nursing practice,* ed 3, St. Louis, 2005, Mosby.

Figure 16-5A From Weston WI, Lane AT: *Color textbook of pediatric dermatology,* ed 3, St. Louis, 2002, Mosby.

Figure 16-5B From Habif TP: *Clinical dermatology: a color atlas guide to diagnosis and therapy,* ed 3, St. Louis, 1996, Mosby.

Figures 16-5C and 16-10A From Habif TP: *Clinical dermatology: a color atlas guide to diagnosis and therapy,* ed 4, St. Louis, 2004, Elsevier.

Figures 16-7, 16-8, 16-9, and 16-10C From Noble J, editor: *Textbook of primary care medicine,* St. Louis, 1996, Mosby.

Figure 16-10B From Ignatavicius DD, Workman ML: *Medical-surgical nursing: critical thinking for collaborative care,* ed 4, Philadelphia, 2002, Saunders

Figure 16-11 From Bork K, Brauninger W: *Skin diseases in clinical practice,* ed 2, Philadelphia, 1999, Saunders.

Figure 16-12 From Habif TP: *Clinical dermatology: a color atlas guide to diagnosis and therapy,* ed 2, St. Louis, 1985, C.V. Mosby.

Figure 16-13 Drawing from Lewis SM, Heitkemper MM, Dirksen SR: *Medical-surgical nursing, assessment and management of clinical problems,* ed 6, St. Louis, 2004, Mosby.

Figure 16-14 From Ignatavicius DD, Workman ML, Mischler MA: *Medical-surgical nursing across the health care continuum,* ed 3, Philadelphia, 1999, Saunders.

Chapter 17

Figure 17-1 Photomicrograph by Bodansky HJ: *Pocket picture guide to diabetes,* London, 1989, Gower Medical Publishing.

Figure 17-6 From Thompson JM, Wilson SF: *Health assessment for nursing practice,* St. Louis, 1996, Mosby.

Figure 17-7 From Dorland NW: *Dorland's illustrated medical dictionary,* ed 30, Philadelphia, 2003, Saunders.

Figure 17-8 From Svane G, Potchen EJ, Sierra A, Azavedo E: *Screening mammography, breast cancer diagnosis in asymptomatic women,* St. Louis, 1993, Mosby.

Figure 17-9 From Zitelli BJ, Davis HW: *Atlas of pediatric physical diagnosis,* ed 4, St. Louis, 2002, Mosby.

Figure 17-10 Courtesy of Ewing Galloway.

Figure 17-11 From Mendeloff AI, Smith DE, editors: Acromegaly, diabetes, hypermetabolism, proteinuria, and heart failure. *Clin Pathol Conf. Am J Med,* 1956, 20:133.

Figure 17-12 From Ignatavicius DD, Workman ML, Mischler MA: *Medical-surgical nursing across the health care continuum,* ed 3, Philadelphia, 1999, Saunders.

Figure 17-13 Courtesy of MiniMed Technologies, Sylmar, CA.